Calculate
WITH
Confidence

First Canadian Edition

Calculate
WITH
Confidence

First Canadian Edition

Deborah C. Gray Morris, RN, BSN, MA, LNC
Professor of Nursing
Department of Nursing and Allied Health Sciences
Bronx Community College of the University of New York (CUNY)
Bronx, New York

Marcia Brown, RN, BScN, MEd, CDE
Professor of Nursing, York University–Seneca College Collaborative BScN Program
Faculty of Applied Arts and Health Sciences
Seneca College of Applied Arts and Technology
Toronto, Ontario

ELSEVIER

ELSEVIER

Notices

Library and Archives Canada Cataloguing in Publication

Morris, Deborah Gray, author
Calculate with confidence / Deborah Gray Morris (RN, BSN, MA, LNC, Professor of Nursing, Department of Nursing and Allied Health Sciences, Bronx Community College of the University of New York (CUNY) Bronx, New York), Marcia Brown (RN, BScN, MEd, CDE Professor of Nursing, York–Seneca Collaborative BScN Program, Faculty of Applied Arts and Health Sciences, Seneca College of Applied Arts and Technology, Toronto, Ontario).—First Canadian edition.

Includes bibliographical references and index.
ISBN 978-1-927406-62-5 (paperback)

1. Pharmaceutical arithmetic. 2. Nursing–Mathematics. I. Brown, Marcia (Professor of Nursing), author II. Title.

RS57.M67 2015   615.1′401513   C2015-906247-0

Vice President, Publishing: Ann Millar
Content Strategist: Roberta A. Spinosa-Millman
Developmental Editor: Theresa Fitzgerald
Publishing Services Manager: Jeffrey Patterson
Senior Project Manager: Mary Pohlman
Copy Editor: Claudia Forgas

Proofreader: Wendy Thomas
Cover Image: antishock
Book Designer: Brian Salisbury
Typesetting and Assembly: Toppan Best-set Premedia Limited
Printing and Binding: Transcontinental Printing

Elsevier Canada
420 Main Street East, Suite 636, Milton, ON Canada L9T 5G3
416-644-7053

Printed in Canada.

4 5 6 7 20 19 18 17

Ebook ISBN: 978-1-927406-60-1

Working together
to grow libraries in
developing countries

www.elsevier.com • www.bookaid.org

To my family, friends, nursing colleagues, and students past
and present, but especially with love to my children,
Cameron, Kimberly, Kanin, and Cory.
You light up my life and have been proud of whatever I do.

To my mother, whose guidance and nurturing
has made me what I am today.
Thanks for always being there to support me.

To current practitioners of nursing and future nurses,
I hope this book will be valuable in teaching the basic
principles of medication administration and will ensure
safe administration of medication to all patients
regardless of the setting.

—Deborah C. Gray Morris

This one is for me.
The next one is for you. Maybe.

—Marcia Brown

About the Authors

Deborah C. Gray Morris

Deborah C. Gray Morris began her nursing education at Bronx Community College, graduating in 1971. In 1973, Deborah earned a bachelor of science in nursing (BSN) from the City College of the City University of New York, followed by a master (MA) in nursing from New York University in 1978. In 1998, Deborah pursued her interest in the legal aspects of nursing and graduated with certification as a legal nurse consultant from Long Island University's Legal Nurse Consultant Program in 1999. Deborah has also earned 12 credits from John Jay College of the City University of New York, including credits in criminal justice and forensic science.

Deborah is currently a full professor and the chairperson of the Department of Nursing and Allied Health Sciences at Bronx Community College, where she teaches dosage calculations in the Registered Nursing and Licensed Practical Nursing Programs. Deborah has held the position of chairperson since 2010; first as acting, then elected to the position in 2011. Prior to becoming chairperson, Deborah served as deputy chairperson for 13 years and as course coordinator for Pharmacology Computations. Her second term as chairperson began in July 2015. Deborah is also a program evaluator for the Accreditation Commission for Education in Nursing (ACEN). Upon request, Deborah provides consultant services to nursing programs in the area of dosage calculation.

Deborah's interest in dosage calculation started with her career at Bronx Community College of the City University of New York in 1978. Her original position at the college was in the capacity of providing nursing students with tutoring in the area of dosage calculation, which had been identified as an area of difficulty for students. She began with the development of a manual to assist students with the subject matter and later developed a course titled Pharmacology Computations, which was approved through the college governance bodies and is currently a required course for students in the Associate Degree Nursing Program. Deborah's very first edition of *Calculate with Confidence* was published in 1994. *Calculate with Confidence* is currently in its 6th U.S. edition and ranks among the top books published by Elsevier in this area.

Deborah is married. She has four children and one grandson.

Marcia Brown

Since achieving an RN diploma, Marcia Brown has acquired additional certification in critical care nursing, educator development, health care education, diabetes education, and creative training techniques. In addition, she has earned a bachelor of science in nursing (BScN) from Laurentian University and a master of education from the Ontario Institute for Studies in Education (OISE) of the University of Toronto. In her doctoral research study she focuses on clinical simulation and its impact on critical thinking and student learning. As a simlab facilitator, Marcia sees a positive correlation between the simulation learning experience and nursing students' ability to engage in higher level thinking during patient delivery.

Marcia has held educator positions in both community hospital and academic institutions. Subject areas taught encompass critical care, leadership, ethics, knowledge of nursing, pharmacology, dosage calculation, clinical simulation, and more. She has presented research work at Registered Nurses' Association of Ontario (RNAO) and Canadian Association of Schools of Nursing (CASN) conferences. Over the years, she has designed and conducted workshops in critical care nursing and diabetes education.

Marcia has been a professor in the York University–Seneca College Collaborative BScN degree program (Seneca College site) since January 2001. Since her tenure at Seneca, she has held several leadership positions, including curriculum coordinator, chair of Theory & Practice Committee, founder and chair of the Curriculum Committee and founder and co-coordinator of the Seneca Nursing Outreach Program, which garnered the Senecans of Distinction Award in November 2014. Her passion is helping students *learn* how to learn, while helping others to be the best they can be. Her mantra for nursing and life: "Do unto others as you would have others do unto you."

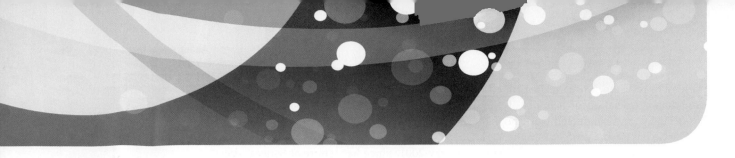

Canadian Reviewers

Renée Anderson, RN, BScN, MN
Senior Lecturer
School of Nursing
Thompson Rivers University
Kamloops, British Columbia

Polina Belts, RN
Nursing Instructor
Bachelor of Nursing
John Abbott College
Sainte-Anne-de-Bellevue, Quebec

Jennifer Black, RN, BScN, MN
Professor and Coordinator
Practical Nursing Program
Fanshawe College—Woodstock/Oxford Regional Campus
Woodstock, Ontario

Terri Burrell, RN, BScN, MSN
Faculty
Saskatchewan Collaborative Bachelor of Science
in Nursing
Saskatchewan Polytechnic
Regina, Saskatchewan

Edward Venzon Cruz, RN, BN, MEdM, MScN, PhD (DentSc)
Professor, Nursing
Coordinator, Bridging to University Nursing (full-time)
School of Community and Health Studies
Centennial College
Toronto, Ontario

Spring Farrell, PhD
Lecturer in Pharmacology
Faculty of Health Professions, School of Nursing
Dalhousie University
Halifax, Nova Scotia

Neemera Jamani, RN, MN
Professor
School of Nursing
York University
Toronto, Ontario

Tina V. Johnston, RN, BScN, MN
Nurse Educator
Langara College School of Nursing
Vancouver, British Columbia

Lisa McKendrick-Calder, RN, BScN, MN
Faculty Member
Bachelor of Science in Nursing Program
MacEwan University
Edmonton, Alberta

Barbara Morrison, RN, BScN, MEd
Simulation Coordinator
Nursing Faculty
Confederation College
Thunder Bay, Ontario

Katherine Poser, RN, BScN, MNEd
Professor
School of Baccalaureate Nursing
St. Lawrence College—Kingston Campus
Kingston, Ontario

Preface to the Instructor

Safety has become a focus and priority in the delivery of health care. To advance patient safety and its importance in health care delivery worldwide, several organizations have become involved in reinforcing the promotion of patient safety in health care, which includes an emphasis on improving safety in medication administration. Canadian organizations include Health Canada, the Canadian Institute for Health Information (CIHI), the Institute for Safe Medication Practices Canada (ISMP Canada), and the Canadian Patient Safety Institute (CPSI). These organizations also collaborate on the Canadian Medication Incident Reporting and Prevention System (CMIRPS). This pan-Canadian program encourages reporting, sharing, and learning about medication incidents in order to help reduce their reoccurrence and create a safer health care system.

The first Canadian edition of *Calculate with Confidence* not only teaches the aspects of dosage calculation but also emphasizes the importance of safety in medication administration. *Calculate with Confidence* is written to meet the needs of current and future practitioners of nursing at any level. This book can be used as a resource for any education program or practice setting that involves dosage calculation and medication administration by health care providers.

Calculate with Confidence, First Canadian Edition, primarily uses the metric system in calculating dosages, but it presents examples that incorporate imperial system (household, apothecary) measurements where applicable. Specifically, you will see the conversion of pounds to kilograms in some examples because weight is still sometimes measured in pounds in the community at large. Therefore it is prudent to include imperial units of measurement in this book.

The first Canadian edition of *Calculate with Confidence* illustrates the standard methods of dosage calculation: the ratio and proportion method, the formula method, and the dimensional analysis method. With the inclusion of all three, instructors have the freedom to decide which method(s) best suit their program, and students have the same freedom to choose the method that facilitates *correct dosage calculations*.

This first Canadian edition responds to evidence-informed practices as they relate to safe medication practices at all levels. Highlights include best practices for the labelling, dispensing, preparing, and administering of medications. With the nursing student in mind, emphasis is placed on critical thinking and clinical reasoning in the prevention of medication errors. Principles of competence and safety are integrated throughout.

Answers to the Practice Problems include rationales to enhance the understanding of principles. In response to the increased need for competency in basic math as an essential prerequisite for dosage calculation, many Practice Problems are included in the basic math section.

The once controversial use of calculators is now a more accepted practice, and they are used on many nursing exams, including the NCLEX. Critical care areas in some health care institutions have policies that require the use of calculators to verify calculations to avoid medication errors. A **basic** calculator is usually sufficient for dosage calculations. Calculator use is not encouraged in the basic math section of this book due to the expectation that students should be able to perform calculations proficiently and independently without their use.

Despite decreased errors in calculating medication dosages due to the availability of better technology, health care providers must continue to use sound clinical reasoning in problem solving to minimize the risk to patient safety.

The first Canadian edition of *Calculate with Confidence* embodies all the standards of nursing practice. It clearly delineates the nurse's responsibility in medication practices, including accurate dosage calculation to optimize safe patient outcomes.

Organization of Content

The first Canadian edition is organized in a progression from simple topics to more complex ones, making content relevant to the needs of students and using realistic Practice Problems to enhance learning and make material clinically applicable.

The 23 chapters are arranged into 5 units.

Unit One includes Chapters 1 through 4. This unit provides a review of basic math skills, including fractions, decimals, ratio and proportion, and percentages. A pre-test and post-test are included. This unit allows students to determine their weaknesses and strengths in math and provides a review. Academic institutions using this book may use these units as independent study for students to review basic math concepts before venturing on to actual dosage calculations.

Unit Two includes Chapters 5 through 7. Chapter 5 introduces students to the metric and imperial (household, apothecary) systems of measurement. Canada's health care providers use the metric system. However, some units of household measurement are discussed because of their continued use, albeit limited. These measurements are pound, ounce, teaspoon, tablespoon, and cup. In Chapter 6, students learn to convert measurements. Chapter 7 presents conversions relating to temperature, length, weight, and international time.

Unit Three includes Chapters 8 through 14. This unit provides essential information that is needed as a foundation for dosage calculation and safe medication administration. Chapter 8 includes an expanded discussion of medication errors, routes of medication administration, equipment used in medication administration, the rights of medication administration, and the nursing role in preventing medication errors. Chapter 9 presents the abbreviations used in medication administration and discusses how to interpret medication orders. Chapter 10 introduces students to medication administration records and the various medication distribution systems. Chapter 11 provides students with the skills necessary to read medication labels to calculate dosages. Chapters 12 through 14 introduce students to the various methods used for dosage calculation followed by Practice Problems illustrating each method.

Unit Four includes Chapters 15 through 18. In Chapter 15, students learn the principles and calculations related to oral medications (solid and liquids). In Chapter 16, students learn about the various types of syringes and skills needed for calculating injectable medications. Chapter 17 introduces students to the calculations associated with reconstituting solutions for injectable and noninjectable medications. Calculations associated with the preparation of noninjectable solutions such as nutritional feedings include determining the strength of a solution and determining the amount of the desired solution. Chapter 18 introduces students to insulin types, insulin equipment, and Canadian Diabetes Association 2013 Clinical Practice Guidelines for the prevention and management of diabetes in Canada.

Unit Five includes Chapters 19 through 23. Chapters 19 and 20 provide students with a discussion of intravenous (IV) fluids and associated calculations related to IV therapy. The recalculation of IV flow rate includes an alternative method to determining the percentage of variation. IV labels have been added throughout the chapter, with a discussion of additives to IV solutions. Chapter 21 focuses on heparin and uses the new heparin labelling. Sample heparin weight-based protocols are used to adjust IV heparin based on activated partial thromboplastin time (aPTT). Chapter 22 discusses the principles of calculating pediatric and adult dosages, with emphasis on calculating dosages based on body weight and body surface area as well as verifying the safety of dosages. Chapter 23 provides students with the skills necessary to calculate critical care IV medications. Determining the titration of IV flow rates for titrated medications includes developing a titration table.

Safety Alerts, Practice Problems, Clinical Reasoning scenarios, and Points to Remember are included throughout the book. A Comprehensive Post-Test is included at the end of the book and covers all 23 chapters.

Features of the First Canadian Edition

- Objectives at the beginning of each chapter to emphasize content to be mastered.
- Canadian medication labels.

- Integration of ISMP Canada recommendations in the book to alert students to the importance of patient safety and reducing medication errors.
- Content related to preventing medication errors, such as the use of Tall Man Lettering, verification of the rights of medication administration, and an examination of the nursing role in preventing medication errors.
- Discussions on preventing medication errors in chapters dealing with high-alert medications (heparin and insulin).
- An up-to-date insulin chapter that reflects the Canadian Diabetes Association 2013 Clinical Practice Guidelines on insulin therapy, which features basal + bolus + correction insulin dosing as well as IV insulin therapy.
- An IV chapter, including IV labels and a discussion of IV additives. Recalculation of IV therapy includes an alternative approach to determining the variation of change using percentages.
- Safety Alert boxes that direct students to common errors and how to avoid them.
- Inclusion of heparin weight-based protocol and problems on adjusting the flow rate based on PTT.
- Critical care discussion on IV flow rates for titrated medications, including how to develop a titration table.
- Calculation of fluid resuscitation for patients with burns as well as daily pediatric fluid maintenance.
- Practice Problems and Chapter Review problems in each chapter.
- An Answer Key at the end of each chapter to provide immediate feedback on solutions to problems.

Ancillaries

Evolve Resources for Calculate with Confidence, First Canadian Edition, are available to enhance student instruction. This online resource can be found at http://evolve.elsevier.com/Canada/GrayMorris/. It corresponds with the chapters of the main book and includes the following:
- TEACH for Nurses
- Test Bank
- PowerPoint Slides
- Image Collection of Drug Labels
- Answer Key from Textbook
- Student Review Questions
- *Drug Calculations Comprehensive Test Bank, Version 4* is a generic test bank that contains more than 700 questions on general mathematics, converting within the same system of measurement, converting between different systems of measurement, oral dosages, parenteral dosages, IV flow rates, pediatric dosages, IV calculations, and more.
- *Drug Calculations Companion, Version 5* is a completely updated, interactive student tutorial that includes an extensive menu of various topic areas within drug calculations, including oral, parenteral, pediatric, and IV calculations. It contains more than 600 Practice Problems covering the ratio and proportion method, the formula method, and the dimensional analysis method.

We hope that this book will be a valuable asset to current and future practitioners. May it help you calculate dosages accurately and with confidence, using calculation and critical thinking skills to ensure that medications are administered safely to all patients, regardless of the setting. This is both a priority and a primary responsibility of the nurse.

Deborah C. Gray Morris and Marcia Brown

Acknowledgements

The very first person I must offer thanks to for her role in the completion of this first Canadian edition of *Calculate with Confidence* is Roberta A. Spinosa-Millman. Your insight has afforded me the opportunity to showcase my work to the nursing community and beyond. Thank you for your courage in believing that I could.

To Elsevier Canada, I say kudos for promoting a culture of equality that offers positive regard and respect in the pursuit of quality in academic resources. This edition became alive through Theresa Fitzgerald, my developmental editor. With "the patience of Job," and with deliberate calm, you focused on my ability to get the work done rather than my inability to meet deadlines. Thank you; greatly appreciated.

Before starting the writing process, Ann Millar offered me the opportunity to speak with previous authors connected with Elsevier. I did. To Sandra A. Pike-MacDonald, Sonja L. Jakubec, and Cheryl L. Pollard, I say a big THANK YOU for responding honestly to my queries about the unknown. The reviewers of the first draft of this edition were anonymous to me. However, I thank them for their critical review of the draft manuscript. Their feedback not only adds value to the text but also underscores the benefits of having blind reviewers as part of the process.

Finally, I thank my three children, Danielle, Ayesha, and Cecilia, in reverse order of arrival. You have all contributed in the capacity that you can at each stage of the project. A special thank you to Ayesha for assisting me at the very first stage with double-checking answers to Practice Problems and Chapter Review problems. To my husband, I say, "Your support of me and family during the writing of this book has been incredible! You have changed me."

—**Marcia Brown**

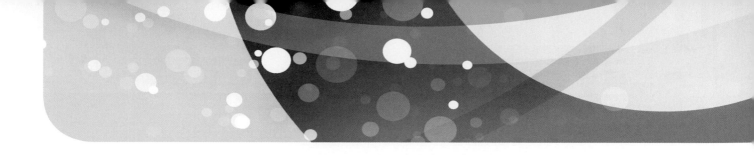

Contents

UNIT ONE

Math Review

An essential role of the nurse is providing safe medication administration to all patients. To accurately perform dosage calculations, the nurse must have knowledge of basic math, regardless of the problem-solving method used in calculation. Knowledge of basic math is a necessary component of dosage calculation that nurses need to know to prevent medication errors and ensure the safe administration of medications to all patients, regardless of the setting. Serious harm to patients can result from a mathematical error during calculation and administration of a medication dosage. The nurse must practise and be proficient in the basic math used in dosage calculations. Knowledge of basic math is a prerequisite for the prevention of medication errors and ensures the safe administration of medications.

Although calculators are accessible for basic math operations, the nurse needs to be able to perform the processes involved in basic math. Controversy still exists among educators regarding the use of calculators in dosage calculation. Calculators may indeed be recommended for complex calculations to ensure accuracy and save time; the types of calculations requiring their use are presented later in this text. However, because the basic math required for less complex calculations is often simple and can be done without the use of a calculator, it is a realistic expectation that each practitioner should be competent in the performance of basic math operations without its use. Performing basic math operations enables the nurse to think logically and critically about the dosage ordered and the dosage calculated.

PRE-TEST

This test is designed to evaluate your ability in the basic math areas reviewed in Unit One. The test consists of 62 questions. If you are able to complete the pre-test with 100% accuracy, you may want to bypass Unit One. Any problems answered incorrectly should be used as a basis for what you might need to review. The purposes of this test and the review that follows are to build your confidence in basic math skills and to help you avoid careless mistakes when you begin to perform dosage calculations.

Reduce the following fractions to lowest terms.

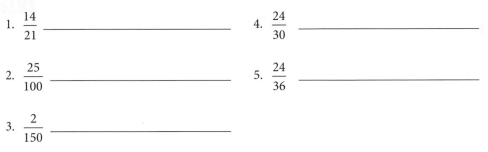

1. $\dfrac{14}{21}$ _____   4. $\dfrac{24}{30}$ _____

2. $\dfrac{25}{100}$ _____   5. $\dfrac{24}{36}$ _____

3. $\dfrac{2}{150}$ _____

Perform the indicated operations; reduce to lowest terms where necessary.

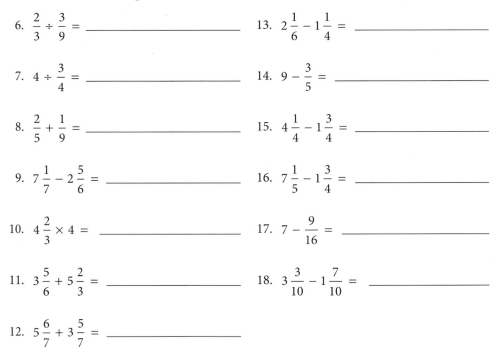

6. $\dfrac{2}{3} \div \dfrac{3}{9} =$ _____   13. $2\dfrac{1}{6} - 1\dfrac{1}{4} =$ _____

7. $4 \div \dfrac{3}{4} =$ _____   14. $9 - \dfrac{3}{5} =$ _____

8. $\dfrac{2}{5} + \dfrac{1}{9} =$ _____   15. $4\dfrac{1}{4} - 1\dfrac{3}{4} =$ _____

9. $7\dfrac{1}{7} - 2\dfrac{5}{6} =$ _____   16. $7\dfrac{1}{5} - 1\dfrac{3}{4} =$ _____

10. $4\dfrac{2}{3} \times 4 =$ _____   17. $7 - \dfrac{9}{16} =$ _____

11. $3\dfrac{5}{6} + 5\dfrac{2}{3} =$ _____   18. $3\dfrac{3}{10} - 1\dfrac{7}{10} =$ _____

12. $5\dfrac{6}{7} + 3\dfrac{5}{7} =$ _____

Change the following fractions to decimals; express your answer to the nearest tenth.

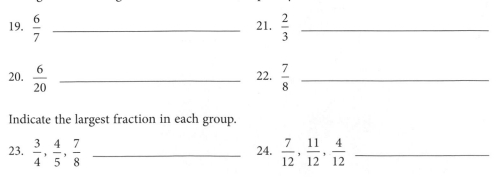

19. $\dfrac{6}{7}$ _____   21. $\dfrac{2}{3}$ _____

20. $\dfrac{6}{20}$ _____   22. $\dfrac{7}{8}$ _____

Indicate the largest fraction in each group.

23. $\dfrac{3}{4}, \dfrac{4}{5}, \dfrac{7}{8}$ _____   24. $\dfrac{7}{12}, \dfrac{11}{12}, \dfrac{4}{12}$ _____

Perform the indicated operations with decimals. Provide the exact answer; do not round off.

25. $20.1 + 67.35 =$ _____

26. $0.008 + 5 =$ _____

27. $4.6 \times 8.72 =$ _____

28. $56.47 - 8.7 =$ _____

Divide the following decimals; express your answer to the nearest tenth.

29. $7.5 \div 0.004 =$ _____

30. $45 \div 1.9 =$ _____

31. $84.7 \div 2.3 =$ _____

Indicate the largest decimal in each group.

32. $0.674, 0.659$ _____

33. $0.375, 0.37, 0.38$ _____

34. $0.25, 0.6, 0.175$ _____

Solve for x, the unknown value.

35. $82 = 48 : x$ _____

36. $x : 300 = 1 : 150$ _____

37. $\dfrac{1}{10} : x = \dfrac{1}{2} : 15$ _____

38. $0.4 : 1 = 0.2 : x$ _____

Round off to the nearest tenth.

39. 0.43 _____

40. 0.66 _____

41. 1.47 _____

Round off to the nearest hundredth.

42. 0.735 _____

43. 0.834 _____

44. 1.227 _____

Complete the table below, expressing the measures in their equivalents where indicated. Reduce to lowest terms where necessary.

	Percentage	Decimal	Ratio	Fraction
45.	6%	_____	_____	_____
46.	_____	_____	$7:20$	_____
47.	_____	_____	_____	$5\dfrac{1}{4}$
48.	_____	0.015	_____	_____

Find the following percentages. Express your answer to the hundredths place as indicated.

49. 5% of 95 _____   52. 20 is what % of 100 _____

50. $\frac{1}{4}$% of 2 000 _____   53. 30 is what % of 164 _____

51. 2 is what % of 600 _____

54. A patient is instructed to take 7.5 millilitres (mL) of a cough syrup 3 times a day. How many mL of cough syrup will the patient take each day? _____

55. A tablet contains 0.75 milligrams (mg) of a medication. A patient receives 3 tablets a day for 5 days. How many mg of the medication will the patient receive in 5 days? _____

56. A patient took 0.44 micrograms (mcg) of a medication every morning and 1.4 mcg each evening for 5 days. What is the total amount of medication taken? _____

57. Write a ratio that represents that every tablet in a bottle contains 0.5 mg of a medication. _____

58. Write a ratio that represents 60 mg of a medication in 1 mL of a liquid. _____

59. A patient takes 10 mL of a medication 3 times a day. How long will 120 mL of medication last? _____

60. A patient weighed 125 kilograms (kg) before dieting. After dieting, the patient weighed 113.6 kg. What is the percentage of change in the patient's weight? _____

61. A patient was prescribed 10 mg of a medication for a week. After a week, the health care provider reduced the medication to 7 mg. What was the percentage of decrease in medication? _____

62. A patient received 22.5 mg of a medication in tablet form. Each tablet contained 4.5 mg of medication. How many tablets were given to the patient? _____

Answers on page 5.

✴ ANSWERS

1. $\dfrac{2}{3}$

2. $\dfrac{1}{4}$

3. $\dfrac{1}{75}$

4. $\dfrac{4}{5}$

5. $\dfrac{4}{6} = \dfrac{2}{3}$

6. 2

7. $5\dfrac{1}{3}$

8. $\dfrac{23}{45}$

9. $4\dfrac{13}{42}$

10. $18\dfrac{2}{3}$

11. $9\dfrac{3}{6} = 9\dfrac{1}{2}$

12. $8\dfrac{11}{7} = 9\dfrac{4}{7}$

13. $\dfrac{11}{12}$

14. $8\dfrac{2}{5}$

15. $2\dfrac{2}{4} = 2\dfrac{1}{2}$

16. $5\dfrac{9}{20}$

17. $6\dfrac{7}{16}$

18. $1\dfrac{6}{10} = 1\dfrac{3}{5}$

19. 0.9

20. 0.3

21. 0.7

22. 0.9

23. $\dfrac{7}{8}$

24. $\dfrac{11}{12}$

25. 87.45

26. 5.008

27. 40.112

28. 47.77

29. 1 875

30. 23.7

31. 36.8

32. 0.674

33. 0.38

34. 0.6

35. $x = 12$

36. $x = 2$

37. $x = 3$

38. $x = 0.5$ or $\dfrac{1}{2}$

39. 0.4

40. 0.7

41. 1.5

42. 0.74

43. 0.83

44. 1.23

Percentage	Decimal	Ratio	Fraction
45. 6%	0.06	3:50	$\dfrac{3}{50}$
46. 35%	0.35	7:20	$\dfrac{7}{20}$
47. 525%	5.25	21:4	$5\dfrac{1}{4}$
48. 1.5%	0.015	3:200	$\dfrac{3}{200}$

49. 4.75

50. 5

51. 0.33%

52. 20%

53. 18.29%

54. 22.5 mL

55. 11.25 mg

56. 9.2 mcg

57. 0.5 mg : 1 tablet

58. 60 mg : 1 mL

59. 4 days

60. 9%

61. 30%

62. 5 tablets

CHAPTER 1
Fractions

Objectives

After reviewing this chapter, you should be able to:
1. Compare the size of fractions
2. Add fractions
3. Subtract fractions
4. Divide fractions
5. Multiply fractions
6. Reduce fractions to lowest terms

Health care providers need to have an understanding of fractions. Fractions may be seen in medical orders, patient records, prescriptions, documentation relating to care given to patients, and literature related to health care. Nurses often encounter fractions in dosage calculation.

Some methods of solving dosage calculations rely on expressing relationships in a fraction format. Therefore, proficiency with fractions can be beneficial in a variety of situations.

A fraction is used to indicate a part of a whole number (Figure 1-1). It is a division of a whole into units or parts (Figure 1-2). A fraction is composed of two parts: an upper number referred to as the **numerator** and a lower number called the **denominator.** The numerator and denominator are separated by a horizontal line. A fraction may also be read as the numerator divided by the denominator.

Example: $\dfrac{1}{2}$ is a whole divided into two equal parts.

$$\frac{\text{Numerator}}{\text{Denominator}} : \frac{\text{how many parts of the whole are considered}}{\text{how many equal parts the whole is divided into}}$$

Example: In the fraction $\dfrac{5}{6}$, the whole is divided into 6 equal parts (denominator), and five parts (numerator) are considered.

$\dfrac{5}{6}$ = 5 parts of 6 parts, or $\dfrac{5}{6}$ of the whole.

The fraction $\dfrac{5}{6}$ may also be read as 5 divided by 6.

Figure 1-1 Diagram representing fractions of a whole. Five parts shaded out of the six parts represent:

$$\frac{5}{6} \quad \frac{\text{Numerator}}{\text{Denominator}}$$

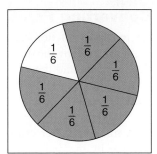

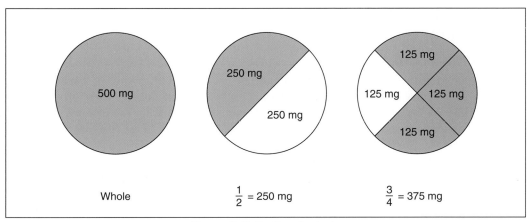

Figure 1-2 Fraction pie charts.

Types of Fractions

Proper Fraction: Numerator is less than the denominator, and the fraction has a value of less than 1.

Examples: $\frac{1}{8}, \frac{5}{6}, \frac{7}{8}, \frac{1}{150}$

Improper Fraction: Numerator is larger than, or equal to, the denominator, and the fraction has a value of 1 or greater than 1.

Examples: $\frac{3}{2}, \frac{7}{5}, \frac{300}{150}, \frac{4}{4}$

Mixed Number: Whole number and a proper fraction in which the total value of the mixed number is greater than 1.

Examples: $3\frac{1}{3}, 5\frac{1}{8}, 9\frac{1}{6}, 25\frac{7}{8}$

Complex Fraction: Numerator, denominator, or both are fractions. The value may be less than, greater than, or equal to 1.

Examples: $\frac{3\frac{1}{2}}{2}, \frac{\frac{1}{3}}{\frac{1}{2}}, \frac{2}{1\frac{1}{4}}, \frac{2}{\frac{1}{150}}$

Whole Numbers: Have an unexpressed denominator of one (1).

Examples: $1 = \frac{1}{1}, 3 = \frac{3}{1}, 6 = \frac{6}{1}, 100 = \frac{100}{1}$

Converting Fractions

An improper fraction can be changed to a mixed number or whole number by dividing the numerator by the denominator. If there is a remainder, that number is placed over the denominator, and the answer is reduced to lowest terms.

Examples: $\dfrac{6}{5} = 6 \div 5 = 1\dfrac{1}{5},\ \dfrac{100}{25} = 100 \div 25 = 4,\ \dfrac{10}{8} = 10 \div 8 = 1\dfrac{2}{8} = 1\dfrac{1}{4}$

A mixed number can be changed to an improper fraction by multiplying the whole number by the denominator, adding it to the numerator, and placing the sum over the denominator.

Example: $5\dfrac{1}{8} = \dfrac{(5 \times 8) + 1}{8} = \dfrac{41}{8}$

Comparing Fractions

Comparing the size of fractions is important in the administration of medications. It helps the new practitioner learn the value of medication dosages early on. Fractions can be compared if the numerators are the same by comparing the denominators or if the denominators are the same by comparing the numerators. These rules are presented in Box 1-1.

BOX 1-1 Rules for Comparing the Size of Fractions
Here are some basic rules to keep in mind when comparing fractions.   1. If the numerators are the same, the fraction with the smaller denominator has the greater value.   Example: $\dfrac{1}{2}$ is larger than $\dfrac{1}{3}$ Example: $\dfrac{1}{150}$ is larger than $\dfrac{1}{300}$ 2. If the denominators are the same, the fraction with the larger numerator has the greater value.   Example: $\dfrac{3}{4}$ is larger than $\dfrac{1}{4}$ Example: $\dfrac{3}{100}$ is larger than $\dfrac{1}{100}$

Two or more fractions with different denominators can be compared by changing both fractions to fractions with the same denominator (see Box 1-1). This is done by finding the lowest common denominator (LCD), or the lowest number evenly divisible by the denominators of the fractions being compared.

Example: Which is larger, $\dfrac{3}{4}$ or $\dfrac{4}{5}$?

NOTE
LCD = 20

Solution: The LCD is 20, because it is the smallest number that can be divided by both denominators evenly. Change each fraction to the same terms by dividing the LCD by the denominator and multiplying that answer by the numerator. The answer obtained from this is the new numerator. The numerators are then placed over the LCD.

For the fraction $\dfrac{3}{4}$, $20 \div 4 = 5$; $5 \times 3 = 15$; therefore $\dfrac{3}{4}$ becomes $\dfrac{15}{20}$.

For the fraction $\dfrac{4}{5}$, $20 \div 5 = 4$; $4 \times 4 = 16$; therefore $\dfrac{4}{5}$ becomes $\dfrac{16}{20}$.

Therefore $\dfrac{4}{5}\left(\dfrac{16}{20}\right)$ is larger than $\dfrac{3}{4}\left(\dfrac{15}{20}\right)$.

Box 1-2 presents fundamental rules of fractions.

BOX 1-2   Fundamental Rules of Fractions

When working with fractions, there are some fundamental rules that we need to remember.

1. When the numerator and denominator of a fraction are both multiplied or divided by the same number, the value of the fraction remains unchanged.

Examples:
$$\frac{1}{2} = \frac{1 \times (2)}{2 \times (2)} = \frac{2}{4} = \frac{2 \times (25)}{4 \times (25)} = \frac{50}{100} \text{, etc.}$$

$$\frac{50}{100} = \frac{50 \div (10)}{100 \div (10)} = \frac{5}{10} = \frac{5 \div (5)}{10 \div (5)} = \frac{1}{2} \text{, etc.}$$

As shown in the examples, common fractions can be written in various forms, provided that the numerator, divided by the denominator, always yields the same number (quotient). The particular form of a fraction that has the smallest possible whole number for its numerator and denominator is called the *fraction in its lowest terms.* In the example, therefore, $\frac{50}{100}$, $\frac{5}{10}$, or $\frac{2}{4}$ is $\frac{1}{2}$ in its lowest terms.

2. To change a fraction to its lowest terms, divide its numerator and its denominator by the largest whole number that will divide both evenly.

Example: Reduce $\frac{128}{288}$ to lowest terms.

$$\frac{128}{288} = \frac{128 \div 32}{288 \div 32} = \frac{4}{9}$$

Note: When you do not see the largest number that can be divided evenly at once, the fraction may have to be reduced by using repeated steps.

Example:
$$\frac{128}{288} = \frac{128 \div 4}{288 \div 4} = \frac{32}{72} = \frac{32 \div 8}{72 \div 8} = \frac{4}{9}$$

Note: If both the numerator and denominator cannot be divided evenly by a whole number, the fraction is already in lowest terms. Fractions should always be expressed in their lowest terms.

3. The LCD is the smallest whole number that can be divided evenly by all of the denominators within the problem.

Example: $\frac{1}{3}$ and $\frac{5}{12}$: 12 is evenly divisible by 3; therefore 12 is the LCD.

$\frac{3}{7}$, $\frac{2}{14}$, and $\frac{2}{28}$: 28 is evenly divisible by 7 and 14; therefore 28 is the LCD.

✛ ➖ ➗ ✖ PRACTICE **PROBLEMS**

Circle the fraction with the lesser value in each of the following sets.

1. $\frac{6}{30}$ $\frac{4}{5}$ 6. $\frac{4}{8}$ $\frac{1}{8}$ $\frac{3}{8}$

2. $\frac{5}{4}$ $\frac{6}{8}$ 7. $\frac{1}{40}$ $\frac{1}{10}$ $\frac{1}{5}$

3. $\frac{1}{75}$ $\frac{1}{100}$ $\frac{1}{150}$ 8. $\frac{1}{300}$ $\frac{1}{200}$ $\frac{1}{175}$

4. $\frac{6}{18}$ $\frac{7}{18}$ $\frac{8}{18}$ 9. $\frac{4}{24}$ $\frac{5}{24}$ $\frac{10}{24}$

5. $\frac{4}{5}$ $\frac{7}{5}$ $\frac{3}{5}$ 10. $\frac{4}{3}$ $\frac{1}{2}$ $\frac{1}{6}$

Circle the fraction with the greater value in each of the following sets.

11. $\dfrac{6}{8}$ $\dfrac{5}{9}$

16. $\dfrac{2}{5}$ $\dfrac{6}{5}$ $\dfrac{3}{5}$

12. $\dfrac{7}{6}$ $\dfrac{2}{3}$

17. $\dfrac{1}{8}$ $\dfrac{4}{6}$ $\dfrac{1}{4}$

13. $\dfrac{1}{72}$ $\dfrac{6}{12}$ $\dfrac{1}{24}$

18. $\dfrac{7}{9}$ $\dfrac{5}{9}$ $\dfrac{8}{9}$

14. $\dfrac{1}{10}$ $\dfrac{1}{6}$ $\dfrac{1}{8}$

19. $\dfrac{1}{10}$ $\dfrac{1}{50}$ $\dfrac{1}{150}$

15. $\dfrac{1}{75}$ $\dfrac{1}{125}$ $\dfrac{1}{225}$

20. $\dfrac{2}{15}$ $\dfrac{1}{15}$ $\dfrac{6}{15}$

Answers on page 21.

Reducing Fractions

Fractions should always be reduced to their lowest terms.

> **RULE**
>
> To reduce a fraction to its lowest terms, the numerator and denominator are each divided by the largest number by which they are both evenly divisible.

Example: Reduce the fraction $\dfrac{6}{20}$.

Solution: Both numerator and denominator are evenly divisible by 2.

$$\frac{6}{20} \div \frac{2}{2} = \frac{3}{10}$$

$$\frac{6}{20} = \frac{3}{10}$$

Example: Reduce the fraction $\dfrac{75}{100}$.

Solution: Both numerator and denominator are evenly divisible by 25.

$$\frac{75}{100} \div \frac{25}{25} = \frac{3}{4}$$

$$\frac{75}{100} = \frac{3}{4}$$

+−÷× PRACTICE **PROBLEMS**

Reduce the following fractions to their lowest terms.

21. $\dfrac{10}{15} =$ _____

22. $\dfrac{7}{49} =$ _____

23. $\dfrac{64}{128}$ = _____

30. $\dfrac{9}{27}$ = _____

24. $\dfrac{100}{150}$ = _____

31. $\dfrac{9}{9}$ = _____

25. $\dfrac{20}{28}$ = _____

32. $\dfrac{15}{45}$ = _____

26. $\dfrac{14}{98}$ = _____

33. $\dfrac{124}{155}$ = _____

27. $\dfrac{10}{18}$ = _____

34. $\dfrac{12}{18}$ = _____

28. $\dfrac{24}{36}$ = _____

35. $\dfrac{36}{64}$ = _____

29. $\dfrac{10}{50}$ = _____

Answers on page 21.

Adding Fractions

RULE

To add fractions with the same denominator, add the numerators, place the sum over the denominator, and reduce to lowest terms.

Example:
$$\frac{1}{6} + \frac{4}{6} = \frac{5}{6}$$

Example:
$$\frac{1}{6} + \frac{3}{6} + \frac{4}{6} = \frac{8}{6}$$

$$\frac{8}{6} = \frac{4}{3} = 1\frac{1}{3}$$

NOTE

In addition to reducing to lowest terms in the second Example, the improper fraction was changed to a mixed number.

RULE

To add fractions with different denominators, change fractions to their equivalent fraction with the LCD, add the numerators, write the sum over the common denominator, and reduce if necessary.

Example: $\dfrac{1}{4} + \dfrac{1}{3}$

Solution: The LCD is 12. Change to equivalent fractions.

$$\frac{1}{4} = \frac{3}{12}$$
$$+\frac{1}{3} = \frac{4}{12}$$
$$\overline{\qquad \frac{7}{12}}$$

Example:
$$\frac{1}{2} + 1\frac{1}{3} + \frac{2}{4}$$

Solution: Change the mixed number $1\frac{1}{3}$ to $\frac{4}{3}$. Find the LCD, change fractions to equivalent fractions, add, and reduce if necessary.
The LCD is 12.

$$\frac{1}{2} = \frac{6}{12}$$

$$\frac{4}{3} = \frac{16}{12}$$

$$+\frac{2}{4} = \frac{6}{12}$$

$$\frac{28}{12} = 2\frac{4}{12} = 2\frac{1}{3}$$

Subtracting Fractions

> **RULE**
>
> To subtract fractions with the same denominator, subtract the numerators, and place this amount over the denominator. Reduce to lowest terms if necessary.

Example: $\dfrac{5}{4} - \dfrac{3}{4} = \dfrac{2}{4} = \dfrac{1}{2}$

Example: $2\dfrac{1}{6} - \dfrac{5}{6}$

Solution: Change the mixed number $2\frac{1}{6}$ to $\frac{13}{6}$

$$\frac{13}{6} - \frac{5}{6} = \frac{8}{6} = \frac{4}{3} = 1\frac{1}{3}$$

> **RULE**
>
> To subtract fractions with different denominators, find the LCD, change to equivalent fractions, subtract the numerators, and place the sum over the common denominator. Reduce to lowest terms if necessary.

Example: $\dfrac{15}{6} - \dfrac{3}{5}$

Solution: The LCD is 30. Change to equivalent fractions, and subtract.

$$\frac{15}{6} = \frac{75}{30}$$

$$-\frac{3}{5} = \frac{18}{30}$$

$$\frac{57}{30} = 1\frac{27}{30} = 1\frac{9}{10}$$

Example: $2\dfrac{1}{5} - \dfrac{4}{3}$

Solution: Change the mixed number $2\frac{1}{5}$ to $\frac{11}{5}$. Find the LCD, change to equivalent fractions, subtract, and reduce if necessary.

The LCD is 15.

$$
\begin{array}{r}
\dfrac{11}{5} = \dfrac{33}{15} \\[2mm]
-\dfrac{4}{3} = \dfrac{20}{15} \\[2mm]
\hline
\dfrac{13}{15}
\end{array}
$$

Subtracting a Fraction from a Whole Number

RULE

To subtract a fraction from a whole number, follow these steps:

1. Borrow 1 from the whole number, and change it to a fraction, creating a mixed number.
2. Change the fraction so it has the same denominator as the fraction to be subtracted.
3. Subtract the fraction from the mixed number.
4. Reduce if necessary.

Example: Subtract $\dfrac{7}{12}$ from 6

$$
6 = 5 + \dfrac{1}{1} = 5\dfrac{12}{12}
$$

$$
\begin{array}{r}
-\dfrac{7}{12} = \dfrac{7}{12} \\[2mm]
\hline
5\dfrac{5}{12}
\end{array}
$$

Subtracting Fractions Using Borrowing

RULE

To subtract fractions using borrowing, use the following steps:

1. Change both fractions to the same denominator if necessary.
2. Borrow 1 from the whole number and change it to the same denominator as the fraction in the mixed number. Add the two fractions together.
3. Subtract the fractions and the whole numbers.
4. Reduce if necessary.

Example: $5\dfrac{1}{4} - 3\dfrac{3}{4}$

In the above example, because $\dfrac{3}{4}$ is larger than $\dfrac{1}{4}$, subtraction of the fractions is not possible. Both fractions have the same denominator; no changes need to be made. Therefore, borrow 1 from the whole number part (5), and add the 1 to the fractional part $\left(\dfrac{1}{4}\right)$.

The result is $5\dfrac{1}{4} = 4 + \dfrac{1}{1} + \dfrac{1}{4} = 4 + \dfrac{4}{4} + \dfrac{1}{4} = 4\dfrac{5}{4}$

$$
\begin{array}{r}
5\dfrac{1}{4} = 4\dfrac{5}{4} \\[2mm]
3\dfrac{3}{4} = 3\dfrac{3}{4} \\[2mm]
\hline
1\dfrac{5-3}{4} = 1\dfrac{2}{4} = 1\dfrac{1}{2}
\end{array}
$$

Example: Subtract $4\dfrac{3}{4}$ from $9\dfrac{2}{3}$

Both fractions need to be changed to the same denominator of 12:

$$9\dfrac{2}{3} = 9\dfrac{8}{12} \text{ and } 4\dfrac{3}{4} = 4\dfrac{9}{12}$$

Subtraction of the fractions is not possible because $\dfrac{9}{12}$ is larger than $\dfrac{8}{12}$.

Therefore, borrow 1 from 9.

$$9\dfrac{8}{12} = 8 + \dfrac{1}{1} + \dfrac{8}{12} = 8 + \dfrac{12}{12} + \dfrac{8}{12} = 8\dfrac{20}{12}$$

Now subtract:

$$9\dfrac{2}{3} = 9\dfrac{8}{12} = 8\dfrac{20}{12}$$
$$-\ 4\dfrac{3}{4} = 4\dfrac{9}{12} = 4\dfrac{9}{12}$$
$$\rule{4cm}{0.4pt}$$
$$4\dfrac{11}{12}$$

Multiplying Fractions

> **RULE**
> 1. Cancel terms if possible.
> 2. Multiply the numerators, multiply the denominators.
> 3. Reduce the result (product) to the lowest terms, if necessary.

NOTE
If fractions are not in lowest terms, reduction can be done before multiplication. This can make the calculation simple because you are working with smaller numbers.

Notice in this example that the numerator and denominator of any of the fractions involved in multiplication may be cancelled when they can be divided by the same number (cross-cancellation).

Example 1: $\dfrac{3}{\cancel{4}_{2}} \times \dfrac{\cancel{2}^{1}}{5} = \dfrac{3}{10}$

Example 2: $\dfrac{2}{4} \times \dfrac{3}{4}$

Solution: Reduce $\dfrac{2}{4}$ to $\dfrac{1}{2}$ and then multiply.

$$\dfrac{1}{2} \times \dfrac{3}{4} = \dfrac{3}{8}$$

Example 3: $6 \times \dfrac{5}{6}$

NOTE
The whole number 6 is expressed as a fraction here by placing 1 as the denominator, as shown in Example 3, then cross-cancellation is done because the numerator and denominator of the fractions can be divided by the same number.

$$\dfrac{\cancel{6}^{1}}{1} \times \dfrac{5}{\cancel{6}_{1}} = 5$$

or

$$\dfrac{6 \times 5}{6} = \dfrac{30}{6} = 5$$

Example 4: $3\dfrac{1}{3} \times 2\dfrac{1}{2}$

Solution: Change the mixed numbers to improper fractions. Proceed with multiplication.

$$3\frac{1}{3} = \frac{10}{3}; \ 2\frac{1}{2} = \frac{5}{2}$$

$$\frac{10}{3} \times \frac{5}{2} = \frac{50}{6} = 8\frac{2}{6} = 8\frac{1}{3}$$

or

$$\frac{\overset{5}{\cancel{10}}}{3} \times \frac{5}{\underset{1}{\cancel{2}}} = \frac{25}{3} = 8\frac{1}{3}$$

Dividing Fractions

RULE

1. To divide fractions, invert (turn upside down) the second fraction (divisor); change ÷ to ×.
2. Cancel terms, if possible.
3. Multiply fractions.
4. Reduce if necessary.

Example:

$$\frac{3}{4} \div \frac{2}{3}$$

Solution:

$$\frac{3}{4} \times \frac{3}{2} = \frac{9}{8} = 1\frac{1}{8}$$

Example:

$$1\frac{3}{5} \div 2\frac{1}{10}$$

Solution: Change the mixed numbers to improper fractions. Proceed with the steps of division.

$$1\frac{3}{5} = \frac{8}{5}; \ 2\frac{1}{10} = \frac{21}{10}$$

$$\frac{8}{\underset{1}{\cancel{5}}} \times \frac{\overset{2}{\cancel{10}}}{21} = \frac{16}{21}$$

Example:

$$5 \div \frac{1}{2}$$

Solution:

$$5 \times \frac{2}{1} = \frac{10}{1} = 10$$

or

$$\frac{5}{1} \times \frac{2}{1} = \frac{10}{1} = 10$$

When doing dosage calculations that involve division, the fractions may be written as follows: $\dfrac{\frac{1}{4}}{\frac{1}{2}}$. In this case, $\dfrac{1}{4}$ is the numerator and $\dfrac{1}{2}$ is the denominator. Therefore, the problem is set up as $\dfrac{1}{4} \div \dfrac{1}{2}$, which becomes $\dfrac{1}{\underset{2}{\cancel{4}}} \times \dfrac{\overset{1}{\cancel{2}}}{1} = \dfrac{1}{2}$.

👆 PRACTICE **PROBLEMS**

Change the following improper fractions to mixed numbers, and reduce to lowest terms.

36. $\dfrac{18}{5}$ = _____   39. $\dfrac{35}{12}$ = _____

37. $\dfrac{60}{14}$ = _____   40. $\dfrac{112}{100}$ = _____

38. $\dfrac{13}{8}$ = _____

Change the following mixed numbers to improper fractions.

41. $1\dfrac{4}{25}$ = _____   44. $3\dfrac{3}{8}$ = _____

42. $4\dfrac{2}{8}$ = _____   45. $15\dfrac{4}{5}$ = _____

43. $4\dfrac{1}{2}$ = _____

Add the following fractions and mixed numbers, and reduce fractions to lowest terms.

46. $\dfrac{2}{3} + \dfrac{5}{6}$ = _____   49. $7\dfrac{2}{5} + \dfrac{2}{3}$ = _____

47. $2\dfrac{1}{8} + \dfrac{2}{3}$ = _____   50. $12\dfrac{1}{2} + 10\dfrac{1}{3}$ = _____

48. $2\dfrac{3}{10} + 4\dfrac{1}{5} + \dfrac{2}{3}$ = _____

Subtract and reduce fractions to lowest terms.

51. $\dfrac{4}{3} - \dfrac{3}{7}$ = _____   55. $\dfrac{1}{8} - \dfrac{1}{12}$ = _____

52. $3\dfrac{3}{8} - 1\dfrac{3}{5}$ = _____   56. $14 - \dfrac{5}{9}$ = _____

53. $\dfrac{15}{16} - \dfrac{1}{4}$ = _____   57. $3\dfrac{3}{10} - 1\dfrac{7}{10}$ = _____

54. $2\dfrac{5}{6} - 2\dfrac{3}{4}$ = _____

Multiply the following fractions and mixed numbers, and reduce to lowest terms.

58. $\dfrac{2}{3} \times \dfrac{4}{5}$ = _____   59. $\dfrac{6}{25} \times \dfrac{3}{5}$ = _____

60. $\dfrac{1}{50} \times 3 =$ _____

61. $2\dfrac{5}{8} \times 2\dfrac{3}{4} =$ _____

62. $\dfrac{5}{12} \times \dfrac{4}{9} =$ _____

Divide the following fractions and mixed numbers and reduce to lowest terms.

63. $2\dfrac{6}{8} \div 1\dfrac{2}{3} =$ _____

64. $\dfrac{1}{60} \div \dfrac{1}{2} =$ _____

65. $6 \div \dfrac{2}{5} =$ _____

66. $\dfrac{7}{8} \div \dfrac{7}{8} =$ _____

67. $3\dfrac{1}{3} \div 1\dfrac{7}{12} =$ _____

Answers on page 21.

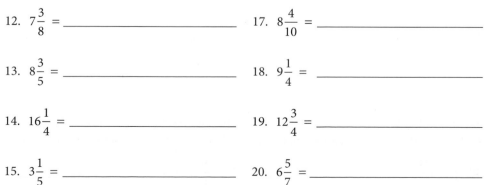

CHAPTER **REVIEW**

Change the following improper fractions to mixed numbers, and reduce to lowest terms.

1. $\dfrac{10}{8} =$ _____

2. $\dfrac{30}{4} =$ _____

3. $\dfrac{22}{6} =$ _____

4. $\dfrac{11}{4} =$ _____

5. $\dfrac{59}{14} =$ _____

6. $\dfrac{67}{10} =$ _____

7. $\dfrac{9}{2} =$ _____

8. $\dfrac{11}{5} =$ _____

9. $\dfrac{64}{15} =$ _____

10. $\dfrac{100}{13} =$ _____

Change the following mixed numbers to improper fractions.

11. $2\dfrac{1}{2} =$ _____

12. $7\dfrac{3}{8} =$ _____

13. $8\dfrac{3}{5} =$ _____

14. $16\dfrac{1}{4} =$ _____

15. $3\dfrac{1}{5} =$ _____

16. $2\dfrac{3}{5} =$ _____

17. $8\dfrac{4}{10} =$ _____

18. $9\dfrac{1}{4} =$ _____

19. $12\dfrac{3}{4} =$ _____

20. $6\dfrac{5}{7} =$ _____

Add the following fractions and mixed numbers. Reduce to lowest terms.

21. $\dfrac{2}{5} + \dfrac{1}{3} + \dfrac{7}{10} =$ _____

26. $\dfrac{15}{47} + \dfrac{15}{47} =$ _____

22. $\dfrac{1}{4} + \dfrac{1}{6} + \dfrac{1}{8} =$ _____

27. $10\dfrac{1}{6} + 12\dfrac{4}{6} =$ _____

23. $20\dfrac{1}{2} + \dfrac{1}{4} + \dfrac{5}{4} =$ _____

28. $101\dfrac{3}{4} + 33\dfrac{1}{4} + 5\dfrac{1}{4} =$ _____

24. $\dfrac{1}{2} + \dfrac{1}{5} =$ _____

29. $55\dfrac{1}{3} + 51\dfrac{5}{9} =$ _____

25. $6\dfrac{1}{4} + \dfrac{2}{9} + \dfrac{1}{36} =$ _____

30. $1\dfrac{4}{5} + 7\dfrac{9}{10} + 3\dfrac{1}{2} =$ _____

Subtract the following fractions and mixed numbers. Reduce to lowest terms.

31. $\dfrac{4}{9} - \dfrac{3}{9} =$ _____

39. $\dfrac{8}{5} - \dfrac{1}{3} =$ _____

32. $2\dfrac{1}{4} - 1\dfrac{1}{2} =$ _____

40. $\dfrac{4}{7} - \dfrac{1}{3} =$ _____

33. $2\dfrac{3}{4} - \dfrac{1}{4} =$ _____

41. $\dfrac{5}{6} - \dfrac{7}{12} =$ _____

34. $\dfrac{4}{5} - \dfrac{1}{6} =$ _____

42. $39\dfrac{5}{8} - 13\dfrac{1}{3} =$ _____

35. $\dfrac{6}{4} - \dfrac{1}{2} =$ _____

43. $48\dfrac{6}{11} - 24 =$ _____

36. $\dfrac{4}{5} - \dfrac{1}{4} =$ _____

44. $12\dfrac{1}{2} - \dfrac{3}{10} =$ _____

37. $\dfrac{4}{6} - \dfrac{3}{8} =$ _____

45. $39\dfrac{11}{18} - 8\dfrac{3}{6} =$ _____

38. $4\dfrac{1}{6} - 1\dfrac{1}{3} =$ _____

Multiply the following fractions and mixed numbers. Reduce to lowest terms.

46. $\dfrac{1}{3} \times \dfrac{4}{12} =$ _____

49. $15 \times \dfrac{2}{3} =$ _____

47. $2\dfrac{7}{8} \times 3\dfrac{1}{4} =$ _____

50. $36 \times \dfrac{3}{4} =$ _____

48. $8 \times 1\dfrac{3}{4} =$ _____

51. $\dfrac{5}{4} \times \dfrac{2}{4} =$ _____

52. $\dfrac{2}{5} \times \dfrac{1}{6} =$ _____

53. $\dfrac{3}{10} \times \dfrac{4}{12} =$ _____

54. $\dfrac{1}{9} \times \dfrac{7}{3} =$ _____

55. $\dfrac{10}{25} \times \dfrac{5}{3} =$ _____

56. $\dfrac{1}{2} \times \dfrac{3}{4} \times \dfrac{3}{5} =$ _____

57. $\dfrac{3}{5} \times 3\dfrac{1}{8} =$ _____

58. $2\dfrac{2}{5} \times 4\dfrac{1}{6} =$ _____

59. $2 \times 4\dfrac{3}{8} =$ _____

60. $\dfrac{2}{5} \times \dfrac{5}{4} =$ _____

Divide the following fractions and mixed numbers. Reduce to lowest terms.

61. $2\dfrac{1}{3} \div 4\dfrac{1}{6} =$ _____

62. $\dfrac{1}{3} \div \dfrac{1}{2} =$ _____

63. $25 \div 12\dfrac{1}{2} =$ _____

64. $\dfrac{7}{8} \div 2\dfrac{1}{4} =$ _____

65. $\dfrac{6}{2} \div \dfrac{3}{4} =$ _____

66. $\dfrac{4}{6} \div \dfrac{1}{2} =$ _____

67. $\dfrac{3}{10} \div \dfrac{5}{25} =$ _____

68. $3 \div \dfrac{2}{5} =$ _____

69. $\dfrac{15}{30} \div 10 =$ _____

70. $\dfrac{8}{3} \div \dfrac{8}{3} =$ _____

71. $\dfrac{3}{4} \div \dfrac{3}{8} =$ _____

72. $12 \div \dfrac{2}{3} =$ _____

73. $\dfrac{7}{8} \div 14 =$ _____

74. $1\dfrac{1}{2} \div \dfrac{3}{4} =$ _____

75. $\dfrac{15}{8} \div 5 =$ _____

Arrange the following fractions in order from largest to smallest.

76. $\dfrac{3}{16}, \dfrac{1}{16}, \dfrac{5}{16}, \dfrac{14}{16}, \dfrac{7}{16}$ _____

77. $\dfrac{5}{12}, \dfrac{5}{32}, \dfrac{5}{8}, \dfrac{5}{6}, \dfrac{5}{64}$ _____

78. A patient is instructed to drink 600 mL of water within 1 hour. The patient has only been able to drink 360 mL. What portion of the water remains? (Express your answer as a fraction reduced to lowest terms.) _____

79. A child's oral ibuprofen (Motrin) suspension contains 100 mg per 5 mL. What part of the dosage does 20 mg represent? _____

80. A patient is receiving 240 mL of Ensure by mouth as a supplement. The patient consumes 200 mL. What portion of the Ensure remains? (Express your answer as a fraction reduced to lowest terms.) _____

81. A patient takes $1\frac{1}{2}$ tablets of medication 4 times per day for 4 days. How many tablets will the patient have taken at the end of the 4 days? _____

82. A juice glass holds 120 mL. If a patient drinks $2\frac{1}{3}$ glasses, how many mL did the patient consume? _____

83. How many hours are there in $3\frac{1}{2}$ days? _____

84. One tablet contains 200 mg of pain medication. How many mg are in $3\frac{1}{2}$ tablets? _____

85. A bottle of medicine contains 30 doses. How many doses are in $2\frac{1}{2}$ bottles? _____

86. At the beginning of a shift, $5\frac{1}{4}$ bottles of hand sanitizer are available. At the end of the shift, $3\frac{1}{2}$ bottles are left. How much hand sanitizer was used? _____

Apply the principles of borrowing, and subtract the following:

87. $2 - \dfrac{10}{21} =$ _____

88. $9\dfrac{1}{4} - \dfrac{3}{4} =$ _____

89. $5\dfrac{1}{2} - 3\dfrac{3}{4} =$ _____

Answers on page 22.

evolve

For additional practice problems, refer to the Mathematics Review section of the Drug Calculations Companion, Version 5 on Evolve.

✳ ANSWERS

Answers to Practice Problems

1. LCD = 30; therefore $\dfrac{6}{30}$ has the lesser value.

2. LCD = 8; therefore $\dfrac{6}{8}$ has the lesser value.

3. $\dfrac{1}{150}$ has the lesser value; the denominator (150) is larger.

4. $\dfrac{6}{18}$ has the lesser value; the numerator (6) is smaller.

5. $\dfrac{3}{5}$ has the lesser value; the numerator (3) is smaller.

6. $\dfrac{1}{8}$ has the lesser value; the numerator (1) is smaller.

7. $\dfrac{1}{40}$ has the lesser value; the denominator (40) is larger.

8. $\dfrac{1}{300}$ has the lesser value; the denominator (300) is larger.

9. $\dfrac{4}{24}$ has the lesser value; the numerator (4) is smaller.

10. LCD = 6; therefore $\dfrac{1}{6}$ has the lesser value.

11. LCD = 72; therefore $\dfrac{6}{8}$ has the higher value.

12. LCD = 6; therefore $\dfrac{7}{6}$ has the higher value.

13. LCD = 72; therefore $\dfrac{6}{12}$ has the higher value.

14. $\dfrac{1}{6}$ has the higher value; the denominator (6) is smaller.

15. $\dfrac{1}{75}$ has the higher value; the denominator (75) is smaller.

16. $\dfrac{6}{5}$ has the higher value; the numerator (6) is larger.

17. LCD = 24; therefore $\dfrac{4}{6}$ has the higher value.

18. $\dfrac{8}{9}$ has the higher value; the numerator (8) is larger.

19. $\dfrac{1}{10}$ has the higher value; the denominator (10) is smaller.

20. $\dfrac{6}{15}$ has the higher value; the numerator (6) is larger.

21. $\dfrac{10 \div 5}{15 \div 5} = \dfrac{2}{3}$

22. $\dfrac{7 \div 7}{49 \div 7} = \dfrac{1}{7}$

23. $\dfrac{64 \div 2}{128 \div 2} = \dfrac{32}{64} = \dfrac{1}{2}$

24. $\dfrac{100 \div 2}{150 \div 2} = \dfrac{50}{75} = \dfrac{2}{3}$

25. $\dfrac{20 \div 4}{28 \div 4} = \dfrac{5}{7}$

26. $\dfrac{14 \div 2}{98 \div 2} = \dfrac{7}{49} = \dfrac{1}{7}$

27. $\dfrac{10 \div 2}{18 \div 2} = \dfrac{5}{9}$

28. $\dfrac{24 \div 12}{36 \div 12} = \dfrac{2}{3}$

29. $\dfrac{10 \div 10}{50 \div 10} = \dfrac{1}{5}$

30. $\dfrac{9 \div 9}{27 \div 9} = \dfrac{1}{3}$

31. $\dfrac{9 \div 9}{9 \div 9} = \dfrac{1}{1} = 1$

32. $\dfrac{15 \div 15}{45 \div 15} = \dfrac{1}{3}$

33. $\dfrac{124 \div 31}{155 \div 31} = \dfrac{4}{5}$

34. $\dfrac{12 \div 6}{18 \div 6} = \dfrac{2}{3}$

35. $\dfrac{36 \div 4}{64 \div 4} = \dfrac{9}{16}$

36. $3\dfrac{3}{5}$

37. $4\dfrac{2}{7}$

38. $1\dfrac{5}{8}$

39. $2\dfrac{11}{12}$

40. $1\dfrac{3}{25}$

41. $\dfrac{29}{25}$

42. $\dfrac{34}{8}$

43. $\dfrac{9}{2}$

44. $\dfrac{27}{8}$

45. $\dfrac{79}{5}$

46. $1\dfrac{1}{2}$

47. $2\dfrac{19}{24}$

48. $7\dfrac{1}{6}$

49. $8\dfrac{1}{15}$

50. $22\dfrac{5}{6}$

51. $\dfrac{19}{21}$

52. $1\dfrac{31}{40}$

53. $\dfrac{11}{16}$

54. $\dfrac{1}{12}$

55. $\dfrac{1}{24}$

56. $13\dfrac{4}{9}$

57. $1\dfrac{3}{5}$

58. $\dfrac{8}{15}$

59. $\dfrac{18}{125}$

60. $\dfrac{3}{50}$

61. $7\dfrac{7}{32}$

62. $\dfrac{5}{27}$

63. $1\dfrac{13}{20}$

64. $\dfrac{1}{30}$

65. 15

66. 1

67. $2\dfrac{2}{19}$

Answers to Chapter Review

1. $1\dfrac{2}{8} = 1\dfrac{1}{4}$

2. $7\dfrac{2}{4} = 7\dfrac{1}{2}$

3. $3\dfrac{4}{6} = 3\dfrac{2}{3}$

4. $2\dfrac{3}{4}$

5. $4\dfrac{3}{14}$

6. $6\dfrac{7}{10}$

7. $4\dfrac{1}{2}$

8. $2\dfrac{1}{5}$

9. $4\dfrac{4}{15}$

10. $7\dfrac{9}{13}$

11. $\dfrac{5}{2}$

12. $\dfrac{59}{8}$

13. $\dfrac{43}{5}$

14. $\dfrac{65}{4}$

15. $\dfrac{16}{5}$

16. $\dfrac{13}{5}$

17. $\dfrac{84}{10}$

18. $\dfrac{37}{4}$

19. $\dfrac{51}{4}$

20. $\dfrac{47}{7}$

21. LCD = 30; $1\dfrac{13}{30}$

22. LCD = 24; $\dfrac{13}{24}$

23. LCD = 4; $\dfrac{88}{4} = 22$

24. LCD = 10; $\dfrac{7}{10}$

25. LCD = 36;

$\dfrac{234}{36} = 6\dfrac{18}{36} = 6\dfrac{1}{2}$

26. $\dfrac{30}{47}$

27. $22\dfrac{5}{6}$

28. $140\dfrac{1}{4}$

29. LCD = 9; $106\dfrac{8}{9}$

30. LCD = 10; $13\dfrac{2}{10} = 13\dfrac{1}{5}$

31. $\dfrac{1}{9}$

32. LCD = 4; $\dfrac{3}{4}$

33. $2\dfrac{2}{4} = 2\dfrac{1}{2}$

34. LCD = 30; $\dfrac{19}{30}$

35. LCD = 4; 1

36. LCD = 20; $\dfrac{11}{20}$

37. LCD = 24; $\dfrac{7}{24}$

38. LCD = 6; $\dfrac{17}{6} = 2\dfrac{5}{6}$

39. LCD = 15; $\dfrac{19}{15} = 1\dfrac{4}{15}$

40. LCD = 21; $\dfrac{5}{21}$

41. LCD = 12; $\dfrac{3}{12} = \dfrac{1}{4}$

42. LCD = 24; $26\dfrac{7}{24}$

43. $24\dfrac{6}{11}$

44. LCD = 10; $12\dfrac{1}{5}$

45. LCD = 18; $31\dfrac{1}{9}$

46. $\dfrac{4}{36} = \dfrac{1}{9}$

47. $9\dfrac{11}{32}$

48. 14

49. 10

50. 27

51. $\dfrac{10}{16} = \dfrac{5}{8}$

52. $\dfrac{2}{30} = \dfrac{1}{15}$

53. $\dfrac{12}{120} = \dfrac{1}{10}$

54. $\dfrac{7}{27}$

55. $\dfrac{50}{75} = \dfrac{2}{3}$

56. $\dfrac{9}{40}$

57. $1\dfrac{7}{8}$

58. 10

59. $8\dfrac{3}{4}$

60. $\dfrac{1}{2}$

61. $\dfrac{42}{75} = \dfrac{14}{25}$

62. $\dfrac{2}{3}$

63. 2

64. $\dfrac{7}{18}$

65. 4

66. $1\dfrac{1}{3}$

67. $1\dfrac{25}{50} = 1\dfrac{1}{2}$

68. $7\dfrac{1}{2}$

69. $\dfrac{15}{300} = \dfrac{1}{20}$

70. 1

71. 2

72. 18

73. $\dfrac{1}{16}$

74. 2

75. $\dfrac{3}{8}$

76. $\dfrac{14}{16}, \dfrac{7}{16}, \dfrac{5}{16}, \dfrac{3}{16}, \dfrac{1}{16}$

77. $\dfrac{5}{6}, \dfrac{5}{8}, \dfrac{5}{12}, \dfrac{5}{32}, \dfrac{5}{64}$

78. $\dfrac{2}{5}$ of water remains

79. $\dfrac{1}{5}$ of the dosage

80. $\dfrac{1}{6}$ of Ensure remains

81. 24 tablets

82. 280 mL

83. 84 hours

84. 700 mg

85. 75 doses

86. $1\dfrac{3}{4}$ bottles

87. $1\dfrac{11}{21}$

88. $8\dfrac{2}{4} = 8\dfrac{1}{2}$

89. $1\dfrac{3}{4}$

CHAPTER 2
Decimals

Objectives

After reviewing this chapter, you should be able to:

1. Read decimals
2. Write decimals
3. Compare the size of decimals
4. Convert fractions to decimals
5. Convert decimals to fractions
6. Add decimals
7. Subtract decimals
8. Multiply decimals
9. Divide decimals
10. Round decimals to the nearest tenth
11. Round decimals to the nearest hundredth

Medication dosages and other measurements in the health care system use metric measures, which are based on the decimal system. An understanding of decimals is crucial to the calculation of dosages. In the administration of medications, nurses calculate dosages that contain decimals (e.g., levothyroxine 0.075 mg).

Decimal points in dosages have been cited as a major source of medication errors. A misunderstanding of the value of a dosage expressed as a decimal or the omission of a decimal point can result in a serious medication error. Decimals should be written with great care to prevent misinterpretation. A clear understanding of the importance of decimal points and their value will assist the nurse in the prevention of medication errors.

Example: Digoxin 0.125 mg

Example: Carvedilol 3.125 mg

A decimal is a fraction that has a denominator that is a multiple of 10. A decimal fraction is written as a decimal by the use of a decimal point (.). The decimal point is used to indicate place value. Some examples are as follows:

Fraction	Decimal Number
$\frac{3}{10}$	0.3
$\frac{18}{100}$	0.18
$\frac{175}{1000}$	0.175

The decimal point represents the centre. Notice that the numbers written to the right of the decimal point are decimal fractions with a denominator of 10 or a multiple of 10 and represent a value that is less than 1 or part of 1. Numbers written to the left of the decimal point are whole numbers, or have a value of 1 or greater.

The easiest way to understand decimals is to memorize the place values (Box 2-1).

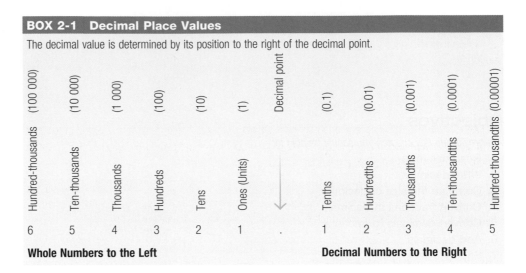

BOX 2-1 Decimal Place Values

The decimal value is determined by its position to the right of the decimal point.

Hundred-thousands (100 000)	Ten-thousands (10 000)	Thousands (1 000)	Hundreds (100)	Tens (10)	Ones (Units) (1)	Decimal point	Tenths (0.1)	Hundredths (0.01)	Thousandths (0.001)	Ten-thousandths (0.0001)	Hundred-thousandths (0.00001)
6	5	4	3	2	1	.	1	2	3	4	5

Whole Numbers to the Left   **Decimal Numbers to the Right**

The **first** place to the right of the decimal is tenths.
The **second** place to the right of the decimal is hundredths.
The **third** place to the right of the decimal is thousandths.
The **fourth** place to the right of the decimal is ten-thousandths.

In the calculation of medication dosages, it is necessary to **consider only three figures after the decimal point (thousandths) (e.g., 0.375 mg).**

> ! **SAFETY ALERT!**
>
> When there is no whole number before a decimal point, it is important to place a zero (0) to the left of the decimal point to emphasize that the number is a decimal fraction and has a value less than 1. This will emphasize its value and prevent errors in interpretation and avoid errors in dosage calculation. This zero does not change the value of the number. This point has been emphasized by the Institute for Safe Medication Practices Canada (ISMP Canada). The ISMP Canada (2006a) official "Do Not Use" list prohibits the writing of a decimal fraction that is less than 1 without a zero before a decimal point.

> **NOTE**
> ISMP Canada is an independent national nonprofit organization dedicated to promoting safe medication practices in Canada.

The source of many medication errors is misplacement of a decimal point or incorrect interpretation of a decimal value.

Reading and Writing Decimals

Once you understand the place value of decimals, reading and writing them are simple.

> → **RULE**
>
> To read a decimal number:
>
> 1. Read the whole number;
> 2. Read the decimal point as "and"; and
> 3. Read the decimal fraction.
>
> Notice that the words for all decimal fractions end in th(s).

Example 1: The number 0.001 is read as "one thousandth."

Example 2: The number 4.06 is read as "four and six hundredths."

Example 3: The number 0.4 is read as "four tenths."

RULE

When there is only a zero (0) to the left of the decimal, as in Examples 1 and 3, the zero is not read aloud.

TIPS FOR CLINICAL PRACTICE

An exception to this rule is in an emergency situation when a nurse must take a verbal order over the phone from a prescriber. When repeating back an order for a medication involving a decimal, the zero should be read aloud to prevent a medication error.

Example: "Zero point 4" would be the verbal interpretation of Example 3. In addition to repeating the order back, the receiver of the order should write down the complete order or enter it into a computer, then read it back, and receive confirmation of the order from the individual giving the order.

RULE

To write a decimal number:

1. Write the whole number (if there is no whole number, write zero [0]);
2. Write the decimal point to indicate the place value of the rightmost number; and
3. Write the decimal portion of the number.

Example: Written, seven and five tenths = 7.5

Example: Written, one hundred twenty-five thousandths = 0.125

Example: Written, five tenths = 0.5

RULE

When writing decimals, placing a zero after the last digit of a decimal fraction does not change its value.

Example: 0.37 mg = 0.370 mg

SAFETY ALERT!

When writing decimals, unnecessary zeros should not be placed at the end of the number to avoid misinterpretation of a value and the overlooking of a decimal point. ISMP Canada (2006b) also makes this recommendation. ISMP Canada discourages the use of trailing zeros for medication orders or other medication-related documentation. Exception: A trailing zero may be used only when required to demonstrate the level of precision of the value being reported, such as for laboratory results, imaging studies that report the size of lesions, or catheter/tube sizes.

Because the last zero does not change the value of the decimal, it is not necessary. The preferred notation, as in the example shown here, is 0.37 mg, not 0.370 mg.

PRACTICE **PROBLEMS**

Write each of the following numbers in word form.

1. 8.35 _____

2. 11.001 _____

3. 4.57 _____

4. 5.0007 _____

5. 10.5 _____

6. 0.163 _____

Write each of the following in decimal form.

7. four tenths _____

8. eighty-four and seven hundredths _____

9. seven hundredths _____

10. two and twenty-three hundredths _____

11. five hundredths _____

12. nine thousandths _____

Answers on page 38.

Comparing the Value of Decimals

> **RULE**
> Zeros added before or after the decimal point of a decimal number change its value.

Example: 0.375 mg ≠ (is not equal to) 0.0375 mg

Example: 2.025 mg ≠ 20.025 mg

Example: However, .7 = 0.7 and 12.625 = 12.6250;
But you should write 0.7 (with a leading zero) and 12.625 (without a trailing zero).

> **SAFETY ALERT!**
> Understanding which decimal is of greater or lesser value is important in the calculation of dosage problems. This knowledge helps to prevent errors in dosage and gives the nurse an understanding of the size of a dosage (e.g., 0.5 mg, 0.05 mg). Understanding the value of decimals prevents errors of misinterpretation. There is an appreciable difference between 0.5 mg and 0.05 mg. In fact, 0.5 mg is 10 times larger than 0.05 mg. A misinterpretation of the value of decimals can result in serious consequences in dosage calculations.

> **RULE**
> When decimal numbers contain whole numbers, the whole numbers are compared to determine which is greater.

Example: 4.8 is greater than 2.9

Example: 11.5 is greater than 7.5

Example: 7.37 is greater than 6.94

> **RULE**
> If the whole numbers being compared are the **same** (e.g., 5.6 and 5.2) or if there is **no whole number** (e.g., 0.45 and 0.37), then the number in the **tenths place** determines which decimal is greater.

Example: 0.45 is greater than 0.37

Example: 1.75 is greater than 1.25

> **RULE**
> If the whole numbers are the same or zero and the numbers in the **tenths place** are the **same,** then the decimal with the higher number in the **hundredths place** has the greater value, and so forth.

Example: 0.67 is greater than 0.66

Example: 0.17 is greater than 0.14

Example: 0.2 is the same as 0.2000, 0.20

Example: 4.4 is the same as 4.40, 4.400

PRACTICE **PROBLEMS**

Circle the decimal with the largest value in the following:

13. 0.5   0.15   0.05   16. 0.175   0.1   0.05

14. 2.66   2.36   2.87   17. 7.02   7.15   7.35

15. 0.125   0.375   0.25   18. 0.067   0.087   0.077

Answers on page 38.

Adding and Subtracting Decimals

> **RULE**
> To add or subtract decimals, place the numbers in columns so the decimal points are lined up directly under one another and add or subtract from right to left. Zeros may be added at the end of the decimal fraction, making all decimals of equal length, but unnecessary zeros should be eliminated in the final answer.

> **! SAFETY ALERT!**
> Eliminate unnecessary zeros in the final answer to avoid confusion and prevent errors of misinterpretation.

Example: Add 16.4 + 21.8 + 13.2

$$
\begin{array}{r}
16.4 \\
21.8 \\
+\ 13.2 \\
\hline
51.4
\end{array} = 51.4
$$

Example: Add 2.25 + 1.75

$$
\begin{array}{r}
2.25 \\
+\ 1.75 \\
\hline
4.00 = 4
\end{array}
$$

Example: Subtract 2.6 from 18.6

$$
\begin{array}{r}
18.6 \\
-\ 2.6 \\
\hline
16.0 = 16
\end{array}
$$

Example: Add 11.2 + 16

$$
\begin{array}{r}
11.2 \\
+\ 16.0 \\
\hline
27.2 = 27.2
\end{array}
$$

Example: Subtract 3.78 from 12.84

$$
\begin{array}{r}
12.84 \\
-\ 3.78 \\
\hline
9.06 = 9.06
\end{array}
$$

Example: Subtract 0.007 from 0.05

$$
\begin{array}{r}
0.050 \\
-\ 0.007 \\
\hline
0.043 = 0.043
\end{array}
$$

Example: Add 6.54 + 2.26

$$
\begin{array}{r}
6.54 \\
+\ 2.26 \\
\hline
8.80 = 8.8
\end{array}
$$

Example: Add 0.7 + 0.75 + 0.23 + 2.324

$$
\begin{array}{r}
0.700 \\
0.750 \\
0.230 \\
+\ 2.324 \\
\hline
4.004 = 4.004
\end{array}
$$

Example: Subtract 0.2 from 0.375

$$
\begin{array}{r}
0.375 \\
-\ 0.200 \\
\hline
0.175 = 0.175
\end{array}
$$

⊕–÷× PRACTICE **PROBLEMS**

Add the following decimals.

19. $4.7 + 5.3 + 8.4 =$ _____

20. $38.52 + 0.029 + 1.9 =$ _____

21. $0.7 + 3.25 =$ _____

22. $2.2 + 1.67 =$ _____

Subtract the following decimals.

23. $3.67 - 0.75 =$ _____

24. $64.3 - 21.2 =$ _____

25. $0.08 - 0.045 =$ _____

26. $6.75 - 0.87 =$ _____

Answers on page 38.

Multiplying Decimals

⊘ **SAFETY ALERT!**
When multiplying decimals, be sure the decimal is placed in the correct position in the answer (product). Misplacement of decimal points can lead to a critical medication error.

→ **RULE**
To multiply decimals, multiply as with whole numbers. In the answer (product), count off from right to left as many decimal places as there are in the numbers being multiplied. Zeros may also be added to the left if necessary.

Example 1: 1.2×3.2

$$
\begin{array}{r}
1.2 \quad \text{(1 decimal place)} \\
\times 3.2 \quad \text{(1 decimal place)} \\
\hline
24 \\
36 \\
\hline
384. \\
\end{array}
$$

Answer: 3.84

In Example 1, 1.2 has one number after the decimal, and 3.2 also has one. Therefore, you will need to place the decimal point two places to the left in the answer (product).

→ **RULE**
When there are insufficient numbers in the answer for correct placement of the decimal point, add as many zeros as needed to the left of the answer.

Example 2: 1.35×0.65

$$
\begin{array}{r}
1.35 \quad \text{(2 decimal places)} \\
\times 0.65 \quad \text{(2 decimal places)} \\
\hline
675 \\
810 \\
\hline
8775. \\
\end{array}
$$

Answer: 0.8775

In Example 2, 1.35 has two numbers after the decimal, and 0.65 also has two. Therefore, you will need to place the decimal point four places to the left in the answer (product), and add a zero before the decimal point.

Example 3: $\qquad$ 0.11×0.33

$$
\begin{array}{r}
0.11 \quad \text{(2 decimal places)} \\
\times 0.33 \quad \text{(2 decimal places)} \\
\hline
33 \\
33 \\
\hline
0363. \\
\end{array}
$$

Answer: 0.0363

In Example 3, four decimal places are needed (two numbers after each decimal in 0.11 and 0.33), but there are only three numbers in the product. A zero must be placed to the left of these numbers for correct placement of the decimal point. Place a zero before the decimal point.

Example 4: $\qquad$ 1.6×0.05

$$
\begin{array}{r}
1.6 \quad \text{(1 decimal place)} \\
\times 0.05 \quad \text{(2 decimal places)} \\
\hline
080. \\
\end{array}
$$

Answer: $0.080 = 0.08$

In Example 4, three decimal places are needed (1.6 has one number after the decimal and 0.05 has two), so a zero has to be placed between the decimal point and 8 to allow for enough places. The unnecessary zero is eliminated in the final answer, and a zero is placed before the decimal point.

Multiplication by Decimal Movement

> **RULE**
>
> This method may be preferred when doing metric conversions because it is based on the decimal system. Multiplying by 10, 100, 1 000, and so forth can be done by moving the decimal point to the right the same number of places as there are zeros in the number by which you are multiplying.

When multiplying by 10, move the decimal one place to the right; by 100, two places to the right; by 1 000, three places to the right; and so forth.

Example: $1.6 \times 10 = 16$ (The multiplier 10 has 1 zero; the decimal point is moved 1 place to the right.)

Example: $5.2 \times 100 = 520$ (The multiplier 100 has 2 zeros; the decimal point is moved 2 places to the right.)

NOTE
Add zeros as necessary to complete the operation.

Example: $0.463 \times 1\,000 = 463$ (The multiplier 1 000 has 3 zeros; the decimal point is moved 3 places to the right.)

Example: $6.64 \times 10 = 66.4$ (The multiplier 10 has 1 zero; the decimal point is moved one place to the right.)

PRACTICE **PROBLEMS**

Multiply the following decimals.

27. $3.15 \times 0.015 =$ _____

28. $3.65 \times 0.25 =$ _____

29. $9.65 \times 1\,000 =$ _____

30. $8.9 \times 0.2 =$ _____

31. $14.001 \times 7.2 =$ _____

Answers on page 38.

Dividing Decimals

Division of decimals is done in the same manner as division of whole numbers except for placement of the decimal point. Incorrect placement of the decimal point changes the numerical value and can cause errors in calculation. Errors made in the division of decimals are commonly caused by improper placement of the decimal point, incorrect placement of numbers in the quotient, and omission of necessary zeros in the quotient.

The parts of a division problem are as follows:

$$\text{Divisor} \overline{)\text{Dividend}}^{\text{Quotient}}$$

The number being divided is called the **dividend,** the number being divided into the dividend is the **divisor,** and the answer is the **quotient.**

Symbols used to indicate division are as follows:

1. $\overline{)}$

   Example: $9\overline{)27}$ Read as 27 divided by 9.

2. $\div$

   Example: $27 \div 9$ Read as 27 divided by 9.

3. The horizontal bar with the dividend on the top and the divisor on the bottom

   Example: $\dfrac{27}{9}$ Read as 27 divided by 9.

4. The slanted bar with the dividend to the left and the divisor to the right

   Example: $^{27}\!/_9$ Read as 27 divided by 9.

Dividing a Decimal by a Whole Number

> **RULE**
>
> To divide a decimal by a whole number, place the decimal point in the quotient directly above the decimal point in the dividend. Proceed to divide as with whole numbers.

Example: Divide 17.5 by 5.

$$\begin{array}{r} 3.5 \\ 5\overline{)17.5} \\ -\;15 \\ \hline 25 \\ -\;25 \\ \hline 0 \end{array}$$

Answer: 3.5

Dividing a Decimal or a Whole Number by a Decimal

> **RULE**
>
> To divide a decimal by a decimal, the decimal point in the divisor is moved to the right until the number is a whole number. The decimal point in the dividend is moved the same number of places to the right, and zeros are added as necessary. Proceed to divide as with whole numbers.

Example: Divide 6.96 by 0.3.

Step 1: $6.96 \div 0.3 = 0.3\overline{)6.9\,6}$

$3\overline{)69.6}$ (after moving decimals in the divisor the same number of places as the dividend)

Step 2:

$$\begin{array}{r} 23.2 \\ 3\overline{)69.6} \\ -\;6 \\ \hline 9 \\ -\;9 \\ \hline 6 \\ -\;6 \\ \hline 0 \end{array}$$

Answer: 23.2

Division by Decimal Movement

> **RULE**
>
> To divide a decimal by 10, 100, or 1 000, move the decimal point to the **left** the same number of places as there are zeros in the divisor.

Example: $0.46 \div 10 = 0.046$ (The divisor 10 has 1 zero; the decimal point is moved 1 place to the left.)

Example: $0.07 \div 100 = 0.0007$ (The divisor 100 has 2 zeros; the decimal point is moved 2 places to the left.)

Example: $0.75 \div 1\,000 = 0.00075$ (The divisor 1 000 has 3 zeros; the decimal point is moved 3 places to the left.)

Rounding Off Decimals

The determination of how many places to carry your division when calculating dosages is based on the equipment being used. Some syringes are marked in **tenths** and some in

hundredths. As you become familiar with the equipment used in dosage calculation, you will learn how far to carry your division and when to round off. To ensure accuracy, most calculation problems require that you carry your division at least **two decimal places (hundredths place)** and **round off to the nearest tenth.**

NOTE

In some instances, such as critical care or pediatrics, it may be necessary to compute decimal calculations to thousandths (three decimal places) and round to hundredths (two decimal places). These areas may require this accuracy.

> **RULE**
>
> To express an answer to the nearest tenth, carry the division to the hundredths place (two places after the decimal). If the number in the hundredths place **is 5 or greater, add** one to the tenths place. If the number **is less than 5, drop** the number to the right of the desired decimal place.

Example: Express 4.15 to the nearest tenth.

Answer: 4.2 (The number in the hundredths place is 5, so the number in the tenths place is increased by one. 4.1 becomes 4.2.)

Example: Express 1.24 to the nearest tenth.

Answer: 1.2 (The number in the hundredths place is less than 5, so the number in the tenths place does not change. The 4 is dropped.)

> **RULE**
>
> To express an answer to the nearest hundredth, carry the division to the thousandths place (three places after the decimal). If the number in the thousandths place **is 5 or greater, add** one to the hundredths place. If the number **is less than 5, drop** the number to the right of the desired decimal place.

Example: Express 0.176 to the nearest hundredth.

Answer: 0.18 (The number in the thousandths place is 6, so the number in the hundredths place is increased by one. 0.17 becomes 0.18.)

Example: Express 0.554 to the nearest hundredth.

Answer: 0.55 (The number in the thousandths place is less than 5, so the number in the hundredths place does not change.)

> **SAFETY ALERT!**
>
> When rounding for dosage calculations, unnecessary zeros should not be added. Zeros are not necessary to clarify the number.

Example: 0.98 (round to tenths) = 1.0 = 1

Example: 0.40 (round to hundredths) = 0.4

PRACTICE **PROBLEMS**

Divide the following decimals. Carry division to the hundredths place where necessary. Do not round off.

32. 2 ÷ 0.5 = _____   35. 39.6 ÷ 1.3 = _____

33. 1.4 ÷ 1.2 = _____   36. 1.9 ÷ 3.2 = _____

34. 63.8 ÷ 0.9 = _____

Express the following decimals to the nearest tenth.

37. 3.57 _____   39. 1.98 _____

38. 0.95 _____

Express the following decimals to the nearest hundredth.

40. 3.550 _____   42. 0.738 _____

41. 0.607 _____

Divide the following decimals.

43. 0.005 ÷ 10 = _____   44. 0.004 ÷ 100 = _____

Multiply the following decimals.

45. 58.4 × 10 = _____   46. 0.5 × 1 000 = _____

Answers on page 38.

Changing Fractions to Decimals

> **RULE**
> To change a fraction to a decimal, divide the numerator by the denominator and add zeros as needed. If the numerator does not divide evenly into the denominator, carry division three places.

Example:

$$\frac{2}{5} = 5\overline{)2} = 5\overline{)2.0}^{\,0.4}$$

Example:

$$\frac{3}{8} = 8\overline{)3} = 8\overline{)3.000}^{\,0.375}$$

Changing fractions to decimals can also be a method of comparing fraction size. The fractions being compared are changed to decimals, and the rules relating to comparing decimals are then applied. (See Comparing the Value of Decimals, page 26.)

Example: Which fraction is larger, $\frac{1}{3}$ or $\frac{1}{6}$?

Solution: $\frac{1}{3} = 0.333$ ... as a decimal

$\frac{1}{6} = 0.166$ ... as a decimal

Answer: $\frac{1}{3}$ is therefore the larger fraction.

Changing Decimals to Fractions

> **RULE**
> To change a decimal to a fraction, write the decimal number as a whole number in the numerator of the fraction, and express the denominator of the fraction as a power of 10. Place the number 1 in the denominator of the fraction, and add as many zeros as there are places to the right of the decimal point. Reduce to lowest terms if necessary. (See Reading and Writing Decimals, page 24.)

Example: 0.4 is read "four tenths" and written $\frac{4}{10}$, which $= \frac{2}{5}$ when reduced.

Example: 0.65 is read "sixty-five hundredths" and written $\frac{65}{100}$, which $= \frac{13}{20}$ when reduced.

Example: 0.007 is read "seven thousandths" and written $\frac{7}{1\,000}$.

Notice that the number of places to the right of the decimal point is the same as the number of zeros in the denominator of the fraction.

+−÷× PRACTICE **PROBLEMS**

Change the following fractions to decimals, and carry the division three places as indicated. Do not round off.

47. $\frac{3}{4}$ _____

49. $\frac{1}{2}$ _____

48. $\frac{5}{9}$ _____

Change the following decimals to fractions, and reduce to lowest terms.

50. 0.75 _____

52. 0.04 _____

51. 0.0005 _____

Answers on page 39.

POINTS TO **REMEMBER**

- Read decimals carefully.
- When the decimal fraction is **not** preceded by a whole number (e.g., .12), **always place a "0"** to the left of the decimal (0.12) to avoid interpretation errors and to avoid overlooking the decimal point.
- Never follow a whole number with a decimal point and zero. This could result in a medication error because of misinterpretation (e.g., 3, not 3.0).
- Add zeros to the right as needed for making decimals of equal spacing for addition and subtraction. These zeros do not change the value.
- Note that adding zeros at the end of a decimal (except when called for to create decimals of equal length for addition or subtraction) can result in error (e.g., 1.5, not 1.50).
- Note that adding zeros before the decimal point can change the value (e.g., 1.5 is not equal to 1.05, nor is it the same number).
- To convert a fraction to a decimal, divide the numerator by the denominator.
- To convert a decimal to a fraction, write the decimal number as a whole number in the numerator and the denominator as a power of 10. Reduce to lowest terms (e.g., $0.05 = \frac{5}{100} = \frac{1}{20}$).
- Double-check your work to avoid errors.

◄ CHAPTER **REVIEW**

Identify the decimal with the largest value in the following sets.

1. 0.4, 0.44, 0.444 _____

2. 0.8, 0.7, 0.12 _____

3. 1.32, 1.12, 1.5 _____

5. 0.725, 0.357, 0.125 _____

4. 0.1, 0.05, 0.2 _____

Arrange the following decimals from smallest to largest:

6. 0.5, 0.05, 0.005 _____

9. 5.15, 5.05, 5.55 _____

7. 0.123, 0.1023, 1.23 _____

10. 0.73, 0.307, 0.703 _____

8. 0.64, 4.6, 0.46 _____

Perform the indicated operations. Give exact answers.

11. $3.005 + 4.308 + 2.47 =$ _____

14. $8.17 - 3.05 =$ _____

12. $20.3 + 8.57 + 0.03 =$ _____

15. $3.8 - 1.3 =$ _____

13. $5.886 - 3.143 =$ _____

Solve the following equations. Carry division to the hundredths place where necessary.

16. $5.7 \div 0.9 =$ _____

19. $0.15 \times 100 =$ _____

17. $3.75 \div 2.5 =$ _____

20. $15 \times 2.08 =$ _____

18. $1.125 \div 0.75 =$ _____

21. $472.4 \times 0.002 =$ _____

Express the following decimals to the nearest tenth.

22. 1.75 _____

23. 0.13 _____

Express the following decimals to the nearest hundredth.

24. 1.427 _____

25. 0.147 _____

Change the following fractions to decimals. Carry division three decimal places as necessary.

26. $\dfrac{8}{64}$ _____

28. $6\dfrac{1}{2}$ _____

27. $\dfrac{3}{50}$ _____

Change the following decimals to fractions, and reduce to lowest terms.

29. 1.01 _____

30. 0.065 _____

Add the following decimals.

31. You are to give a patient one tablet labelled 0.15 milligrams (mg) and one labelled 0.025 mg. What is the total dosage of these two tablets? _____

32. If you administer two tablets labelled 0.04 mg, what total dosage will you administer? _____

33. You have two tablets, one labelled 0.025 mg and the other 0.1 mg. What is the total dosage of these two tablets? _____

34. You have just administered three tablets with a dose strength of 1.5 mg each. What was the total dosage? _____

35. If you administer two tablets labelled 0.6 mg, what total dosage will you administer? _____

Multiply the following numbers by moving the decimal.

36. $0.08 \times 10 =$ _____ 39. $2.34 \times 10 =$ _____

37. $5.65 \times 100 =$ _____ 40. $0.002 \times 100 =$ _____

38. $0.849 \times 1\,000 =$ _____

Divide the following numbers, and round to the nearest hundredth.

41. $6.45 \div 10 =$ _____ 44. $4 \div 4.1 =$ _____

42. $37.5 \div 100 =$ _____ 45. $5 \div 14.3 =$ _____

43. $0.13 \div 0.25 =$ _____

Round the following decimals to the nearest thousandth.

46. 4.2475 _____ 49. 7.8393 _____

47. 0.5673 _____ 50. 5.8333 _____

48. 2.3249 _____

51. A patient's water intake is 1.05 litres (L), 0.65 L, 2.05 L, and 0.8 L. What is the total intake in L? _____

52. A patient's blood glucose level on admission was 13.8 millimoles/litre (mmol/L). By discharge the blood glucose level dropped 2.2 mmol/L. What is the patient's current blood glucose level? _____

53. A baby weighed 4.85 kilograms (kg) at birth and now weighs 7.9 kg. How many kg did the baby gain? _____

54. A patient is taking $\dfrac{1}{15}$ of a liquid medication containing 0.375 mg of medication every day. How many mg will the patient take in 4 days? _____

55. A patient's sodium intake at one meal was the following: 0.002 grams (g) and 0.35 g. How many grams of sodium did the patient consume? _____

56. True or false? 2.4 g = 2.04 g. _____

57. True or false? 5.5 L = 5.500 L. _____

58. An order has been placed for 0.7 mg of a medication. The recommended maximum dosage of the medication is 0.35 mg, and the minimum recommended dosage is 0.175 mg. Is the dosage ordered within the allowable limits? _____

59. Which of the following decimals is largest? 0.125, 0.01, 0.4 _____

60. Which of the following decimals is smallest? 0.855, 0.8, 0.085 _____

61. A patient received a series of injections of medication in millilitres (mL): 1.5 mL, 2.3 mL, and 2.1 mL. What was the total amount of mL the patient received? _____

62. A patient weighed 85.4 kg in January. In February, the patient gained 1.8 kg. In March, the patient gained 2.3 kg. How much did the patient weigh in March? _____

63. If a dosage of medication is 2.5 mL, how much medication is needed for 25 dosages? _____

64. A patient received 17.5 mg of a medication in tablet form. Each tablet contained 3.5 mg of medication. How many tablets were given to the patient? _____

Answers on page 39.

ANSWERS

Answers to Practice Problems

1. eight and thirty-five hundredths
2. eleven and one thousandth
3. four and fifty-seven hundredths
4. five and seven ten thousandths
5. ten and five tenths
6. one hundred sixty-three thousandths
7. 0.4
8. 84.07
9. 0.07
10. 2.23
11. 0.05
12. 0.009
13. 0.5
14. 2.87
15. 0.375
16. 0.175
17. 7.35
18. 0.087
19. 18.4
20. 40.449
21. 3.95
22. 3.87
23. 2.92
24. 43.1
25. 0.035
26. 5.88
27. 0.04725
28. 0.9125
29. 9 650
30. 1.78
31. 100.8072
32. 4
33. 1.16
34. 70.88
35. 30.46
36. 0.59
37. 3.6
38. 1
39. 2

evolve

For additional practice problems, refer to the Mathematics Review section of the Drug Calculations Companion, Version 5 on Evolve.

40. 3.55

41. 0.61

42. 0.74

43. 0.0005

44. 0.00004

45. 584

46. 500

47. 0.75

48. 0.555

49. 0.5

50. $\dfrac{3}{4}$

51. $\dfrac{1}{2\,000}$

52. $\dfrac{1}{25}$

Answers to Chapter Review

1. 0.444

2. 0.8

3. 1.5

4. 0.2

5. 0.725

6. 0.005, 0.05, 0.5

7. 0.1023, 0.123, 1.23

8. 0.46, 0.64, 4.6

9. 5.05, 5.15, 5.55

10. 0.307, 0.703, 0.73

11. 9.783

12. 28.9

13. 2.743

14. 5.12

15. 2.5

16. 6.33

17. 1.5

18. 1.5

19. 15

20. 31.2

21. 0.9448

22. 1.8

23. 0.1

24. 1.43

25. 0.15

26. 0.125

27. 0.06

28. 6.5

29. $1\dfrac{1}{100}$

30. $\dfrac{13}{200}$

31. 0.175 mg

32. 0.08 mg

33. 0.125 mg

34. 4.5 mg

35. 1.2 mg

36. 0.8

37. 565

38. 849

39. 23.4

40. 0.2

41. 0.65

42. 0.38

43. 0.52

44. 0.98

45. 0.35

46. 4.248

47. 0.567

48. 2.325

49. 7.839

50. 5.833

51. 4.55 L

52. 11.6 mmol/L

53. 3.05 kg

54. 0.1 mg

55. 0.352 g

56. False

57. True

58. No, 0.7 mg is outside the allowable limits of the safe dosage range of 0.175 mg to 0.35 mg. It is twice the allowable maximum dosage.

59. 0.4

60. 0.085

61. 5.9 mL

62. 89.5 kg

63. 62.5 mL

64. 5 tablets

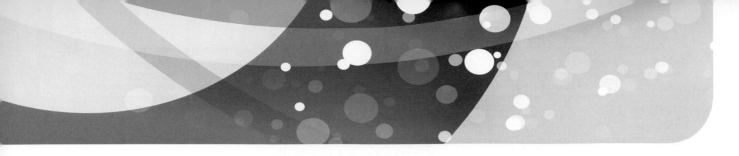

CHAPTER 3
Ratio and Proportion

Objectives

After reviewing this chapter, you should be able to:

1. Define *ratio* and *proportion*
2. Define *means* and *extremes*
3. Calculate problems for a missing term (*x*) using ratio and proportion

Ratio and proportion is one logical method for calculating medications. It can be used to calculate all types of medication problems. Nurses use ratios to calculate and to check medication dosages. Some medications express the strength of the solution by using a ratio. Example: An epinephrine label may state 1:1000. Ratios are used in hospitals to determine the patient to nurse ratio. Example: If there are 28 patients and 4 nurses on a unit, the ratio of patients to nurses is 28:4 or "28 to 4" or 7:1. As with fractions, ratios should be stated in lowest terms. Like a fraction, which indicates the division of two numbers, a ratio indicates the division of two quantities. The use of ratio and proportion is a logical approach to calculating medication dosages.

Ratios

A ratio is used to indicate a relationship between two numbers. These numbers are separated by a colon (:).

Example: 3:4

The colon indicates division; therefore a ratio is a fraction.

> **RULE**
> The numbers or terms of the ratio are the numerator and the denominator. The numerator is always to the left of the colon, and the denominator is always to the right of the colon. Like fractions, ratios should be stated in lowest terms.

Example: 3:4 (3 is the numerator, 4 is the denominator, and the expression can be written as $\frac{3}{4}$).

Example: In a nursing class, if there are 25 male students and 75 female students, what is the ratio of male students to female students? 25 male students to 75 female students = 25 male students per 75 female students = $\frac{25}{75} = \frac{1}{3}$. This is the same as a ratio of 25:75 or 1:3.

Ratio Measures in Solutions

Some medications express the strength of the solution by using a ratio. Ratio measures are commonly seen in solutions. Ratios represent parts of medication per parts of solution; for example, 1:10 000 (this means 1 part medication to 10 000 parts solution).

Example: A 1:5 solution contains 1 part medication in 5 parts solution.

Example: A solution that is 1 part medication in 2 parts solution would be written as 1:2.

Ratio strengths are always expressed in lowest terms.

> ### TIPS FOR CLINICAL PRACTICE
>
> The more solution a medication is dissolved in, the less potent the strength becomes. For example, a ratio strength of 1:1 000 (1 part medication to 1 000 parts solution) is more potent than a ratio strength of 1:10 000 (1 part medication to 10 000 parts solution). A misunderstanding of these numbers and what they represent can have serious consequences.

Proportions

A proportion is an equation of two ratios of equal value. The terms of the first ratio have a relationship to the terms of the second ratio. A proportion can be written in any of the following formats:

Example: 3:4 = 6:8 (separated with an equal sign)

Example: 3:4::6:8 (separated with a double colon)

Example: $\dfrac{3}{4} = \dfrac{6}{8}$ (written as a fraction)

Read as follows: 3 is to 4 equals 6 is to 8; 3 is to 4 as 6 is to 8; or, as a fraction, three fourths equals six eighths.

Proving that ratios are equal and that the proportion is true can be done mathematically.

Example:

$$5:25 = 10:50$$

or

$$5:25::10:50$$

The terms in a proportion are called the *means* and *extremes*. Confusion of these terms can result in an incorrect answer. To avoid confusion of terms in proportions, remember **m** for the middle terms (**means**) and **e** for the end terms (**extremes**) of the proportion. Let's refer to our example to identify these terms.

The extremes are the outer or end numbers (previous example: 5, 50), and the means are the inner or middle numbers (previous example: 25, 10).

Example:

means
⌐‾‾‾⌐
5:25 = 10:50
└‾‾‾‾‾‾‾‾‾┘
extremes

In other words, the answers obtained when you multiply the means and extremes are equal.

Example:

$$5 : 25 = 10 : 50$$

$$25 \times 10 = 50 \times 5$$

means   extremes

$$250 = 250$$

To verify that the two ratios in a proportion are equal and that the proportion is true, multiply the numerator of each ratio by its opposite denominator. The products should be equal. The numerator of the first fraction and the denominator of the second fraction are the extremes. The numerator of the second fraction and the denominator of the first fraction are the means.

Example:

$$5 : 25 = 10 : 50$$

$$\frac{5}{25} = \frac{10}{50} \quad \text{(proportion written as a fraction)}$$

$$\frac{5\,(\textbf{extreme})}{25\,(\textbf{mean})} \times \frac{10\,(\textbf{mean})}{50\,(\textbf{extreme})}$$

Solving for x in Ratio and Proportion

Because the product of the means always equals the product of the extremes, if three numbers of the two ratios are known, the fourth number can be found. The unknown quantity may be any of the four terms. In a proportion problem, the unknown quantity is represented by x. After multiplying the means and extremes, the unknown x is usually placed on the left side of the equation. Begin with the product containing the x, which will result in the x being isolated on the **left** and the answer on the **right**.

Example: $12 : 9 = 8 : x$

Steps: $12x = 72$

1. Multiply the extremes and then the means. (This results in x being placed on the left side of the equation.)

$$\frac{12x}{12} = \frac{72}{12}$$
$$x = \frac{72}{12}$$
$$x = 6$$

2. Divide both sides of the equation by the number preceding the x, in this instance 12, without changing the relationship. The number used for division should always be the number preceding the unknown (x), so that when this step is completed, the unknown (x) will stand alone on the left side of the equation.

Proof: Place the value obtained for x in the equation, and multiply to be certain that the product of the means equals the product of the extremes.

$$12:9 = 8:6$$
$$9 \times 8 = 12 \times 6$$
$$72 = 72$$

Solving for x with a proportion in a fraction format can be done by cross-multiplication to determine the value of x.

Example: $\dfrac{4}{3} = \dfrac{12}{x}$

Steps:

$4x = 36$

1. Cross-multiply to obtain the product of the means and extremes.

$\dfrac{4x}{4} = \dfrac{36}{4}$

$x = \dfrac{36}{4}$

2. Divide both sides by the number preceding x (in this example, 4) to obtain the value of x.

$x = 9$

Proof: Place the value obtained for x in the equation; the cross-products should be equal.

$$\frac{4}{3} = \frac{12}{9}$$
$$4 \times 9 = 12 \times 3$$
$$36 = 36$$

Solving for x in proportions that involve decimals in the equation can be done using the same process.

Example: $25:5 = 1.5:x$

Steps:

$25x = 5 \times 1.5$

1. Multiply the extremes and then the means. (The x will be placed on the left side of the equation.)

$\dfrac{25x}{25} = \dfrac{7.5}{25}$

$x = \dfrac{7.5}{25}$

2. Divide both sides by the number preceding x (in this example, 25) to obtain the value of x.

$x = 0.3$

Proof:

$$25:5 = 1.5:0.3$$
$$25 \times 0.3 = 5 \times 1.5$$
$$7.5 = 7.5$$

Solving for x in proportions that involve fractions in the equation can be done using the same process.

Example: $\dfrac{1}{2}:x = \dfrac{1}{5}:1$

Steps:

$\dfrac{1}{5} \times x = \dfrac{1}{2} \times 1$

1. Multiply the means and then the extremes. (The x will be placed on the left side of the equation.)

$$\frac{1}{5}x = \frac{1}{2}$$

$$\frac{\frac{1}{5}x}{\frac{1}{5}} = \frac{\frac{1}{2}}{\frac{1}{5}}$$

$$x = \frac{1}{2} \div \frac{1}{5}$$

$$x = \frac{1}{2} \times \frac{5}{1}$$

$$x = \frac{5}{2} = 2.5 \text{ or } 2\frac{1}{2}$$

2. Divide *both* sides by the number preceding x (in this example, $\frac{1}{5}$).

Division of the two fractions becomes multiplication, and the second fraction is inverted. Multiply numerators and denominators.

3. Reduce the final fraction to solve for x.

Proof:

$$\frac{1}{2} : 2\frac{1}{2} = \frac{1}{5} : 1$$

$$1 \times \frac{1}{2} = 2\frac{1}{2} \times \frac{1}{5} = \frac{5}{2} \times \frac{1}{5}$$

$$\frac{1}{2} = \frac{5}{10} = \frac{1}{2}$$

$$\frac{1}{2} = \frac{1}{2}$$

> **RULE**
>
> *Note:* If the answer is expressed in fraction format for x, it must be reduced to **lowest terms.** Division should be carried **two decimal places** when an answer does not work out evenly and may have to be **rounded to the nearest tenth** to prove the answer correct.

Applying Ratio and Proportion to Dosage Calculation

Now that we have reviewed the basic definitions and concepts relating to ratio and proportion, let's look at how they might be applied in dosage calculation.

In dosage calculation, ratio and proportion may be used to represent **the weight of a medication that is in tablet or capsule form.**

Example: 1 tab : 0.125 mg *or* $\dfrac{1 \text{ tab}}{0.125 \text{ mg}}$

This may also be expressed by stating the weight of the medication first:

0.125 mg : 1 tab *or* $\dfrac{0.125 \text{ mg}}{1 \text{ tab}}$

This means that 1 tablet contains 0.125 milligrams (mg) or is equal to 0.125 mg of medication.

Example: If a capsule contains a dosage of 500 mg, this dosage could be represented by the following ratio:

1 capsule : 500 mg *or* $\dfrac{1 \text{ capsule}}{500 \text{ mg}}$

This dosage could also be expressed stating the weight of the medication first:

500 mg : 1 capsule *or* $\dfrac{500 \text{ mg}}{1 \text{ capsule}}$

Another use of ratio and proportion in dosage calculation is to express liquid medications used for oral administration and for injection. When stating a dosage of a liquid medication, a ratio expresses the **weight (strength) of a medication in a certain volume of solution.**

Example: A solution that contains 250 mg of medication in each **1 millilitre (mL)** could be written as follows:

$$250 \text{ mg} : \textbf{1 mL} \ \ or \ \ \frac{250 \text{ mg}}{\textbf{1 mL}}$$

1 mL contains 250 mg of medication.

Example: A solution that contains 80 mg of medication in each **2 mL** would be written as follows:

$$80 \text{ mg} : \textbf{2 mL} \ \ or \ \ \frac{80 \text{ mg}}{\textbf{2 mL}}$$

2 mL contains 80 mg of medication.

! **SAFETY ALERT!**

When using ratio and proportion in dosage calculation, do not forget the units of measurement. Including units in the dosage strength will help you to avoid some common errors. For example, imagine that you have two solutions of a medication. One of the solutions contains 1 g of the medication in 25 mL; the other contains 1 mg of the medication in 25 mL. Notice that although both of these solution strengths have a ratio of 1 : 25, they are obviously different from each other. To clearly distinguish between them and avoid error, the unit of measurement should be included. The first solution is written as 1 g : 25 mL. The second solution is written as 1 mg : 25 mL.

Proving mathematically that ratios are equal and the proportion is true is important with medications. This point can be illustrated by using the previous medication strength examples.

Example:

$$1 \text{ capsule} : 500 \text{ mg} = 2 \text{ capsules} : 1\ 000 \text{ mg}$$

If 1 capsule contains 500 mg, 2 capsules contain 1 000 mg.

extremes

$$1 \text{ capsule} : 500 \text{ mg} = 2 \text{ capsules} : 1\ 000 \text{ mg}$$

means

$$500 \times 2 = 1\ 000 \times 1$$
$$1\ 000 = 1\ 000$$

Example:

$$2 \text{ mL} : 80 \text{ mg} = 1 \text{ mL} : 40 \text{ mg}$$
$$80 \times 1 = 2 \times 40$$
$$80 = 80$$

POINTS TO REMEMBER

- Proportions represent two ratios that are equal and have a relationship to each other.
- When three values are known, the fourth can be easily calculated.
- When solving for the unknown (x), regardless of which term of the equation is the unknown, the unknown value (x) is usually placed on the left side. Begin with the product containing x, so x can be isolated on the left side and the answer on the right side.
- Proportions can be stated using an equal (=) sign, a double colon (::), or a fraction format.
- Ratio can be used to state the amount of medication contained in a volume of solution, a tablet, or a capsule. When using ratio and proportion in dosage calculation, include the units of measurement in the dosage strength.
- Proportions are solved by multiplying the means and extremes.
- Ratios are always stated in their lowest terms.
- Double-check your work.

PRACTICE **PROBLEMS**

Express the following solution strengths as ratios.

1. 1 part medication to 100 parts solution _____

2. 1 part medication to 3 parts solution _____

Identify the strongest solution in each of the following:

3. $1:2$, $1:20$, $1:200$ _____

4. $1:1\,000$, $1:5\,000$, $1:10\,000$ _____

5. Assume that the ratio of patients to nurses is 15 to 2. Express the ratio in fraction and colon format. _____

Express the following dosages as ratios. Include the unit of measurement and the numerical value.

6. An injectable liquid that contains 100 mg in each 0.5 mL _____

7. A tablet that contains 0.25 mg of medication _____

8. An oral liquid that contains 1 gram (g) in each 10 mL _____

9. A capsule that contains 500 mg of medication _____

Determine the value of x in the following problems. Express your answer to the nearest tenth as indicated.

10. $12.5:5 = 24:x$ _____

11. $1.5:1 = 4.5:x$ _____

12. $\dfrac{750}{3} = \dfrac{600}{x}$ _____

13. $\dfrac{1}{300}:3 = \dfrac{1}{120}:x$ _____

14. $x:12 = 9:6$ _____

Answers on page 49.

CHAPTER **REVIEW**

Express the following fractions as ratios. Reduce to lowest terms.

1. $\dfrac{2}{3}$ _____

2. $\dfrac{1}{9}$ _____

3. $\dfrac{6}{8}$ _____

4. $\dfrac{1}{5}$ _____

5. $\dfrac{5}{10}$ _____

6. $\dfrac{2}{10}$ _____

Express the following ratios as fractions. Reduce to lowest terms.

7. 3:7 _____   10. 8:6 _____

8. 4:6 _____   11. 3:4 _____

9. 1:7 _____

Solve for x in the following proportions. Carry division two decimal places as necessary.

12. $20:40 = x:10$ _____   24. $\dfrac{1}{x} = \dfrac{10}{6}$ _____

13. $\dfrac{1}{4}:\dfrac{1}{2} = 1:x$ _____   25. $0.5:0.15 = 0.3:x$ _____

14. $0.12:0.8 = 0.6:x$ _____   26. $\dfrac{5}{7} = \dfrac{x}{35}$ _____

15. $\dfrac{1}{250}:2 = \dfrac{1}{150}:x$ _____   27. $\dfrac{2}{x} = \dfrac{13}{52}$ _____

16. $x:9 = 5:10$ _____   28. $\dfrac{16}{40} = \dfrac{22}{x}$ _____

17. $\dfrac{1}{4}:1.6 = \dfrac{1}{8}:x$ _____   29. $\dfrac{x}{48} = \dfrac{7}{8}$ _____

18. $\dfrac{1}{2}:2 = \dfrac{1}{3}:x$ _____   30. $20:40 = x:15$ _____

19. $125:0.4 = 50:x$ _____   31. $2:26 = 4:x$ _____

20. $x:1 = 0.5:5$ _____   32. $1:x = 5:200$ _____

21. $\dfrac{1}{4}:16 = \dfrac{1}{8}:x$ _____   33. $\dfrac{x}{26} = \dfrac{10.1}{13}$ _____

22. $15:20 = x:30$ _____   34. $12:1 = x:5.5$ _____

23. $\dfrac{2.2}{x} = \dfrac{8.8}{5}$ _____   35. $\dfrac{60}{1} = \dfrac{x}{2\frac{1}{4}}$ _____

Set up the following problems as a proportion and solve. Include labels in the set up and on the answer.

36. If 150 mg of medication is in 2 capsules, how many mg of medication is in 10 capsules?
_____

37. If 60 mg of a medication is in 500 mL, how many mL of solution contain 36 mg of medication? _____

38. If 1 kilogram (kg) equals 2.2 pounds (lb), how many kg are in 61.6 lb? _____

39. If 1 glass of milk contains 280 mg of calcium, how many mg of calcium are in $2\frac{1}{2}$ glasses of milk? _____

40. The prescriber orders 0.25 mg of a medication. The medication is available in 0.125 mg tablets. How many tablets will you give? _____

Express the following dosages as ratios. Be sure to include the units of measure and numerical value.

41. An injectable solution that contains 1 000 units in each mL _____

42. A tablet that contains 0.2 mg of medication _____

43. A capsule that contains 250 mg of medication _____

44. An oral solution that contains 125 mg in each 5 mL _____

45. An injectable solution that contains 40 mg in each mL _____

46. An injectable solution that contains 1 000 micrograms (mcg) in each 2 mL _____

47. An injectable solution that contains 1 g in each 3.6 mL _____

48. A tablet that contains 0.4 mg of medication _____

49. A capsule that contains 1 g of medication _____

50. An oral liquid that contains 0.5 mg in each mL _____

Express the following strengths as ratios.

51. 1 part medication to 2 000 parts solution _____

52. 1 part medication to 400 parts solution _____

53. 1 part medication to 50 parts solution _____

Identify the weakest solution in each of the following:

54. 1:50, 1:500, 1:5 000 _____

55. 1:3, 1:6, 1:60 _____

Set up the following word problems as proportions and solve. Include units in the set up and in the answer.

56. The prescriber orders 15 mg of a medication for every 10 lb of a patient's weight. How many mg of medication will be given for a person who weighs 120 lb? _____

57. There are 40 mg of a medication in every 5 mL of liquid. How much liquid is required to administer 120 mg of medication? _____

58. 15 g of a medication is dissolved in 300 mL of solution. If 45 g of the medication is needed, how many mL of the solution are needed? _____

59. A tablet contains 325 mg of medication. How many tablets contain 975 mg of medication? _____

60. The ratio of male to female patients in a nursing facility is 3 to 5. If there are 40 women in the facility, how many men are there? _____

Answers on pages 49–50.

evolve

For additional practice problems, refer to the Mathematics Review section of the Drug Calculations Companion, Version 5 on Evolve.

✳ ANSWERS

Answers to Practice Problems

1. $1:100$

2. $1:3$

3. $1:2$

4. $1:1\,000$

5. $\dfrac{15}{2}$, $15:2$

6. $100\text{ mg}:0.5\text{ mL}$, $0.5\text{ mL}:100\text{ mg}$,
   $\dfrac{100\text{ mg}}{0.5\text{ mL}}$, $\dfrac{0.5\text{ mL}}{100\text{ mg}}$

7. $0.25\text{ mg}:1\text{ tab}$, $1\text{ tab}:0.25\text{ mg}$,
   $\dfrac{0.25\text{ mg}}{1\text{ tab}}$, $\dfrac{1\text{ tab}}{0.25\text{ mg}}$

8. $1\text{ g}:10\text{ mL}$, $10\text{ mL}:1\text{ g}$,
   $\dfrac{1\text{ g}}{10\text{ mL}}$, $\dfrac{10\text{ mL}}{1\text{ g}}$

9. $500\text{ mg}:1\text{ capsule}$,
   $1\text{ capsule}:500\text{ mg}$,
   $\dfrac{500\text{ mg}}{1\text{ capsule}}$, $\dfrac{1\text{ capsule}}{500\text{ mg}}$

10. $x = 9.6$

11. $x = 3$

12. $x = 2.4$

13. $x = 7.5$

14. $x = 18$

Answers to Chapter Review

1. $2:3$

2. $1:9$

3. $3:4$

4. $1:5$

5. $1:2$

6. $1:5$

7. $\dfrac{3}{7}$

8. $\dfrac{2}{3}$

9. $\dfrac{1}{7}$

10. $1\dfrac{1}{3}$

11. $\dfrac{3}{4}$

12. $x = 5$

13. $x = 2$

14. $x = 4$

15. $x = 3.33$

16. $x = 4.5$

17. $x = 0.8$

18. $x = 1.33$

19. $x = 0.16$

20. $x = 0.1$

21. $x = 8$

22. $x = 22.5$

23. $x = 1.25$

24. $x = 0.6$

25. $x = 0.09$

26. $x = 25$

27. $x = 8$

28. $x = 55$

29. $x = 42$

30. $x = 7.5$

31. $x = 52$

32. $x = 40$

33. $x = 20.2$

34. $x = 66$

35. $x = 135$

36. $150\text{ mg}:2\text{ capsules} = x\text{ mg}:10\text{ capsules}$ *or*

   $$\dfrac{150\text{ mg}}{2\text{ capsules}} = \dfrac{x\text{ mg}}{10\text{ capsules}}$$
   $$x = 750\text{ mg}$$

37. $60\text{ mg}:500\text{ mL} = 36\text{ mg}:x\text{ mL}$ *or*

   $$\dfrac{60\text{ mg}}{500\text{ mL}} = \dfrac{36\text{ mg}}{x\text{ mL}}$$
   $$x = 300\text{ mL}$$

38. 1 kg : 2.2 lb = x kg : 61.6 lb *or*

$$\frac{1 \text{ kg}}{2.2 \text{ lb}} = \frac{x \text{ kg}}{61.6 \text{ lb}}$$

$x = 28$ kg

39. 1 glass : 280 mg = $2\frac{1}{2}$ glasses : x mg *or*

$$\frac{1 \text{ glass}}{280 \text{ mg}} = \frac{2\frac{1}{2} \text{ glasses}}{x \text{ mg}}$$

$x = 700$ mg

40. 0.125 mg : 1 tab = 0.25 mg : x tab *or*

$$\frac{0.125 \text{ mg}}{1 \text{ tab}} = \frac{0.25 \text{ mg}}{x \text{ tab}}$$

$x = 2$ tabs

41. 1 000 units : 1 mL *or* 1 mL : 1 000 units

$$\frac{1\,000 \text{ units}}{1 \text{ mL}} \quad or \quad \frac{1 \text{ mL}}{1\,000 \text{ units}}$$

42. 0.2 mg : 1 tab *or* 1 tab : 0.2 mg

$$\frac{0.2 \text{ mg}}{1 \text{ tab}} \quad or \quad \frac{1 \text{ tab}}{0.2 \text{ mg}}$$

43. 250 mg : 1 capsule *or* 1 capsule : 250 mg

$$\frac{250 \text{ mg}}{1 \text{ capsule}} \quad or \quad \frac{1 \text{ capsule}}{250 \text{ mg}}$$

44. 125 mg : 5 mL *or* 5 mL : 125 mg

$$\frac{125 \text{ mg}}{5 \text{ mL}} \quad or \quad \frac{5 \text{ mL}}{125 \text{ mg}}$$

45. 40 mg : 1 mL *or* 1 mL : 40 mg

$$\frac{40 \text{ mg}}{1 \text{ mL}} \quad or \quad \frac{1 \text{ mL}}{40 \text{ mg}}$$

46. 1 000 mcg : 2 mL *or* 2 mL : 1 000 mcg

$$\frac{1\,000 \text{ mcg}}{2 \text{ mL}} \quad or \quad \frac{2 \text{ mL}}{1\,000 \text{ mcg}}$$

47. 1 g : 3.6 mL *or* 3.6 mL : 1 g

$$\frac{1 \text{ g}}{3.6 \text{ mL}} \quad or \quad \frac{3.6 \text{ mL}}{1 \text{ g}}$$

48. 0.4 mg : 1 tab *or* 1 tab : 0.4 mg

$$\frac{0.4 \text{ mg}}{1 \text{ tab}} \quad or \quad \frac{1 \text{ tab}}{0.4 \text{ mg}}$$

49. 1 g : 1 capsule *or* 1 capsule : 1 g

$$\frac{1 \text{ g}}{1 \text{ capsule}} \quad or \quad \frac{1 \text{ capsule}}{1 \text{ g}}$$

50. 0.5 mg : 1 mL *or* 1 mL : 0.5 mg

$$\frac{0.5 \text{ mg}}{1 \text{ mL}} \quad or \quad \frac{1 \text{ mL}}{0.5 \text{ mg}}$$

51. 1 : 2 000

52. 1 : 400

53. 1 : 50

54. 1 : 5 000

55. 1 : 60

56. 15 mg : 10 lb = x mg : 120 lb *or*

$$\frac{15 \text{ mg}}{10 \text{ lb}} = \frac{x \text{ mg}}{120 \text{ lb}}$$

$x = 180$ mg

57. 40 mg : 5 mL = 120 mg : x mL *or*

$$\frac{40 \text{ mg}}{5 \text{ mL}} = \frac{120 \text{ mg}}{x \text{ mL}}$$

$x = 15$ mL

58. 15 g : 300 mL = 45 g : x mL *or*

$$\frac{15 \text{ g}}{300 \text{ mL}} = \frac{45 \text{ g}}{x \text{ mL}}$$

$x = 900$ mL

59. 325 mg : 1 tab = 975 mg : x tab *or*

$$\frac{325 \text{ mg}}{1 \text{ tab}} = \frac{975 \text{ mg}}{x \text{ tab}}$$

$x = 3$ tabs

60. 3 males : 5 females = x males : 40 females *or*

$$\frac{3 \text{ males}}{5 \text{ females}} = \frac{x \text{ males}}{40 \text{ females}}$$

$x = 24$ males

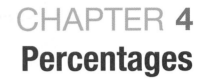

CHAPTER 4
Percentages

Objectives

After reviewing this chapter, you should be able to:

1. Define *percentage*
2. Convert percentages to fractions
3. Convert percentages to decimals
4. Convert percentages to ratios
5. Convert fractions to percentages
6. Convert decimals to percentages
7. Convert fractions to ratios
8. Determine the percentage of change

Percentage is a commonly used word. Sales tax is a *percentage* of the sale price; a final examination is a certain *percentage* of the final grade; interest on a home mortgage represents a *percentage* of the balance owed; interest on a savings account is expressed as a *percentage*. **Health care providers see percentages written with medications** (e.g., magnesium sulphate 50%, lidocaine 2%). Intravenous (IV) solutions and topical creams may also be expressed in percentages. For example, normal saline is 0.9% sodium chloride.

In current practice, percentage solutions are prepared by the hospital or community pharmacy. In the community, people can purchase solutions or components of the solutions over the counter. Understanding percentages provides the foundation for preparing and calculating dosages for medications that are ordered in percentages.

The term *percent* (%) means parts per hundred. A percentage is the same as a fraction in which the denominator is 100, and the numerator indicates the part of 100 that is being considered.

The symbol used to indicate a percent (%) is placed after the number, as in 40%. The example 40% means 40 out of 100. Percentages can be more than 100% (such as 200%) or less than 1% (0.1%). A percentage may also contain a decimal (0.6%), a fraction ($\frac{1}{2}$%), or a mixed number ($14\frac{1}{2}$%).

Example: $$4\% = 4 \text{ percent} = \frac{4}{100} \,(4 \text{ per } 100) = 0.04$$

Percentage Measures

IV (which means given directly into a person's vein) **solutions are ordered in percentage strengths, and nurses need to be familiar with their meaning** (e.g., 1 000 millilitres [mL] 5% dextrose and water). **Percentage solution means the number of grams (g) of solute per 100 mL of diluent.**

Example: 1 000 mL IV of 5% dextrose and water contains 50 g of dextrose

$$\% = g \text{ per } 100 \text{ mL; therefore } 5\% = 5 \text{ g per } 100 \text{ mL}$$
$$5 \text{ g} : 100 \text{ mL} = x \text{ g} : 1\,000 \text{ mL}$$
$$x = 50 \text{ g dextrose}$$

Example: 250 mL IV of 10% dextrose contains 25 g of dextrose

$$\% = g \text{ per } 100 \text{ mL; therefore } 10\% = 10 \text{ g per } 100 \text{ mL}$$
$$10 \text{ g} : 100 \text{ mL} = x \text{ g} : 250 \text{ mL}$$
$$x = 25 \text{ g dextrose}$$

In addition to encountering percentage strengths with IV solutions, the nurse and other health care providers may see percentages used with a variety of other medications, including eye and topical (for external use) ointments and creams. For example, triamcinolone acetonide cream is available in 0.1% and 0.5%. Timolol ophthalmic solution is available in 0.25% and 0.5%.

! SAFETY ALERT!

The higher the percentage strength, the stronger the solution or ointment. A misunderstanding of these numbers (%) can have serious consequences.

Example: 10% IV solution is more potent than 5%. A solution of 5% is more potent than 0.9%. **Always check the percentage of IV solution prescribed.**

+−÷× PRACTICE **PROBLEMS**

Determine the number of grams of medication and dextrose as indicated in the following solutions.

1. How many grams of medication will 500 mL of a 10% solution contain?

   _____

2. How many grams of dextrose will 1 000 mL of a 10% solution contain?

   _____

3. How many grams of dextrose will 250 mL of a 5% solution contain?

   _____

4. How many grams of medication will 100 mL of a 50% solution contain?

   _____

5. How many grams of dextrose will 150 mL of a 5% solution contain?

   _____

Identify the strongest solution or ointment in each of the following:

6. Ophthalmic solution 0.1%, 0.5%, 1% _____

7. Ointment 0.025%, 0.3%, 0.5% _____

8. Cream 0.02%, 0.025%, 0.25% _____

Answers on page 63.

Converting Percentages to Fractions, Decimals, and Ratios

> **RULE**
>
> To convert a percentage to a fraction:

1. Drop the percent sign.
2. Write the number as the numerator (top number in a fraction).
3. Write 100 as the denominator (bottom number in a fraction).
4. Reduce the fraction to lowest terms.

Example: $8\% = \dfrac{8}{100}$, reduced it is $\dfrac{2}{25}$

Example: $\dfrac{1}{4}\% = \dfrac{1}{4} \div 100 = \dfrac{1}{4} \times \dfrac{1}{100} = \dfrac{1}{400}$

PRACTICE **PROBLEMS**

Convert the following percentages to fractions, and reduce to lowest terms.

9. 1% _____

10. 2% _____

11. 50% _____

12. 80% _____

13. 3% _____

Answers on page 63.

> **RULE**
>
> To convert a percentage to a decimal:

1. Drop the percent sign.
2. Divide the number by 100; this is the same as moving the decimal point two places to the left (add zeros as needed).

Example 1: $25\% = \dfrac{25}{100} = 25 \div 100 = .25 = 0.25$

Example 2: $1.4\% = \dfrac{1.4}{100} = 1.4 \div 100 = .014 = 0.014$

Example 3: $75\% = \dfrac{75}{100} = \dfrac{3}{4}$ (lowest terms).

Divide the numerator of the fraction (3) by the denominator (4).

$$4\overline{)3.00} = 0.75 \quad (0.75)$$

> **NOTE**
> Example 3 is an alternative method. Drop the percent sign. Write the remaining number as the numerator. Write "100" as the denominator. Reduce the result to lowest terms. Divide the numerator by the denominator to obtain a decimal.

PRACTICE **PROBLEMS**

Convert the following percentages to decimals. Round to two decimal places, as indicated.

14. 10% _____

15. 35% _____

16. 50% _____

17. 14.2% _____

18. $\dfrac{6}{7}$% _____

Answers on page 63.

> ### → RULE
>
> To convert a percentage to a ratio:
>
> 1. Drop the percent sign.
> 2. Write the number as a fraction (place it in the numerator).
> 3. Write 100 as the denominator.
> 4. Reduce the fraction to lowest terms.
> 5. Place the numerator as the first term of the ratio and the denominator as the second term.
> 6. Separate the two terms with a colon (:).

Example:
$$10\% = \frac{10}{100} = \frac{1}{10} = 1:10$$

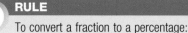 PRACTICE **PROBLEMS**

Convert the following percentages to ratios. Express in lowest terms.

19. 25% _____

20. 11% _____

21. 75% _____

22. 4.5% _____

23. $\dfrac{2}{5}$% _____

Answers on page 63.

Converting Fractions, Decimals, and Ratios to Percentages

> ### → RULE
>
> To convert a fraction to a percentage:
>
> 1. Multiply the fraction by 100.
> 2. Reduce if necessary.
> 3. Add the percent sign (%).
>
>   OR
>
> 1. Convert the fraction to a decimal.
> 2. Multiply the decimal by 100, which is the same as moving the decimal point two places to the right.
> 3. Add the percent sign (%).

Example: $\dfrac{3}{4}$ converted to a percentage is   *or* $\dfrac{3}{4}$ converted to a decimal is

$$\frac{3}{4} \times \frac{100}{1} = \frac{300}{4} = \frac{75}{1} = 75$$

$$\begin{array}{r} 0.75 \\ 4\overline{)3.00} \end{array}$$

$$0.75 \times 100 = 0.75 = 75$$

Add the percent sign: 75%   Add the percent sign: 75%

Example: $5\dfrac{1}{2}$ converted to a percentage is

Change to an improper fraction: $\dfrac{11}{2}$ *or*   Change to an improper fraction: $\dfrac{11}{2}$

$$2\overline{)11.0}^{\,5.5}$$

$\dfrac{11}{2} \times \dfrac{100}{1} = \dfrac{1100}{2} = \dfrac{550}{1}$ $5.5 \times 100 = 5.50 = 550$

Add the percent sign: 550%   Add the percent sign: 550%

✏ PRACTICE **PROBLEMS**

Convert the following fractions to percentages.

24. $\dfrac{2}{5}$ _____   27. $\dfrac{1}{4}$ _____

25. $\dfrac{11}{4}$ _____   28. $\dfrac{7}{10}$ _____

26. $\dfrac{1}{2}$ _____

Answers on page 63.

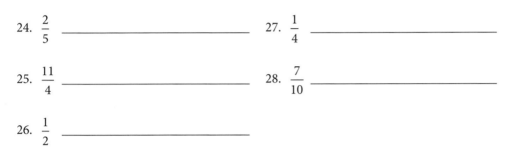

→ **RULE**

To convert a decimal to a percentage:

1. Multiply the decimal number by 100, which is the same as moving the decimal point two places to the right. Add zeros if necessary.
2. Add the percent sign (%).

Example: Convert 0.45 to %.

Move the decimal point two places to the right.

Add the percent sign:

$0.45 = 45\%$

Example: Convert 2.35 to %.

Move the decimal point two places to the right.

Add the percent sign:

$2.35 = 235\%$

→ **RULE**

A decimal may also be converted to a percentage by the following procedure:

1. Change the decimal to a fraction, then follow the steps to convert a fraction to a percentage.
2. If the percentage does not end as a whole number, express the percentage with the remainder as a fraction, to the nearest whole percent, or to the nearest tenth of a percent.

Example: $0.625 = \dfrac{625}{1\,000} = \dfrac{5}{8} = 62\dfrac{1}{2}\%,\ 63\%,\ \text{or}\ 62.5\%$

$$\dfrac{625}{1\,000} = \dfrac{5}{8}; \dfrac{5}{8} \times \dfrac{100}{1} = \dfrac{500}{8} = 62.5\%$$

→ **RULE**

To convert a ratio to a percentage:

1. Convert the ratio to a fraction, and proceed with the steps for changing a fraction to a percentage.

   OR

1. Convert the ratio to a fraction.
2. Convert the fraction to a decimal.
3. Convert the decimal to a percentage.

Example: $1:4 = \dfrac{1}{4}, \dfrac{1}{4} \times \dfrac{100}{1} = 25\ or$ $1:4 = \dfrac{1}{4}$

$$4\overline{)1.00}^{\,0.25}$$

$$0.25 \times 100 = 0.25 = 25$$

Add the percent sign: 25%   Add the percent sign: 25%

➕➖➗✖ PRACTICE **PROBLEMS**

Convert the following ratios to percentages.

29. 1:25 _____   32. 1:100 _____

30. 3:4 _____   33. 1:2 _____

31. 1:10 _____

Convert the following decimals to percentages.

34. 1.32 _____   37. 2.3 _____

35. 0.02 _____   38. 0.013 _____

36. 0.8 _____

Answers on page 63.

Comparing Percentages and Ratios

Nurses as well as other health care providers administer solutions that may be expressed as percentages or ratios. IV solutions come in varying percentages (e.g., 0.45%, 5%). It is important to be clear on the numbers and quantities they represent. An IV solution that is 5% is more potent or concentrated than an IV solution that is 0.45%. Converting percentages and ratios to equivalent decimals can clarify values so health care providers can compare concentrations.

Example: $0.45\% = \dfrac{0.45}{100} = 0.45 \div 100 = \underset{\smile}{00}.45 = 0.0045$

Example: $5\% = \dfrac{5}{100} = 5 \div 100 = \underset{\smile}{05}. = 0.05 \, (\text{greater value, stronger concentration})$

Compare solution concentrations expressed as a ratio, such as 1:1000 and 1:10 000.

Example: $1:1000 = \dfrac{1}{1000} = 0.001 \, (1:1000 \text{ is a stronger concentration})$

Example: $1:10\,000 = \dfrac{1}{10\,000} = 0.0001$

Determining the Percentage of a Quantity

> **RULE**
>
> To determine a given percentage of a number:
>
> 1. First convert the percentage to a decimal or fraction.
> 2. Multiply the decimal or fraction by the number.

Nurses may find it necessary to determine a given percentage or part of a quantity.

Example: A patient reports that he drank 25% of his cup (240 mL) of tea. Determine what amount 25% of 240 mL is.

Solution: Convert the percentage to a decimal:

$$25\% = \dfrac{25}{100} = \underset{\smile}{.25} = 0.25$$

Multiply the decimal by the number:

$$0.25 \times 240 \ \text{mL} = 60 \ \text{mL}$$

Therefore 25% of 240 mL = 60 mL

Example: 40% of 90

Solution:

$$40\% = \dfrac{40}{100} = \underset{\smile}{.40} = 0.4$$
$$0.4 \times 90 = 36$$
$$\text{Therefore } 40\% \text{ of } 90 = 36$$

Determining What Percentage One Number Is of Another

> **RULE**
>
> To determine what percentage one number is of another, it is necessary to make a fraction with the numbers.
>
> 1. The **denominator** (bottom number) of the fraction is the number following the word "of" in the problem.
> 2. The other number is the **numerator** (top number) of the fraction.
> 3. Convert the fraction to a decimal, and then convert to a percentage.

Example: 12 is what percentage of 60? *or* What percentage of 60 is 12?

Solution: Make a fraction using the two numbers:

$$\frac{12}{60}$$

Convert the fraction to a decimal:

$$60\overline{)12.0}^{\,0.2}$$

Convert the decimal to a percentage:

$$0.2 \times 100 = 0.20 = 20\%$$

Therefore 12 = 20% of 60 or 20% of 60 = 12

Example: 1.2 is what percentage of 4.8? *or* What percentage of 4.8 is 1.2?

Solution: Make a fraction using the two numbers:

$$\frac{1.2}{4.8}$$

Convert the fraction to a decimal:

$$4.8\overline{)1.200}^{\,0.25}$$

Convert the decimal to a percentage:

$$0.25 \times 100 = 0.25 = 25\%$$

Therefore 1.2 = 25% of 4.8 *or* 25% of 4.8 = 1.2

Example: $3\frac{1}{2}$ is what percentage of 8.5? *or* What percentage of 8.5 is $3\frac{1}{2}$?

Solution: Make a fraction using the two numbers:

$$\frac{3\frac{1}{2}}{8.5} = \frac{3.5}{8.5}$$

Convert the fraction to a decimal:

$$
\begin{array}{r}
0.411 \\
8.5\overline{)3.5000} \\
-340 \\
\hline
100 \\
-85 \\
\hline
150
\end{array}
$$

Convert the decimal to a percentage:

$$0.411 \times 100 = 0.411 = 41.1\%$$

Therefore $3\frac{1}{2}$ = 41.1% of 8.5 or 41.1% of 8.5 = $3\frac{1}{2}$

✛−÷✕ PRACTICE **PROBLEMS**

Perform the indicated operations. Round decimals to the hundredths place.

39. 60% of 30 _____

40. 20% of 75 _____

41. 2 is what percentage of 200? _____

42. 50 is what percentage of 500? _____

43. 40 is what percentage of 1 000? _____

44. 3% of 842 _____

45. 0.7% of 60 _____

46. 75% of 165 _____

47. 25 is what percentage of 40? _____

48. 1.3 is what percentage of 5.2? _____

49. $\frac{1}{4}$% of 68 _____

50. What percentage of 8.4 is $3\frac{1}{2}$? _____

Answers on page 63.

Calculating the Percentage of Change

It may be useful to determine a percentage of change (increase or decrease). For example, you might want to know if an increase or decrease in a patient's weight is a significant increase or decrease.

> **RULE**
>
> To determine the percentage of change:
>
> 1. Make a fraction of change $= \dfrac{\textbf{change}}{\textbf{old}}$
> 2. Multiply the fraction by 100 to convert the fraction to a percentage OR convert the fraction to a decimal and multiply the decimal by 100, which is the same as moving the decimal point two places to the right.
> 3. Add the percent sign.

Example: A patient's weight before surgery was 80 kilograms (kg). Following 2 weeks of bed rest, the patient's weight was 84 kg. What is the percentage increase in the patient's weight?

Solution: The increase = 84 kg − 80 kg = 4 kg

$$\text{Fraction of change} = \frac{4}{80}$$

$$\frac{4}{80} \times 100 = \frac{400}{80} = 5\%$$

or

Convert the fraction to a decimal and multiply by 100.

$$\text{Fraction of change} = \frac{4}{80}$$

$$\frac{4}{80} = 0.05 \qquad 0.05 \times 100 = 0.05 = 5\%$$

The percentage increase in the patient's weight was 5%.

Example: A patient was drinking 1 200 mL of water per day, but this amount was reduced by 300 mL per day. What is the percentage of change?

Solution: The decrease = 1 200 mL − 900 mL = 300 mL

$$\text{Fraction of change} = \frac{300}{1\,200} = 25\%$$

$$\frac{300}{1\,200} \times 100 = \frac{30\,000}{1\,200} = 25\%$$

or

Convert the fraction to a decimal and multiply by 100.

$$\text{Fraction of change} = \frac{300}{1\,200}$$

$$1200\overline{)300.00} = 0.25 \times 100 = 0.25 = 25\%$$
$$\underline{2400}$$
$$6000$$

with quotient 0.25

> **NOTE**
> Reducing the fraction, when possible, before solving can simplify the problem.

PRACTICE **PROBLEMS**

51. A patient's weight before dieting was 136.4 kg. After one month of dieting, the patient's weight is 109 kg. What is the percentage decrease in the patient's weight? _____

52. A patient was taking 400 milligrams (mg) of a pain medication. The doctor increased the dosage to 600 mg. What is the percentage increase in the dosage? _____

53. Physical therapy increases a patient's pulse rate. The patient's rate before the physical therapy was 60 beats per minute. At the completion of physical therapy, the rate is 75 beats per minute. What is the percentage increase in the pulse rate? _____

54. The number of nurses on the night shift has increased from 4 to 6. What is the percentage increase of nurses on the night shift? _____

55. The population at a small assisted-living facility dropped from 150 to 135 residents. What is the percentage decrease in population? _____

Answers on page 63.

CHAPTER **REVIEW**

Complete the table below. Express each of the following measures in their equivalents where indicated. Reduce fractions and ratios to lowest terms; round decimals to hundredths.

	Percentage	Ratio	Fraction	Decimal
1.	52%	_____	_____	_____
2.	71%	_____	_____	_____
3.	_____	_____	$\dfrac{7}{100}$	_____

Percentage	Ratio	Fraction	Decimal
4. _____	1 : 50	_____	_____
5. _____	_____	_____	0.06
6. _____	_____	$\dfrac{3}{8}$	_____
7. _____	_____	$\dfrac{61}{100}$	_____
8. _____	7 : 1 000	_____	_____
9. 5%	_____	_____	_____
10. 2.5%	_____	_____	_____

Perform the indicated operations.

11. A patient reports that he drank 40% of his 355 mL can of ginger ale. How many mL did the patient drink? _____

12. 40% of 140 _____   14. $\dfrac{1}{2}$ is what percentage of 60? _____

13. 100 is what percentage of 750? _____   15. 15% of 250 _____

16. What percentage of 6.4 is 1.6? _____

17. Which of the following solutions is strongest: 0.0125%, 0.25%, 0.1%?

    _____

Convert the following percentages to ratios, and reduce to lowest terms.

18. 16% _____   19. 45% _____

20. A patient is on a 1 000 mL fluid restriction per 24 hours. At breakfast and lunch the patient consumed 40% of the fluid allowance. How many mL did the patient consume?

    _____

21. A patient drank 75% of a 355 mL can of ginger ale. How many mL did the patient drink? _____

22. A patient consumes 55% of a bowl of chicken broth at lunch. The bowl holds 180 mL. How many mL did the patient consume? _____

23. In a class of 30 students, 6 students did not pass an exam. What percentage of the students did not pass the exam? _____

24. At the first prenatal visit a patient weighed 64 kg. At the second visit the patient had a 5% weight increase. How many kg did the patient gain? _____

25. An infant consumed 55% of a 240 mL bottle of formula. How many mL of formula did the infant consume? _____

26. In a portion of turkey that is 100 g, there are 23 g of protein and 4 g of fat.

    What percentage of the portion is protein? _____

    What percentage is fat? _____

27. A nursing review test has 130 questions, and you answer 120 correctly. What is your score, as a percentage? _____

28. A patient's intake for the day was 2 000 calories, and 600 of the calories came from fat. What percentage of the patient's intake came from fat? _____

29. A patient began receiving 325 mg of a medication. The prescriber increased the dosage of medication by 10%. What will the new dosage be? _____

30. The recommended daily allowance (RDA) of a vitamin is 14 mg. If a multivitamin provides 55% of the RDA, how many mg of the vitamin would the patient receive from the multivitamin? _____

31. A patient's pulse rate decreases from 80 beats per minute to 72 beats per minute. What is the percentage decrease? _____

32. A patient's medication is increased from 400 mg to 500 mg. What is the percentage increase in the dosage? _____

33. A patient's weight increased from 120 pounds (lb) to 132 lb. What is the percentage increase in body weight? _____

34. A patient's intake decreased from 2 500 mL per day to 2 000 mL per day. What is the percentage decrease in the patient's intake? _____

35. The number of capsules a patient received each day has decreased from 3 capsules per day to 2 capsules per day. What is the percentage decrease in capsules? _____

Convert the following percentages to decimals.

36. 4.4% _____   37. 103% _____

Convert the following decimals to percentages.

38. 0.32 _____   39. 0.06 _____

Identify the strongest in each of the following.

40. 1:10, 1:100, 1:200 _____   41. 1:25, $\dfrac{1}{5}$, 0.02% _____

Answers on page 63.

evolve

For additional practice problems, refer to the Mathematics Review section of the Drug Calculations Companion, Version 5 on Evolve.

✳ ANSWERS

Answers to Practice Problems

1. 50 g
2. 100 g
3. 12.5 g
4. 50 g
5. 7.5 g
6. 1%
7. 0.5%
8. 0.25%
9. $\frac{1}{100}$
10. $\frac{1}{50}$
11. $\frac{1}{2}$

12. $\frac{4}{5}$
13. $\frac{3}{100}$
14. 0.1
15. 0.35
16. 0.5
17. 0.14
18. 0.86
19. 1:4
20. 11:100
21. 3:4
22. 4.5:100

23. 0.4:100
24. 40%
25. 275%
26. 50%
27. 25%
28. 70%
29. 4%
30. 75%
31. 10%
32. 1%
33. 50%
34. 132%

35. 2%
36. 80%
37. 230%
38. 1.3%
39. 18
40. 15
41. 1%
42. 10%
43. 4%
44. 25.26
45. 0.42
46. 123.75

47. 62.5%
48. 25%
49. 0.17
50. 41.67%
51. 20%
52. 50%
53. 25%
54. 50%
55. 10%

Answers to Chapter Review

Percentage	Ratio	Fraction	Decimal
1. 52%	13:25	$\frac{13}{25}$	0.52
2. 71%	71:100	$\frac{71}{100}$	0.71
3. 7%	7:100	$\frac{7}{100}$	0.07
4. 2%	1:50	$\frac{1}{50}$	0.02
5. 6%	3:50	$\frac{3}{50}$	0.06
6. 37.5%	3:8	$\frac{3}{8}$	0.38
7. 61%	61:100	$\frac{61}{100}$	0.61
8. 0.7%	7:1000	$\frac{7}{1000}$	0.007
9. 5%	1:20	$\frac{1}{20}$	0.05
10. 2.5%	1:40	$\frac{1}{40}$	0.03

11. 142 mL
12. 56
13. 13.3%
14. 0.83%
15. 37.5
16. 25%
17. 0.25%
18. 4:25
19. 9:20
20. 400 mL
21. 266.25 mL
22. 99 mL
23. 20%
24. 3.2 kg
25. 132 mL
26. 23% protein, 4% fat

27. 92.3%
28. 30%
29. 357.5 mg
30. 7.7 mg
31. 10%
32. 25%
33. 10%
34. 20%
35. 33.3% or $33\frac{1}{3}$%
36. 0.044
37. 1.03
38. 32%
39. 6%
40. 1:10
41. $\frac{1}{5}$

POST-TEST

After completing Unit One of this text, you should be able to complete this test. The test consists of a total of 65 questions. If you miss any questions in any section, review the chapter relating to that content.

Reduce the following fractions to lowest terms.

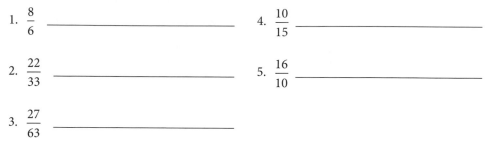

1. $\dfrac{8}{6}$ _____

2. $\dfrac{22}{33}$ _____

3. $\dfrac{27}{63}$ _____

4. $\dfrac{10}{15}$ _____

5. $\dfrac{16}{10}$ _____

Perform the indicated operations with fractions; reduce to lowest terms where needed.

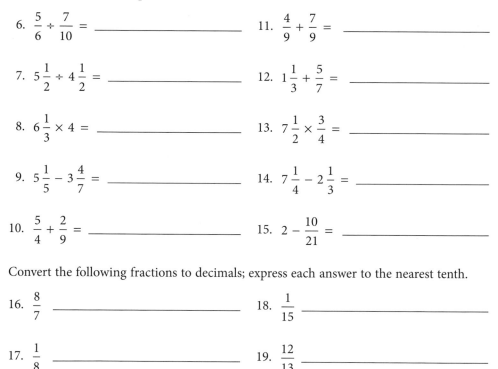

6. $\dfrac{5}{6} \div \dfrac{7}{10} =$ _____

7. $5\dfrac{1}{2} \div 4\dfrac{1}{2} =$ _____

8. $6\dfrac{1}{3} \times 4 =$ _____

9. $5\dfrac{1}{5} - 3\dfrac{4}{7} =$ _____

10. $\dfrac{5}{4} + \dfrac{2}{9} =$ _____

11. $\dfrac{4}{9} + \dfrac{7}{9} =$ _____

12. $1\dfrac{1}{3} + \dfrac{5}{7} =$ _____

13. $7\dfrac{1}{2} \times \dfrac{3}{4} =$ _____

14. $7\dfrac{1}{4} - 2\dfrac{1}{3} =$ _____

15. $2 - \dfrac{10}{21} =$ _____

Convert the following fractions to decimals; express each answer to the nearest tenth.

16. $\dfrac{8}{7}$ _____

17. $\dfrac{1}{8}$ _____

18. $\dfrac{1}{15}$ _____

19. $\dfrac{12}{13}$ _____

Indicate the largest fraction in each group.

20. $\dfrac{1}{2}, \dfrac{2}{3}, \dfrac{5}{9}$ _____

21. $\dfrac{3}{4}, \dfrac{7}{10}, \dfrac{5}{8}$ _____

Perform the indicated operations with decimals. Provide exact answers.

22. $16.7 + 21 =$ _____

23. $0.007 + 17.4 =$ _____

24. $10.57 \times 10 =$ _____

25. $36.8 - 3.86 =$ _____

Divide the following decimals; express each answer to the nearest tenth.

26. $67.8 \div 0.8 =$ _____   28. $5.01 \div 10 =$ _____

27. $9 \div 0.4 =$ _____

Indicate the largest decimal in each group.

29. 0.85, 0.085 _____   31. 0.478, 0.445, 0.493 _____

30. 3.002, 0.39, 0.399 _____

Solve for x, the unknown value.

32. $10:20 = x:8$ _____   34. $0.3:x = 1.8:0.6$ _____

33. $500:x = 200:1$ _____   35. $\dfrac{1}{4}:x = \dfrac{1}{8}:2$ _____

Round off to the nearest tenth.

36. 0.57 _____   38. 1.42 _____

37. 0.99 _____

Round off to the nearest hundredth.

39. 0.677 _____   41. 1.222 _____

40. 0.832 _____

Complete the table below. Express each of the measures in their equivalents where indicated. Reduce fractions and ratios to lowest terms; round decimals to hundredths.

	Percentage	Decimal	Ratio	Fraction
42.	_____	_____	1:10	_____
43.	60%	_____	_____	_____
44.	$66\dfrac{2}{3}\%$	_____	_____	_____
45.	25%	_____	_____	_____

Find the percentage.

46. 9% of 200 _____   49. 5 is what percentage of 2 000? _____

47. 2.5% of 750 _____   50. 25 is what percentage of 65? _____

48. 30 is what percentage of 45? _____

Express the following solution strengths as ratios.

51. 1 part medication to 80 parts solution _____

52. 1 part medication to 300 parts solution _____

53. 1 part medication to 20 parts solution _____

Identify the strongest solution in each of the following:

54. 1:80, 1:800, 1:8000 _____   55. 1:1000, 1:2000, 1:5000 _____

56. A patient who weighed 81.5 kg lost 3.75 kg. How much does the patient weigh now? _____

57. A patient's weight increased from 79.5 kg to 95.5 kg. What is the percentage increase in the patient's weight? _____

58. A patient is receiving 0.6 mg of a medication 4 times a day. How many mg would the patient receive after $2\frac{1}{2}$ days? _____

59. If 180 mL of medication must be mixed with 450 mL of water, how many mL of water is needed for 120 mL of medication? _____

60. A patient is taking 2 tablets twice a day for 14 days. The tablet contains 2.2 mg. How much medication did the patient receive? _____

61. A patient should have received 3.25 g of medication. In error the nurse administered 32.5 g. How much more medication did the patient receive? _____

62. Write a ratio that represents 20 mg of a medication in 100 mL of liquid. _____

63. A patient's weight decreased from 68.2 kg to 60 kg. What is the percentage decrease in the patient's weight? _____

64. A patient receives a total of 13.5 mg from 9 tablets. What is the dosage strength of each tablet? _____

65. Write a ratio that represents each capsule in a bottle contains 0.75 mg. _____

Answers on page 67.

✳ ANSWERS

1. $1\frac{1}{3}$

2. $\frac{2}{3}$

3. $\frac{3}{7}$

4. $\frac{2}{3}$

5. $1\frac{3}{5}$

6. $1\frac{4}{21}$

7. $1\frac{2}{9}$

8. $25\frac{1}{3}$

9. $1\frac{22}{35}$

10. $1\frac{17}{36}$

11. $\frac{11}{9} = 1\frac{2}{9}$

12. $2\frac{1}{21}$

13. $5\frac{5}{8}$

14. $4\frac{11}{12}$

15. $1\frac{11}{21}$

16. 1.1

17. 0.1

18. 0.1

19. 0.9

20. $\frac{2}{3}$

21. $\frac{3}{4}$

22. 37.7

23. 17.407

24. 105.7

25. 32.94

26. 84.8

27. 22.5

28. 0.5

29. 0.85

30. 3.002

31. 0.493

32. $x = 4$

33. $x = 2.5$ or $2\frac{1}{2}$

34. $x = 0.1$ or $\frac{1}{10}$

35. $x = 4$

36. 0.6

37. 1

38. 1.4

39. 0.68

40. 0.83

41. 1.22

	Percentage	Decimal	Ratio	Fraction
42.	10%	0.1	1:10	$\frac{1}{10}$
43.	60%	0.6	3:5	$\frac{3}{5}$
44.	$66\frac{2}{3}\%$	0.67	67:100	$\frac{67}{100}$
45.	25%	0.25	1:4	$\frac{1}{4}$

46. 18

47. 18.75

48. $66\frac{2}{3}\%$ *or* 66.7% *or* 67%

49. 0.25%

50. 38.46% *or* 38.5% *or* 38%

51. 1:80

52. 1:300

53. 1:20

54. 1:80

55. 1:1 000

56. 77.75 kg

57. 20%

58. 6 mg

59. 300 mL

60. 123.2 mg

61. 29.25 g

62. 20 mg:100 mL or 1 mg:5 mL

63. 12%

64. 1.5 mg

65. 0.75 mg:1 capsule

UNIT TWO

Systems of Measurement

The two main systems of measurement are the metric system and the imperial system. The metric system of measurement is used in Canada. The United States continues to use the imperial system, which includes apothecary, household, and Roman numeral measurements. Although the Canadian health care system uses metric measurements for dosage calculations, it is crucial for those who are administering medications to be knowledgeable about common measurements of the imperial system used in the United States: health care providers and students in Canada read literature containing these measurements, they may come across these measurements in community health care practice, or they may see them in work assignments in the United States or other countries. Pounds, ounces, tablespoons, and teaspoons are measurements that are still used in everyday living in Canada despite the adaptation of the metric system.

In addition, as of January 2015, the same National Council Licensure Examination for registered Nurses (NCLEX-RN) is used for Canadian and U.S. entry to nursing practice (National Council of State Boards of Nursing [NCSBN], 2015, p. 2). "NCLEX exam items currently include a combination of metric, international systems of units (SI) and imperial measurement used in the nursing profession" (NCSBN, 2015, p. 2). For these reasons, selected measurements from the imperial system are discussed in this unit and addressed in other chapters as appropriate.

CHAPTER 5
Metric, Apothecary, Household, and Other Systems

Objectives

After reviewing this chapter, you should be able to:

1. Express metric measures correctly using rules of the metric system
2. State common equivalents in the metric system
3. Convert measures within the metric system
4. Identify reasons for non-use of the imperial (apothecary) measures and symbols
5. State the common household equivalents
6. Define other measures used in medication administration:
   - units
   - international units
   - millimoles (mmol)

To administer medications safely to patients, it is important to have a thorough knowledge of the system of measurements used in medication administration. Understanding common equivalents of measurement used in medication administration will help in the prevention of **medication errors** related to incorrect dosages.

Historically, two different systems of measurement have been used in medication administration: the imperial and metric systems. The metric system is the preferred system of measurement for medications and measurements used in the health care setting. For example, newborn weights are recorded in grams (g) and kilograms (kg); centimetres (cm) are used in obstetrics to express fundal height (upper portion of the uterus) and to measure incisions.

The metric system is an international decimal system of weights and measures that was introduced in France in the late seventeenth and early eighteenth centuries. It is also referred to as the *International System of Units,* abbreviated as SI, taken from the French *Système International d'Unités.* The benefit of the metric system lies in its simplicity and accuracy because it is based on the decimal system.

Prescribers should use the metric system for prescribing medications to prevent medication errors. Over the years, several organizations in Canada have collaborated to work toward reducing and preventing medication incidents. For example, the Canadian Medication Incident Reporting and Prevention System (CMIRPS) is a collaborative pan-Canadian program of Health Canada, the Canadian Institute for Health Information (CIHI), the Institute for Safe Medication Practices Canada (ISMP Canada), and the Canadian Patient Safety Institute (CPSI) (Canadian Medication Incident Reporting and Prevention System, 2011). This program is based on the premise that reporting, sharing, and learning about medication incidents will help to reduce their reoccurrence and help create a safer health care system, which is the fundamental goal of CMIRPS. The program also underscores the importance of using the metric system when prescribing and preparing medications for administration to help prevent medication errors.

Metric System

1. The metric system is based on the decimal system, in which divisions and multiples of 10 are used. Therefore, a lot of the math can be done by decimal point movement.
2. Three basic units of measurement are used in the metric system, as shown in Table 5-1. Dosages are calculated by using metric measurements that relate to weight and volume. Metre, which is used for linear (length) measurement, is not used in the calculation of dosages. Linear measurements (metre, centimetre) are commonly used to measure the height of an individual and to determine growth patterns, serial abdominal girth (the circumference of the abdomen, usually measured at the umbilicus), the circumference of an infant's head, the length of an amount of a medicated paste, and the dimensions of pressure ulcers. These are important measures that can be seen in the health care setting.

TABLE 5-1	Basic Units of Metric Measurement	
Table of Measure	**Basic Unit**	**Abbreviation**
Weight (solid)	Gram	g
Volume (liquid)	Litre	L
Length	Metre	m

3. Common prefixes in this system denote the numerical value of the unit being discussed. Memorization of these prefixes is necessary for quick and accurate calculations. The prefixes in bold in Table 5-2 are the ones used most often in health care for dosage calculations. However, some of the prefixes may be used to express other values, such as laboratory values. *Kilo* is a common prefix used to identify a measure larger than the basic unit. The other common prefixes used in medication administration are smaller units: *centi, milli,* and *micro.*

TABLE 5-2	Common Prefixes Used in Health Care	
Prefix	**Numerical Value**	**Meaning**
Kilo*	1 000	one thousand times
Hecto	100	one hundred times
Deka	10	ten times
Deci	0.1	one tenth
Centi*	0.01	one hundredth part of
Milli*	0.001	one thousandth part of
Micro*	0.000 001	one millionth part of

*Prefixes used most often in medication administration.

Let's look at the following example to see how the prefixes may be used.

Example: 67 milligrams (mg)

Prefix—*milli*—means measure in thousandths of a unit.
Gram is a unit of weight.
Therefore 67 milligrams = 67 thousandths of a gram.

4. Regardless of the size of the unit, the name of the basic unit is incorporated into the measure. This allows easy recognition of the unit of measurement.

Example: milli**litre**—The word *litre* indicates you are measuring volume (*milli* indicates $\frac{1}{1\,000}$ of that volume).

Example: kilo**gram**—The word *gram* indicates you are measuring weight (*kilo* indicates 1 000 of that weight; 1 kilogram = 1 000 grams).

Example: micro**gram**—The word *gram* indicates you are measuring weight (*micro* indicates $\dfrac{1}{1\,000\,000}$ of that weight). 1 microgram = 1 millionth of a gram.

> **SAFETY ALERT!**
> Do not confuse units of measurement in the metric system for weight, volume, and length that have similar names. Milligram is a unit of weight; millilitre is a unit of volume; and millimetre is a unit of length.

> **POINTS TO REMEMBER**
> It is important to memorize the prefixes and the amounts they represent. A mnemonic to help remember the important metric prefixes order from largest measurement to smallest is **K**itty **H**awk **D**oesn't **D**rink **C**anned **M**ilk **M**uch.
> **kilo, hecto, deka, deci, centi, milli, micro.**

5. The abbreviation for a unit of measurement in the metric system is often the first letter of the word. Lowercase letters are used more often than capital letters.

Example: g = gram

Example: m = metre

The exception to this rule is litre, for which a capital letter is used.

Example: litre = L

6. When prefixes are used in combination with the basic unit, the first letter of the prefix and the first letter of the unit of measurement are written together in lowercase letters.

Example: Milligram—abbreviated as **mg.** The *m* is taken from the prefix *milli* and the *g* from *gram,* the unit of weight.

Example: Microgram—abbreviated as **mcg.** Microgram is also written using the symbol μ in combination with the letter *g* from the basic unit *gram* (μg). However, use of the abbreviation μg should be avoided when writing orders. It can be mistaken for "mg" when handwritten and result in an error when orders are transcribed.

> **SAFETY ALERT!**
> The abbreviation μg for microgram is listed on the official "Do Not Use" list of ISMP Canada (2006a) Confusion of the symbol used for microgram with the abbreviation for milligram could cause a critical error in dosage calculation. These units differ from each other in value by 1 000.

Although the symbol for microgram is no longer approved for use when writing medication orders, it may be seen on some medication labels (e.g., digoxin [Lanoxin] tablets, digoxin injectable, digoxin elixir for pediatric use), and you should be familiar with the meaning.

Example: Millilitre—abbreviated as **mL.** Note that when *L (litre)* is used in combination with a prefix, it **remains capitalized.**

SAFETY ALERT!

You may see gram abbreviated as Gm or gm, litre as lowercase l, or millilitre as ml. These abbreviations are outdated and can lead to misinterpretation. Use only the standardized SI abbreviations. Use **g** for gram, **L** for litre, and **mL** for millilitre. Cubic centimetre, abbreviated as cc, was used interchangeably for mL. Using cc for mL should not be done. It has been misinterpreted for zeros (00) or units (U). The use of the abbreviation U is prohibited and must be spelled out (unit). It has been mistaken for zero (0) and the number 4 (four). When in doubt about an abbreviation being used, never assume; ask the prescriber for clarification.

SAFETY ALERT!

It is critical to differentiate between the SI abbreviations for milligram (mg) and millilitre (mL). At a quick glance these abbreviations appear similar; however, confusing these two units can result in lethal consequences for a patient.

Box 5-1 lists the common metric abbreviations.

BOX 5-1   **Common Metric Abbreviations**
gram = g
microgram = mcg
milligram = mg
kilogram = kg
litre = L
decilitre = dL*
millilitre = mL

*May be seen in the expression of laboratory values that originate from the United States (e.g., hemoglobin, creatinine levels).

Rules of the Metric System

Certain rules specific to the metric system are important to remember (Box 5-2). **These rules are critical to the prevention of errors and ensure accurate interpretation of metric notations when used in medication orders. [Never assume.]** Ask for clarification if you are not sure of the abbreviation or notation to prevent an error.

SAFETY ALERT!

To enhance patient safety, ISMP Canada (2006b) published guidelines for the use of leading and trailing zeros. When the quantity is less than 1, always place a zero before the decimal point (leading zero). When the quantity is a decimal preceded by a whole number, do not place an extra zero after the last digit to the right of the decimal point (trailing zero). These rules are critical to preventing misinterpretation and medication errors. Always double-check the placement of decimals and zeros.

Example: .52 mL is written as 0.52 mL to **reinforce the decimal** and avoid being misread as 52 mL. Lack of a leading zero before the decimal point could result in the decimal point being missed and cause a critical error in dosage interpretation.

Example: 2.5 mL is written as 2.5 mL, not 2.50 mL. **Addition of unnecessary zeros can lead to errors in reading;** 2.50 mL may be misread as 250 mL instead of 2.5 mL. Unnecessary zeros can also result in the decimal point being missed and cause a critical error in dosage interpretation.

BOX 5-2 Metric System Rules

1. Use Arabic numerals (0, 1, 2, 3, etc.) to express quantities in this system.

   Example: 1, 1 000, 0.5

2. Express parts of a unit or fractions of a unit as decimals.

   Example: 0.4 g, 0.5 L $\left(\text{not } \frac{2}{5} \text{ g, } \frac{1}{2} \text{ L} \right)$

3. Always write the quantity, whether in whole numbers or in decimals, before the abbreviation or symbol for a unit of measurement.

   Example: 1 000 mg, 0.75 mL (not mg 1 000, mL 0.75)

4. Use a full space between the numeral and abbreviation.

   Example: 2 mL, 1 L (not 2mL, 1L)

5. Always place a leading zero to the left of the decimal point if the quantity is less than one. Eliminate trailing zeros to the right of the decimal point.

   Example: 0.4 mL, 2 mg (not .4 mL, 2.0 mg)

6. Do not use the abbreviation μg for microgram; it might be mistaken for mg. Remember mg is 1 000 times larger.

7. Do not use the abbreviation *cc* for mL. This abbreviation can be misinterpreted as zeros.

   Example: 2 mL (not 2 cc)

8. Avoid using a period after the abbreviation for a unit of measurement to prevent the possibility of it being misread for the number 1 in a poorly handwritten order.

   Example: mg (not mg.)

9. Place a space between groups of three digits in a number.

   Example: 100 000 units (not 100000 units)

10. Do not add "s" on a unit of measurement to make it plural; this could lead to misinterpretation.

    Example: mg (not mgs)

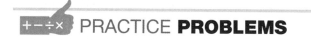

PRACTICE **PROBLEMS**

Applying the guidelines relating to the use of leading and trailing zeros, express the following values correctly.

1. .750 g _____   4. 7.0 kg _____

2. 1.70 mL _____   5. .002 mg _____

3. .68 L _____   **Answers on page 83.**

Units of Measurement

Understanding common equivalents in the metric system can assist the nurse in preventing medication errors related to incorrect dosage.

Weight

The gram is the basic unit of weight. Medications may be ordered in grams or fractions of a gram, such as milligram or microgram.

1. The milligram is 1 000 times smaller than a gram:

$$1 g = 1 000 mg$$

2. The microgram is 1 000 times smaller than a milligram and 1 million times smaller than a gram. The word *micro* also means tiny or small. Micrograms are tiny parts of a gram (i.e., 1 000 mcg = 1 mg). A milligram is 1 000 times larger than a microgram. It takes 1 million mcg to make 1 g.
3. The kilogram is very large and is not used for measuring medications. A kilogram is 1 000 times larger than a gram (i.e., 1 kg = 1 000 g). This measure is often used to denote weights of patients, on which medication dosages are based. This is the only unit you will see used to identify a unit larger than the basic unit.

Box 5-3 presents the metric units of measurement used most often for dosage calculations and measurement of health status. This text uses the standardized abbreviations for metric units throughout.

BOX 5-3 **Metric Equivalents to Memorize**	
Weight	**Volume**
1 kilogram (kg) = 1 000 grams (g) 1 gram (g) = 1 000 milligrams (mg) 1 milligram (mg) = 1 000 micrograms (mcg)	1 litre (L) = 1 000 millilitres (mL) 1 millilitre (mL) = 0.001 litre (L)
	Length 1 metre (m) = 100 centimetres (cm) = 1 000 mm 1 millimetre (mm) = 0.001 metre (m) = 0.1 cm

Volume

1. The **litre** is the basic unit.

$$1\,L = 1\,000\,mL$$

2. The **millilitre** is 1 000 times smaller than a litre. It is abbreviated as mL.

$$1\,mL = 0.001\,L$$

3. As previously stated **cubic centimetre** (cc) should not be used because of misinterpretation. The cubic centimetre is the amount of space that 1 mL of liquid occupies. Remember, mL is the correct term for volume. The use of cc for mL is currently prohibited by many health care organizations. ISMP Canada (2006a) has suggested that institutions prohibit the use of cc and includes this abbreviation in its "Do Not Use" list. Figure 5-1 shows metric measures that may be seen on a medication cup.

Figure 5-1 Medicine cup showing volume measure in millilitres (mL) and ounces (oz). (From Ogden, S. J., & Fluharty, L. K. (2012). *Calculation of drug dosages* (9th ed.). St. Louis: Mosby.)

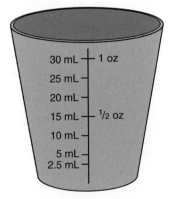

Conversions between Metric Units

Because the metric system is based on the decimal system, conversions between one metric system unit and another can be done by moving the decimal point. The number of places to move the decimal point depends on the equivalent. In health care, each unit of measurement in common use for purposes of medication administration differs by 1 000. In the metric system the most common terms used are the kilogram, gram, milligram, microgram, litre, millilitre, and centimetre. To **convert** or make a **conversion** means to change from one unit to another. This converting can be simply changing a measure to its equivalent in the same system. Changing from grams to milligrams illustrates a metric measure changed to another metric measure. Each metric unit in common use for *medication administration* differs from the next by a factor of 1 000. Metric conversions can therefore be made by dividing or multiplying by **1000**. Knowledge of the size of a unit is important when converting by moving the decimal because this determines whether division or multiplication is necessary to make the conversion.

> Nurses often make conversions within the metric system when administering medications, for example, from grams to milligrams.

To make conversions within the metric system, remember the common conversion factors (1 kg = 1 000 g, 1 g = 1 000 mg, 1 mg = 1 000 mcg, and 1 L = 1 000 mL) and the following rules:

> **RULE**
>
> To convert a **smaller** unit to a **larger** one, **divide** by moving the decimal point **three places to the left**.

Example: 100 mL = ___ L   (conversion factor: 1 000 mL = 1 L)
             (smaller)   (larger)

100 mL = .100 = 0.1 L   (**Placing zero in front of the decimal is important.**)

Example: 50 mg = ___ g   (conversion factor: 1 000 mg = 1 g)
             (smaller)   (larger)

50 mg = .050 = 0.05 g   (**Placing zero in front of the decimal is important.**)

> **RULE**
>
> To convert a **larger** unit to a **smaller** one, **multiply** by moving the decimal **three places to the right**.

> **NOTE**
>
> Answers to conversions should be labelled with the unit of measurement.

Example: 0.75 g = ___ mg   (conversion factor: 1 g = 1 000 mg)
             (larger)   (smaller)

0.75 g = 0.750 = 750 mg

Example: 0.04 kg = ___ g   (conversion factor: 1 kg = 1 000 g)
             (larger)   (smaller)

0.04 kg = 0.040 = 40 g

> **SAFETY ALERT!**
>
> When converting quantities from one unit of measurement to another within the metric system, pay close attention to the decimal point. Moving the decimal point incorrectly (i.e., in the wrong direction) can result in a dangerous error.

PRACTICE **PROBLEMS**

Convert the following metric measures by moving the decimal.

6. 300 mg = _____ g   16. 529 mg = _____ g

7. 6 mg = _____ mcg   17. 645 mcg = _____ mg

8. 0.7 L = _____ mL   18. 347 L = _____ mL

9. 180 mcg = _____ mg   19. 238 g = _____ mcg

10. 0.02 mg = _____ mcg   20. 3 500 mL = _____ L

11. 4.5 L = _____ mL   21. 0.04 kg = _____ g

12. 4.2 g = _____ mg   22. 658 kg = _____ g

13. 0.9 g = _____ mg   23. 51 mL = _____ L

14. 3 250 mL = _____ L   24. 1.6 mg = _____ mcg

15. 42 g = _____ kg   25. 28 mL = _____ L

Answers on page 83.

POINTS TO REMEMBER

- Note that the litre and the gram are the basic units used for medication administration.
- Memorize the common conversion factors to be able to make conversions. The common conversion factors in the metric system are 1 kg = 1 000 g, 1 g = 1 000 mg, 1 mg = 1 000 mcg, and 1 L = 1 000 mL (mL is the correct term to use in relation to volume, rather than cc).
- Apply the following rules of the metric system:
  1. Express fractional metric units as decimal numbers.
  2. Place a leading zero in front of the decimal point when the quantity is less than 1 to prevent potential dosage error.
  3. Omit trailing zeros to avoid misreading a value and to prevent a potential error in dosage.
  4. Place the abbreviation for a measure after the quantity.
  5. Place a full space between the numeral and abbreviation.
  6. Use standard SI abbreviations.
- Convert common metric units used in medication administration from one unit to another by multiplying or dividing by 1 000.
- Write the quantity with the unit of measurement.
- Use a space between groups of three digits in a number (1 000; 1 000 000).
- Never guess at the meaning of a metric notation. Ask for clarification.

Apothecary System (Imperial)

The apothecary system of measurement is an English system that is considered to be one of the oldest systems of measure. Many notations in this system are confusing. However, those that will be discussed in this chapter are shown under the **household system**. To help reduce medication errors and improve patient safety, ISMP Canada has recommended that all medications be prescribed and calculated with metric measures.

Roman Numeral System (Imperial)

The Roman numeral system dates back to ancient Roman times and uses letters to designate amounts. Roman numerals (I, II, III, etc.) are still used in countries that continue to use the apothecary system of measurement for writing medication dosages. For example, they are seen on medication labels that are considered to be controlled substances in the United States. The labels of these substances in Canada do not carry Roman numerals. However, these numerals are still used on objects that indicate time (e.g., watches, clocks) and for clotting factors. In Canada, it is best practice to use Arabic numerals for medication dosages. Please refer to Appendix A for Roman numeral equivalents of Arabic numerals.

Household System (Imperial)

The household system is an old system and the **least accurate** system of measure. It is a modified system designed for everyday use at home and includes approximate equivalents. Many of the household measures originated as **apothecary** measures. Although Canadian health care uses the metric system, measures like *pounds* may still be used for weight while *cups, ounces, tablespoons, teaspoons,* and *drops* may still be used for volume in some cases. For this reason, these measures are briefly discussed in this chapter to enhance knowledge and understanding should health care providers have to work with these measurements in community settings or abroad. Conversions between household and metric measures are based on approximate equivalents. Capacities of utensils such as a teaspoon, a tablespoon, and a cup vary; therefore, liquid measures are approximate. Because of the increase in nursing care provided at home (home care, visiting nurses), it is important that nurses know how to convert from one system to another. The nurse should be able to calculate equivalents for adaptation in the home, if necessary, even though medication administration droppers and medication measuring cups (Figure 5-2) are available.

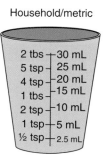

Household/metric

1-ounce medicine cup (30 mL)

Figure 5-2 Medicine cup showing household/metric measurements. *tbs,* tablespoon; *tsp,* teaspoon; *mL,* millilitres.

> **! SAFETY ALERT!**
> Although household utensils may be most familiar to patients, they may invite inaccuracies with medication dosages. Using ordinary household utensils may constitute a safety risk because ordinary household utensils do not come in standard sizes. Therefore, patients and their families should be advised to use the measuring device provided with the medication or purchase calibrated devices from the pharmacy as opposed to using their kitchen teaspoon, for example.

> **✎ NOTE**
> Anything less than a teaspoon should be measured in a syringe-type device that has no needle, not in a measuring cup.

See Box 5-4 for household measures and metric equivalents.

Particulars of the Household System

1. There are no standard rules for expressing household measures, which accounts for variations in their use.
2. Standard cookbook abbreviations are used in this system.
3. Arabic numerals and fractions are used to express quantities.
4. The smallest unit of measurement in the household system is the drop (gtt).
5. The unit ounce used to measure liquid is sometimes referred to as *fluid ounce.*

> **! SAFETY ALERT!**
> Drops should never be used as a measure for medications because the size of drops varies according to the diameter of the utensil and therefore can be inaccurate. When drops are used as a measure for medications, they should be calibrated or used only when associated with a dropper size, as in intravenous (IV) flow rates.

BOX 5-4   Household/Metric Equivalents

Unit	Abbreviation	Equivalent	Metric Equivalent
teaspoon	t (tsp)	—	5 mL
tablespoon	T (tbsp)	1 T = 3 t	15 mL
ounce (fluid)	oz	1 oz = 2 T	30 mL
cup (standard measuring)	C	1 C = 8 oz	240 mL
pound (weight)	lb	1 lb = 16 oz	2.2 lb = 1 kg (1 000 g)

Other Measurements Used in Dosage Calculation

Other measurements that may be used to indicate the strength or potency of certain medications include units, international unit, and milliequivalent. The quantity or amount is expressed using Arabic numerals, with the unit of measurement following.

- **Units** express the amount of medication present in 1 mL of solution and are specific to the medication for which they are used. Units measure a medication in terms of its action. Medications such as heparin, penicillin, and insulin are some examples of medications expressed in units.
- **International unit** represents a unit of potency used to measure things such as vitamins and chemicals. These international units represent the amount of medication needed to produce a certain effect and are standardized by international agreement.
- **Millimoles (mmol)** are used to measure electrolytes (e.g., potassium) and the ionic activity of a medication. The millimole is a unit of metric measurement that is equal to one thousandth ($\frac{1}{1\,000}$) of a gram-molecule. Other electrolytes measured in millimoles include calcium, magnesium, and sodium.

Units, international units, millimoles, or milliequivalents are not converted to other measures; medications that are prescribed in these measurements are prepared and administered in the same system. Figure 5-3 shows sample labels of medications in millimoles and units.

> **NOTE**
> Milliequivalents (mEq) are also used to measure electrolytes and may still be seen on some medication labels. In Canada, the preferred measurement for electrolytes is the millimole.

> **! SAFETY ALERT!**
> The abbreviations U (units) and IU (international units) are prohibited and must be written out. The abbreviations U and IU are included in the "Do Not Use" list published by ISMP Canada (2006a).

> **POINTS TO REMEMBER**
> - Teaspoon and tablespoon are measures that may be used in the household system.
> - For safety, patients should be encouraged to use the measuring device that comes with the medication.
> - There are no rules for stating household measures.
> - The household system uses fractions and Arabic numerals.
> - Conversions between metric and household measures are approximate equivalents.
> - Dosages less than a teaspoon should be measured with a syringe-type device that does not have a needle attached.
> - When possible, household measures should be converted to metric measures.
> - When in doubt about an unfamiliar unit or one that is not used often, it is best to consult a reference or an equivalency table.
> - No conversion is necessary for unit, international unit, and milliequivalent. Medications prescribed in these measures are available in the same system.

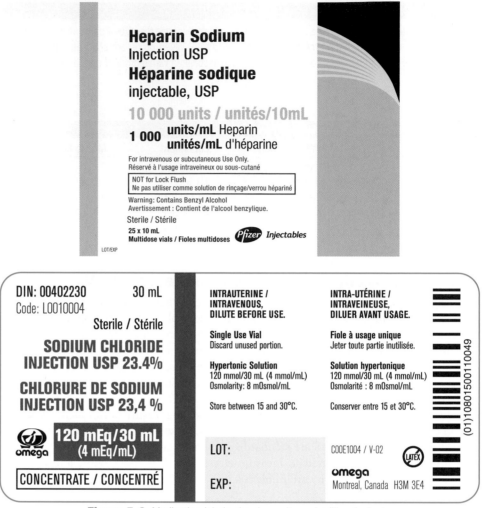

Figure 5-3 Medication labels showing units and milliequivalents.

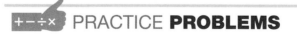 PRACTICE **PROBLEMS**

Write the abbreviations for the following measures.

26. ounce _____

27. tablespoon _____

28. teaspoon _____

29. pound _____

Use Box 5-4 to determine the following equivalents.

30. $\frac{1}{2}$ oz = _____ mL

31. 2 tsp = _____ mL

32. 45 mL = _____ tbsp

33. 90 mL = _____ oz

34. 8 oz = _____ cup

35. 1 oz = _____ T

36. 3 tbsp = _____ mL

Write the following amounts correctly using Arabic numerals and abbreviations.

37. 10 ounces _____

38. Fifteen units _____

39. Sixty-five pounds _____

40. Twenty milliequivalents _____

41. Two and one half teaspoons _____

42. Fourteen and one quarter ounces ____

43. Ten tablespoons _____

44. What household measure might be used to give a $\frac{1}{2}$ ounce of cough syrup?

    _____

45. The nurse encouraged a patient with diarrhea to drink 40 ounces of water per day. How many cups does this represent?

    _____

46. Medications such as penicillin and insulin are commonly measured in

    _____

47. The unit used to measure the concentration of serum electrolytes such as potassium and sodium is the

    _____ and is

    abbreviated as _____.

Answers on page 84.

CHAPTER **REVIEW**

1. List the three basic units of measurement used in the metric system.

   a. _____   c. _____

   b. _____

2. Which is larger, a kg or an mg? _____

3. 1 mL = _____ L

4. What units of measurement are used in the metric system for the following:

   a. liquid capacity? _____   b. weight? _____

5. 1 000 mg = _____ g   7. 1 000 mcg = _____ mg

6. 1 L = _____ mL   8. 1 000 mL = _____ L

9. The abbreviation for litre is _____   13. The abbreviation for kilogram is ____

10. The abbreviation for microgram is ____   14. The prefix *kilo* means _____

11. The abbreviation for millilitre is _____   15. The prefix *milli* means _____

12. The abbreviation for gram is _____

Using abbreviations and the rules of the metric system, express the following quantities correctly.

16. Six tenths of a gram _____   17. Fifty kilograms _____

18. Four tenths of a milligram _____   22. Six hundredths of a gram _____

19. Four hundredths of a litre _____   23. Two and six tenths millilitres _____

20. Four and two tenths micrograms ____   24. One hundred millilitres _____

21. Five thousandths of a gram _____   25. Three hundredths of a millilitre _____

Convert the following metric measures by moving the decimal.

26. 950 mcg = _____ mg   46. 400 g = _____ kg

27. 58.5 L = _____ mL   47. 0.024 L = _____ mL

28. 130 mL = _____ L   48. 100 mg = _____ g

29. 276 g = _____ mg   49. 150 g = _____ mg

30. 550 mL = _____ L   50. 85 mcg = _____ mg

31. 56.5 L = _____ mL   51. 1.25 L = _____ mL

32. 205 g = _____ kg   52. 0.05 mg = _____ mcg

33. 0.025 kg = _____ g   53. 120 mg = _____ g

34. 1 L = _____ mL   54. 475 mL = _____ L

35. 0.015 g = _____ mg   55. 4.5 g = _____ mg

36. 250 mcg = _____ mg   56. 8.6 mg = _____ mcg

37. 8 kg = _____ g   57. 250 000 mcg = _____ mg

38. 2 kL = _____ L   58. 40 mg = _____ g

39. 5 L = _____ mL   59. 0.65 kg = _____ g

40. 0.75 L = _____ mL   60. 37.5 mcg = _____ mg

41. 0.33 g = _____ mg   61. 0.026 mg = _____ mcg

42. 750 mg = _____ g   62. 36 000 mg = _____ g

43. 6.28 kg = _____ g   63. 0.125 g = _____ mg

44. 36.5 mg = _____ g   64. 5 524 g = _____ kg

45. 2.2 mg = _____ g   65. 8 500 mcg = _____ mg

Which of the following is stated correctly using metric abbreviations and rules?

66. .5 g, 0.5 gm, .5 gm, 0.5 g _____ _____

67. 4 KG, 4.0 Kg, Kg 04, 4 kg _____ _____

68. Furosemide (Lasix) 20.0 mg, Furosemide (Lasix) 20 mg, Furosemide (Lasix) 20 MG, Furosemide (Lasix) mg 20 _____

69. Gentamicin $1\frac{1}{2}$ mL, gentamicin 1.5 ml, gentamicin 1.5 mL, gentamicin $1\frac{1}{2}$ ml

_____

70. Ampicillin 500 mg, ampicillin 500.0 mg, ampicillin 500 MG, ampicillin mg 500

_____

Express the following using Arabic numerals and abbreviations.

71. One-third ounce _____   74. Ten thousand units _____

72. Three million units _____   75. Forty-five millimoles _____

73. Five and one-quarter teaspoons _____   76. Five ounces _____

Complete the following sentences.

77. Pound is a unit of _____.   81. 1 t = _____ mL

78. The abbreviation for drop is _____.   82. 1 oz = _____ mL

79. T is the abbreviation for _____.   83. 1 cup = _____ oz

80. The abbreviation t is used for _____.   84. 1 tbsp = _____ mL

Express the following notations in words.

85. $8\frac{1}{4}$ oz _____   87. $15\frac{1}{2}$ lb _____

86. 30 mmol _____   88. 8 tbsp _____

89. True or false? The household system of measurement is used for patient dosages at home. _____

90. True or false? Units can be abbreviated as U. _____

91. True or false? Household measures are approximate equivalents. _____

Answers on page 84.

✳ ANSWERS

Answers to Practice Problems

1. 0.75 g	4. 7 kg	7. 6000 mcg	10. 20 mcg	13. 900 mg
2. 1.7 mL	5. 0.002 mg	8. 700 mL	11. 4500 mL	14. 3.25 L
3. 0.68 L	6. 0.3 g	9. 0.18 mg	12. 4200 mg	15. 0.042 kg

evolve

For additional practice problems, refer to the Drug Measures section of the Drug Calculations Companion, Version 5 on Evolve.

16. 0.529 g

17. 0.645 mg

18. 347 000 mL

19. 238 000 000 mcg

20. 3.5 L

21. 40 g

22. 658 000 g

23. 0.051 L

24. 1 600 mcg

25. 0.028 L

26. oz

27. T, tbsp

28. t, tsp

29. lb

30. 15 mL

31. 10 mL

32. 3 tbsp

33. 3 oz

34. 1 cup

35. 2 T

36. 45 mL

37. 10 oz

38. 15 units

39. 65 lb

40. 20 mEq

41. $2\frac{1}{2}$ t, $2\frac{1}{2}$ tsp

42. $14\frac{1}{4}$ oz

43. 10 tbsp; 10 T

44. 1 tbsp; 1 T

45. 5 cups

46. units

47. millimole; mmol

Answers to Chapter Review

1. gram (g), litre (L), metre (m)

2. kilogram

3. 0.001 L

4. a. L, mL
   b. g, mg, mcg, kg

5. 1 g

6. 1 000 mL

7. 1 mg

8. 1 L

9. L

10. mcg

11. mL

12. g

13. kg

14. thousand times

15. the thousandth part of

16. 0.6 g

17. 50 kg

18. 0.4 mg

19. 0.04 L

20. 4.2 mcg

21. 0.005 g

22. 0.06 g

23. 2.6 mL

24. 100 mL

25. 0.03 mL

26. 0.95 mg

27. 58 500 mL

28. 0.13 L

29. 276 000 mg

30. 0.55 L

31. 56 500 mL

32. 0.205 kg

33. 25 g

34. 1 000 mL

35. 15 mg

36. 0.25 mg

37. 8 000 g

38. 2 000 L

39. 5 000 mL

40. 750 mL

41. 330 mg

42. 0.75 g

43. 6 280 g

44. 0.036 5 g

45. 0.002 2 g

46. 0.4 kg

47. 24 mL

48. 0.1 g

49. 150 000 mg

50. 0.085 mg

51. 1 250 mL

52. 50 mcg

53. 0.12 g

54. 0.475 L

55. 4 500 mg

56. 8 600 mcg

57. 250 mg

68. 0.04 g

59. 650 g

60. 0.0375 mg

61. 26 mcg

62. 36 g

63. 125 mg

64. 5.524 kg

65. 8.5 mg

66. 0.5 g

67. 4 kg

68. Furosemide (Lasix) 20 mg

69. Gentamicin 1.5 mL

70. Ampicillin 500 mg

71. $\frac{1}{3}$ oz

72. 3 000 000 units

73. $5\frac{1}{4}$ tsp; $5\frac{1}{4}$ t

74. 10 000 units

75. 45 mmol

76. 5 oz

77. weight

78. gtt

79. tablespoon

80. teaspoon

81. 5 mL

82. 30 mL

83. 8 oz

84. 15 mL

85. eight and one quarter ounces

86. thirty millimoles

87. fifteen and one half pounds

88. eight tablespoons

89. True

90. False

91. True

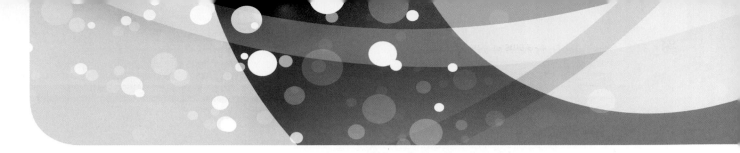

CHAPTER 6

Converting Within and Between Systems

Objectives

After reviewing this chapter, you should be able to:

1. State the metric and household approximate equivalents
2. Convert a unit of measurement to its equivalent within the same system
3. Convert a unit from one system of measurement to its equivalent in another system of measurement

Equivalents among Metric and Household Systems

As noted in earlier chapters dealing with the systems of measurement, some measures in one system have equivalents in another system; however, some equivalents are not exact measures, and there are discrepancies. Several tables illustrating equivalents/conversions are available in books and online. Sometimes pharmaceutical companies use different equivalents for a measurement.

In the health care system, nurses should be able to convert among the different systems of measurement. Nurses have become more involved in discharge planning and are responsible for ensuring that the patient can safely self-administer medications in the correct dosage. Table 6-1 lists some of the equivalents you may need to convert between systems.

Converting

The term *convert* means to change from one form to another. Converting can mean changing a unit of measurement to its equivalent in the same system or changing a measurement from one system to another system, which is called *converting between systems*. The measurement obtained when converting between systems is **approximate, not exact.** Thus, certain conversion factors have been established to ensure continuity.

One of the most important skills needed for calculating dosages is the ability to make conversions when necessary to administer the ordered amount of medication. Therefore, the nurse must understand the system of measurement and be able to convert within the same system and from one system to another with accuracy.

Before beginning the actual process of converting, the nurse should know the approximate equivalents presented in Table 6-1.

TABLE 6-1 Approximate Equivalents
1 tsp = 5 mL
1 tbsp = 3 tsp = 15 mL
1 oz = 30 mL (2 tbsp)
1 cup (measuring) = 8 oz (240 mL)
16 oz = 1 lb
2.2 lb = 1 kg (1 000 g)
1 in = 2.5 cm

POINTS TO REMEMBER

1. Think of equivalents/conversions as essential conversion factors, or as ratios.

   Example: 1 000 mg = 1 g is called a conversion factor.

   1 000 mg : 1 g is a ratio.

2. Follow basic math principles, regardless of the conversion method used.
3. Express answers applying the specific rules that relate to the system to which you are converting.

   Example: The metric system uses decimals; the household system uses fractions.

4. THINK CRITICALLY—select the appropriate equivalent to make conversions (see Table 6-1).

Methods of Converting
Moving the Decimal Point

Moving the decimal point is discussed in Chapter 5. Because the metric system is based on the decimal system, conversions within the metric system can be done easily by moving the decimal point. This method cannot be applied in the household system because decimal points are not often used in the system (with the exception of pounds [lb]). **Remember the following two rules for moving decimal points:**

RULE

To convert a smaller unit to a larger one in the metric system, divide or move the decimal point three places to the left.

Example:

$$350 \, \text{mg} = \underline{\hspace{1cm}} \text{g}$$
(smaller)   (larger)

Solution: After determining that milligrams (mg) is the smaller unit and that you are converting to the larger unit of grams (g), recall the conversion factor that allows you to change milligrams to grams (1 g = 1 000 mg). Therefore, 350 is divided by 1 000 by moving the decimal point three places to the left, indicating 350 mg = 0.35 g.

$$350 \, \text{mg} = .350 = 0.35 \, \text{g}$$

Note: The final answer is expressed in decimal form. Remember to always place a zero (0) in front of the decimal point to indicate a value that is less than 1.

RULE

To convert a larger unit to a smaller one in the metric system, multiply or move the decimal point three places to the right.

Example:

$$0.85 \, \text{L} = \underline{\hspace{1cm}} \text{mL}$$
(larger)   (smaller)

Solution: After determining that litre (L) is the larger unit and that you are converting to the smaller unit of millilitres (mL), recall the conversion factor that allows you to change litres to millilitres (1 L = 1 000 mL). Therefore, 0.85 is multiplied by 1 000 by moving the decimal point three places to the right, indicating 0.85 L = 850 mL.

$$0.850 \text{ L } = \ 0.850 \ = \ 850 \text{ mL}$$

Note the addition of a zero here to allow movement of the decimal point the correct number of places.

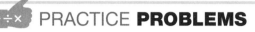 PRACTICE **PROBLEMS**

For additional practice in converting by decimal movement, convert the following metric measures to the equivalent units indicated.

1. 600 mL = _____ L

2. 0.016 g = _____ mg

3. 4 kg = _____ g

4. 3 mcg = _____ mg

5. 0.3 mg = _____ g

6. 0.01 kg = _____ g

7. 1.9 L = _____ mL

8. 0.5 g = _____ kg

9. 0.07 mg = _____ mcg

10. 650 mL = _____ L

11. 0.04 g = _____ mg

12. 0.12 g = _____ kg

13. 180 mg = _____ g

14. 1 700 mL = _____ L

15. 15 kg = _____ g

16. 3.5 g = _____ mg

17. 0.16 kg = _____ g

18. 0.004 L = _____ mL

19. 1 mL = _____ L

20. 8 mg = _____ g

21. 0.5 g = _____ mg

22. 300 g = _____ kg

23. 25 mg = _____ g

24. 65 kg = _____ g

25. 0.006 mg = _____ mcg

Answers on page 102.

Rather than remembering the right-to-left rule or left-to-right rule, you might find it easier to use ratio and proportion as a method of conversion.

Using Ratio and Proportion

Using ratio and proportion is one of the easiest ways to make conversions, whether within the same system or between systems. The basics on how to state ratios and proportions and how to solve them when looking for one unknown are presented in Chapter 3. To make conversions using ratio and proportion, a proportion that expresses a numerical relationship between the two systems must be set up. A proportion may be written in colon format or as a fraction when making conversions. Regardless of the format used, there are some basic rules to follow when using this method.

Rules for Ratio and Proportion

1. State the conversion first.
2. Add the incomplete ratio on the other side of the equals sign, making sure the units of measurement are written in the same sequence.

    Example: mg : g = mg : g

3. Label all terms in the proportion, including x. (These labels are not carried when multiplying or dividing.)
4. Solve the problem by using the rule for solving ratios and proportions (the product of the means equals the product of the extremes).
5. Label the final answer for x with the appropriate unit of measurement (i.e., the desired unit).

When using the method of ratio and proportion to make conversions, stating the proportion in the fraction format may be a way of avoiding confusion with the terms (means and extremes). However, regardless of the format used, the terms must correspond to each other in value and have a relationship. Division should always be carried at least two decimal places to ensure accuracy.

Example: 8 mg = ___ g

Solution: State the conversion factor first, then add the incomplete ratio, making sure the units are in the same sequence. Label all the terms in the proportion, including x.

$$1\,000\,\text{mg} : 1\,\text{g} \quad = \quad 8\,\text{mg} : x\,\text{g}$$
$$\text{(conversion factor)} \qquad \text{(unknown)}$$

Read as "1 000 mg is to 1 g as 8 mg is to x g."

Place the "x" product on the left side of the equation.

NOTE

The terms of the proportion are in the same sequence (mg : g = mg : g), and there is a correspondence in the ratio: small : large = small : large.

Result:

$$\begin{array}{c}\overbrace{\phantom{1\,000\,\text{mg} : 1\,\text{g}}}^{\text{means}}\\1\,000\,\text{mg} : 1\,\text{g} = 8\,\text{mg} : x\,\text{g}\\\underbrace{\phantom{1\,000\,\text{mg} : 1\,\text{g} = 8\,\text{mg}}}_{\text{extremes}}\end{array}$$

$$1 \times 8 = 1\,000 \times x$$
$$\frac{1\,000x}{1\,000} = \frac{8}{1\,000}$$
$$x = \frac{8}{1\,000}$$
$$x = 0.008\,\text{g}$$

Because the measurement you are converting to is metric, the fraction is changed to a decimal by dividing 8 by 1 000 to obtain an answer of 0.008 g. However, because the measures are metric in this example, perhaps moving the decimal point would be the preferred method as opposed to actual division.

Example: 8 mg = ___ g

1. Note that conversion is going from smaller to larger; thus, division or moving the decimal point to the left is indicated.

2. Note that the unit is going from milligrams to grams, thus changing by a factor of 1 000.

3. The decimal point will be moved three places to the left to complete this conversion: 8 mg = 0.008 g.

An alternate way of stating the same problem would be to express it as a fraction and cross-multiply to solve for x.

$$\frac{1\,000\text{ mg}}{1\text{ g}} \bowtie \frac{8\text{ mg}}{x\text{ g}}$$

$$1\,000x = 8$$

$$\frac{1\,000x}{1\,000} = \frac{8}{1\,000}$$

$$x = 0.008\text{ g}$$

Another way of writing a ratio and proportion to eliminate errors is to set up the conversion problem in a fraction format.

Place the conversion factor above (the numerator), and place the problem underneath, matching up the units (the denominator); then cross-multiply to solve for x.

Example: 8 mg = ___ g

$$\frac{1\,000\text{ mg}}{8\text{ mg}} \bowtie \frac{1\text{ g}}{x\text{ g}}$$

$$1\,000x = 8$$

$$\frac{1\,000x}{1\,000} = \frac{8}{1\,000}$$

$$x = 0.008\text{ g}$$

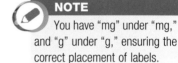

NOTE
You have "mg" under "mg," and "g" under "g," ensuring the correct placement of labels.

The remainder of this chapter will show examples of the methods used in converting within the same system and between systems.

Converting Within the Same System

Converting within the same system is often seen with metric measures. However, converting can be done using the household system of measurement; that is, one household measurement can be converted to an equivalent within the household system. Any one of the methods discussed can be used, but movement of decimal points is limited to the metric system. Ratio and proportion can be used for all systems.

Example: (metric)   (metric)
                 0.6 mg = ___ mcg

Solution: Conversion factor: 1 000 mcg = 1 mg

A milligram is larger than a microgram (mcg); the answer is obtained by moving the decimal point three places to the right (multiplying).

Answer: 600 mcg

Alternative: Set up the problem as a proportion, in fraction or colon format.

Example: (metric) (metric)
                 40 g = ___ kg

Solution: Conversion factor: 1 kg = 1 000 g

A gram is smaller than a kilogram (kg); the answer is obtained by moving the decimal three places to the left (dividing).

Answer: 0.04 kg (Note the placement of the zero before the decimal point.)

Alternative: Set up the problem using ratio and proportion, in fraction or colon format.

> The principles for solving ratio and proportion problems (see Chapter 3) can be applied to solving for *x* in a conversion problem that is presented in colon or fraction format.

Dimensional Analysis. Dimensional analysis is a conversion method that is used in chemistry and other sciences and will be discussed in more detail in Chapter 14. Dimensional analysis involves the manipulation of units to get the desired unit. This method can be used for conversion in all systems. As with other methods discussed, you must know the conversion factor.

Steps:
1. Identify the desired unit you are converting to.
2. Write the conversion factor in fraction format, so that the desired unit is in the numerator of the fraction. This is written first in the equation, followed by a multiplication sign (×). (Notice that the unit in the numerator is the same as the unit you desire.)
3. Write the unit in the successive numerator to match the unit of measurement in the previous denominator.
4. Cancel the alternate denominator/numerator units to leave the unit desired (being calculated).
5. Perform the mathematical process indicated.

Example: (metric)   (metric)

0.12 kg   to grams

Solution: You want to cancel the kilograms and obtain the equivalent amount in grams. Begin by identifying the unknown, in this case, grams. Because 1 kg = 1 000 g, the fraction that will allow you to cancel kilograms is $\dfrac{1\,000\,g}{1\,kg}$.

$$x\,g = \frac{1\,000\,g}{1\,kg} \times \frac{0.12\,kg}{1}$$

Note: The unit you want to cancel is always written in the denominator of the fraction. Then proceed by placing as the next numerator the same label as the first denominator, in this case, kg.

Note: Placing a 1 under a number does not change its value.

$$\text{Cancel the units } x\,g = \frac{1\,000\,g}{1\,\cancel{kg}} \times \frac{0.12\,\cancel{kg}}{1}$$

$$1\,000 \times 0.12 = 120\,g$$
$$x = 120\,g$$

Answer: 0.12 kg is equivalent to 120 g

PRACTICE **PROBLEMS**

Convert the following measures to the equivalent units indicated.

26. 500 mL = _____ L   27. 4 kg = _____ g

28. 1.4 L = _____ mL

29. 45 mL = _____ oz

30. 4.5 mg = _____ mcg

31. $3\frac{1}{2}$ oz = _____ mL

32. 6.5 L = _____ mL

33. 60 g = _____ kg

34. 600 mg = _____ g

35. 0.736 mg = _____ mcg

36. 1 600 mL = _____ L

37. 0.015 L = _____ mL

38. 0.18 g = _____ mg

39. 25 mcg = _____ mg

40. 5.2 g = _____ kg

Answers on page 102.

Converting between Systems

The methods presented previously can be used to convert a unit of measurement in one system to its equivalent in another, or the conversion factor method can be used. This method requires that you consider the size of units. To convert from a larger to a smaller unit of measurement, you multiply by the conversion factor (as shown in Example 1). To convert from a smaller to a larger unit of measurement, you divide by the conversion factor (as shown in Examples 2 and 3).

Example 1:

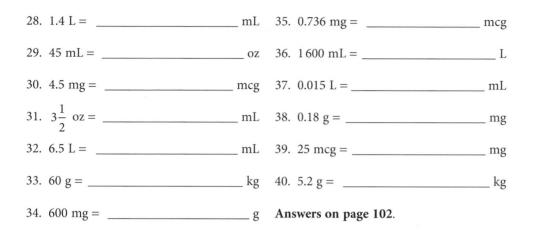

           (household) (metric)

          4 oz = ___ mL

          (large)   (small)

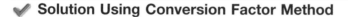

✔ Solution Using Conversion Factor Method

Conversion factor: 1 oz = 30 mL

An ounce (oz) is larger than a millilitre.

Multiply 4 by 30

Answer: 120 mL

Alternative: Express the conversion in proportion format and solve for x. (One way to remember this method is as the "known or have : want to know or have" method.)

✔ Solution Using Ratio and Proportion

$$1\,oz : 30\,mL = 4\,oz : x\,mL$$
$$x = 30 \times 4 = 120$$
$$x = 120\,mL$$
or
$$\frac{1\,oz}{30\,mL} = \frac{4\,oz}{x\,mL}$$
$$x = 4 \times 30 = 120$$
$$x = 120\,mL$$
or
$$\frac{1\,oz}{4\,oz} = \frac{30\,mL}{x\,mL}$$

✔ Solution Using Dimensional Analysis

Here you want to cancel ounces to find the equivalent amount in millilitres. Because $1 \text{ oz} = 30 \text{ mL}$, the fraction that will allow you to cancel ounces is $\dfrac{30 \text{ mL}}{1 \text{ oz}}$.

Therefore:
$$x \text{ mL} = \frac{30 \text{ mL}}{1 \text{ oz}} \times 4 \text{ oz}$$
$$x = 30 \times 4 = 120$$
$$x = 120 \text{ mL}$$

120 mL is equivalent to 4 oz

Example 2:   (household) (metric)
$$110 \text{ lb} = \underline{\quad} \text{ kg}$$

✔ Solution Using Conversion Factor Method

Conversion factor: $1 \text{ kg} = 2.2 \text{ lb}$

A pound is smaller than a kilogram.

Divide 110 by 2.2.

Answer: 50 kg

✔ Solution Using Ratio and Proportion

$$1 \text{ kg} : 2.2 \text{ lb} = x \text{ kg} : 110 \text{ lb}$$
$$\frac{2.2x}{2.2} = \frac{110}{2.2}$$
$$x = 50 \text{ kg}$$

or

$$\frac{1 \text{ kg}}{2.2 \text{ lb}} = \frac{x \text{ kg}}{110 \text{ lb}}$$

or

$$\frac{1 \text{ kg}}{x \text{ kg}} = \frac{2.2 \text{ lb}}{110 \text{ lb}}$$

✔ Solution Using Dimensional Analysis

Here you want to cancel pounds to find the equivalent amount in kilograms. Because $1 \text{ kg} = 2.2 \text{ lb}$, the fraction that will allow you to cancel pounds is $\dfrac{1 \text{ kg}}{2.2 \text{ lb}}$.

Therefore:
$$x \text{ kg} = \frac{1 \text{ kg}}{2.2 \text{ lb}} \times \frac{110 \text{ lb}}{1}$$
$$x = \frac{110}{2.2}$$
$$x = 50 \text{ kg}$$

Example 3:   (metric)   (household)
$$55 \text{ cm} = \underline{\quad} \text{ in}$$

✔ Solution Using Conversion Factor Method

Conversion factor: 1 in = 2.5 cm

A centimetre (cm) is smaller than an inch (in); divide 55 by 2.5.

Answer: 22 in

✔ Solution Using Ratio and Proportion

$$2.5 \text{ cm} : 1 \text{ in} = 55 \text{ cm} : x \text{ in}$$

$$\frac{2.5x}{2.5} = \frac{55}{2.5}$$

$$x = 22 \text{ in}$$

or

$$\frac{2.5 \text{ cm}}{2.5} = \frac{55 \text{ cm}}{x \text{ in}}$$

or

$$\frac{2.5 \text{ cm}}{55 \text{ cm}} = \frac{1 \text{ in}}{x \text{ in}}$$

✔ Solution Using Dimensional Analysis

Here you want to cancel centimetres to find the equivalent amount in inches. Because 2.5 cm = 1 in, the fraction that will allow you to cancel centimetres is $\dfrac{1 \text{ in}}{2.5 \text{ cm}}$.

Therefore:
$$x \text{ in} = \frac{1 \text{ in}}{2.5 \, \cancel{\text{cm}}} \times \frac{55 \, \cancel{\text{cm}}}{1}$$

$$x = \frac{55}{2.5}$$

$$x = 22 \text{ in}$$

22 in is equivalent to 55 cm

Calculating Intake and Output

The nurse often converts between systems to calculate a patient's **intake and output.** Intake and output is abbreviated as **I&O.** *Intake* refers to the monitoring of fluid a patient takes orally (PO), by feeding tube, or parenterally. Oral intake includes fluids and solids that become liquid at body and room temperature, such as gelatin and Popsicles. Intake also includes water, broth, and juice. Intake does not include solids, such as bread, cereal, or meats. Liquid *output* refers to fluids that exit the body, such as diarrhea, vomitus, gastric suction, and urine. A patient's intake and output are usually recorded on a special form called an intake and output flow sheet or record (or I&O flow sheet or record) (Figure 6-1), which varies from institution to institution. A variety of patients require I&O monitoring, such as those whose fluids are restricted and those who are receiving diuretic or intravenous (IV) therapy.

Intake and output is recorded in millilitres. The preferred term for volume is millilitres. Millilitres will be used throughout this text. When measuring output, the nurse uses a graduated receptacle calibrated in metric measures (mL), and conversions are not necessary. Oral intake usually must be converted from household measures to metric measures before it can be recorded. Each time a patient takes oral liquids, even those administered with medications, the amount and time are recorded on the appropriate form. The total intake and output are recorded at the end of each shift and also totalled for a 24-hour period.

				INTAKE			OUTPUT				
	ORAL			IV						OTHER	
TIME	TYPE	AMT	TIME	TYPE	AMOUNT ABSORBED	TIME	URINE	STOOL			
8A	Juice	60 mL									
	Coffee	120 mL									
	Milk	180 mL									

Juice glass   – 180 mL   Jello cup   – 150 mL
Water glass   – 210 mL   Ice cream   – 120 mL
Coffee cup   – 240 mL   Creamer   – 30 mL
Soup bowl   – 180 mL
Small water
   cup   – 120 mL

Date **October 30, 2016**

Addressograph with Client Information

Figure 6-1 Sample I&O flow sheet.

Conversion of a patient's intake is usually required when recording measurements such as a bowl or coffee cup. Each employer usually has an I&O flow sheet with a ledger that indicates the standard measurement for the utensils used in its facility. For example, it may indicate that a standard juice glass is 6 oz or that a coffee cup is 240 mL. A patient's oral intake is calculated in the same manner as other conversion problems. After each item is converted, the items are added together for the total intake. Intake and output are based on the conversion factor 1 oz = 30 mL.

Example: Calculate the patient's intake for breakfast in millilitres. Assume that the glass holds 6 oz and the cup holds 8 oz. The patient had the following for breakfast at 8:00 AM:

> **NOTE**
> Two sausages and one boiled egg are not part of fluid intake.

Items	Conversion Factors
$\frac{1}{3}$ glass of apple juice	1 oz = 30 mL
2 sausages	1 cup = 8 oz
1 boiled egg	1 glass = 6 oz
$\frac{1}{2}$ cup of coffee	
$\frac{3}{4}$ cup of milk	

Solution:

1. $\frac{1}{3}$ glass of apple juice

$$1\,\text{glass} = 6\,\text{oz}; \frac{1}{3} \text{ of } 6\,\text{oz} = 2\,\text{oz}$$

Therefore, 1 oz = 30 mL, 2 oz × 30 mL = 60 mL

✔ Solution Using Ratio and Proportion

1 oz : 30 mL = 2 oz : x mL, x = 60 mL

✔ Solution Using Dimensional Analysis

$$x\,\text{mL} = \frac{30\,\text{mL}}{1\,\cancel{\text{oz}}} \times \frac{2\,\cancel{\text{oz}}}{1}$$

2. $\frac{1}{2}$ cup of coffee

$$1\,\text{cup} = 8\,\text{oz}; \frac{1}{2} \text{ of } 8\,\text{oz} = 4\,\text{oz}$$

Therefore, 4 oz × 30 mL = 120 mL

✔ Solution Using Ratio and Proportion

1 oz : 30 mL = 4 oz : x mL, x = 120 mL

✔ Solution Using Dimensional Analysis

$$x\,\text{mL} = \frac{30\,\text{mL}}{1\,\cancel{\text{oz}}} \times \frac{4\,\cancel{\text{oz}}}{1}$$

3. $\frac{3}{4}$ cup of milk

$$1\,\text{cup} = 240\,\text{mL}; \frac{3}{4} \text{ of } 240\,\text{mL} = 180\,\text{mL}$$

4. Total mL = 60 mL + 120 mL + 180 mL = 360 mL

Another solution would be to total the number of ounces (6 oz in this example). Convert ounces to millilitres, and add the amount of milk (expressed in millilitres).

✔ Solution Using Ratio and Proportion

$$1\,\text{oz} : 30\,\text{mL} = 6\,\text{oz} : x\,\text{mL}$$
$$x = 180\,\text{mL}$$
$$180\,\text{mL} + 180\,\text{mL} = 360\,\text{mL}$$

✔ Solution Using Dimensional Analysis

$$x\,\text{mL} = \frac{30\,\text{mL}}{1\,\cancel{\text{oz}}} \times \frac{6\,\cancel{\text{oz}}}{1}$$

Juice glass	– 180 mL	Small water cup	– 120 mL
Water glass	– 210 mL	Jello cup	– 150 mL
Coffee cup	– 240 mL	Ice cream	– 120 mL
Soup bowl	– 180 mL	Creamer	– 30 mL

Client information

Date: _September 21, 2016_

INTAKE					OUTPUT				
Time	Type	Amt	Time	IV/ blood type	Amount absorbed	Time	Urine	Stool	Other
			7A	D5W 1000 mL	850 mL				
8 hr total					850 mL				
			3P	D5W 150 mL TBA					

Figure 6-2 Charting IV fluids on an I&O flow sheet. *TBA*, to be absorbed.

The conversions are recorded on an I&O flow sheet (or record) next to the time ingested. The I&O flow sheet in Figure 6-1 is filled out with the data for this sample problem:

8:00 AM   juice, 60 mL   coffee, 120 mL   milk, 250 mL

In addition to oral intake, if a patient is receiving IV therapy, the amount of IV fluid given is also recorded on the I&O flow sheet. When an IV bottle or bag is hung or added, the nurse indicates the time and the type and amount of fluid in the appropriate column on the flow sheet. When the IV fluid has infused or the IV is changed, the nurse records the actual amount of fluid **infused,** or **absorbed.**

In a situation in which a bag or bottle of IV fluid is not completed by the end of the shift, the nurse beginning the next shift is informed of how much fluid is left in the bag. At some institutions, the amount is also indicated on the I&O flow sheet with the abbreviation TBA (to be absorbed).

Example: The nurse hangs a 1 000-mL bag of D5W (dextrose 5% solution) at 7:00 AM. At 3:00 PM, 150 mL is left in the bag. The nurse records 850 mL was absorbed and indicates that 150 mL is TBA. Refer to the sample I&O flow sheet in Figure 6-2, which shows how this example is charted.

I&O flow sheets usually have a place for recording oral or by mouth (PO) intake and IV intake and a column or columns for output. Figure 6-3 shows a sample 24-hour I&O flow sheet illustrating the charting of intake and output.

The most commonly measured output is urine. After a patient's output is recorded in the I&O flow sheet, sometimes the nurse needs to compute an average. The most important average nurses compute in most health care settings is the hourly urine output. The **hourly** urine output for an adult to maintain proper renal function is 30 mL/h to 50 mL/h. Usually, the hourly amount is more significant than each voiding. To find the hourly average of urinary output, take the total and divide by the number of hours.

Juice glass   – 180 mL   Small water cup – 120 mL
Water glass – 210 mL   Jello cup   – 150 mL
Coffee cup   – 240 mL   Ice cream – 120 mL
Soup bowl   – 180 mL   Creamer   – 30 mL

Date: _September 21, 2016_

Client information

INTAKE					OUTPUT				
Time	Type	Amt	Time	IV/ blood type	Amount absorbed	Time	Urine	Stool	Other
8A	juice	240 mL	7A	D5W 1 000 mL	850 mL	8A	300 mL		
	milk	120 mL				10A	200 mL		
	coffee	200 mL				1³⁰/P	425 mL		
9³⁰/A	water	60 mL							
12P	broth	180 mL							
	juice	120 mL							
1P	water	120 mL							
8 hr total		1 040 mL			850 mL		925 mL		
5P	tea	100 mL	3P	TBA D5W 150 mL	150 mL	4p	425 mL		
	broth	360 mL	5P	D5W 1000 mL	750 mL	7p	350 mL		
	ice-cream	120 mL				9³⁰/P	200 mL		
9 P	water	240 mL							
8 hr total		820 mL			900 mL		975 mL		
1A	water	120 mL	11P	TBA D5W 250 mL	250 mL				
5A	tea	200 mL	3A	D5W 1000 mL	600 mL	2A	350 mL		
						5A	150 mL		
8 hr total		320 mL			850 mL		500 mL		
24 hr total		2 180 mL			2600 mL		2400 mL		

Total intake 24 hr: _(4 780 mL)_   (2 180 mL + 2 600 mL)

Total output 24 hr: _(2 400 mL)_   (925 mL + 975 mL + 500 mL)

Figure 6-3 I&O flow sheet (completed over 24 hours). *TBA*, to be absorbed.

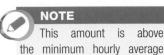

NOTE

This amount is above the minimum hourly average (30 mL/h) for adequate kidney function in the adult.

Example:

$$\frac{400 \text{ mL of urine}}{8 \text{ h}} = 50 \text{ mL of urine/h}$$

The charting of I&O varies at each institution. Always check the policies to ensure adherence with a particular institution.

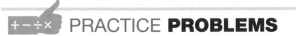 PRACTICE **PROBLEMS**

Convert the following amounts to the equivalent measures indicated.

41. 60 lb = _____ kg   47. 178.2 lb = _____ kg

42. 187.5 cm = _____ in   48. 20 mL = _____ tsp

43. 66 lb = _____ kg   49. 3 oz = _____ T

44. 7 oz = _____ mL   50. 72 kg = _____ lb

45. 45 mL = _____ tbsp   51. 3 in = _____ cm

46. 10 cm = _____ in   52. 2.4 L = _____ mL

Compute how much IV fluid you would document on an I&O flow sheet as being absorbed from a 1000-mL bag if the following amounts remain.

53. 300 mL _____   55. 100 mL _____

54. 450 mL _____

Compute the average hourly urinary output in the following situations (round your answer to the nearest whole number).

56. 650 mL in 8 h _____   58. 1000 mL in 24 h _____

57. 250 mL in 8 h _____   59. 1240 mL in 24 h _____

60. A patient's output for the 3:00 to 11:00 PM shift was as follows:

    325 mL of urine at 4:00 PM
     75 mL of vomitus at 7:00 PM
    225 mL of urine at 8:00 PM
    200 mL of nasogastric (NG) drainage at 11:00 PM
     50 mL of wound drainage at 11:00 PM
    What is the total output in mL? _____

61. What is the patient's output in L in question 60? _____

62. If 375 mL of a 500-mL bag of IV solution were absorbed on the 3:00 to 11:00 PM shift, the nurse records that 375 mL was absorbed. How many mL are recorded to be absorbed (TBA)? _____

Answers on page 102.

POINTS TO REMEMBER

- **Reduce** answers stated in fraction format as necessary.
- When more than one equivalent is learned for a unit, use the **most common equivalent** for the measurement or use the number that divides equally without a remainder.
- Carry out division to the hundredths place or two decimal places to ensure accuracy, and do not round the number.
- Use decimal point movement as a method for converting in the metric system; use ratio and proportion, dimensional analysis, and the conversion factor method for converting in all systems of measurement.
- Convert oral intake before placing data on an I&O flow sheet (or record). The amount is usually recorded in cubic centimetres at many institutions; however, millilitre is the correct unit for volume. Conversion factor for I&O is 1 oz = 30 mL.
- Always check the policy of the institution regarding I&O and the charting of it.
- Keep in mind that the most common units of measurement used to calculate dosages are metric units of measurement.

CHAPTER **REVIEW**

Convert the following amounts to the equivalent measures indicated.

1. 0.007 g = _____ mg

2. 1 mg = _____ g

3. 6 000 g = _____ kg

4. 5 mL = _____ L

5. 0.45 L = _____ mL

6. 75 mL = _____ oz

7. 1.8 mg = _____ mcg

8. 23 g = _____ kg

9. 6.5 mcg = _____ mg

10. 1 200 mL = _____ oz

11. 1.6 L = _____ mL

12. 47 kg = _____ lb

13. 3 mL = _____ L

14. 75 lb = _____ kg

15. 0.008 g = _____ mg

16. 0.25 mg = _____ mcg

17. 82 kg = _____ g

18. 6 172 g = _____ kg

19. 200 mL = _____ tsp

20. 102 lb = _____ kg

21. 204 g = _____ kg

22. 1.5 L = _____ mL

23. 200 mcg = _____ mg

24. 48.6 L = _____ mL

25. 0.7 L = _____ mL

26. $6\frac{1}{2}$ oz = _____ mL

27. 4 tsp = _____ mL

28. 1.8 mg = _____ g

29. 2 tbsp = _____ mL

30. 67.5 mL = _____ t

31. 66.25 cm = _____ in

32. 16 t = _____ mL

33. 20 oz = _____ mL

34. 16 mcg = _____ mg

35. 75 tsp = _____ mL

36. 255 mL = _____ oz

37. 4 kg = _____ lb   42. 4 g = _____ mg

38. 3.25 mg = _____ mcg   43. 36 mg = _____ g

39. 10 mL = _____ oz   44. 0.8 g = _____ mg

40. $9\frac{1}{2}$ oz = _____ tbsp   45. 142.5 mL = _____ tbsp

41. 6.653 g = _____ mg

Calculate the fluid intake in millilitres. Use the following conversion factors for the problems below: 1 cup = 8 oz, 1 glass = 6 oz.

46. A patient had the following at lunch:
    4 oz fruit cocktail
    1 tuna fish sandwich
    $\frac{1}{2}$ cup of tea
    $\frac{1}{2}$ glass of milk

    Total mL = _____

47. Calculate the following individual items and give the total number of millilitres:
    3 Popsicles (3 oz each)
    3 glasses of iced tea
    $1\frac{1}{2}$ glasses of water
    12 oz of soft drink

    Total mL = _____

48. A patient had the following:
    8 oz of milk
    6 oz of orange juice
    4 oz of water with medication

    Total mL = _____

49. A patient had the following:
    10 oz of coffee
    8 oz of water
    6 oz of vegetable broth

    Total mL = _____

50. A patient had the following:
    $\frac{3}{4}$ glass of milk
    4 oz of water
    2 oz of beef broth

    Total mL = _____

51. A patient had the following at lunch:
    $\frac{1}{4}$ glass of apple juice
    8 oz of chicken broth
    6 oz of gelatin dessert
    $1\frac{3}{4}$ cups of coffee

    Total mL = _____

Convert the following amounts of fluid to millilitres.

52. $3\frac{1}{2}$ oz = _____ mL   53. $\frac{3}{4}$ C (8 oz cup) = _____ mL

Compute how much IV fluid you would document on an I&O flow sheet as being absorbed from a 1 000-mL bag if the following amounts are left in the bag.

54. 275 mL _____   56. 75 mL _____

55. 550 mL _____

Compute the average hourly urinary output in each of the following situations (round your answer to the nearest whole number).

57. 500 mL in 8 h _____   59. 700 mL in 8 h _____

58. 640 mL in 24 h _____

Compute how much IV fluid you would document on an I&O flow sheet as being absorbed from a 500-mL bag if the following amounts are left in the bag.

60. 125 mL _____   61. 225 mL _____

62. A patient received 1 750 mL of IV fluid. How many L of IV fluid did the patient receive? _____

63. A patient has an order for 125 mcg of digoxin. How many mg will you administer to the patient? _____

64. The prescriber directs a patient to take 15 oz of the laxative agent GoLYTELY. The cup holds 6 oz. How many cups will the patient have to drink? _____

65. A patient has an order for 1 500 mL of water by mouth every 24 hours. How many oz is this? _____

66. A patient had an output of 1.1 L. How many mL is this? _____

67. The prescriber orders 2 oz of a liquid medication for a patient. How many tbsp should the patient take? _____ tbsp

68. A patient is given a prescription for 7.5 mL of a cough suppressant every 4 hours. The patient will be using a measuring device that is calibrated in tsp. How much medication should the patient take for each dose? _____ tsp

69. A patient weighed 95 kg on the initial visit to the clinic. When the patient reported for the subsequent visit the patient reported losing 11 lb. What is the patient's current weight in kg? _____ kg

70. An infant's head circumference is 45 cm. The parents ask for the equivalent in inches. You tell the parents their infant's head circumference is _____ in.

71. A patient drank 24 oz of water. How many cups did the patient drink? _____ cups

72. A patient needs to drink $1\frac{1}{2}$ oz of an elixir per day. How many tbsp would this be equivalent to? _____ tbsp

73. Calculate the total fluid intake in mL for 24 h.

Breakfast: 5 oz milk
　　　　　　2 oz orange juice
　　　　　　4 oz water with medication

Lunch: 12 oz ginger ale

Snack: 10 oz hot tea
　　　　　2 oz gelatin dessert

Dinner: 4 oz water
　　　　　6 oz apple juice
　　　　　3 oz chicken broth

Snack: 3 oz Jell-O
　　　　　8 oz iced tea
　　　　　6 oz water with medication

Total = _____ mL

Answers on page 102.

evolve

For additional practice problems, refer to the Drug Measures section of the Drug Calculations Companion, Version 5 on Evolve.

✳ ANSWERS

Answers to Practice Problems

1. 0.6 L
2. 16 mg
3. 4000 g
4. 0.003 mg
5. 0.0003 g
6. 10 g
7. 1900 mL
8. 0.0005 kg
9. 70 mcg
10. 0.65 L
11. 40 mg
12. 0.00012 kg
13. 0.18 g
14. 1.7 L
15. 15000 g
16. 3500 mg
17. 160 g
18. 4 mL
19. 0.001 L
20. 0.008 g
21. 500 mg
22. 0.3 kg
23. 0.025 g
24. 65000 g
25. 6 mcg
26. 0.5 L
27. 4000 g
28. 1400 mL
29. $1\frac{1}{2}$ oz
30. 4500 mcg
31. 105 mL
32. 6500 mL
33. 0.06 kg
34. 0.6 g
35. 736 mcg
36. 1.6 L
37. 15 mL
38. 180 mg
39. 0.025 mg
40. 0.0052 kg
41. 27.27 kg
42. 75 in
43. 30 kg
44. 210 mL
45. 3 tbsp
46. 4 in
47. 81 kg
48. 4 tsp
49. 6 T
50. 158.4 lb *or* $158\frac{2}{5}$ lb
51. 7.5 cm
52. 2400 mL
53. 700 mL
54. 550 mL
55. 900 mL
56. 81 mL/h
57. 31 mL/h
58. 42 mL/h
59. 52 mL/h
60. 875 mL
61. 0.875 L
62. 125 mL

Answers to Chapter Review

1. 7 mg
2. 0.001 g
3. 6 kg
4. 0.005 L
5. 450 mL
6. $2\frac{1}{2}$ oz
7. 1800 mcg
8. 0.023 kg
9. 0.0065 mg
10. 40 oz
11. 1600 mL
12. 103.4 lb, $103\frac{2}{5}$ lb
13. 0.003 L
14. 34.09 kg
15. 8 mg
16. 250 mcg
17. 82000 g
18. 6.172 kg
19. 40 tsp
20. 46.36 kg
21. 0.204 kg
22. 1500 mL
23. 0.2 mg
24. 48600 mL
25. 700 mL
26. 195 mL
27. 20 mL
28. 0.0018 g
29. 30 mL
30. $13\frac{1}{2}$ tsp
31. $26\frac{1}{2}$ in
32. 80 mL
33. 600 mL
34. 0.016 mg
35. 375 mL
36. $8\frac{1}{2}$ oz
37. 8.8 lb, $8\frac{4}{5}$ lb
38. 3250 mcg
39. $\frac{1}{3}$ oz
40. 19 T
41. 6653 mg
42. 4000 mg
43. 0.036 g
44. 800 mg
45. $9\frac{1}{2}$ T
46. 210 mL
47. 1440 mL
48. 540 mL
49. 720 mL
50. 315 mL
51. 885 mL
52. 105 mL
53. 180 mL
54. 725 mL
55. 450 mL
56. 925 mL
57. 63 mL/h
58. 27 mL/h
59. 88 mL/h
60. 375 mL
61. 275 mL
62. 1.75 L
63. 0.125 mg
64. $2\frac{1}{2}$ cups
65. 50 oz
66. 1100 mL
67. 4 tbsp
68. $1\frac{1}{2}$ tsp
69. 90 kg
70. 18 in
71. 3 cups
72. 3 tbsp
73. 1950 mL

CHAPTER 7

Additional Conversions Useful in the Health Care Setting

Objectives

After reviewing this chapter, you should be able to:

1. Convert between Celsius and Fahrenheit
2. Convert between units of length: inches, centimetres, and millimetres
3. Convert between units of weight: pounds and kilograms, pounds and ounces to kilograms
4. Convert between traditional and military (international) time

Converting between Celsius and Fahrenheit

In the Canadian health care environment, the Celsius scale is used when measuring a patient's temperature. Many electronic digital temperature thermometers instantly convert between the two scales. However, such devices do not eliminate the need for the nurse to understand the important difference between Celsius and Fahrenheit. Converting between the two scales is discussed in this chapter to enhance that understanding. Let us look first at some general information that will help you understand the formulas used.

Differentiating between Celsius and Fahrenheit

To differentiate which scale is being used (Fahrenheit or Celsius), the temperature reading is followed by an *F* indicating Fahrenheit, and *C* indicating Celsius. (*Note:* Celsius was formerly known as *centigrade.*)

Examples: 98°F

36°C

The freezing point of water on the Fahrenheit scale is **32°F**, and the boiling point is **212°F.** The freezing point of water on the Celsius scale is **0°C**, and the boiling point is **100°C.**

The difference between the freezing and boiling points on the Fahrenheit scale is **180°**, whereas the difference between these points on the Celsius scale is **100°.**

The differences between Fahrenheit and Celsius in relation to the freezing and boiling points led to the development of appropriate conversion formulas. Figure 7-1 shows two thermometers reflecting the relationship of pertinent values between the two scales. Figure 7-2 shows medically important Celsius and Fahrenheit temperature ranges.

The **32° difference** between the freezing point on the scales is used for converting temperature from one scale to the other. As mentioned above, there is a **180°** difference

103

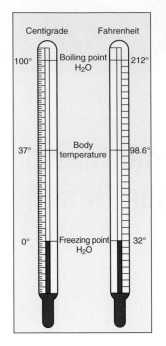

Figure 7-1 Celsius and Fahrenheit temperature scales. *Note:* The glass thermometers pictured here are for demonstration purposes only. Electronic digital temperature devices are more commonly used in health care settings. (From Clayton, B. D., & Willihnganz, M. (2013). *Basic pharmacology for nurses* (16th ed.). St. Louis: 2013, Mosby.)

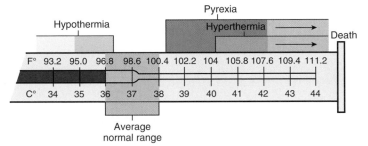
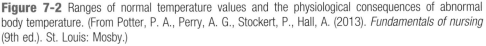

Figure 7-2 Ranges of normal temperature values and the physiological consequences of abnormal body temperature. (From Potter, P. A., Perry, A. G., Stockert, P., Hall, A. (2013). *Fundamentals of nursing* (9th ed.). St. Louis: Mosby.)

between the boiling and freezing points on the Fahrenheit thermometer and **100°** between the boiling and freezing points on the Celsius scale. These differences can be set as a ratio, 180 : 100. Therefore, consider the following:

$$180:100 = \frac{180}{100} = \frac{9}{5}$$

The fraction $\frac{9}{5}$ expressed as a decimal is 1.8; therefore, you will see this constant used in temperature conversions.

Formulas for Converting between Fahrenheit and Celsius Scales

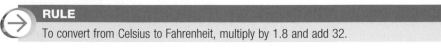

RULE

To convert from Celsius to Fahrenheit, multiply by 1.8 and add 32.

$$°F = 1.8(°C) + 32$$

or

$$°F = \frac{9}{5}(°C) + 32$$

NOTE
Your preference for one of these formulas is based on whether you find it easier to work with decimals or fractions.

Example: Convert 37.5°C to °F.

$$°F = 1.8(37.5) + 32 \qquad\qquad °F = \frac{9}{5}(37.5) + 32$$

$$°F = 67.5 + 32 \qquad or \qquad °F = 67.5 + 32$$

$$°F = 99.5° \qquad\qquad °F = 99.5°$$

RULE

To convert from Fahrenheit to Celsius, subtract 32 and divide by 1.8.

$$°C = \frac{°F - 32}{1.8} \qquad or \qquad °C = (°F - 32) \div \frac{9}{5}$$

Example: Convert 68°F to °C.

$$°C = \frac{68 - 32}{1.8} \qquad\qquad °C = (68 - 32) \div \frac{9}{5}$$

$$°C = \frac{36}{1.8} \qquad or \qquad °C = 36 \div \frac{9}{5}$$

$$°C = (36) \times \frac{5}{9}$$

$$°C = 20° \qquad\qquad °C = 20°$$

NOTE

When converting between Fahrenheit and Celsius, if necessary, carry the math process to hundredths and round to the nearest tenth.

PRACTICE **PROBLEMS**

Convert the following temperatures as indicated (round your answer to the nearest tenth).

1. 4°C = _____ °F   4. 101.3°F = _____ °C

2. 101°F = _____ °C   5. 37.5°C = _____ °F

3. 38.1°C = _____ °F

Change the given temperatures in the following statements to their corresponding equivalents in Celsius or Fahrenheit.

6. Store medication at room temperature: 20°C to 25°C. _____ °F

7. Notify health care provider for temperature greater than 101°F. _____ °C

8. Store vaccine serum at 7°F. _____ °C

9. Normal adult body temperature is 37°C. _____ °F

10. Do not store intravenous (IV) solutions at less than 46°F. _____ °C

Answers on page 115.

In addition to temperature conversions, other measures that may be encountered in the health care setting relate to linear measurement. As with temperature conversion, even though there are devices that instantly convert these measures, nurses need to understand the process. For the purpose of this chapter, we will focus on millimetres (mm) and centimetres (cm).

Converting Measures of Length

Metric measures of length are most commonly used in health care settings. The diameter of the pupil of the eye may be described in millimetres; the normal diameter of pupils is 3 to 7 mm. Charts may show pupillary size in millimetres. Accommodation of pupils is tested by asking a patient to gaze at a distant object (e.g., a far wall) and then at a test object (e.g., a finger or pencil) held by the examiner approximately 10 cm from the bridge of the patient's nose.

A baby's head and chest circumference are expressed in centimetres. Gauze for dressings is available in different size squares measured in centimetres and sometimes inches (in).

Example: 10×10 cm (4×4 in); 5×5 cm (2×2 in)

Also, incisions may be expressed in millimetres or centimetres (refer to the conversions in Box 7-1).

Now let us try some conversions of length.

Example 1: A patient's incision measures 25 mm. How many centimetres is this?

Conversion factor: 1 cm = 10 mm

Solution: Think: You are converting from a smaller unit (mm) to a larger unit (cm). Divide by 10, or move the decimal point one place to the left.

$$25 \div 10 = 2.5 \text{ cm } or\ 25. = 2.5 \text{ cm}$$

Answer: 2.5 cm

Example 2: Convert 30 cm to in.

Conversion factor: 1 in = 2.5 cm

Solution: Think: smaller to larger (divide).

$$30 \div 2.5 = 12 \text{ in}$$

Answer: 12 in

> **NOTE**
> In Example 2, you cannot get the answer by decimal movement. You are converting to inches, which is a household measurement.

Example 3: An infant's head circumference is 35.5 cm. How many millimetres is this?

Conversion factor: 1 cm = 10 mm

Solution: Think: You are converting from a larger unit (cm) to a smaller unit (mm). Multiply by 10, or move the decimal point one place to the right.

$$35.5 \times 10 = 355 \text{ mm } or\ 35.5 = 355 \text{ mm}$$

Answer: 355 mm

> **NOTE**
> Any of the methods presented in Chapter 6 may be used for conversion. Remember, however, that decimal movement is limited to conversions from one metric measurement to another, and the number of places the decimal is moved is based on the conversion factor. If necessary, review Chapter 6.

BOX 7-1   Conversions Relating to Length
1 cm = 10 mm
1 in = 2.54 cm*

*The approximate conversion of 1 in = 2.5 cm is used for conversions.

✋ PRACTICE **PROBLEMS**

Convert the following to the equivalent indicated.

11. A gauze pad for a dressing is

    10 cm _____ in

12. A patient's incision measures

    45 mm _____ cm

13. An infant's head circumference is

    37.5 cm _____ mm

14. A newborn's length is $20\frac{1}{2}$ in

    _____ cm

15. 14.8 in = _____ cm

16. 6.5 cm = _____ in

17. 100 in = _____ cm

18. An infant's chest circumference is

    32 cm _____ in

19. An infant's head circumference is

    38 cm _____ in

20. A newborn's length is 20 in

    _____ cm

Answers on page 115.

Converting between Units of Weight

Determination of body weight is important for calculating dosages in adults, children, and, because of the immaturity of their systems, even more so in infants and neonates. This chapter focuses on converting weights for adults and children. Medications such as heparin are more therapeutic when based on weight in kilograms (kg). The most frequently used calculation method for pediatric medication administration is milligrams (mg) per kilogram. Some medications are calculated in micrograms (mcg) per kilogram.

Because medication dosages in drug references are usually based on kilograms, it is essential to be able to convert from pounds (lb) to kilograms. However, the nurse also needs to know how to do the opposite (convert from kilograms to pounds). In addition, because a child's weight may be in pounds and ounces (oz), conversion of these units to kilograms is also important. Weight conversion is an important part of general nursing knowledge. The nurse must be able to explain conversions to others to determine and administer medication doses accurately and safely.

Converting Pounds to Kilograms

Conversion factor: 2.2 lb = 1 kg
To convert pounds to kilograms, divide by 2.2 (think smaller to larger).
The answer is rounded to the nearest tenth.

Example: A child weighs 65 lb. Convert to kilograms.

$$65 \div 2.2 = 29.54 = 29.5 \, kg$$

Example: An adult weighs 135 lb. Convert to kilograms.

$$135 \div 2.2 = 61.36 = 61.4 \, kg$$

Converting Pounds and Ounces to Kilograms

Step 1:   Convert the ounces to the nearest tenth of a pound, and **add** this to the total pounds.

           Conversion factor: 16 oz = 1 lb

Step 2:   Convert the total pounds to kilograms, and round to the nearest tenth.

Conversion factor: 2.2 lb = 1 kg

Example: A child's weight is 10 lb, 2 oz.

Think: smaller to larger.

2 oz ÷ 16 = 0.12 = 0.1 lb

10 lb + 0.1 lb = 10.1 lb

Think: smaller to larger.

10.1 ÷ 2.2 = 4.59 = 4.6 kg

Example: A child's weight is 7 lb, 4 oz.

4 oz ÷ 16 = 0.25 = 0.3 lb

7 lb + 0.3 lb = 7.3 lb

7.3 ÷ 2.2 = 3.31 = 3.3 kg

PRACTICE **PROBLEMS**

Convert the following weights to kilograms (round your answer to the nearest tenth).

21. 6 lb, 5 oz = _____ kg   23. 10 lb, 4 oz = _____ kg

22. 12 lb, 2 oz = _____ kg   24. 7 lb, 12 oz = _____ kg

Convert the following weights in pounds to kilograms (round your answer to the nearest tenth where indicated).

25. 20 lb = _____ kg   28. 121 lb = _____ kg

26. 64 lb = _____ kg   29. 85 lb = _____ kg

27. 22 lb = _____ kg   **Answers on page 115.**

Converting Kilograms to Pounds

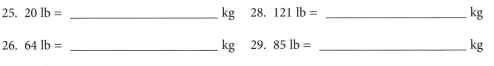

> **RULE**
>
> Conversion factor: 2.2 lb = 1 kg
> To convert kilograms to pounds, multiply by 2.2. (Think: larger to smaller.)
> The answer is rounded to the nearest tenth.

NOTE
Any of the methods presented in Chapter 6 for converting could also be used to convert from pounds to kilograms and kilograms to pounds, except for decimal movement.

Example: A child weighs 24.7 kg. Convert to pounds.

24.7 × 2.2 = 54.34 = 54.3 lb

Example: An adult weighs 72.2 kg. Convert to pounds.

72.2 × 2.2 = 158.84 = 158.8 lb

PRACTICE **PROBLEMS**

Convert the following weights in kilograms to pounds (round your answer to the nearest tenth where indicated).

30. 20 kg = _____ lb   33. 10.4 kg = _____ lb

31. 46 kg = _____ lb   34. 34.9 kg = _____ lb

32. 98.2 kg = _____ lb 35. 5.8 kg = _____ lb

Answers on page 115.

Converting between Traditional and Military (International) Time

The nurse must also know how to convert time on a traditional 12-hour clock to time on a 24-hour clock. The 24-hour clock is commonly referred to as **military time, international time,** or **24-hour time.** Although some watches are manufactured with traditional time and military time visible on the face of the watch to eliminate confusion, learning the conversion of time is the best method for avoiding errors.

The traditional 12-hour clock is a potential source for error in medication administration. On the traditional 12-hour clock, each time occurs twice a day. For example, the hour 7:00 is recorded as both 7:00 AM and 7:00 PM. The abbreviation "AM" means ante meridian, or before noon; "PM" means post meridian, or after noon. The times 7 AM and 7 PM may look very similar if the A and P are not clear; the patient could receive medication at the wrong time.

Military (international) time is a 24-hour clock (Figure 7-3). The main advantage of using military time is that it prevents errors in documentation and medication errors because numbers are not repeated. Each time occurs once per day. In military time, 7:00 AM is written as 0700, whereas 7:00 PM is written as 1900.

In military time, you write a four-digit number without the colon and AM and PM are omitted. The first two digits represent the hour; the last two digits, the minutes. The AM or PM notations are the only things that differentiate traditional time.

Military hours start at 1 AM or 0100 in the morning and end at 12 midnight, which is 0000 or 2400. The time 0000 is commonly used by the military and read as "zero hundred." 2400 is read as "twenty-four hundred." Although still referred to as military time, a more accurate term is "international time."

Many health care facilities use military (international) time in documentation such as nursing notes, medication administration records, and the documentation of treatments. Use of military (international) time prevents misinterpretation about when a therapeutic measure is due, such as medications, and is less problematic.

Rules for Converting to Military (International) Time

RULE

To convert AM time to military (international) time: omit the colon and AM and ensure that a four-digit number is written, adding a zero in the beginning as needed.

Example: 8:45 AM = 0845

RULE

To convert PM time to military (international) time: omit the colon and PM; add 1200 to the time.

Example: 7:50 PM = 750 + 1200 = 1950

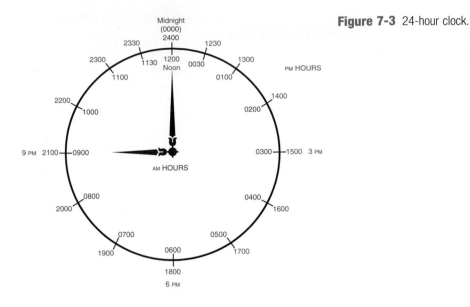

Figure 7-3 24-hour clock.

Rules for Converting to Traditional Time

> **RULE**
> To convert military (international) time to AM time: insert a colon, add AM, and delete any zero in front of the number.

Example: 0845 = 8:45 AM

> **RULE**
> To convert military (international) time to PM time: subtract 1200, insert a colon, and add PM.

Example: 1950 = 1950 − 1200 = 7:50 PM

＋－÷✕ PRACTICE **PROBLEMS**

Convert the following traditional times to military (international) time.

36. 7:30 AM = _____   41. 6:20 AM = _____

37. 10:30 AM = _____   42. 1:30 PM = _____

38. 8:10 PM = _____   43. 11:45 AM = _____

39. 5:45 PM = _____   44. 11:58 PM = _____

40. 12:16 AM = _____   45. 2:10 AM = _____

Convert the following military (international) times to traditional (AM/PM) time.

46. 0207 = _____   51. 0525 = _____

47. 1743 = _____   52. 1620 = _____

48. 0004 = _____   53. 1050 = _____

49. 0240 = _____   54. 1830 = _____

50. 1259 = _____   55. 1200 = _____

Answers on page 115.

Calculating Completion Times

As you will see in Chapter 20, the nurse can determine the time an IV bag will be completed or empty using military (international) time or traditional time (the time used depends on institutional policy). Now that we have discussed the conversion of time, we will briefly look at how the addition of times (traditional and military) can be used. This will be discussed in more detail in Chapter 20.

Military (International) Time Calculations

Example: An IV started at 0300 is to be completed in 3 h 30 min. Determine the completion time.

- Add the 3 h 30 min infusion time to the 0300 start time.

$$
\begin{array}{r}
0300 \\
+\ 330 \\
\hline
0630
\end{array}
$$

- The completion time is 0630.

Example: An IV started at 0650 is to be completed in 4 h 10 min. Determine the completion time.

- Add the 4 h 10 min infusion time to the 0650 start time.

$$
\begin{array}{r}
0650 \\
+\ 410 \\
\hline
1060
\end{array}
$$

- Change the 60 min in "1060" to 1 h, and add to 1000 to equal 1100.

Traditional Time Calculations

Example: An IV medication will infuse in 30 minutes. It is now 6:15 PM. Determine the completion time.

- Add the 30-min infusion time to the 6:15 PM start time.

$$6{:}15\ \text{PM} + 30\ \text{min} = 6{:}45\ \text{PM}$$

- The completion time is 6:45 PM.

Example: An IV with an infusion time of 12 h is started at 2:00 AM. Determine the completion time.

- Add the 12-h infusion time to the 2:00 AM start time.

$$
\begin{array}{r}
2{:}00\ \text{AM} \\
+\ 12{:}00 \\
\hline
14{:}00
\end{array}
$$

- Subtract 12 h to make the time 2:00 PM.

+−÷× PRACTICE **PROBLEMS**

Calculate the following completion times in military (international) time.

56. An IV started at 0215 will infuse in 2 h 30 min. _____

57. An IV started at 0250 will infuse in 5 h 10 min. _____

Calculate the following completion times in traditional time.

58. An IV started at 6:30 AM has an infusion time of 45 min. _____

59. An IV started at 9:00 AM has an infusion time of 6 h 30 min. _____

60. An IV started at 7:05 PM has an infusion time of 8 h. _____

Answers on page 115.

POINTS TO REMEMBER

Conversions Relating to Temperature

- Use the following formulas to convert between Fahrenheit and Celsius temperature:

  - To convert from °C to °F: $°F = 1.8(°C) + 32$ *or* $\frac{9}{5}(°C) + 32$.

  - To convert from °F to °C: $°C = \frac{°F - 32}{1.8}$ *or* $(°F - 32) \div \frac{9}{5}$.

- When converting between Fahrenheit and Celsius, carry the math process to hundredths and round to the nearest tenth.

Conversions Relating to Length

- To convert from one length to another, use any of the methods presented in Chapter 6; however, use decimal movement only when converting between metric measures.

$$1\,cm = 10\,mm$$
$$1\,in = 2.5\,cm$$

Conversions Relating to Weight

$$2.2\,lb = 1\,kg$$
$$16\,oz = 1\,lb$$

- Note that weight conversion of pounds to kilograms is done most often because many medications are based on kilograms of body weight.
- Note that body weight is **essential** for determining dosages in infants and neonates.
- To convert pounds to kilograms, divide by 2.2. Round the answer to the nearest tenth.
- To convert pounds and ounces to kilograms, convert the ounces to the nearest tenth of a pound; add this number to the total pounds. Convert the total pounds to kilograms and round the answer to the nearest tenth.
- To convert kilograms to pounds, multiply by 2.2. Round the answer to the nearest tenth.

Conversions Relating to Time

- Note that the 24-hour clock is also referred to as *military time*, *international time*, or *24-hour time*.
- To convert AM time to military (international) time: omit the colon and AM and ensure that a four-digit number is written, adding a zero in the beginning as needed.
- To convert PM time to military (international) time: omit the colon and PM, and add 1200 to the time.
- To convert military (international) time to AM time: insert a colon and add AM, and delete any zero in front of the number.
- To convert military (international) time to PM time: subtract 1200, insert a colon, and add PM.
- Note that use of military (international) time decreases the possibility of errors in administering medications and the possibility of misinterpreting when a therapy is due or actually was done because no two times are expressed by the same number.

CHAPTER **REVIEW**

For each of the following statements, change the given temperature to its corresponding equivalent in Celsius or Fahrenheit (round your answer to the nearest tenth).

1. Notify health care provider for temperature greater than 101.4°F. _____ °C

2. Store medication at room temperature, 77°F. _____ °C

3. Store medication within temperature range of 15°C to 30°C. _____ °F

4. An infant has a body temperature of 36.5°C. _____ °F

5. Store vaccine at 6°C. _____ °F

6. A nurse reports a temperature of 37.8°C. _____ °F

7. Do not expose a medication to temperatures greater than 84°F. _____ °C

8. A medication contains a crystalline substance with a melting point of about 186°C.

   _____ °F

9. Store vaccine at 4°C. _____ °F

10. Do not expose medication to temperatures greater than 88°F. _____ °C

Convert temperatures as indicated (round your answer to the nearest tenth).

11. −10°C = _____ °F   18. 64.4°F = _____ °C

12. 0°F = _____ °C   19. 35°C = _____ °F

13. 102.8°F = _____ °C   20. 50°F = _____ °C

14. 29°C = _____ °F   21. 39.8°C = _____ °F

15. 106°C = _____ °F   22. 86°F = _____ °C

16. 70°F = _____ °C   23. 41°C = _____ °F

17. 39.6°C = _____ °F

Convert the following to the equivalent indicated.

24. 18 in = _____ cm   30. 4 in = _____ cm

25. 31 cm = _____ in   31. 36.6 cm = _____ mm

26. 44.5 cm = _____ mm   32. 6.2 in = _____ cm

27. 32 in = _____ cm   33. 350 mm = _____ in

28. 3 cm = _____ mm   34. $21\frac{1}{2}$ in = _____ cm

29. 7.9 cm = _____ mm   35. 2 in = _____ mm

Convert the following weights in pounds to kilograms (round your answer to the nearest tenth where indicated).

36. 63 lb = _____ kg   39. 81 lb = _____ kg

37. 150 lb = _____ kg   40. 27 lb = _____ kg

38. 78 lb = _____ kg

Convert the following weights in kg to lb (round your answer to the nearest tenth).

41. 77.3 kg = _____ lb   44. 9 kg = _____ lb

42. 7 kg = _____ lb   45. 56.1 kg = _____ lb

43. 4.5 kg = _____ lb

46. A child weighs 70 lb during a pediatric clinic visit. How many kg does the child weigh? (Round your answer to the nearest tenth.) _____

47. A patient's wound measures 41 mm. How many cm is the wound? _____ cm

48. A patient weighs 99.2 kg. How many lb does the patient weigh? (Round your answer to the nearest tenth.) _____ lb

49. An infant's head circumference is 40 cm. How many inches is the circumference? _____ in

50. An infant's head circumference is 40.6 cm. How many mm is the circumference? _____ mm

Convert the following weights to kg. (Round your answer to the nearest tenth.)

51. 7 lb, 1 oz = _____ kg   54. 8 lb, 10 oz = _____ kg

52. 9 lb, 3 oz = _____ kg   55. 5 lb, 5 oz = _____ kg

53. 10 lb, 12 oz = _____ kg

Convert the following military (international) times to traditional times (AM/PM).

56. 0032 = _____   59. 1345 = _____

57. 0220 = _____   60. 2122 = _____

58. 1650 = _____

Convert the following traditional times to military (international) times.

61. 5:20 AM = _____   64. 4:30 PM = _____

62. 12:00 midnight = _____   65. 1:35 PM = _____

63. 12:05 AM = _____

State whether AM or PM is represented by the following times.

66. 0154 _____

67. 1450 _____

68. If a patient had IV therapy for 8 h, ending at 1100, when on the 24-h clock was the IV

   started? _____

State the following completion times as indicated.

69. An IV started at 11:50 PM with an infusion time of 3 h 30 min _____
   (traditional time).

70. An IV started at 0025 with an infusion time of 1 h 15 min _____ (military
   [international] time).

Answers on page 116.

ANSWERS

Answers to Practice Problems

1. 39.2°F	13. 375 mm	25. 9.1 kg	37. 1030	49. 2:40 AM
2. 38.3°C	14. 51.25 cm	26. 29.1 kg	38. 2010	50. 12:59 PM
3. 100.6°F	15. 37 cm	27. 10 kg	39. 1745	51. 5:25 AM
4. 38.5°C	16. 2.6 in	28. 55 kg	40. 0016	52. 4:20 PM
5. 99.5°F	17. 250 cm	29. 38.6 kg	41. 0620	53. 10:50 AM
6. 68°F to 77°F	18. 12.8 in	30. 44 lb	42. 1330	54. 6:30 PM
7. 38.3°C	19. 15.2 in	31. 101.2 lb	43. 1145	55. 12:00 PM (noon)
8. −13.9°C	20. 50 cm	32. 216 lb	44. 2358	56. 0445
9. 98.6°F	21. 2.9 kg	33. 22.9 lb	45. 0210	57. 0800
10. 7.8°C	22. 5.5 kg	34. 76.8 lb	46. 2:07 AM	58. 7:15 AM
11. 4 in	23. 4.7 kg	35. 12.8 lb	47. 5:43 PM	59. 3:30 PM
12. 4.5 cm	24. 3.5 kg	36. 0730	48. 12:04 AM	60. 3:05 AM

---

evolve

For additional information, refer to the Drug Measures section of the Drug Calculations Companion,
Version 5 on Evolve.

Answers to Chapter Review

1. 38.6°C
2. 25°C
3. 59°F to 86°F
4. 97.7°F
5. 42.8°F
6. 100°F
7. 28.9°C
8. 366.8°F
9. 39.2°F
10. 31.1°C
11. 14°F
12. −17.8°C
13. 39.3°C
14. 84.2°F
15. 222.8°F

16. 21.1°C
17. 103.3°F
18. 18°C
19. 95°F
20. 10°C
21. 103.6°F
22. 30°C
23. 105.8°F
24. 45 cm
25. 12.4 in
26. 445 mm
27. 80 cm
28. 30 mm
29. 79 mm
30. 10 cm

31. 366 mm
32. 15.5 cm
33. 14 in
34. 53.75 cm
35. 50 mm
36. 28.6 kg
37. 68.2 kg
38. 35.5 kg
39. 36.8 kg
40. 12.3 kg
41. 170.1 lb
42. 15.4 lb
43. 9.9 lb
44. 19.8 lb
45. 123.4 lb

46. 31.8 kg
47. 4.1 cm
48. 218.2 lb
49. 16 in
50. 406 mm
51. 3.2 kg
52. 4.2 kg
53. 4.9 kg
54. 3.9 kg
55. 2.4 kg
56. 12:32 AM
57. 2:20 AM
58. 4:50 PM
59. 1:45 PM
60. 9:22 PM

61. 0520
62. 2400 (0000 used in military)
63. 0005
64. 1630
65. 1335
66. AM
67. PM
68. 0300
69. 3:20 AM
70. 0140

UNIT THREE

Methods of Administration and Calculation

Note: The safe and accurate administration of medications to a patient is an important and a primary responsibility of a nurse. Being able to read and interpret an order correctly and calculate medication dosages is necessary for accurate administration.

CHAPTER 8
Medication Administration

Objectives

After reviewing this chapter, you should be able to:

1. State the consequences of medication errors
2. Identify the causes of medication errors
3. Identify the role of the nurse in preventing medication errors
4. Identify the different organizations involved in the prevention of medication errors in Canada
5. Define *critical thinking*
6. Explain the importance of critical thinking in medication administration
7. Identify important critical thinking skills necessary in medication administration
8. Identify factors that influence medication dosages
9. Identify special considerations relating to the older adult and medication administration
10. Discuss the importance of patient teaching
11. State 15 rights of medication administration
12. Identify the common routes for medication administration

Medication Errors

Medications are therapeutic measures aimed at improving a patient's health. Medication administration is a basic nursing skill, but it is one of the most critical functions of nursing practice. All medication dosages must be prepared, dispensed, and administered safely (Cohen, 2010; Institute of Safe Medication Practices Canada [ISMP Canada], 2000–2016). According to Health Canada (2015), patient safety is a significant concern and challenge facing health care systems worldwide today. Health Canada (2015) also reports that medication safety is a significant part of patient safety and that the leading cause of patient injury globally is medication incidents. As the federal regulator for the pharmaceutical industry through the *Food and Drugs Act* and *Food and Drug Regulations,* Health Canada has a key role to play in managing and preventing medication incidents. Medication safety requires a collaborative approach among all health care stakeholders, including patients (whose safety is the primary focus for all health care providers). The critical role that nurses play in medication safety is a primary focus of this text and is based on the knowledge and understanding of careful, correct, and safe medication administration.

When medication errors occur, they can result in grave consequences for patients and legal repercussions for the nurses involved. Outcomes for the patient may include increased hospital stay, acute or chronic disability, and even death. Ramifications for the nurse may include job loss, licence revocation, or even criminal charges. Safety in medication administration involves more than calculating dosages and verifying the "rights" of medication administration. In the abridged edition of *Medication Errors,* Cohen (2010, p. 3) states that "even when practitioners believe they have verified these 'rights,' errors, including fatal ones, occur."

The number of preventable medication errors that take place each year is astonishing. For example, the Institute of Medicine (IOM) (2006) estimated that at least 400 000 medication errors a year, resulting in $3.5 billion in annual costs, occur in U.S. hospitals and could have been prevented. Cohen (2010) identifies reasons for increased risks of error, including a lack of pediatric formulations, dosage forms, and guidelines; confusion between adult and pediatric formulations; confusion among concentrations of oral liquids; calculation errors; and errors with measuring devices. Safety involving pediatric dosages will be discussed in more detail in Chapter 22. Box 8-1 presents the websites for several organizations actively involved in reporting, sharing, and learning about medication incidents in order to reduce their reoccurrence and help create a safer health care system.

BOX 8-1   Websites for Some Organizations Involved in Patient Safety

Canadian Medication Incident Reporting and Prevention System (CMIRPS): http://www.cmirps-scdpim.ca
Institute for Safe Medication Practices Canada (ISMP Canada): https://www.ismp-canada.org
Canadian Patient Safety Institute (CPSI): http://www.patientsafetyinstitute.ca
Health Canada: http://www.hc-sc.gc.ca
Canadian Institute for Health Information (CIHI): https://www.cihi.ca

---

Accreditation Canada (2013) also supports patient safety. This independent, nonprofit organization has been improving health quality through accreditation of health care facilities, community health programs, provincial health authorities, and health care systems. Through its standards and accreditation programs, Accreditation Canada works with health care organizations to help them improve quality, safety, and efficiency so that they can offer optimum care and service, including the prevention of medication errors. Accreditation Canada, the Canadian Institute for Health Information (CIHI), the Canadian Patient Safety Institute (CPSI), and the Institute for Safe Medication Practices Canada (2012) produced the report *Medication Reconciliation in Canada: Raising the Bar—Progress to Date and the Course Ahead.* The intent of medication reconciliation is to prevent medication errors at transition points in patient care, and this joint report underscores the need for vigilance to prevent patient harm as a result of medication errors.

In an effort to increase medication safety, ISMP Canada and the CPSI headed a national collaboration to implement standardized bar codes on pharmaceutical products that have been approved for use in Canada (ISMP Canada, 2013b). Bar codes are used with a barcode–scanning system and a computerized database. The bar code must contain the drug identification number (DIN). Hospitals have bar-code scanners that are linked to a hospital's electronic medical records. The bar coding allows the health care provider to scan the patient's bar code prior to administering medications, which allows access to the patient's medication record. Each medication is scanned prior to administration to the patient, letting the computer know what medication is being administered. The information is then compared with the patient's database and alerts the health care provider if there is a problem requiring investigation.

Bar-code technology has reduced the frequency of certain medication errors. However, this computer technology cannot replace human intellect or negate the need to follow various steps in medication administration to ensure patient safety.

Medication errors can occur anywhere in the distribution process, and when an error occurs, the cause can involve multiple factors, including dosage calculation mistakes, miscommunication of medication orders, errors in computer order entry, and multiple distractions during medication administration.

! SAFETY ALERT!

Focus solely on the task at hand, medication administration (when the actual act of medication administration occurs). Distractions can result in error during medication administration, jeopardize the patient's safety, and may cause harm.

Certain medications, referred to as *high-alert medications,* have also been identified as contributing to harmful errors. The medications on this list include concentrated electrolyte solutions, such as potassium chloride. Other medications that are associated with harmful errors include heparin, insulin, morphine, neuromuscular medications, and chemotherapy medications. Although advances in technology such as automatic dispensing cabinets (ADC), computerized provider order entry (CPOE), and bar-code medication administration have decreased the number of medication errors, these advances are useful *only* if they are properly applied and if the systems are effective and efficient.

The reasons for medication errors are not limited to those presented here and are not necessarily nursing errors alone. However, the nurse is accountable for being knowledgeable about the action, uses, adverse effects, expected response, contraindications, and range of dosage for the medication being administered.

> **SAFETY ALERT!**
> Failure to think about what you are doing and why you are doing it and failure to assess a patient can result in errors. You are accountable for your actions.

Critical Thinking and Medication Administration

Critical thinking has numerous definitions. The best way to define *critical thinking* is as a process of thinking that includes being reasonable and rational. Thinking is based on reason. Critical thinking is important in all phases of nursing, but it is particularly important to the discussion of medication administration. Critical thinking is necessary to the development of clinical reasoning skills and clinical judgment. Critical thinking encompasses several skills relevant to medication administration. One such skill is the ability to identify an organized approach to the task at hand. For example, in medication administration, calculating dosages in an organized, systematic manner (e.g., formula, ratio and proportion, dimensional analysis) decreases the likelihood of errors.

A second skill of critical thinking is the ability to be an autonomous thinker—for example, challenging a medication order that is written incorrectly rather than passively accepting the order. Critical thinking also involves the ability to distinguish irrelevant from relevant information. For example, when reading a medication label, the nurse is able to decipher from the label the information necessary for calculating the correct dosage. Critical thinking involves reasoning and the application of concepts—for example, choosing the correct type of syringe to administer a dose, and using concepts learned to decide the appropriateness of a dose. Critical thinking also involves asking for clarification of what is not understood and not making assumptions. Clarifying a medication order and dosage indicates critical thinking. Checking the accuracy and reliability of information decreases the chance of medication errors. The ability to validate information requires a high level of thinking and decreases the chance of medication errors that could be harmful to the patient.

Critical thinking is essential to the safe administration of medications. This process allows a nurse to think before doing, translate knowledge into practice, and make appropriate judgments. To safely administer medication, the nurse must base decisions on rational thinking and thorough knowledge of medication administration. Proper medication administration involves evaluation of the patient and the medication's effects, both of which require critical thinking and skills of assessment. A nurse who administers medication in a routine manner, rather than with thought and reasoning, is not using critical thinking skills.

> **TIPS FOR CLINICAL PRACTICE**
> Remember that the nurse who administers a medication is accountable for any medication error, regardless of the reason for the error.

Factors That Influence Medication Dosages and Action

Several factors influence medication dosages and the way they act, including the following:
- Route of administration
- Time of administration
- Age of the patient

- Nutritional status of the patient
- Absorption and excretion of the medication
- Health status of the patient
- Gender of the patient
- Ethnicity and culture of the patient
- Genetics

All of these factors affect pharmacokinetics, so the nurse must be cognizant of the patient's overall medical condition in order to evaluate medication therapeutic effectiveness.

Special Considerations for Older Adults

The older adult (age 65 and older) population can be considered high-risk medication consumers. Approximately two thirds of older adults use both prescription and nonprescription medications, and one third of all prescriptions are written for older adults. With the number of individuals over the age of 65 rapidly increasing, the use of medications in this age group will also increase. According to Statistics Canada (2014), on July 1, 2014, 15.7% of Canada's population (nearly one in six Canadians) was age 65 and older. The most recent population projections estimate that by 2016, the number of older adults will be greater than children under 15 years of age. In addition, in the next 50 years, the number of older adults will be between 24 and 28% of the entire Canadian population.

People are now living longer, and older adults tend to use health care services more often. Special consideration should be given to patients who are over 65 years of age. With the aging process come physiological changes that have a direct effect on medications and their action in older adults. Aging causes the slowing down of the body's functions. Other physiological changes include a decrease in circulation, slower absorption, a slower metabolism, a decrease in excretory functions, and a decrease in the ability to respond to stress such as the stress of medications on the system. Other changes with aging may include a decrease in body weight, which can affect the dosage of medications, and changes in mental status, possibly caused by the effects of physical illness or physiological changes in the neurological system that can occur with aging. These physiological changes can cause unexpected medication reactions and make older adults more sensitive to the effects of many medications.

The growing older adult population consumes more medication than any other age group. This amounts to approximately 20 to 40% of all prescription medications and over 40% of over the counter (OTC) medications (Lilley, Harrington, Snyder et al., 2011). An estimated 25 to 30% of hospital admissions of older patients are linked to medication-related problems. Because older adults are often taking more than one medication concurrently (referred to as *polypharmacy*), problems such as medication interactions, severe adverse reactions, medication and food interactions, and an increase in medication errors occur. As the older adult population continues to increase, so too will the need to focus on reducing medication errors in this group.

As a rule, older adult patients require smaller dosages of medications (as dosage size increases, the number of adverse effects and their severity increase), and the dosages should be given farther apart to prevent accumulation of medications and toxic effects.

With aging, visual and hearing problems may develop. Special attention must be given when teaching patients about their medications to help prevent medication errors. Develop a relationship with the patient; building rapport and trust is important for older adults. Take time and talk to these patients, listen to what they have to say, and never assume that they do not know how much or what medications they are taking. Ascertain that all instructions are written as clearly as possible, choosing fonts that are friendly to older eyes. Make sure the patient has appropriate measuring devices to facilitate ease and accuracy when measuring (e.g., a dropper or measuring cup with calibrated lines to indicate small doses [0.2 mg, 0.4 mg, etc.]). To lessen the chance of taking too much medication or forgetting a dosage, try to establish specific times compatible with the patient's routine for taking medications.

Omission of medications is a common cause of error for older adults at home. This omission may be due to the cost of medication or due to forgetfulness. Establishing medication times when possible to coincide with the patient's routine, and engaging a family member or friend if possible in the teaching process may help in preventing omission of medications. Help the patient recognize tablets by the name on the bottle, not by tablet colour. If the print on medications is too small for the patient to read, encourage the use of a magnifying glass. Other measures might include providing a simple chart that outlines the medications to be taken, the times they are to be taken, and special instructions if needed. Such a chart should be geared to the patient's visual ability and comprehension level. Encourage the older adult patient to request that childproof containers not be used for their prescription medications; some older adults have difficulty opening child-resistant containers. Recommend medication aids for the patient, such as special medication containers divided into separate compartments for storing daily or weekly medication dosages. (Figure 8-1 shows examples of medication containers.)

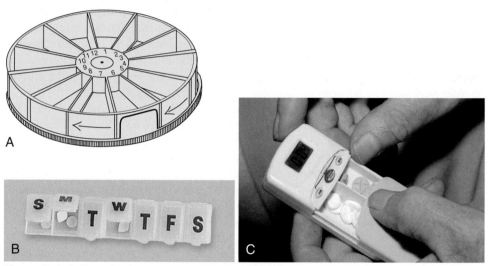

Figure 8-1 A, Example of a container that holds a day's medications, stored by hour of administration. **B,** Container that holds a week's medications. **C,** A pill timer beeps, flashes, and automatically resets every time it is closed. (**A,** From Ogden, S. G., & Floharty, L. K. (2012). *Calculation of drug dosages* (9th ed.). St. Louis: Mosby. **B,** From Perry, A. G., Potter P. A., & Elkin, M. K. (2012). *Nursing interventions and clinical skills* (5th ed.). St. Louis: Mosby. **C,** © Stefan Sollfors / Alamy Stock Photo.)

The Rights of Medication Administration

The **rights** of medication administration are a set of safety checks that serve as guidelines for the practising nurse to follow when administering medications to prevent errors and ensure patient safety. From the various publications that include "the rights" of medication administration, it is clear that there is no universal set number of rights that is conclusive. Historically, most nursing governing bodies followed five basic rights as guidelines or standards of nursing practice: the right medication, the right dose, the right patient, the right route, and the right time. Today, the literature varies on the number of rights, but up to 15 are documented. They are listed in Box 8-2 (in no particular order).

BOX 8-2	The Rights of Medication Administration
1. The right medication	9. The right documentation
2. The right dose	10. The right education
3. The right patient	11. The right technique
4. The right route	12. The right approach
5. The right time	13. The right assessment
6. The right frequency	14. The right evaluation
7. The right site	15. The right to refuse
8. The right reason	

Some of these rights overlap. It may be argued, for example, that **frequency** involves **time** or that **site** is a part of **route**, or even that **assessment** is similar to **reason.** So, the language used in naming a particular right depends on the choice of the author or publisher. In Canada, all nursing regulatory bodies that publish medication *rights* maintain the traditional five rights and add a variation of the others. For example, the College of Registered Nurses of British Columbia (n.d.) **practice standards** of medication administration include seven rights that a nurse should adhere to when administering medications: right medication, right patient, right dose, right time, right route, right reason, and right documentation. Similarly, the College of Registered Nurses of Nova Scotia (2015) establishes 10 rights of medication administration that include the traditional five along with right reason/assessment, right education, right evaluation, right documentation, and right to refuse (p. 13).

The College of Nurses of Ontario (CNO) revised its 2014 medication standard, which was founded on eight rights, to a new **principle-based medication practice standard.** In the CNO (2015) medication practice standard, three principles outline the expectations of nurses in relation to medication practices that promote safe and ethical nursing care: **authority, competence,** and **safety.** First, nurses must have the necessary **authority** to administer medication. Authority is governed by the regulatory body, legislation, and the practice setting. If authorized, nurses are accountable and responsible for ensuring that medication orders are clear, complete, and appropriate for patients. Second, nurses must have the knowledge, skill, and judgment needed to administer medication safely and that their medication practices are evidenced informed. Third, nurses promote safe care and contribute to a culture of safety within their practice environment when administering medication. Safety expectations involve patient education, patient advocacy, and health team collaboration to enhance patient safety in medication practices. Essentially, the CNO medication practice standard requires nurses to incorporate all nursing standards and guidelines as well as evidenced-informed practice and critical inquiry in their medication practices. In this model, the rights of medication administration are not listed as a separate entity because they are considered to be part of the principles of competency and safety.

Since most nursing organizations and nursing literature use the rights of medication administration (see Box 8-2) as guidelines, we discuss those rights in detail below. Safe and competent medication practice requires using the rights of medication administration as established by the provincial governing body for nursing practice. Omission of one or more of these rights in the medication administration process may result in a medication error.

1. **The right medication**—When medications are ordered, the nurse should compare the medication administration record (MAR) or computer record with the actual order. When administering medications, the nurse should check the label on the medication container against the order. Medications should be checked three times: before preparing, after preparing, and before replacing the container. With unit doses (i.e., each medication dose is prepared in the prescribed dose, packaged, labelled, and ready to use), the label should still be checked three times. Remember, regardless of the medication distribution system, the medication label should be checked three times. Errors frequently occur because of similarity in medication names and similar packaging.

   According to Health Canada (2015) poorly designed health product names, labels, and packages can contribute to or cause medication incidents. For example, look-alike and sound-alike (LA/SA) health product names (products whose names share similar spellings or pronunciations or both) have been known to increase the risk of product "mix-ups." Health Canada endorses the "ISMP's List of Confused Drug Names," which is issued by the Institute for Safe Medication Practices (ISMP, 2015), in the United States. The list can be found at http://www.ismp.org/tools/confuseddrugnames.pdf.

   ISMP (2011a) suggests using "Tall Man" lettering to alert health care providers to the potential for error with look-alike names. In this approach, a medication name includes mixed case or enlarged, bolded, or italic letters to distinguish the differing portion of its name from similarly named medications. Tall Man lettering is used at many institutions. Figure 8-2 shows part of the Food and Drug Administration (FDA) list of look-alike medication names with recommended Tall Man lettering. A complete list, including the ISMP Tall Man list, can be found at https://www.ismp.org/tools/tallmanletters.pdf.

Table 1. FDA-Approved List of Generic Drug Names with Tall Man Letters*	
Drug Name with Tall Man Letters	**Confused with**
acetaZOLAMIDE	acetoHEXAMIDE
acetoHEXAMIDE	acetaZOLAMIDE
buPROPion	busPIRone
busPIRone	buPROPion
chlorproMAZINE	chlorproPAMIDE
chlorproPAMIDE	chlorproMAZINE
clomiPHENE	clomiPRAMINE
clomiPRAMINE	clomiPHENE
cycloSERINE	cycloSPORINE
cycloSPORINE	cycloSERINE
DAUNOrubicin	DOXOrubicin
dimenhyDRINATE	diphenhydrAMINE
diphenhydrAMINE	dimenhyDRINATE
DOBUTamine	DOPamine
DOPamine	DOBUTamine

Figure 8-2 Tall Man lettering. *Report medication errors or near misses to the ISMP Medication Errors Reporting Program (MERP) at 1-800-FAIL-SAF(E) or online at www.ismp.org. (© 2011 ISMP. Used with permission from the Institute for Safe Medication Practices.)

> ⓘ **TIPS** FOR **CLINICAL PRACTICE**
>
> Administer only medications that you have prepared and that are clearly labelled. Check that the medication has not expired. Avoid distractions when preparing medications. Some institutions have instituted "no interruption zones" in areas such as the medication room to prevent distractions.

> ⚠ **SAFETY ALERT!**
>
> If the medication name is not clear or the medication does not seem to be appropriate for the patient, question the order. Always double-check that you have the correct medication. If you are unfamiliar with a medication, refer to your nursing drug reference to ensure that you have the correct medication and prevent errors.

2. **The right dose**—Always perform and check calculations carefully, without ignoring decimal points. If you misread a decimal point, the patient could receive a dose significantly different from the one ordered. Risk of harm from dosage errors in the pediatric population is great. Caution should be taken when administering medications to children. Errors can occur because of the frequency of weight-based calculations, the need for decimal points, and fractional dosages (ISMP Canada & Healthcare Insurance Reciprocal of Canada, 2012). Many errors have occurred with infusion pumps and calculations involving administration of parenteral fluids and medications. Electronic infusion pumps have reduced medication errors. Although infusion pump technology has increased administration safety, the nurse cannot rely fully on it. It is a nursing responsibility to be trained in the use of infusion pumps and to be alert for potential problems.

To ensure the right dose of medication, interpret abbreviations correctly. Factors such as illegible handwriting, miscalculation of the amount, and use of inappropriate abbreviations can result in administration of the wrong dose. Always have someone else check a dosage that causes concern. In some organizations, certain medication dosages are required to be checked by two nurses (e.g., insulin, heparin). These medications have been a common source of errors in administration. If a dosage or abbreviation in a written order is not clear, call the prescriber for verification; do not assume.

Computer entry does not eliminate the use of incorrect dosing symbols. Nurses should always consult a drug reference to confirm the dosage when in doubt. Cohen (2010) cites that doses of more than two or three tablets, capsules, or vials are unusual and nurses should question all orders that exceed that number.

3. **The right patient**—Failure to correctly identify the right patient has been cited as one of the three most common causes of medication errors. Patients should be identified

with at least two unique patient identifiers (e.g., name, birth date, identification number). It is permissible to check the two identifiers with the patient's arm band, medication administration record, or chart and ask the patient to state his or her name.

In many institutions, you may be required to scan the bar code on the patient's identification bracelet as well as on the medication being administered. In basic nursing education programs, emphasis is placed on establishing the correct identification of the patient prior to medication administration. Students are required to compare two patient-specific identifiers with the patient's armband, MAR, or chart and by asking the patient to state her or his name (as a third identifier). To avoid administering medications to the wrong patient, the steps identified need to be consistently implemented regardless of how familiar the nurse is with the patient. Always know and use the unique identifiers recognized and required by the facility. Advanced technology does not eliminate your responsibility to correctly identify a patient. Misidentification can result in a patient receiving the wrong medication.

> ## ⚠ SAFETY ALERT!
>
> Always verify your patient's identity by using the two identifiers designated by your institution each time medications are administered. This will help to ensure you have the right patient and avoid an error.

4. **The right route**—*Route* refers to how a medication is administered (e.g., by mouth, by injection). A medication intended for one route is unsafe if administered by another route. Oral medications (e.g., tablets, capsules, caplets) are administered by mouth. Nurses should always consult a reliable reference to confirm the correct route for a medication that is unfamiliar. The route of the medication should be stated on the order. Do not assume which route is appropriate. Orders to administer medications by a feeding tube that should not be crushed (e.g., enteric coated tablets) require that the nurse seek clarification of the order or have the order changed by the prescriber to ensure safe medication administration. For definitions of different routes of medication, see the "Routes of Medication Administration" section later in the chapter.

5. **The right time**—Medications should be given at the correct time of day and interval (e.g., 3 times a day [TID] or every 6 hours [q6h]). If several medications are ordered to be administered at the same time, use sound clinical judgment and critical thinking to prioritize sequence, based on the patient, the medication, the route, and the frequency. For example, a patient may be receiving a diuretic twice a day (BID), and the institution may have BID as 9:00 AM and 9:00 PM. The nurse will need to know that the diuretic should not be given in the late afternoon, so that the individual is not going to the bathroom all night. The nurse must know whether a time schedule can be altered or requires judgment in determining the proper time to be administered.

  In most cases, the right time means the medication must be administered within 30 minutes of the scheduled time. This is referred to as the "30-minute rule" (ISMP, 2011b), which requires that medications be given within 30 minutes before or 30 minutes after their scheduled time. ISMP's survey of nurses in response to the 30-minute rule reveals that many nurses developed unsafe practices that threatened patient safety and increased the potential for medication errors. Some of the unsafe practices that resulted from time pressures included taking risky shortcuts such as deception (e.g., medication documented as being given at a certain time when it was delayed or given beforehand); administering medications without performing assessments and/or checking vital signs, lab values, weight and allergy status; skipping bar-code scanning; and skipping important double checks to save time.

  Canadian hospitals and health institutions establish their own policies and guidelines for the timing of medication. Nurses should become familiar with these policies and incorporate critical thinking in making decisions about timing of scheduled medication that may differ depending on the medication, the route, the patient, and the practice environment (ISMP, 2011b).

  Before administering prn (when necessary) medications, check to ascertain that adequate time has passed since the previous dose, or severe consequences may occur because the medication was administered to the patient too soon.

6. **The right frequency**—All medication orders should include the frequency that a medication is to be administered. Administration of a medication at the prescribed time or right time is important to maximize the therapeutic effect and maintain therapeutic blood levels. Errors have occurred in medication administration because of misinterpretation of time and frequency in medication orders. ISMP Canada (2006a) has taken steps to prevent errors by prohibiting the use of certain abbreviations related to dosing frequency (e.g., QOD and QD have been mistaken for each other; instead of QOD, write "every other day" and instead of QD write "daily" or "every day").

7. **The right site**—Some organizations include "the right site" as a right of medication administration. Others argue that the right route incorporates the right site. However, if the patient is prescribed eye drops or ear drops, it is crucial that the correct eye or ear is treated if the order is not for both areas. Hence, the right site is not always the same as the right route. For topical medications such as ointments and creams, the right site for application (such as a wound on a left arm as opposed to the right arm that has no wound) is not the same as route.

8. **The right reason**—This right involves confirming the rationale for the prescribed medication. The nurse must know why the patient is taking the medication. What is the patient's medical history? Is the patient on the medication for its general indication for use? Or is the patient on the medication for a particular "off-label" use that the medication is known for treating? Knowing the **right reason** for a medication to be administered can help the nurse prevent medication errors. If the nurse understands the reason for a prescribed medication, he or she is in a better position to identify when to hold or not give a medication that may cause harm if administered.

9. **The right documentation**—The right documentation was one of the first rights to be added to the traditional five in the general nursing literature. Medications should be documented accurately as soon as they are given—on the right patient's medication record, under the right date, and next to the right time. If a medication is declined, it should be documented as such with a notation on the medication record or in the nurse's notes. Never chart a medication as given before administering it or without documentation as to why it was not given. Follow the policy of the institution when documenting. All documentation should be legible. Unintentional overmedication of a patient could result if a nurse fails to document a medication that was given and a nurse on a following shift also gives the medication to the patient.

Documentation of medications administered is done on the patient's MAR, which is a paper form or electronic record that tracks the medications a patient receives. A computerized record is used as a working document that records medications as they are administered and is referred to as an electronic medication administration record (eMAR). This system allows electronic tracking of medications administered to help reduce errors. With some of the electronic medication systems, the medication bar code and the patient's identification band is scanned, and the information is documented into the patient's eMAR. **Remember: "If it's not documented, it's not done."**

10. **The right education**—All adult patients have a right to be educated about the medication they are taking. Patients are more likely to take their medication if they understand why they are taking it, and education allows them to make an informed decision.

To ensure patient safety and prevent the occurrence of medication errors, Accreditation Canada, ISMP Canada, and the CPSI propose that health care providers generate a list of all medications a patient is taking, including herbals, vitamins, and nonprescription products. Patients and families may not accurately report all their medications and dosages, as well as home remedies. This lack of information can lead to errors in medication administration as well as adverse effects. Nurses need to get a thorough history of medications being taken by a patient to prevent medication interactions that may be fatal to the patient.

11. **The right technique**—It is important to use proper technique for the type and route of medication being administered. For example, administer subcutaneous insulin at a 90-degree angle and do not aspirate.

12. **The right approach**—This right includes areas such as undertaking proper hand hygiene, knowing how to position a child when administering different medications, and choosing the correct method when administering oral medication.

13. **The right assessment**—Several medications require specific assessment prior to administration. For example, a patient's apical pulse rate must be assessed before digoxin is administered, and blood pressure should be assessed prior to antihypertensive medication. The prescriber may also include specific parameters for a medication, such as "Hold if systolic BP [blood pressure] is less than 100 or diastolic BP is less than 60."

14. **The right evaluation**—The nurse is responsible for evaluating the effect of the medication administered in a timely manner. Did the medication have the therapeutic effect expected? If not, what are the possible reasons? For example, an analgesic was administered to a patient for postoperative pain measuring 8 out of 10 on the pain scale 1.5 hours ago. The patient reports that the pain level is the same as before the analgesic. The nurse should inform the prescriber after additional assessment of the pain regarding the ineffectiveness of the medication dosage. Perhaps the patient requires a higher dose or a more effective analgesic.

15. **The right to refuse**—Adult patients have the right to refuse a medication. When a refusal occurs, the nurse has the responsibility to ensure that the patient is informed of any potential consequences of declining to take the medication. The nurse should also inform the prescriber and document all communications surrounding the refusal on the patient record. The need for additional patient teaching should also be determined.

    The right to refuse may be denied to the patient who has a mental illness. A patient deemed to be dangerous to self or others can be taken to court and mandated to take medication.

    In Ontario, although a patient has the right to refuse medication or treatment, *Brian's Law* may provide some exception to that right. *Brian's Law* was added to the Ontario *Mental Health Act* on December 1, 2000, to address public fears about patients with severe mental health concerns living in the community. It was designed to protect the public and potentially dangerous patients who have a mental illness by ensuring that such patients receive treatment safely and effectively. *Brian's Law* includes community treatment orders (CTOs), which allow physicians or psychiatrists to legally compel a patient to take treatment in the community after leaving a psychiatric facility (Ontario Ministry of Health and Long Term Care, 2000). Under this legislation, if a patient fails to comply with the treatment plan that was agreed upon, a physician or psychiatrist can contact police to have the patient escorted to a treatment facility.

    Nurses should always be aware of the provincial laws, policies, and procedures for their jurisdiction relative to the administration of medications to patients who decline them. It is extremely important for nurses to check frequently for adverse effects related to medications and to listen carefully to patient complaints. The reason for the refusal of medications should be carefully analyzed and documented in all cases. Patient education and a reassuring therapeutic relationship can assist in diminishing a patient's refusal.

All of these rights of medication administration should be consistently followed when administering medications. In addition to these rights, the nurse should always view the patient receiving medications as an important and valuable asset in the prevention of medication errors. Always listen to concerns raised by the patient when administering medication, regardless of the checks that you have performed before administration. For instance, if a patient states, "I have never taken this pill before," the nurse should consider what the patient says as correct and investigate concerns before administering the medication; doing so can be valuable in preventing medication errors.

⚠ SAFETY ALERT!

When a patient questions a medication, **STOP** and **LISTEN.** It may be the opportunity to identify an error before a patient is harmed.

Medication Reconciliation

A high proportion of adverse events are medication-related (Accreditation Canada, the Canadian Institute for Health Information, the Canadian Patient Safety Institute, and the Institute for Safe Medication Practices Canada, 2012). Medication reconciliation can help to reduce these events.

Canada has implemented a national medication implementation strategy to "ensure accurate communication at care transition points, for example, when patients enter a hospital, transition to another service or provider or are discharged home" (Accreditation Canada, the Canadian Institute for Health Information, the Canadian Patient Safety Institute, and the Institute for Safe Medication Practices Canada, 2012, p. 5). This national patient safety strategy requires hospitals to reconcile medications across the continuum of care. Medication reconciliation is to be applied in any setting or service where medications are to be used or the patient's response to treatment or service could be affected by medications that the patient has been taking.

In the context of this strategy, reconciliation is the process of comparing the medications that the patient (or resident) has been taking before the time of admission or entry into a new setting with the medications that the organization is about to provide. The purpose of the reconciliation is to avoid errors of transcription, omission, duplication of therapy, or medication-medication and medication-disease interactions.

Medication reconciliation is an important step in the prevention of medication errors and can assist in obtaining accurate medication histories and ensure continuity of appropriate therapy. This process should begin on admission; discharge orders should be compared and reconciled with the most recent inpatient medication orders and the original list of medications taken at home. Nurses can play a major role in the reconciliation process. Medication reconciliation must be an important focus to prevent errors and misunderstanding regarding medications that a patient may be taking, especially when discharged. Ensuring patient knowledge regarding prehospital medications and post-hospital medications may be a step in preventing errors and medication interactions. For additional information about medication reconciliation, refer to the ISMP Canada website: http://www.ismp-canada.org.

Other Aspects of the Nurse's Role in Medication Error Prevention

According to *Preventing Medication Errors* (IOM, 2006), another effective way to reduce medication errors is through a strong patient–health care provider partnership. To establish this partnership, nurses should emphasize open communication between themselves and patients; that is, communication should include talking to as well as listening to patients. Health care institutions can also improve communication between nurses and patients by displaying brochures and posters encouraging patients to use strategies to avoid medication mistakes. Brochures and posters could include tips such as check your medications; ask questions; and make sure your doctors, nurses, and other caregivers check your wristband and ask your name before giving you medicine (Figure 8-3).

Nurses need to use reliable information sources that provide vital information related to medication errors and preventing their occurrence (e.g., ISMP Canada). Reducing and preventing errors also requires nurses to adhere to the safety standards prescribed by their governing body and organizations such as ISMP Canada and the CPSI. When medication errors do occur, they should be reported following the organization's procedure for reporting.

Routes of Medication Administration

Route refers to how a medication is administered. Medications come in several forms for administration.

Oral (PO). Oral medication is administered by mouth (e.g., tablets, capsules, caplets, liquid solutions).

Sublingual (SL). Sublingual medications are placed under the tongue and designed to be readily absorbed through the blood vessels in this area. They should not be swallowed. Nitroglycerin is an example of a medication commonly administered by the sublingual route.

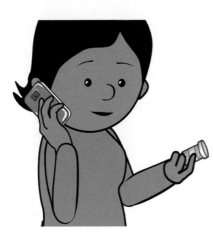

Julie says:

"Read the label on your medicine to make sure it's yours. If something doesn't seem right or if you don't understand, Speak Up!"

Watch the Speak Up™ videos online
at www.jointcommission.org/speakup.

The Joint Commission

Figure 8-3 Sample of a speak-up message. (© The Joint Commission, 2015. Reprinted with permission.)

Sustained-release (SR), extended-release (XL), or delayed-release (DR) tablets or capsules release medication into the bloodstream over a period of time at specific intervals. Therefore, these forms of medication should not be opened, chewed, or crushed.

Buccal. Buccal tablets are placed in the mouth against the mucous membranes of the cheek where the medication will dissolve. The medication is absorbed from the blood vessels of the cheek. Patients should be instructed not to chew or swallow the medication and not to take any liquids with it. Medications administered by the oral route will be discussed in more detail in Chapter 15.

Parenteral. Parenteral medications are administered by a route other than by mouth or gastrointestinal tract. Parenteral routes include intravenous (IV), intramuscular (IM), subcutaneous (SUBCUT), and intradermal (ID). Parenteral routes will be discussed in more detail in Chapter 16.

Insertion. Medication is placed into a body cavity, where the medication dissolves at body temperature (e.g., suppositories). Vaginal medications, creams, and tablets may also be inserted by using special applicators provided by the manufacturer.

Instillation. Medication is introduced in liquid form into a body cavity. It can also include placing an ointment into a body cavity, such as erythromycin eye ointment, which is placed in the conjunctiva of the eye. Nose drops and ear drops are also instillation medications.

Inhalation. Medication is administered into the respiratory tract, for example, through nebulizers used by patients for asthma. Bronchodilators and corticosteroids may be administered by inhalation through the mouth using an aerosolized, pressurized metered-dose inhaler (MDI). In some institutions, these medications are administered to the patient with special equipment, such as positive pressure breathing equipment or the aerosol mask. Other medications in inhalation form include pentamidine, which is used to treat *Pneumocystis jiroveci*, a type of pneumonia found in patients with acquired immunodeficiency syndrome (AIDS). Devices such as "spacers" or "extenders" have been designed for use with inhalers to allow all of the metered dose to be inhaled, particularly in patients who have difficulty using inhalers.

Intranasal. A medicated solution is instilled into the nostrils. This method is used to administer corticosteroids, the antidiuretic hormone vasopressin, and a nasal mist influenza vaccine.

Topical. The medication is applied to the external surface of the skin. It can be in the form of lotion, ointment, or paste.

Percutaneous. Medications are applied to the skin or mucous membranes for absorption. This includes ointments, powders, and lotions for the skin; instillation of solutions onto the mucous membranes of the mouth, ear, nose, or vagina; and inhalation of aerosolized liquids for absorption through the lungs. The primary advantage is that the action of the medication, in general, is localized to the site of application.

Transdermal. Transdermal medication, which is becoming more popular, is contained in a patch or disk and applied topically. The medication is slowly released and absorbed through the skin and enters the systemic circulation. These topical applications may be applied for 24 hours or for as long as 7 days and have systemic effects. Examples include nitroglycerin for chest pain, nicotine transdermal (Habitrol) for smoking cessation, clonidine for hypertension, fentanyl (Duragesic) for persistent pain, and birth control patches.

Forms of oral medications (tablets, capsules), oral solutions, and routes for parenteral medications are discussed in more detail in Chapters 15 to 17.

Some medications are supplied in multiple forms and therefore can be administered by a variety of routes. For example, promethazine hydrochloride is supplied as a tablet, syrup, suppository, and solution for injection.

Equipment Used for Medication Administration

Medicine Cup. Equipment used for oral administration includes a 30-mL medication cup made of plastic, used to measure most liquid medications. The cup has measurements in two systems of measurement (Figure 8-4).

Soufflé Cup. A soufflé cup is a small paper cup or a small translucent plastic cup used for solid forms of medication, such as tablets and capsules (Figure 8-5).

Calibrated Dropper. A calibrated dropper may be used to administer small amounts of medication to an adult or a child (Figure 8-6). The calibrations are usually in millilitres but can be in drops. Droppers (and squeeze drop bottles) are also designed for and used to dispense eye, nose, and ear medications. The amount of the drop (gtt) varies according to the diameter of the opening at the tip of the dropper. For this reason, it is important to remember

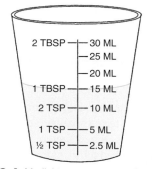

Figure 8-4 Medicine cup. (Modified from Mulholland, J. M. (2011). *The nurse, the math, the meds: Drug calculations using dimensional analysis* (2nd ed.). St. Louis: Mosby.)

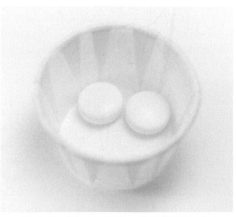

Figure 8-5 Soufflé cup. (Willow Hood/Shutterstock.com.)

that droppers should not be used as a medication measure unless they are calibrated. Because of variation, a properly calibrated dropper is often packaged with the medication (see Figure 8-6) and calibrated for the specified dose. The calibration allows for accurate dosing. Medications that use calibrated droppers include children's vitamins; nystatin oral solution; and furosemide oral solution. The calibration allows for accurate dosing. Use the calibrated dropper only with the medicine it is designed for and packaged with.

Nipple. An infant feeding nipple with additional holes may be used for administering oral medications to infants (Figure 8-7).

Oral Syringe. An oral syringe may be used to administer liquid medications orally to adults and children. No needle is attached (Figure 8-8).

Parenteral Syringe. A parenteral syringe is used for IM, SUBCUT, ID, and IV medications. These syringes come in various sizes and are marked in millilitres or units. The specific types of syringes are discussed in more detail in Chapter 16. The barrel of the syringe holds the medication and has calibrations on it. The needle is attached to the tip. The plunger pushes the medication out (Figure 8-9). The size of the needle depends on how the medication is given (e.g., SUBCUT or IM), the viscosity of the medication, and the size of the patient. See Figure 8-10 for samples of the types of syringes.

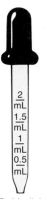

Figure 8-6 Medicine dropper. (Modified from Clayton, B. D., & Willihnganz, M. (2013). *Basic pharmacology for nurses* (16th ed.). St. Louis: Mosby.)

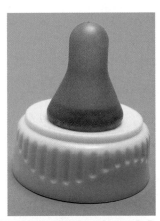

Figure 8-7 Nipple. (Modified from Clayton B. D., & Willihnganz, M. (2013). *Basic pharmacology for nurses* (16 ed.). St. Louis: Mosby.)

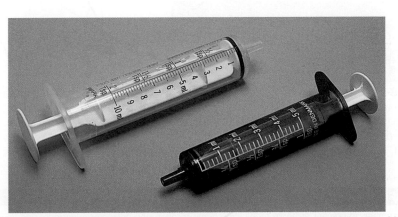

Figure 8-8 Oral syringes. (Courtesy of Chuck Dresner. From Clayton, B. D., & Willihnganz, M. (2013). *Basic pharmacology for nurses* (16th ed.). St. Louis: Mosby.)

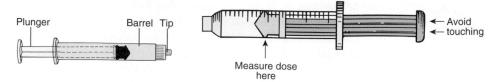

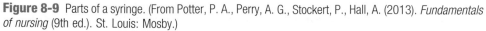

Figure 8-9 Parts of a syringe. (From Potter, P. A., Perry, A. G., Stockert, P., Hall, A. (2013). *Fundamentals of nursing* (9th ed.). St. Louis: Mosby.)

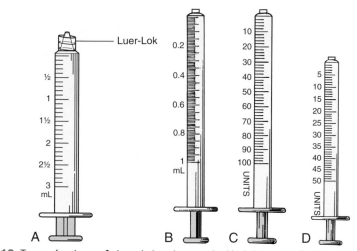

Figure 8-10 Types of syringes. **A,** Luer-Lok syringe marked in 0.1 (tenths). **B,** Tuberculin syringe marked in 0.01 (hundredths) for doses of less than 1 mL. **C,** Insulin syringe marked in units (100). **D,** Insulin syringe marked in units (50). (From Potter, P. A., Perry, A. G., Stockert, P., Hall, A. (2013). *Fundamentals of nursing* (9th ed.). St. Louis: Mosby.)

Equipment for Administering Oral Medications to a Child. Various types of calibrated equipment are available for administering medications to children. Most of this equipment is for oral use. Caregivers should be instructed to always use a calibrated device when administering medications to a child. Figure 8-11 presents samples of equipment used to administer oral medications to a child.

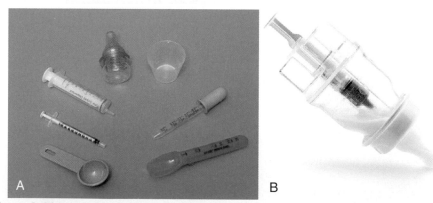

Figure 8-11 A, Acceptable devices for measuring and administering oral medication to children *(clockwise)*: measuring spoon, plastic syringes, calibrated nipple, plastic medicine cup, calibrated dropper, hollow-handled medicine spoon. **B,** Medibottle used to deliver oral medication via a syringe. (**A,** From Hockenberry, M. J., & Wilson, D. (2011). *Wong's nursing care of infants and children* (9th ed.). St. Louis: Mosby. **B,** Courtesy Savi Baby.)

> **! SAFETY ALERT!**
>
> Remember: to prevent errors in medication administration, the device or equipment you use must be calibrated for the dose you need to administer in order to accurately measure the dose.

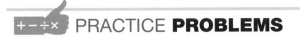 PRACTICE **PROBLEMS**

Answer the following questions by filling in the correct word or words to complete the sentence.

1. A dose for oral use that is less than 5 mL should not be measured in a

   _____.

2. _____ and _____ need special considerations regarding medication dosages.

3. _____ refers to the way in which a medication is administered.

4. Children and older adults usually require _____ dosages.

5. A _____ cup is used for dispensing solid forms of medication.

6. Application of medication to the external surface of the skin is referred to as

   _____ route.

7. Being an autonomous thinker is an example of _____.

8. _____ droppers should be used for medication administration.

9. When medications are placed next to the cheek, they are administered by the

   _____ route.

Answers on page 135.

⚙ POINTS TO REMEMBER

- The rights of medication administration serve as guidelines for administering medications.
- The nurse should know about the medication being administered. Patient rights include the right to refuse and the right to be educated.
- Medication administration includes using critical thinking and the nursing process.
- Medication errors can occur for numerous reasons.
- Medication errors can harm patients physically and economically and can be fatal.
- The nurse who administers a medication is accountable for any medication error, regardless of the reason for the error.
- The nurse is responsible for ensuring the patient's safety when administering medication.
- The nurse can play a major role in the medication reconciliation process.
- The nurse plays a critical role in the prevention of medication errors.
- Talking to and listening to patients can prevent errors. Patient questions should be encouraged.
- Knowing the policy of the institution regarding the timely administration of medications is important.
- The goal of CMIRPS is to reduce and prevent harmful medication incidents in Canada.
- Older adults and children require special considerations with medication administration.
- A calibrated dropper should be used when administering medications with a dropper.
- A medication cup has the capacity of 30 mL. A soufflé cup is used to dispense solid forms of medications.
- Medications are administered by various routes.

CHAPTER **REVIEW**

1. Name the 15 rights of medication administration discussed in this chapter.

   Right _____   Right _____

   Right _____   Right _____

   Right _____   Right _____

   Right _____   Right _____

   Right _____   Right _____

   Right _____   Right _____

   Right _____   Right _____

   Right _____

2. Patients should be identified using _____ patient identifiers, neither of which can be the _____.

3. A medication label should be read _____ times.

4. Medications should be charted _____ you have administered them.

5. Name three routes of medication administration. _____

6. The medicine cup has a _____ capacity.

7. Droppers are calibrated to administer standardized drops, regardless of what type of dropper is used. True or false? _____

8. The syringe used to administer a dose by mouth is referred to as a (an) _____.

9. Volume on a syringe is indicated by _____.

10. A full 25 to 30% of admissions to the hospital for older adults are because of _____.

11. ISMP is the abbreviation for _____.

12. CPSI is the abbreviation for _____.

13. The route by which medicated solutions are instilled into the nostrils is _____.

14. Examples of medications that have been identified as high-alert medications are _____ potassium chloride, _____, _____, and _____.

15. True or false? Medication calculations that are incorrect are an example of a medication error. _____

16. True or False? Safe medication administration is the responsibility of only the nurse.

_____

For questions 17 to 20, read the statements carefully and indicate which right of medication administration has been violated.

17. The medication label indicated for optic use, and the medication was instilled into the patient's ears. Violated right: _____

18. The prescriber ordered Glipizide and the patient received Glyburide. Violated right:

_____

19. The nurse charted all her medications on the medication record before she administered them. Violated right: _____

20. The nurse administers a medication at 10:00 PM that was scheduled for 10:00 AM.

Violated right: _____

21. When a nurse is unfamiliar with a medication that has been ordered, the nurse should

consult a _____

Answers on page 135.

✳ ANSWERS

Answers to Practice Problems

1. medicine cup
2. Older adults; children
3. Route
4. smaller
5. soufflé
6. topical
7. critical thinking
8. Calibrated
9. buccal

Answers to Chapter Review

1. the right medication, dose, patient, route, time, frequency, site, reason, documentation, education, technique, approach, assessment, evaluation, to refuse

2. two unique; patient's room number

3. three

4. after

5. parenteral, oral, inhalation, insertion, topical, percutaneous, intranasal, instillation, sublingual, buccal, transdermal

6. 30 mL
7. False
8. oral syringe
9. mL
10. medication-related problems
11. Institute for Safe Medication Practices
12. Canadian Patient Safety Institute
13. intranasal

14. heparin; insulin; morphine; neuromuscular medications; chemotherapy medications
15. True
16. False
17. Route
18. Medication
19. Documentation
20. Time
21. Reputable drug reference

evolve

For additional information, refer to the Drug Measures section of the Drug Calculations Companion, Version 5 on Evolve.

CHAPTER 9
Understanding and Interpreting Medication Orders

Objectives

After reviewing this chapter, you should be able to:

1. Identify the meanings of standard abbreviations used in medication administration
2. Identify abbreviations, acronyms, and symbols recommended by ISMP Canada's "Do Not Use" list
3. Identify the components of a medication order
4. Interpret a given medication order
5. Read and write medical notations correctly

Before a nurse can administer any medication, there must be a written order for it. Medication orders can be written by physicians, dentists, physician's assistants, nurse midwives, or nurse practitioners, depending on provincial/territorial law. Health care providers use medication orders to convey the therapeutic plan for a patient. Medication orders are used by health care providers to communicate to the nurse or designated health care worker which medication to administer to a patient. Medication orders can be oral or written.

Regardless of the mechanism used for a medication order, the nurse has responsibilities relating to the order to ensure safe administration. The nursing responsibilities include interpreting the order, selecting the correct medication and dosage, and administering the medication safely. **It is important to remember that the nurse who administers a medication to a patient is the one ultimately responsible for any resulting injury, even if the order was incorrect.**

Verbal Orders

It is expected that health care providers who are authorized to prescribe medication will write these orders whenever possible. However verbal medication orders that are stated directly in person or by telephone from a licensed physician or other qualified practitioner can be accepted by a nurse when it is in the best interest of a patient and there is no reasonable alternative (College of Registered Nurses of Nova Scotia [CRNNS], 2015). CRNNS also states the circumstances under which verbal orders are appropriate:

- Urgent or emergency situations when it is impractical for a prescriber to interpret patient care and write the medication order
- When a prescriber is not present and direction is urgently required by a registered nurse to provide appropriate patient care (CRNNS, 2015, p. 15)

Cohen (2010) cites that errors can occur when verbal orders are incomplete and the nurse makes assumptions about the prescriber's intention. Any questions or concerns relating to the order should be clarified during the conversation. In addition, the order must be repeated back to the prescriber for final confirmation. A verbal order must contain the same elements as a written order: the date of the order, the name and dose of the medication, the route, the frequency, any special instructions, the name of the individual giving the order. A verbal order must also include a note that the order was given in person or by telephone as well as the signature of the nurse taking the order. Many institutions require that the order must be signed by the prescriber within 24 hours. All institutions should have established protocols for verbal orders that should be followed to enhance patient safety.

> **(i) TIPS FOR CLINICAL PRACTICE**
>
> It is important to be familiar with specific policies regarding medication orders and responsibilities because they vary according to the institution or health care facility.

> **(!) SAFETY ALERT!**
>
> Acceptance of a verbal order is a major responsibility and can lead to medication errors. Accept a verbal order only in an emergency situation. If you accept a verbal order, follow the policy of the institution. Always clarify questions about the order during the conversation. If you are unsure of the medication or the spelling, spell it back to the prescriber and get confirmation. **NEVER ASSUME.**

The medication order indicates the treatment plan or medication the health care provider has ordered for a patient. Depending on the institution, the medication order may be written on a sheet labelled "physician's order sheet" or "order sheet." After the medication order has been written, the nurse (or in some institutions a trained unit clerk) transcribes the order. This means the order is written on the medication administration record (MAR). In a situation in which the nurse does not transcribe the order, the nurse is still accountable for what is written and for verifying the order, initialling it, and checking it before administering.

At some institutions, computers are used for processing medication orders. Medication orders are either electronically transmitted or manually entered directly into the computer from an order form. The use of the computer allows immediate transmission of the order to the pharmacy. The computerized medication record can be seen directly on the computer screen or on a printed copy. Medication orders done by computer entry allow the prescriber to make changes if indicated, and the orders are signed by the prescriber with an assigned electronic code. Once the medication is received on the unit, the medication order is implemented and the patient receives the medication.

Computerized provider order entry (CPOE), according to Cohen (2010), could prevent many problems that occur with written orders such as dosing mistakes from illegible handwriting. Despite the advent of technology, some institutions still have handwritten orders and nurses must be familiar with the transcription of orders. In some institutions, fax transmission of orders may be used to avoid telephone orders. Faxed orders, however, may not be clearly legible and can also cause errors in interpretation.

Transcription of Medication Orders

The incorrect transcription of medication orders is one of the main causes of medication errors.

Before transcribing an order or preparing a dose, the nurse must be familiar with reading and interpreting an order. To interpret a medication order, the nurse must know the components of a medication order and the standard abbreviations used in writing a medication order as well as those abbreviations and symbols that *should not* be used. Knowledge of error-prone abbreviations, symbols, and dose designations will prevent misinterpretation and errors with medication orders, which can be fatal to the patient. The nurse therefore must memorize the abbreviations commonly used in medication orders. The abbreviations include units of measurement, the route, and the frequency for the medication ordered. The common abbreviations used in medication administration are listed in Tables 9-1 and 9-2 and must be committed to memory. The Institute for Safe Medication Practices Canada's (ISMP Canada) "Do Not Use" list appears in Table 9-3. It includes error-prone abbreviations, symbols, and dose designations (2006a).

Cohen (2010) recommends that the arrows used ↑, ↓ (up and down) to indicate increase and decrease should not be used. These symbols can be confused for numbers and letters.

TABLE 9-1 Abbreviations for Units of Measurement Used in Health Care Administration

Abbreviation	Meaning	Abbreviation	Meaning
g	gram	mcg	microgram
gtt	drop	mmol*	millimole
kg	kilogram	mg	milligram
L	litre	mL	millilitre

*mmol (millimole) is a medication measurement in which electrolytes are measured; it expresses the ionic activity of a medication. Milliequivalents (mEq) are also used to measure electrolytes and may still be seen on some medication labels, but mmol is the preferred measurement in Canada.

TABLE 9-2 Commonly Used Health Care Abbreviations

Abbreviation	Meaning	Abbreviation	Meaning
ac	before meals	pc	after meals
ad lib	as desired, freely	per	through or by
am	morning before noon	pm	evening, before midnight
amp	ampule	PO	by mouth, oral
aq	aqueous, water	pr	by rectum
BID	twice a day	prn	when necessary/required, as needed
c̄	with		
cap*	capsule	q	every
CD	controlled dose	q.a.m.	every morning
CR	controlled release	qh	every hour
dil.	dilute	q2h, q4h, q6h, q8h, q12h	every 2 hours, every 4 hours, every 6 hours, every 8 hours, every 12 hours
DS	double strength		
EC	enteric coated		
elix.	elixir	QID	four times a day
fld.	fluid	qs	a sufficient amount/as much as needed
GT	gastrostomy tube		
gtt	drop		
h, hr	hour	rect	rectum
ID	intradermal	SL	sublingual
IM	intramuscular	soln	solution
IV	intravenous	SR	sustained release
IVPB	intravenous piggyback	stat	immediately, at once
KVO	keep vein open (a very slow infusion rate)	SUBCUT	subcutaneous
		supp	suppository
LA	long acting	susp	suspension
LOS	length of stay	syp	syrup
min	minute	tab	tablet
mix	mixture	TID	three times a day
NAS	intranasal	tinct	tincture
NG, NGT	nasogastric tube	ung, oint	ointment
noct	at night	vag	vaginally
NPO	nothing by mouth	XL	long acting
NS, N/S	normal saline	XR	extended release

*It is preferable to avoid using "cap" because it could refer to "capsule" or "caplet."
Note: "Do not use" and dangerous abbreviations identified by ISMP Canada have been removed.

TABLE 9-3   ISMP Canada's "Do Not Use" List*

The abbreviations, symbols, and dose designations found in this table have been reported as being frequently misinterpreted and involved in harmful medication errors. They should NEVER be used when communicating medication information.

Abbreviation	Intended Meaning	Problem	Correction
U	unit	Mistaken for "0" (zero), "4" (four), or cc.	Use "unit."
IU	international unit	IU international unit. Mistaken for "IV" (intravenous) or "10" (ten).	Use "unit."
Abbreviations for medication names		Misinterpreted because of similar abbreviations for multiple medications; e.g., MS, MSO$_4$ (morphine sulphate), MgSO$_4$ (magnesium sulphate) may be confused for one another.	Do not abbreviate medication names.
QD QOD	every day every other day	QD and QOD have been mistaken for each other, or as "qid." The Q has also been misinterpreted as "2" (two).	Use "daily" and "every other day."
OD	every day	Mistaken for "right eye" (OD = oculus dexter).	Use "daily."
OS, OD, OU	left eye, right eye, both eyes	May be confused with one another.	Use "left eye," "right eye," or "both eyes."
D/C	discharge	Interpreted as "discontinue whatever medications follow" (typically discharge medications).	Use "discharge."
cc	cubic centimetre	Mistaken for "u" (units).	Use "mL" or "millilitre."
μg	microgram	Mistaken for "mg" (milligram) resulting in one thousand-fold overdose.	Use "mL" or "millilitre."

Symbol	Intended Meaning	Potential Problem	Correction
@	at	Mistaken for "2" (two) or "5" (five).	Use "at."
>	Greater than	Mistaken for "7" (seven) or the letter "L."	Use "greater than"/"more than"
<	Less than	Confused with each other.	or "less than"/"lower than."

Dose Designation	Intended Meaning	Potential Problem	Correction
Trailing zero	x.0 mg	Decimal point is overlooked resulting in 10-fold dose error.	Never use a zero by itself after a decimal point. Use "**x mg**."
Lack of leading zero	.x mg	Decimal point is overlooked resulting in 10-fold dose error.	Always use a zero before a decimal point. Use "**0.x mg**."

Institute for Safe Medication Practices Canada. (2006). Do not use: Dangerous abbreviations, symbols and dose designations. Retrieved from https://ismp-canada.org. Reprinted with permission from ISMP Canada.

*Adapted from ISMP's List of *Error-Prone Abbreviations, Symbols, and Dose Designations 2006.*

Writing a Medication Order

The health care provider writes a medication order on a form called the *physician's order sheet.* Order sheets vary from institution to institution. The order sheet should have the patient's name on it.

Components of a Medication Order

When a medication order is written, it must contain the following seven components or it is considered invalid or incomplete: (1) patient's full name, (2) date and time the order was written, (3) name of the medication to be administered, (4) dose of the medication, (5) route of administration, (6) time and frequency of administration, and (7) signature of the person writing the order. These parts of the medication order are discussed in detail in the following sections.

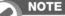
NOTE
Abbreviations may be written with or without the use of periods; this does not alter the meaning.

! SAFETY ALERT!
If any of the components of a medication order are missing, the order is not complete and not a legal medication order.

Patient's Full Name. Using the patient's full name helps to prevent confusion between one patient and another, thereby preventing administration of the wrong medication to a patient. Many institutions use a nameplate to imprint the patient's name and record number on the order sheet; in addition, there is usually a place to indicate allergies. In institutions that use computers, the computer screen may also show identifying information for the patient, such as age and known medication allergies.

Date and Time the Order Was Written. The date and time of the order include the month, day, year, and the time the order was written. This information will help in determining the start and stop of the medication order. In many institutions, the health care provider writing the order is required to include the length of time the medication is to be given (e.g., 7 days); or he or she may use the abbreviation LOS (length of stay), which means the patient is to receive the medication during the entire stay in the hospital. The policy regarding indicating the length of time a medication is to be given varies from institution to institution. At some institutions, if there are no specified days for particular medications, it is assumed to be continued until otherwise stopped by the health care provider. Some medications have automatic stop times according to the facility (e.g., narcotics, certain antibiotics).

Name of the Medication to be Administered. The medication may be ordered by the generic or trade name (Figures 9-1 and 9-2). To avoid confusion with another medication, the name of the medication should be written clearly and spelled correctly.

Trade name—The brand name or proprietary name is the name under which a manufacturer markets the medication. The trade name is followed by the registration symbol ®. The trade name either starts with a capital letter or is all in capital letters on the label.

> **NOTE**
> A record of the time the order was written is preferred in many institutions, but omission of this information does not invalidate the order. This same information is required in computer entry of medication orders.

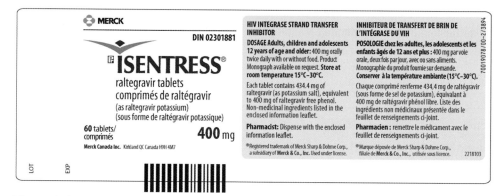

Figure 9-1 Isentress label. Notice the two names. The first, *Isentress,* is the trade name, identified by the registration symbol ®. The name under Isentress in a smaller font is *raltegravir,* the generic or official name.

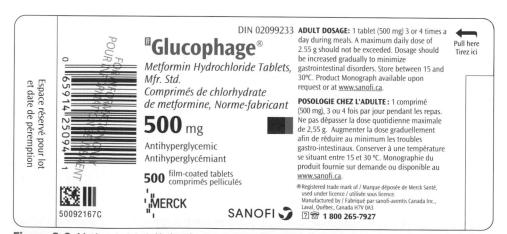

Figure 9-2 Metformin label. Notice the two names. The first, *Glucophage,* is the trade name, identified by the registration symbol ®. The name under Glucophage in a smaller font is *metformin hydrochloride,* the generic or official name.

It is generally the largest printed information on the label. A medication may have several trade names, according to the manufacturer. It is important to note that some medications may not have trade names.

Generic name—The proper name, chemical name, or nonproprietary name of the medication. It is usually designated in lowercase letters or a different typeface. Sometimes the generic name is also placed in parentheses on the medication label. The generic name is usually found under the trade name. Occasionally, only the generic name will appear on the label. Each medication has only one generic name. **By law, the generic name must appear on all medication labels.** Therefore, a medication label must indicate the generic name, and some labels may include a trade name. The prescriber may order medications using the generic name.

> ### ⓘ TIPS FOR CLINICAL PRACTICE
>
> Nurses must be familiar with both the generic name and the trade name for a medication. To ensure correct medication identification, nurses should cross-check trade and generic names as needed with a drug reference.

Checking the names of medications even when they are generic is essential in preventing errors. Some very different medications have similar generic names, such as dimenhydrinate (Gravol), which is used to treat nausea and vomiting, and diphenhydramine (Allerdryl), which is used to treat hay fever. Both of these medications are also classified as antihistamines.

To ensure correct medication information, nurses should cross-check trade and generic names as needed. When reading the name of a medication, never assume. Sometimes orders may be written with abbreviated medication names. This approach has been discouraged unless the abbreviation is common and approved. Some abbreviations used for medications can cause confusion with other medications, such as $MgSO_4$ (intended use: magnesium sulphate) and MSO_4 (intended use: morphine sulphate).

Consider this example, in which the acronym AZT is used: "AZT 100 mg PO " (intended medication order is zidovudine [AZT] [Retrovir], 100 mg, which is used for HIV). The name of the medication could be misread as azathioprine (Imuran), an immunosuppressant. The use of acronyms in writing medication orders is not recommended by ISMP Canada; write the complete medication name to avoid misinterpretation.

> ### ⚠ SAFETY ALERT!
>
> A case of mistaken identity with medications can have tragic results.

Dose of the Medication. The amount and strength of the medication should be written clearly to avoid confusion. Dose indicates the amount or weight provided in the form (e.g., per tablet, per millilitre).

To avoid misinterpretation, "U," which stands for *units,* should not be used when insulin, heparin, or any other medication order that uses units is written. The word *units* should be written out. This would also include "mU" (milliunits). Errors have occurred as a result of confusion of "U" with an "O" in a handwritten order. The abbreviation "U" for units is on ISMP Canada's "Do Not Use" list of "dangerous abbreviations, symbols, and dose designations" (see Table 9-3).

Example: 60 SUBCUT stat of Humulin Regular Insulin. The U is almost completely closed and could be misread as 60 units. Do not use "U." Use the word *units* instead.

Example: The handwritten letters "q.d.," when used in prescription writing, can be misinterpreted as "q.i.d." if the period is raised and the tail of the "q" interferes: domperidone (Motilium) 10 mg *q.d.* Do not use "q.d.," "qd," "QD," or "Q.D." Use the word *daily* instead.

> ### ✎ NOTE
>
> The period can cause confusion with "q.i.d." Use QID for "four times a day" to help reduce the risk of error. The acronym "q.d." should never be used when writing medication orders, regardless of form, in upper or lowercase, with or without periods. Use the word *daily* instead.

Route of Administration. The route of administration is a very important part of a medication order because medications can be administered by several routes. Never assume that you know which route is appropriate. Standard and acceptable abbreviations should be used to indicate the route.

Examples: PO (oral, by mouth)   IM (intramuscular)

ID (intradermal)   IV (intravenous)

> **⚠ SAFETY ALERT!**
>
> Administering a medication by a route other than what the form indicates constitutes a medication error. Regardless of the source of an error, if you administer the wrong dose or give a medication by a route other than what it is intended for, you have made a medication error and are accountable for it.

Time and Frequency of Administration. Standard abbreviations should be used to indicate the times a medication is to be given.

Examples: QID (four times a day), stat (immediately)

The time intervals at which a medication is administered are determined by the institution, and most health care facilities have routine times for administering medications.

Example: TID (three times a day) may be 9:00 AM, 1:00 PM, and 5:00 PM, or 10:00 AM, 2:00 PM, and 6:00 PM.

Factors such as the purpose of the medication, medication interactions, absorption of the medication, and adverse effects should be considered when medication times are scheduled. It is important to realize that when abbreviations such as BID and TID are used, the amount you calculate is for one dose and not for the day's total. The frequency indicates the dose of medication given at a single time.

Signature of the Person Writing the Order. For a medication order to be legal, it must be signed by the health care provider. The health care provider writing the order must include his or her signature on the order, and it should be legible. Orders that are done by computer entry require a signature created by using an assigned electronic code or electronic signature. In addition to the seven required components of a medication order already discussed, any special instructions or parameters for certain medications need to be clearly written.

Examples: 1. Hold if blood pressure (BP) is below 100 systolic.

2. Administer a half hour before meals ($\frac{1}{2}$ hour ac).

Medications ordered as needed or when necessary (prn) should indicate the purpose of administration as well. In addition, a frequency must be written to state the minimum time allowed between doses.

Examples: 1. For chest pain
2. Temperature above 38.5°C
3. For blood pressure (BP) greater than 140 systolic and 90 diastolic

In instances in which specific instructions are not stated, nursing judgment must be used to determine whether it is appropriate to administer a medication.

For dosage calculations, the nurse is usually concerned with the medication name, dose of the medication, route, and time or frequency of administration. This information is necessary in determining a safe and reasonable dosage for a patient.

SAFETY ALERT!
Never make assumptions about what an order states! Clarify an order when in doubt. If an order is not clear, or if essential components are omitted, it is not a legal order and should not be implemented. The nurse is accountable!

Interpreting a Medication Order

Medication orders are written in the following sequence:
1. Name of the medication
2. The dose, expressed in standard abbreviations or symbols
3. Route
4. Frequency

Example: Docusate sodium   100 mg   PO   TID
                  ↓   ↓   ↓   ↓
               name of   dose   route   frequency
              medication

This order means the prescriber wants the patient to receive docusate sodium (name of medication), which is a stool softener, 100 milligrams (dose) by mouth (route), three times a day (frequency). The use of abbreviations in a medication order is a form of shorthand. For the purpose of interpreting orders, it is important for nurses to commit to memory common medical abbreviations as well as abbreviations related to the systems of measurement. Refer to Tables 9-1 and 9-2 for medical abbreviations and symbols used in medication administration. Be systematic when interpreting the order to avoid an error. The medication order follows a specific sequence when it is written correctly (the name of the medication first, followed by the dose, route, and frequency). Interpret the order in this manner as well, and avoid "scrambling the order."

Let's look at some medication orders for practice reading and interpreting.

Example: Buspirone 15 mg PO BID

This order means: Give buspirone 15 milligrams orally (by mouth) two times a day.

Example: Penicillin G 250 000 units IV q6h.

This order means: Give penicillin G 250 000 units by intravenous injection every 6 hours.

Example: Ibuprofen 400 mg PO q6h prn for pain.

This order means: Give ibuprofen 400 milligrams orally (by mouth) every 6 hours when necessary (as required) for pain.

 SAFETY ALERT!
The instruction "prn" must have a frequency that designates the minimum time allowed between doses.

Orders are transcribed in some institutions where unit dose is used. In some institutions, more transcribing may be necessary because the MAR may have the capacity to be used for only a limited period (e.g., 3 days, 5 days). It is therefore necessary to transcribe orders again at the end of the designated period.

In facilities in which computers are used, the medication order is entered into the computer, and a printout lists the currently ordered medications. The computer is able to scan for information such as medication incompatibilities, safe dosage ranges, recommended administration times, and allergies; it can also indicate when a new order for a medication is required.

Computerized order entry and charting do not eliminate the nurse's responsibility for double-checking medication orders before administering. Nurses must be aware that the use of certain abbreviations, acronyms, and symbols has led to actual errors in medication administration that have been harmful to patients. ISMP Canada established its "Do Not Use" list because the abbreviations, acronyms, and symbols it contains are a common source of errors and can be easily misinterpreted.

For the safety of patients and to prevent errors in misinterpretation, prescribers responsible for writing medication orders *must* pay attention to what they write; it could save a life. In addition to knowing correct medication notations, those who administer medications must know the safe dosage and be able to recognize discrepancies in a dosage that can sometimes be caused by misinterpretation of an order.

ⓘ TIPS FOR CLINICAL PRACTICE

Nurses should stay up to date with ISMP Canada's and their health care institution's policies and restrictions regarding medical abbreviations and other medical notations.

⚠ SAFETY ALERT!

The consequences of misinterpreting abbreviations, acronyms, symbols, and dosages may be fatal.

⚙ POINTS TO REMEMBER

- Remember: a primary responsibility of the nurse is the safe administration of medications to a patient.
- Interpret the medication order systematically, following it in the way in which it is written (the name of the medication, the dosage, the route, and frequency).
- Know the seven components of a medication order:
  1. Patient's full name
  2. Date and time the order was written
  3. Name of the medication to be administered
  4. Dose of the medication
  5. Route of administration
  6. Time and frequency of administration
  7. Signature of the person writing the order
- Ensure that all medication orders are legible and include standard abbreviations, acronyms, and symbols.
- Memorize the meaning of standard medical abbreviations, acronyms, and symbols.
- Be aware of acronyms, symbols, and abbreviations that *should not* be used. Their use can increase the potential for errors in medication administration.
- Write down verbal orders, read them back to the prescriber, and confirm with the prescriber that the order is correct.
- If any of the seven components of a medication order are missing or seem incorrect, do not implement the medication order. **Do not assume—clarify the order!**
- If you are in doubt about the meaning of an order, clarify it with the prescriber before administering.
- Always cross-check medications; misidentification can result in a medication error.

+−÷× PRACTICE **PROBLEMS**

Write the meaning of the following abbreviations.

1. pc _____   4. BID _____

2. h _____   5. prn _____

3. q12h _____

Interpret the following orders. Use either *administer* or *give* at the beginning of the sentence and write out medical and measurement abbreviations.

6. Zidovudine 200 mg PO q4h. _____

_____

7. Penicillin G 400 000 units IV q8h. _____

_____

8. Gentamicin sulphate 45 mg IVPB q12h. _____

_____

9. Regular Humulin insulin 5 units SUBCUT, ac at 7:30 AM and at bedtime. _____

_____

10. Vitamin B_{12} 1 000 mcg IM, every other day. _____

_____

11. Omeprazole 20 mg PO BID. _____

_____

12. Imipramine 75 mg PO at bedtime. _____

_____

13. Temazepam 30 mg PO at bedtime. _____

_____

14. Simethicone 30 mL PO q4h prn. _____

_____

15. Levothyroxine 200 mcg PO daily. _____

_____

Answers on page 148.

CHAPTER **REVIEW**

List the seven components of a medication order.

1. _____   5. _____

2. _____   6. _____

3. _____   7. _____

4. _____

Write the meaning of the following abbreviations.

8. ad lib _____   9. SUBCUT _____

10. ac _____   13. syp _____

11. QID _____   14. NPO _____

12. elix. _____   15. SL _____

Give the abbreviations for the following terms.

16. after meals _____   21. intravenous _____

17. three times a day _____   22. immediately _____

18. intramuscular _____   23. ointment _____

19. every eight hours _____   24. millimole _____

20. suppository _____   25. by rectum _____

Interpret the following orders. Use either *administer* or *give* at the beginning of the sentence and write out medical and measurement abbreviations.

26. Dimenhydrinate 50 mg PO q4h prn for nausea. _____

_____

27. Digoxin 0.125 mg PO once a day. _____

_____

28. Regular Humulin insulin 14 units SUBCUT daily at 7:30 AM. _____

_____

29. Meperidine 50 mg IM and atropine 0.4 mg IM on call to the operating room.

_____

30. Ampicillin 500 mg PO stat, and then 250 mg PO QID thereafter. _____

_____

31. Furosemide 40 mg IM stat. _____

_____

32. Lorazepam 1 mg SL q4h prn for anxiety. _____

_____

33. Acetaminophen 650 mg PO q4h prn for pain. _____

_____

34. Simethicone 80 mg PO pc and bedtime. _____

_____

35. Folic acid 1 mg PO daily. _____

_____

36. Lorazepam 1 mg PO at bedtime prn. _____

_____

37. Aspirin 600 mg q4h prn for temperature greater than 38.5°C. _____

_____

38. Phenytoin 100 mg PO TID. _____

_____

39. Prazocin 2 mg PO BID; hold for systolic BP less than 120. _____

_____

40. Ondansetron 8 mg PO q8h prn for nausea and vomiting during chemotherapy.

_____

41. Ampicillin 1 g IVPB q6h for 4 doses. _____

_____

42. Heparin 5 000 units SUBCUT q12h. _____

_____

43. Phenytoin susp 200 mg by NG tube q AM and 300 mg by NG tube at bedtime.

_____

44. Diphenhydramine 50 mg PO stat. _____

_____

45. Epoetin alfa 3 500 units SUBCUT three times a week. _____

_____

46. Magnesium hydroxide 30 mL PO at bedtime prn for constipation. _____

_____

47. Sulfamethoxazole/trimethoprim tab 1 PO daily. _____

_____

48. Neomycin ophthalmic ointment 1% in the right eye TID. _____

_____

49. Sucralfate 1 g via NG tube QID. _____

_____

50. Morphine sulphate 15 mg SUBCUT stat and 10 mg SUBCUT q4h prn for pain.

_____

51. Prednisone 10 mg PO every other day. _____

_____

Identify the missing part from the following medication orders. Assume that the date, time, and signature are included on the orders.

52. Amoxicillin 250 mg QID. _____

53. Levothyroxine 0.05 mg PO. _____

54. Nitrofurantoin PO q6h for 10 days. _____

55. 25 mg PO q12h, hold if BP less than 100 systolic. _____

56. Hydrocortisone sodium succinate 100 q6h. _____

57. Describe what your action would be if the following order was written:

    Omeprazole 20 mg daily. _____

Based on the discussion on medical abbreviations, symbols, and acronyms that should not be used, identify the mistake in the following orders and correct each order.

58. Propranolol 20 mg PO daily. _____

59. Furosemide 10.0 mg PO BID. _____

60. Humulin Regular insulin 4U IV stat. _____

61. Haloperidol .5 mg PO TID _____

Answers on pages 149–150.

✳ ANSWERS

Answers to Practice Problems

1. after meals

2. hour

3. every 12 hours

4. twice daily, twice a day

5. when necessary/required, as needed

6. Give or administer zidovudine 200 milligrams orally (by mouth) every 4 hours.

7. Give or administer penicillin G 400 000 units by intravenous injection every 8 hours.

8. Give or administer gentamicin sulphate 45 milligrams by intravenous piggyback injection every 12 hours.

9. Give or administer regular Humulin insulin 5 units by subcutaneous injection before the morning meal at 7:30 AM and at bedtime.

10. Give or administer vitamin B_{12} 1 000 micrograms by intramuscular injection every other day.

11. Give or administer omeprazole 20 milligrams orally (by mouth) twice a day (two times a day).

12. Give or administer imipramine 75 milligrams orally (by mouth) at bedtime.

13. Give or administer temazepam 30 milligrams orally (by mouth) at bedtime.

14. Give or administer simethicone 30 millilitres orally (by mouth) every 4 hours when necessary (when required).

15. Give or administer levothyroxine 200 micrograms orally (by mouth) daily.

evolve

Answers to Chapter Review

1. Patient's full name
2. Date and time the order was written
3. Name of the medication to be administered
4. Dose of medication
5. Route of administration
6. Time and frequency of administration
7. Signature of the person writing the order
8. as desired
9. subcutaneous
10. before meals
11. four times a day
12. elixir
13. syrup
14. nothing by mouth
15. sublingual
16. pc
17. TID
18. IM
19. q8h
20. supp
21. IV
22. stat
23. ung *or* oint
24. mmol
25. pr

26. Give or administer dimenhydrinate 50 milligrams orally (by mouth) every 4 hours when necessary/required (as needed) for nausea.

27. Give or administer digoxin 0.125 milligrams orally (by mouth) once a day.

28. Give or administer regular Humulin insulin 14 units by subcutaneous injection daily at 7:30 AM.

29. Give or administer meperidine 50 milligrams by intramuscular injection and atropine 0.4 milligrams by intramuscular injection on call to the operating room.

30. Give or administer ampicillin 500 milligrams orally (by mouth) immediately and then 250 milligrams orally (by mouth) four times a day thereafter.

31. Give or administer furosemide 40 milligrams by intramuscular injection immediately (at once).

32. Give or administer lorazepam 1 milligram sublingually (under the tongue) every 4 hours when necessary (when required) for anxiety.

33. Give or administer acetaminophen 650 milligrams orally (by mouth) every 4 hours when necessary (when required) for pain.

34. Give or administer simethicone 80 milligrams orally (by mouth) after meals and at bedtime.

35. Give or administer folic acid 1 milligram orally (by mouth) daily.

36. Give or administer lorazepam 1 milligram orally (by mouth) at bedtime when necessary (when required).

37. Give or administer aspirin 600 milligrams orally (by mouth) every 4 hours when necessary (when required) for temperature greater than 38.5°C.

38. Give or administer phenytoin 100 milligrams orally (by mouth) three times a day.

39. Give or administer prazocin 2 milligrams orally (by mouth) two times a day. Hold for systolic blood pressure less than 120.

40. Give or administer ondansetron 8 milligrams orally (by mouth) every 8 hours when necessary (when required) for nausea and vomiting during chemotherapy.

41. Give or administer ampicillin 1 gram by intravenous piggyback injection every 6 hours for 4 doses.

42. Give or administer heparin 5 000 units by subcutaneous injection every 12 hours.

43. Give or administer phenytoin suspension 200 milligrams by nasogastric tube every morning and 300 milligrams by nasogastric tube at bedtime.

44. Give or administer diphenhydramine 50 milligrams orally (by mouth) immediately (at once).

45. Give or administer epoetin alfa 3 500 units by subcutaneous injection three times a week.

46. Give or administer magnesium hydroxide 30 millilitres orally (by mouth) at bedtime when necessary (when required) for constipation.

47. Give or administer sulfamethoxazole/trimethoprim 1 tablet orally (by mouth) daily.

48. Give or administer neomycin ophthalmic ointment 1% to the right eye three times a day.

49. Give or administer sucralfate 1 gram by nasogastric tube four times a day.

50. Give or administer morphine sulfate 15 milligrams by subcutaneous injection immediately (at once) and 10 milligrams by subcutaneous injection every 4 hours when necessary (when required) for pain.

51. Give or administer prednisone 10 milligrams orally (by mouth) every other day.

52. Route of administration

53. Frequency of administration

54. Dosage of medication

55. Name of medication

56. Dosage of medication and route of administration

57. Notify the prescriber that the order is incomplete; route is missing from the order; do not administer, order not legal. Never assume.

58. Propranolol 20 mg PO daily. There should be adequate spacing between the medication name, dosage, and unit of measurement. Could be misread as 120 mg, which is 6 times the dose ordered.

59. Furosemide 10 mg PO BID. Trailing zeros could cause dose to be interpreted as 100 mg, which is 10 times the intended dose.

60. Humulin Regular Insulin 4 units IV stat. The abbreviation for *units* here could be misread as a zero, which could result in 10 times the dose being administered. Write out *units*.

61. Haloperidol 0.5 mg PO TID. Omission of the zero before the decimal point could result in the dosage being read as 5 mg, which would be 10 times the dose ordered.

CHAPTER 10

Medication Administration Records and Medication Distribution Systems

Objectives

After reviewing the chapter, you should be able to:

1. State the components of a medication order
2. Identify the necessary components of a medication administration record (MAR)
3. Read a MAR and identify medications that are to be administered on a routine basis, including the name of the medication, the dose, the route of administration, and the time of administration
4. Read a MAR and identify medications that are administered, including the name of the medication, the dose, the route of administration, and the time of administration
5. Identify the various medication distribution systems used in health care settings

Medication Orders

Before any medication can be administered or transcribed, there must be an order. Hospitals usually have a special form for recording medication orders. The terms *medication orders* and *doctor's orders* are used interchangeably, and the forms vary from institution to institution. As more and more hospitals transition to electronic medical records, handwritten medication order forms are gradually being replaced by computerized provider order entry (CPOE), which is also referred to as *computerized prescriber order entry*. According to Cancer Care Ontario (2012), CPOE is effective in preventing medication errors and their resulting adverse events.

See Figure 10-1 for a sample CPOE. Notice that in addition to medication orders, other measures related to patient care are also indicated (e.g., strict intake and output, daily weights). The status of the orders is also indicated (e.g., active, discontinued [DC], completed); note that the order for furosemide IV is completed. The medication orders in the CPOE contain all of the components of a medication order. Notice also that the top of the electronic order form has an area for identifying information of the patient.

Medication Administration Record

The medication administration record (MAR) is a form used to document medications a patient has received and is currently receiving. MARs are legal documents that may be handwritten (Figure 10-2) or electronic (Figure 10-3). Electronic medication administration records (eMARs) are viewed and charted on the computer. There is no standard MAR form; the form varies from institution to institution. However, MAR forms across institutions differ in format only; all include the same essential information (the name of each medication, the dose, the route, and the frequency). Whether the MAR is electronic or handwritten, it contains the same information indicated on a medication order and

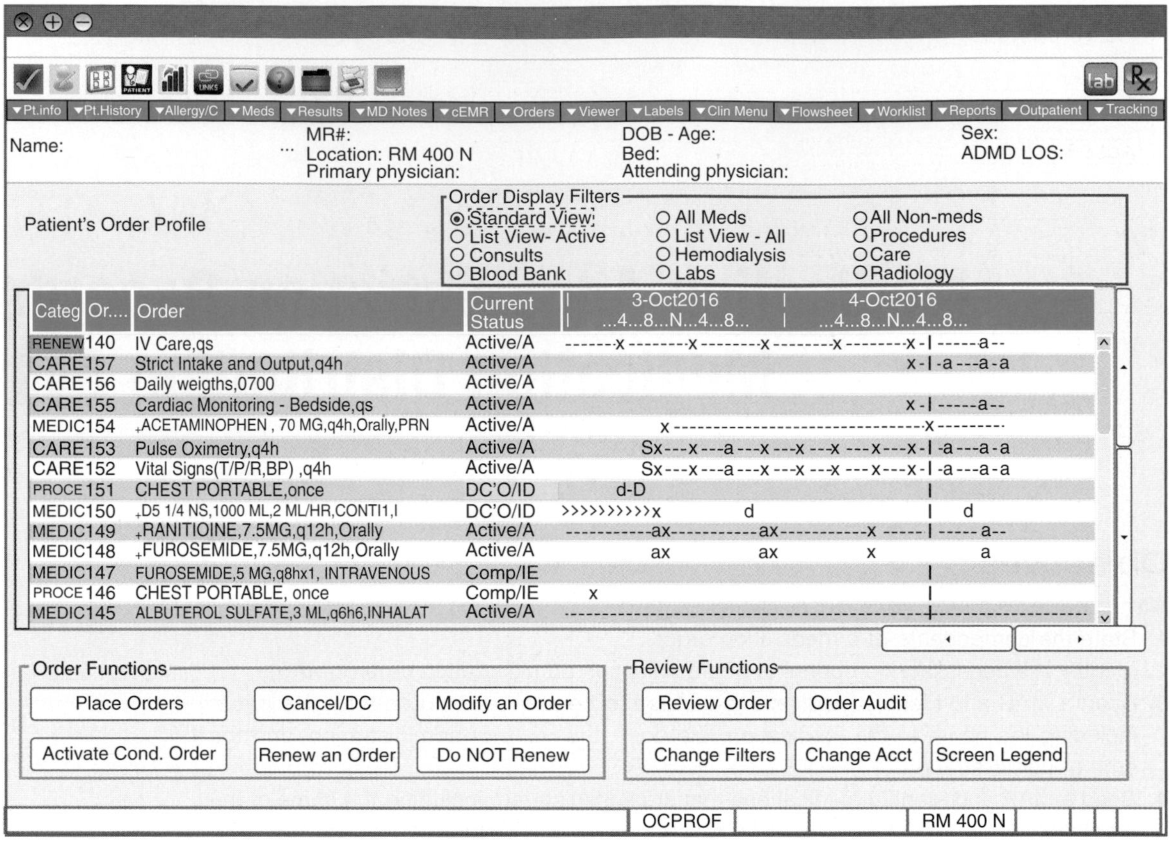

Figure 10-1 Sample computerized provider order entry (CPOE).

specifies the actual time to administer the medication or the actual time of administration. Regardless of the format used to document the administration of medications, the documentation must be accurate, and legally all medications administered must be documented. Documentation should follow the administration of medication and include not only medications administered but also information regarding refusals, delays in administration, and responses to medication administration (including adverse effects). Different forms may be used in the home care setting for the charting of medications that are administered.

> **! SAFETY ALERT!**
>
> Properly and accurately document all medications administered to prevent medication errors caused by overmedication or undermedication.

At some institutions, a complete schedule is written out for all of the administration times for medications given on a continual or routine basis. The method of charting medications on MARs varies from one institution to another (e.g., some require that nurses sign for the day and just put in times given, while others require that nurses note times given and initial each entry). The method of charting medications on eMARs also varies, but each time a dose is given, the nurse records his or her initials next to the time given. Some institutions maintain separate records for routine, intravenous (IV), as-needed (prn) medications (Figure 10-4), and medications administered on a one-time basis, whereas other institutions keep all administered medications on the same record in a designated area.

> **i TIPS FOR CLINICAL PRACTICE**
>
> Regardless of whether the MAR is handwritten or electronic, the nurse uses the MAR to check the medication order, prepare the correct dose, and record the medication administered to a patient.

DEPARTMENT OF NURSING
MEDICATION ADMINISTRATION RECORD

Identifying Client Information (Name,
Room Number, Date of Birth, Medical
Record Number)

Diagnosis:

ALLERGIES: NKDA   Date: 4/2/2016

Order Date	Exp. Date	RN Initial	Medication-Dosage, Frequency, Route	Date 2016	4/2	4/3	4/4	4/5	4/6	4/7	4/8
				Time	Initial	Initial	Initial	Initial	Initial	Initial	Initial
4/2/16	5/2/16	DG	Colace 100 mg PO BID	0900	DG	JN					
				1700	NN	NN					
4/2/16	5/2/16	DG	Furosemide 40 mg PO daily	0900	DG						
4/2/16	5/2/16	DG	K - Dur 10 mmol PO BID	0900	DG	JN					
				1700	NN	NN					
4/2/16	5/2/16	DG	Digoxin 0.125 mg PO daily	0900	DG	JN					
			Check apical pulse (AP)	AP	76	80					
			Hold if less than 60 or above 100 beats per minute (bpm)								

	Initial	Print Name/Title		Initial	Print Name/Title		Initial	Print Name/Title
1	DG	Deborah Gray RN	5			9		
2	NN	Nancy Nurse RN	6			10		
3	JN	Jane Nightingale RN	7			11		
4			8			12		

Figure 10-2 Medication administration record (MAR). *Note:* This MAR is intended to show the basic information that would be included in a MAR.

Essential Components of a Medication Administration Record

If a handwritten MAR is used, the information on the medication record must be legible and transcribed carefully to avoid errors. In addition to patient information (name, date of birth, medical record number, allergies), the following information is necessary on all MARs regardless of the format:

- **Dates.** This information usually includes the date the order was written, the date the medication is to be started (if different from the order date), and when to discontinue it.
- **Medication information.** This information includes the medication's full name, the dose, the route, and the frequency. Abbreviations used on the medication record should be standard abbreviations and follow the guidelines and restrictions of the Institute for Safe Medication Practices (ISMP Canada, 2006b) and the health care institution.
- **Time of administration.** This information is based on the desired administration schedule stated on the order, such as TID (three times a day). The desired administration time is placed on the medication record and converted to time periods based on the institution's time intervals for scheduled or routine medications. Nurses should always become familiar with the hours for medication administration designated by their specific institution. Medication times for prn and one-time dosages are recorded at the time they are administered. Abbreviations for time and frequency should adhere to ISMP Canada guidelines.

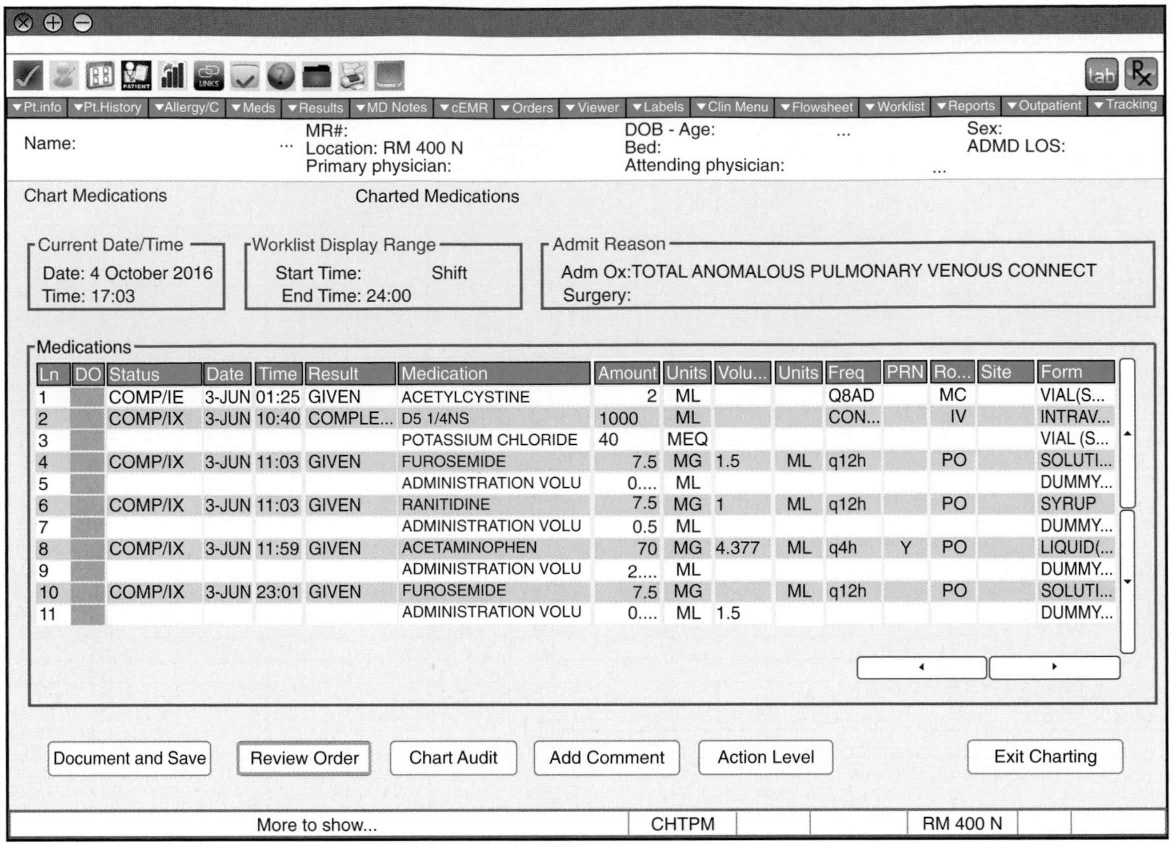

Pt.info | Pt.History | Allergy/C | Meds | Results | MD Notes | cEMR | Orders | Viewer | Labels | Clin Menu | Flowsheet | Worklist | Reports | Outpatient | Tracking

Name: ... MR#: Location: RM 400 N Primary physician: DOB - Age: ... Bed: Attending physician: ... Sex: ADMD LOS:

Chart Medications Charted Medications

Current Date/Time
Date: 4 October 2016
Time: 17:03

Worklist Display Range
Start Time: Shift
End Time: 24:00

Admit Reason
Adm Ox:TOTAL ANOMALOUS PULMONARY VENOUS CONNECT
Surgery:

Medications

Ln	DO	Status	Date	Time	Result	Medication	Amount	Units	Volu...	Units	Freq	PRN	Ro...	Site	Form
1		COMP/IE	3-JUN	01:25	GIVEN	ACETYLCYSTINE	2	ML			Q8AD		MC		VIAL(S...
2		COMP/IX	3-JUN	10:40	COMPLE...	D5 1/4NS	1000	ML			CON...		IV		INTRAV...
3						POTASSIUM CHLORIDE	40	MEQ							VIAL (S...
4		COMP/IX	3-JUN	11:03	GIVEN	FUROSEMIDE	7.5	MG	1.5	ML	q12h		PO		SOLUTI...
5						ADMINISTRATION VOLU	0....	ML							DUMMY...
6		COMP/IX	3-JUN	11:03	GIVEN	RANITIDINE	7.5	MG	1	ML	q12h		PO		SYRUP
7						ADMINISTRATION VOLU	0.5	ML							DUMMY...
8		COMP/IX	3-JUN	11:59	GIVEN	ACETAMINOPHEN	70	MG	4.377	ML	q4h	Y	PO		LIQUID(...
9						ADMINISTRATION VOLU	2....	ML							DUMMY...
10		COMP/IX	3-JUN	23:01	GIVEN	FUROSEMIDE	7.5	MG		ML	q12h		PO		SOLUTI...
11						ADMINISTRATION VOLU	0....	ML	1.5						DUMMY...

Document and Save | Review Order | Chart Audit | Add Comment | Action Level | Exit Charting

More to show... | CHTPM | RM 400 N

Figure 10-3 Electronic medication administration record (eMAR).

- **Initials.** Most medication records have a place for the initials of the person transcribing the medication to the MAR and the person administering the medication. The initials are then written under the signature section to identify who gave the medication. Some forms may request the title as well as the signature of the nurse. The policy regarding initialling after each administration varies by institution and by charting system used. See Figure 10-4 for an example.
- **Special instructions (parameters).** Any special instructions relating to a medication should be indicated on the medication record. For example, "Hold if blood pressure less than 100 systolic" or "prn for pain." Refer to the Percocet and Tylenol order shown on the MAR in Figure 10-4.

In addition to the information listed above, some medication records may include legends, as well as an area for charting to indicate when a medication is omitted or a dose is not given. Other medication records may have an area where the nurse can document the reason for omission of a medication directly on the medication record. Other information may include injection codes so that the nurse may indicate the injection site for parenteral medications. In cases in which no injection codes are indicated, the nurse is still expected to indicate the injection site. Space may also be allotted for charting information such as pulse and blood pressure if this information is relevant to the medication.

> **TIPS FOR CLINICAL PRACTICE**
>
> The nurse must stay alert to the guidelines of ISMP Canada regarding abbreviations and medical notations. Please refer to https://www.ismp-canada.org.

Documentation of Medication Administration

Handwritten MARs include an area for documenting medications administered. After administering the medication, the nurse or other qualified staff member must record his or her initials next to the time the medication was administered. For scheduled medications, a complete schedule is written out, and the initials are recorded next to each given

DEPARTMENT OF NURSING
MEDICATION RECORD

Identifying Client Information (Name, Room Number, Date of Birth, Medical Record Number)

Diagnosis:

ALLERGIES: NKDA Date: 4/9/2016

Order Date	Exp. Date	Initials	PRN MEDICATIONS Med-Dose-Freq-Route								
4/10/16	4/13/16	DG	Percocet 2 tabs PO q4h prn	Date	4/10/16	4/10/16					
			for pain for 3 days	Time	1800	2200					
				Initial	DG	DG					
4/10/16	4/17/16	NN	Tylenol 650 mg PO q4h prn	Date	4/10/16						
			for temp greater than 38.3 C	Time	1400						
				Initial	NN						
4/10/16	4/17/16	JN	Robitussin DM 10 mL PO	Date	4/11/16						
			q12 prn	Time	2200						
				Initial	JN						

	Initial	Print Name/Title		Initial	Print Name/Title		Initial	Print Name/Title
1	DG	Deborah Gray RN	5			9		
2	NN	Nancy Nurse RN	6			10		
3	JN	Jane Nightingale RN	7			11		
4			8			12		

Figure 10-4 Medication administration record (MAR) showing prn medications.

time. As previously mentioned, this practice can vary by institution. With one-time dosages and prn medication, *the time of administration* is written and again initialled by the person administering it. The MAR has a section for the full name of each person administering medications, along with their identifying initials. This section allows for immediate identification of a person's initials.

When medications are not administered, some records have notations, such as an asterisk (*), a circle, or a number corresponding to a legend on the MAR to indicate this, or there may be an area on the back or at the bottom of the MAR for charting medications not given. The type of notation used will depend on the institution.

In addition to notations made on the MAR, most institutions require documentation in the proper section of the patient's chart. Most institutions have a section designated for *Interdisciplinary Progress Notes,* where all members of the interprofessional team document their care identified by the codes used for the discipline. For example, "NUR" beside a section of notes indicates that a nurse has documented those notes.

In institutions in which eMARs are used, the documentation of medications administered is done on a computer. An eMAR also allows the nurse to document comments regarding the medication administration at the computer terminal. Like CPOEs, eMARs are gradually replacing the transcription tasks that were frequently done by nurses and identified as a major contributor to medication errors.

Regardless of whether a handwritten MAR or an eMAR is used, documentation should be done immediately after medications are given. Remember: this practice will prevent forgetting to document, which can result in the administration of the medication by another nurse who thought the medication was not administered. The absence of documentation can be interpreted as medication not being administered.

Computers and Medication Administration

As in other businesses, the use of computers in health care facilities is increasing. As a result of the reported rise in medication errors, many health care facilities have instituted some form of computer-based medication administration.

To improve patient safety and enhance the availability and quality of patient care, Canada Health Infoway has collaborated with every province and territory to support a range of electronic health record (EHR) projects (Canada Health Infoway, 2010). Since 2001, the federal government has provided Infoway with a total of $2.1 billion to develop the health information and communications technology (ICT) needed to create a unified health care system. The total cost associated with this effort is estimated to be between $10 and $12 billion. However, once all of its components are implemented in the health care system, health ICT is expected to lead to savings and efficiencies valued at $6 billion annually.

The health care sector's adoption and use of ICT is central to Canada's digital economy strategy. The level of ICT adoption and use varies across the health care sector. However, the use of health ICT has resulted in improvements in medication management.

The literature supports the fact that one of the causes of medication errors is the incorrect transcription of the original prescriber's order. Many health care facilities have moved away from the written medication order and the transcription of orders on a MAR to a CPOE.

CPOE systems have been consistently identified in the literature as important mechanisms for reducing prescription errors and subsequent patient injury (Cancer Care Ontario, 2012). A prescriber's medication orders are either electronically transmitted or manually entered into the CPOE system. The CPOE system accepts orders in a standard format that conforms to strict criteria. Once the order has been entered into the system, it is transmitted to the pharmacy to be processed. Depending on the institution and the sophistication of the software, information such as medication incompatibilities, medication allergies, range of dosages, and recommended medication times may be part of the system. Information such as medication incompatibilities shows the importance of computers to the safe administration of medication. When a computer is used to process medication orders, orders can be viewed onscreen or in a printout. A corresponding MAR is available at some institutions based on the computerized order entry. An eMAR allows the nurse to chart medications on the computer, as well as any other essential information relating to medication administration. Each institution generates its own medication record according to a specific format.

At some institutions, after the entry of orders into the CPOE system, the computer automatically generates a list of all the medications to be given to patients on a unit and the times the medications are to be given. The computer has become an essential tool for medication administration at some institutions.

Figure 10-3 shows a sample of an eMAR using the bar-code scanned medications charted. Notice that medications administered are indicated by "Given" and the time administered. Another screen on an eMAR would allow for identification of the person who administered the medication. (Note: This eMAR is being shown for educational purposes only; therefore, patient information is not indicated.)

Medication Distribution Systems

The various medication distribution systems available to health care institutions are discussed in the following sections.

Unit-Dose Systems

Many institutions use a system of medication distribution referred to as a *unit dose dispensing system* (UDDS). This system has decreased medication preparation time for nurses because the medications are prepared daily in the pharmacy and sent to the unit.

Figure 10-5 Unit-dose cabinet. (From Clayton, B. D., & Willihnganz, M. (2013). *Basic pharmacology for nurses* (16th ed.). St. Louis: Mosby.)

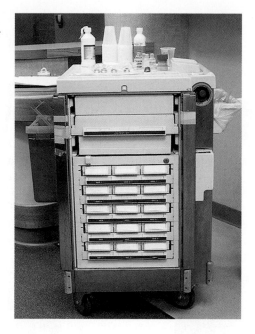

Medications are **dispensed** by the pharmacy in separately wrapped packets that include an individualized dose for a specific patient. Each package is labelled with generic and trade names (and sometimes manufacturer, lot number, and expiration date). Depending on the distribution system, individual packages may be labelled with the patient's name and bar code that matches the bar code of the patient's identification wristband. The medications are placed in a patient-identified drawer in a large unit-dose cabinet at the nurse's station (Figure 10-5). Cohen (2010) points out that not all medications can be dispensed in unit doses. For example, sometimes nurses have to prepare IV doses from floor stock medications to comply with a stat order. Therefore, errors may occur that a fully implemented UDDS could have prevented.

Unit dose is also used as part of another medication system in some institutions (e.g., a computerized unit-dose medication cart). In the computerized unit-dose system, each dose for the patient is released individually and recorded automatically. This system is used for monitoring controlled substances and other items used in the unit (e.g., medications used by the unit in large volumes). The type of medication form used for this system varies from one institution to another. This system has tended to decrease the amount of time spent transcribing orders or eliminated the need for transcription. Some institutions still require the transcription of medication orders to a MAR (see Figure 10-2). In such contexts, the prescriber's orders are written on a separate order sheet and sent to the pharmacy. Other institutions require that the prescriber's order be done by computer entry, eliminating the need for transcription.

Computer-Controlled Dispensing Systems

The use of automated dispensing cabinets (ADCs) is on the rise in health care facilities. The computer-controlled dispensing system is supplied by the pharmacy daily with stock medications. Controlled substances are also kept in the cart, and the system provides a detailed record indicating which controlled substances were used and by whom. The medication order is received by the pharmacy for each patient and then entered into the system. To access medications in this system, the nurse must use a security code and a password or a biometric fingerprint scan.

The three most common computer-controlled dispensing systems are the Pyxis Med Station (Figure 10-6), the Omnicell Omni Rx, and the AcuDose Rx.

The Omnicell system shown in Figure 10-7 is a mobile medication system that assists in providing for the safe and secure transportation of medications from the ADC to the patient's bedside. It allows the nurse to retrieve routine as well as prn medications. The system can record medications administered, along with those wasted, remotely. It also allows nurses to retrieve all medications that are needed for a patient without having to

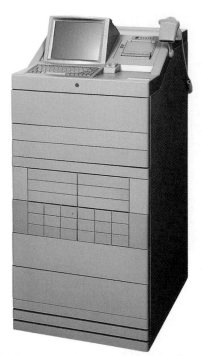

Figure 10-6 Pyxis Med Station System. (From Clayton, B. D., & Willihnganz, M. (2013). *Basic pharmacology for nurses* (16th ed.). St. Louis: Mosby.)

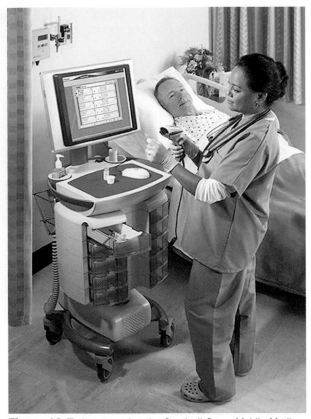

Figure 10-7 A nurse using the Omnicell Savvy Mobile Medication System at the patient's bedside. (Used with permission of Omnicell.)

make multiple trips to the ADC. A controlled substance management system is also part of this mobile unit, and it provides an inventory of controlled substances that are used.

ADCs can store items such as vials and premixed IVs and allow nurses to obtain any medications stocked in the device for any patient and even to override the system in an emergency. However, overrides eliminate verification of medications by the pharmacy, which could result in errors. Currently, almost 90% of all ADCs are linked to pharmacy information systems, thereby decreasing errors by ensuring that the nurse can only access medications for a specific patient.

Some ADCs incorporate bar codes in the medication administration process. At the patient's bedside, the nurse uses a hand-held scanner that records the bar code on the patient's identification wristband and the unit-dose medication packet, linking this information to the patient database. If there is an error, the medication administration process is halted; if the information is correct, the medication is administered and documentation in an eMAR is recorded automatically. Literature supports that the use of ADCs has reduced medication errors by dispensing the correct medication.

Bar-Code Medication Delivery

Bar-code medication delivery is increasing in Canadian health care facilities. *Medication Bar Code System Implementation Planning: A Resource Guide,* published by ISMP Canada (2013c) in collaboration with the Canadian Patient Safety Institute (CPSI) makes a compelling case that this automated system enhances patient safety. This resource guide has garnered excellent feedback from some of Canada's finest health care leaders. For instance, the Canadian Nurses Association (CNA) states that the nursing profession, which is responsible for delivering more care than any other group in the health care system, fully supports the widespread adoption of medication bar-code technology (ISMP Canada, 2013b, p. 6). CNA also asserts that in order for bar coding to improve patient safety, nurses and other health care providers need a clear understanding of how the technology works and how to use it to support their practice.

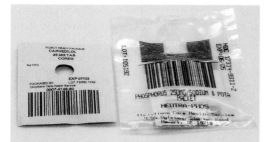

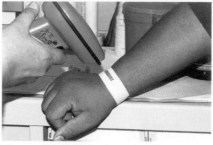

Figure 10-8 Bar code for unit-dose medication. (From Kee, J. L., & Marshall, S. M. (2013). *Clinical calculations: With applications to general and specialty areas* (7th ed.). St. Louis: Saunders.)

Figure 10-9 Bar-code reader. (From Kee, J. L., & Marshall, S. M. (2013). *Clinical calculations: With applications to general and specialty areas* (7th ed.). St. Louis: Saunders.)

The basic system of bar coding verifies that a patient receives the right dose of the right medication by the right route at the right time. This system requires that each patient wear an identification wristband with a unique bar code. Each medication must therefore have a bar code that matches the bar code of a patient. Computers installed at the patient's bedside and/or hand-held devices enable the nurse to scan the bar code on the patient's wristband and the medication to be administered. Once the information has been validated to the patient and the patient's medication profile, the medication given is documented on an eMAR (Figure 10-8 shows a bar code for unit-dose medication, and Figure 10-9 shows a bar-code reader). Bar coding is being added to some medication distribution systems as mentioned in the discussions of unit-dose and computer-controlled dispensing systems. Many pharmacists are using the bar-code system to prepare unit-dose medications. The bar-code medication administration system allows overrides in cases where medications need to be administered in an emergency. However, literature points out that an override bypasses the important step of order verification by the pharmacist.

Additional Technology in Medication Administration

Computer-based drug administration (CBDA) is a technological software system that has been designed to prevent medication errors. The purpose of the software is to automate the medication administration process and improve accuracy and efficiency in documentation. The system comprises the CPOE system, the bar-code medication delivery system, an eMAR, and the pharmacy information system.

When used with the bar-code medication delivery system, an eMAR acts as a stringent safeguard to ensure patient safety in medication administration. An eMAR uses the bar code on the patient's wristband and the bar code on the medication supplied by the pharmacy through CPOE. Before administering medication, bar codes on the patient's wristband and the medication are scanned using the bar-code scanner. The computer then checks the medications against the patient's history (allergies, medication history) and lab results. The computer verifies and confirms that the nurse is administering the right medication to the right patient in the right dose, by the right route, and at the right time. The computer also alerts the nurse to any conditions that should be checked before administering the medication. The pharmacist and the nurse can access the computerized record to confirm medication delivery.

Advantages and Disadvantages of Technology

The nursing literature supports the belief that technology has decreased the number of medication errors; however, the risks of medication errors with technology have also been discussed. Even though the use of technology in the health care system has increased, technology-based medication administration systems are not foolproof.

Technology cannot eliminate all medication errors, but it can provide safeguards that are not possible in manual processes. ISMP Canada (2013b) agrees that the implementation of any new technology requires systematic planning and the preparation of employees to work with the program. Any technology implemented in a health care setting does not substitute for the knowledge of the practitioner or eliminate the need for health care providers to take basic safety precautions. Literature relating to the use of technology in the health care system reinforces the need for nurses and other health care providers to be properly educated on its use to avoid compromising patient safety. Basic safety precautions such as patient identification cannot be eliminated and can help reduce medication errors, even when technology is used. With the influx of new medications and technology in the health care system, nurses must remain competent and accountable for their own actions regarding patient safety.

POINTS TO REMEMBER

- The system used for medication administration plays a role in determining the type of medication record used and whether the transcription of orders is necessary.
- Regardless of the type of medication record used at an institution, the nurse should know the data that are essential for the medication record and understand the importance of accuracy and clarity on medication orders.
- Persons transcribing orders should transcribe them in ink and write legibly to avoid medication errors. All essential notations or instructions should be clearly written on the medication record. Notations should follow ISMP Canada guidelines.
- Documentation of medications administered should be done promptly, accurately, and only by the person administering the medications.
- To avoid errors in administration, the nurse should always check transcribed orders against the prescriber's orders.
- The use of technology has reduced medication errors.
- The nurse must be aware of the different distribution systems in use.
- Regardless of the system used, patient safety is the priority, and the nurse must still follow the process in medication administration of verifying the order and administering the medication according to practice standards and guidelines.

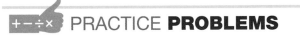 PRACTICE **PROBLEMS**

1. True or false? Illegible prescribers' handwriting is the most common reason for medication errors on handwritten MARs. _____

2. True or false? The use of technology is a foolproof method to prevent medication errors. _____

3. True or false? Medication administration forms have information that is common to all, regardless of the format used. _____

4. The _____ is responsible for the medication administered, regardless of the reason for the error.

5. The Pyxis is an example of _____.

6. The ability to _____ a system eliminates _____ by the pharmacy, which increases the likelihood of a medication error.

7. What is the last step in medication administration? _____

8. CPOE is an abbreviation for _____.

Refer to the handwritten MAR in Figure 10-2 to answer the following questions.

9. How many times a day is furosemide ordered? _____

10. Identify the medications and their doses administered at 0900. _____

11. Potassium chloride 10 mmol is ordered. What does mmol mean?

    _____

12. What action must you take before administering digoxin? _____

13. What is the equivalent of the scheduled administration time for potassium chloride
    (K-Dur) in traditional time? _____

Refer to the eMAR in Figure 10-3 to answer the following questions.

14. What is the ordered route of administration for ranitidine? _____

15. What is the frequency ordered for furosemide? _____

Answers on page 162.

CHAPTER **REVIEW**

1. Who determines medication administration times? _____

2. Do BID and q2h have the same meaning? _____ Explain: _____

   _____

   _____

3. What is the purpose of bar coding? _____

4. The abbreviation *eMAR* stands for _____.

5. Times for medication administration can be indicated in _____ or

   _____.

Refer to the eMAR in Figure 10-3 to answer the following questions.

6. Which medications are indicated as being prn? _____

7. What is the frequency indicated for the prn medications? _____

8. What time and date was the acetaminophen and codeine phosphate (APAP w/codeine)
   administered? (Give date and state time in traditional and international time.)

   _____

Refer to the handwritten MAR in Figure 10-4 to answer the following questions.

9. What would be the next time the patient could receive Percocet if needed? (Give
   date and state time in traditional and international time.) _____

10. When could the patient receive another dose of Robitussin DM if needed? (Give date and state time in traditional and international time.) _____

Answers on page 162.

✳ ANSWERS

Answers to Practice Problems

1. True

2. False

3. True

4. nurse

5. an automated dispensing cabinet (ADC), which is a computer-controlled dispensing system

6. override, verification

7. documentation

8. computerized provider order entry

9. Once a day

10. Colace 100 mg, furosemide 40 mg, K-DUR 10 mEq, digoxin 0.125 mg

11. Millimole

12. Check the patient's apical pulse

13. 9:00 AM, 5:00 PM

14. PO (orally, by mouth)

15. q12h

Answers to Chapter Review

1. hospital, institution, or health care facility

2. No. BID means the order will be given two times in 24 hours, whereas a q2h order would be given 12 times in 24 hours.

3. To ensure dispensing and administration of the correct medication to the right patient

4. Electronic medication administration record

5. traditional time, military time (international time)

6. Acetaminophen, and APAP with codeine

7. q4h (every 4 hours)

8. June 3, 5:38 PM, 1738

9. 4/11/16 2:00 AM, 0200

10. 4/12/16 10:00 AM, 1000

---

evolve

For additional information, refer to the Safety in Medication Administration section of the Drug Calculations Companion, Version 5 on Evolve.

Reading Medication Labels

Objectives

After reviewing this chapter, you should be able to:

1. Identify the generic and trade names of medications
2. Identify the dosage strength of medications
3. Identify the form in which a medication is supplied
4. Identify the total volume of a medication container, where indicated
5. Locate directions for mixing or preparing a medication, where necessary
6. Understand how to read information on a combination medication label

Administering medications safely to a patient begins with the nurse accurately reading and interpreting the information on a medication label. The medication label provides the information needed to perform dosage calculations. It includes the dosage contained in the package, the medication name, form, total volume (for liquid forms of medication), total amount in container (for solid forms of medication), route of administration, warnings, storage requirements, and manufacturing information. In addition, the label includes the expiration date and a Drug Identification Number (DIN). It is important to read a medication label carefully and recognize essential information.

> **! SAFETY ALERT!**
> Always read a medication label carefully. Read the label three times to prevent an error in administration of the wrong medication.

Reading Medication Labels

The nurse should be able to recognize the following pertinent information on a medication label.

Generic Name

Every medication has an official name, which is referred to as the *generic name*. By law, the generic name must be identified on all medication labels. The generic name is given by the manufacturer that first develops the medication. Medications have only one generic name. Prescribers in Canada are encouraged to order medication in the generic name, but nurses need to know both the generic name and the trade name of medication. Pharmacists in health care institutions dispense medications by generic name along with the trade name even if the prescriber orders it by the trade name. On a medication label, the generic name appears directly under the trade name and sometimes is placed inside parentheses.

Sometimes only the generic name appears on a medication label or package. This is common for medications that have been used for many years, are well established, and do not require marketing under a different trade name. An example is heparin (Figure 11-1). Other examples of medications commonly used in the clinical setting and often seen with only the generic name on the label are furosemide (Figure 11-2, *A*) and famciclovir (Figure 11-2, *B*). Lasix is the trade name for furosemide; however, this medication is often seen with the generic name only, furosemide.

> ### ⓘ TIPS FOR CLINICAL PRACTICE
>
> It is important for the nurse to cross-check all medications, whether just the generic name or both the trade and generic names appear on the label, to accurately identify a medication. Failure to cross-check medications could lead to choosing the wrong medication, a violation of the rights of medication administration ("the right medication"; see Chapter 8).

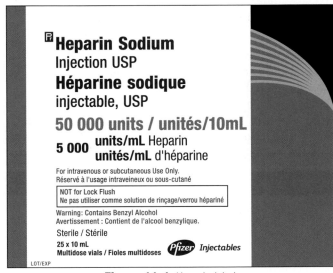

Figure 11-1 Heparin label.

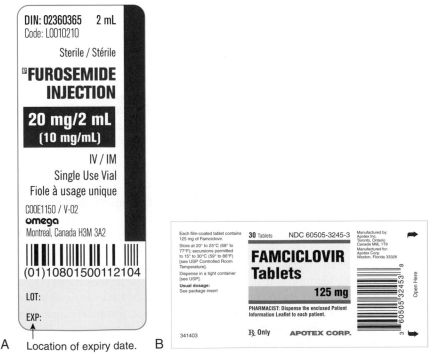

Figure 11-2 A, Furosemide label: 20 mg per 2 mL (10 mg per mL). **B,** Famciclovir label: 125 mg per tablet.

Remember that medications with similar names may have markedly different chemical structures and actions. Consider, for example, buspirone (BuSpar), which is an antianxiety medication, and bupropion (Welbutrin), which is used to treat major depressive disorder. Although the generic names are similar, the action, composition, and use of the medications are different. The U.S. Institute for Safe Medication Practices (ISMP, 2015) has recommended that "Tall Man" lettering be used to distinguish look-alike generic name pairs that are associated with errors. Tall Man lettering uses mixed-case, enlarged, bolded, or italic letters to distinguish the differing portions of similar medication names. The U.S. Food and Drug Administration–approved versions of buspirone and bupropion with Tall Man lettering are bus**PIR**one and bu**PROP**ion. Notice that the letters are bolded and capitalized to indicate the differing portions of the names.

Following their U.S. counterparts, Canadian practitioners have collaborated in various health care disciplines to identify look-alike and sound-alike (LA/SA) medication names that have great potential for patient injury. For example, the Canadian Association of Provincial Cancer Agencies (CAPCA) and the Institute for Safe Medication Practices Canada (ISMP Canada) have recommended that Tall Man lettering be applied to medications used in oncology that have easily confusable names (ISMP Canada, 2010).

Trade Name

The trade name is also referred to as the *brand name* or *proprietary name*; it is the manufacturer's name for the medication. Notice that the brand name is very prominent on the label and is capitalized to market the medication.

In Figures 11-3 and 11-4, note that the trade name is listed before the generic name. A trade name is for the sole use of the company that manufactures the medication. The trade name is identified by a registered trademark ®, a symbol that means the name has been legally registered with a national trademark office (in Canada, the Canadian Intellectual Property Office) and that the owner of the trademark has exclusive rights to its use.

Figure 11-3 shows the label for leuprolide acetate (Lupron). Lupron is the trade name identified by the registered trademark symbol ®. The name below in smaller print,

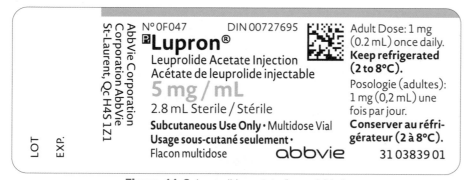

Figure 11-3 Leuprolide acetate (Lupron) label.

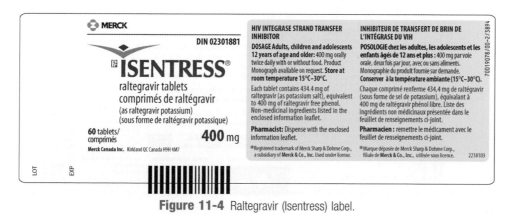

Figure 11-4 Raltegravir (Isentress) label.

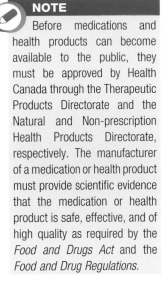

leuprolide acetate, is the generic name of the medication. It is important to remember that the same medication may be manufactured by different manufacturers but is marketed under different trade names.

Notice the registered trademark symbol ® after the name Isentress in Figure 11-4. This indicates that the medication name is a trademark that belongs to the manufacturer. Therefore, the trade name cannot be used by another company. Once the Canadian Intellectual Property Office formally registers an unregistered trademark, the symbol ® will then appear on the medication label. The name below Isentress in smaller print and enclosed in parentheses—raltegravir—is the generic name.

Dosage Strength

Dosage strength refers to the weight or amount of the medication provided in a specific unit of measurement (the weight per tablet [tab], capsule, millilitre [mL], milligram [mg], microgram [mcg], etc.). For solid forms of medications, the dosage strength is the amount of medication per tablet, capsule, or other form. For liquid medications, the dosage strength is the amount of medication present in a certain amount of solution.

Examples: In Figure 11-3, the dosage strength of Lupron is 5 mg (the weight and specific unit of measurement) per mL. In Figure 11-4, the dosage strength of Isentress is 400 mg per tablet (the weight and specific unit of measurement). In Figure 11-5, the dosage strength of oral solution Azithromycin is 200 mg per 5 mL. Some medication labels, such as the label for Apo-Pen-VK oral solution in Figure 11-6, may have two different but equivalent dosage strengths shown on the label. Apo-Pen-VK has a dosage strength of 300 mg (per 5 mL) or 480 000 units (per 5 mL). The prescriber therefore could order the medication in either unit of measurement.

Dosage strength can be expressed in different systems of measurement. Some oral liquids may state household measures (e.g., each 15 mL contains 80 mg).

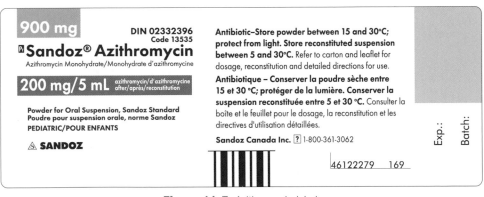

Figure 11-5 Azithromycin label.

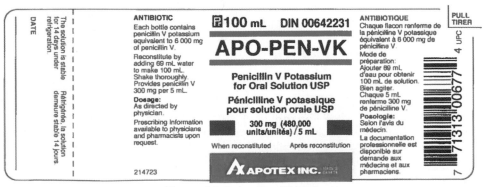

Figure 11-6 Apo-Pen-VK label.

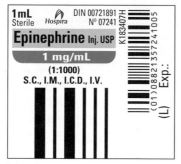

Figure 11-7 Epinephrine label. Epinephrine contains 1 g of medication per 1 000 mL solution (1 : 1 000) and 1 mg per mL.

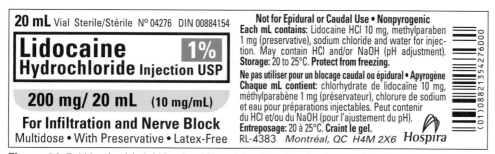

Figure 11-8 Lidocaine label. Lidocaine 1% contains 1 g of medication per 100 mL solution and 10 mg per mL.

Dosage Expressed as a Ratio or Percentage. Sometimes the dosage for a solution is expressed as a ratio or percentage. Refer to the labels in Figures 11-7 and 11-8. Notice that the labels also express the dosage strength in milligrams per millilitres.

> **⚠ SAFETY ALERT!**
>
> ISMP Canada recommends that the slash mark (/) not be used to separate two doses or to indicate *per* because it can be misread and mistaken for the number *1*. Use *per* rather than the slash mark. Example: Use 10 mg per 5 mL. Do not use 10 mg/5 mL, which could be misread as 10 mg and 15 mL. This approach is followed in this text.

Form

The form specifies the type of preparation available in the package.

- Examples of forms are tablets, capsules, liquids, suppositories, and ointments. Solutions may be indicated by millilitres and described as oral suspension or aqueous solution. Some medications are available in powdered or granular form or as patches.

- Labels may also include abbreviations or words that describe the form of the medication. Examples are CR (controlled release), LA (long acting), DS (double strength), SR (sustained release), XL (extended release), and ES (extra strength). Some labels may use abbreviations such as EC (enteric coated) or just indicate "enteric coated"; these medications should not be crushed. Figure 11-9, *D* shows ERYC capsules, which are enteric coated.

- Abbreviations that describe the form of a medication indicate whether the medication has been prepared in a way that allows extended action (or slow release) of the active ingredient. Typically, these medications are given less frequently. Examples are Procardia XL, Inderal LA, Calan SR, and metformin hydrochloride extended-release tablets. These special forms should be swallowed whole and never crushed. Always read labels carefully. Refer to the labels in Figure 11-9, *A–D* for examples of medication labels that indicate special forms. Also note that the label for ERYC in Figure 11-9, *D* indicates that the tablets are delayed release and enteric coated.

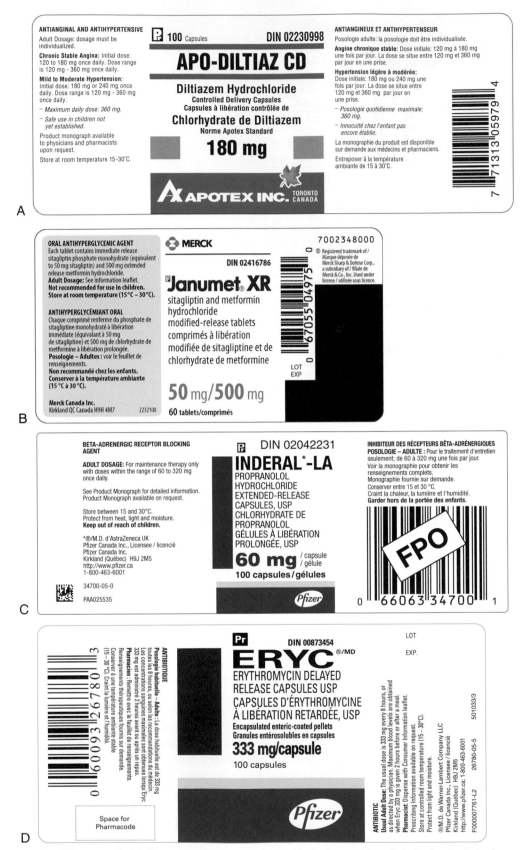

ANTIANGINAL AND ANTIHYPERTENSIVE

Adult Dosage: dosage must be individualized.

Chronic Stable Angina: Initial dose: 120 to 180 mg once daily. Dose range is 120 mg - 360 mg once daily.

Mild to Moderate Hypertension: Initial dose: 180 mg or 240 mg once daily. Dose range is 120 mg - 360 mg once daily.

– Maximum daily dose: 360 mg.

– Safe use in children not yet established.

Product monograph available to physicians and pharmacists upon request.

Store at room temperature 15-30°C.

℞ **100** Capsules   DIN 02230998

APO-DILTIAZ CD

Diltiazem Hydrochloride
Controlled Delivery Capsules
Capsules à libération contrôlée de
Chlorhydrate de Diltiazem
Norme Apotex Standard
180 mg

APOTEX INC. TORONTO CANADA

ANTIANGINEUX ET ANTIHYPERTENSEUR

Posologie adulte: la posologie doit être individualisée.

Angine chronique stable: Dose initiale: 120 mg à 180 mg une fois par jour. La dose se situe entre 120 mg et 360 mg par jour en une prise.

Hypertension légère à modérée: Dose initiale: 180 mg ou 240 mg une fois par jour. La dose se situe entre 120 mg et 360 mg par jour en une prise.

– Posologie quotidienne maximale: 360 mg.

– Innocuité chez l'enfant pas encore établie.

La monographie du produit est disponible sur demande aux médecins et pharmaciens.

Entreposer à la température ambiante de 15 à 30°C.

A

ORAL ANTIHYPERGLYCEMIC AGENT
Each tablet contains immediate release sitagliptin phosphate monohydrate (equivalent to 50 mg sitagliptin) and 500 mg extended release metformin hydrochloride.
Adult Dosage: See information leaflet.
Not recommended for use in children.
Store at room temperature (15°C – 30°C).

ANTIHYPERGLYCÉMIANT ORAL
Chaque comprimé renferme du phosphate de sitagliptine monohydrate à libération immédiate (équivalant à 50 mg de sitagliptine) et 500 mg de chlorhydrate de metformine à libération prolongée.
Posologie – Adultes : voir le feuillet de renseignements.
Non recommandé chez les enfants.
Conserver à la température ambiante (15 °C à 30 °C).

Merck Canada Inc.
Kirkland QC Canada H9H 4M7   2232100

MERCK

7002348000

DIN 02416786

℞ **Janumet XR**
sitagliptin and metformin hydrochloride
modified-release tablets
comprimés à libération modifiée de sitagliptine et de chlorhydrate de metformine

50 mg/500 mg
60 tablets/comprimés

® Registered trademark of / Marque déposée de Merck Sharp & Dohme Corp., a subsidiary of / filiale de Merck & Co., Inc. Used under license / utilisée sous licence.

LOT
EXP

B

BETA-ADRENERGIC RECEPTOR BLOCKING AGENT

ADULT DOSAGE: For maintenance therapy only with doses within the range of 60 to 320 mg once daily.

See Product Monograph for detailed information. Product Monograph available on request.

Store between 15 and 30°C.
Protect from heat, light and moisture.
Keep out of reach of children.

*®/M.D. d'AstraZeneca UK
Pfizer Canada Inc., Licensee / licencié
Pfizer Canada Inc.
Kirkland (Québec) H9J 2M5
http://www.pfizer.ca
1-800-463-6001

34700-05-0

PAA025535

℞   DIN 02042231

INDERAL*-LA
PROPRANOLOL HYDROCHLORIDE EXTENDED-RELEASE CAPSULES, USP
CHLORHYDRATE DE PROPRANOLOL GÉLULES À LIBÉRATION PROLONGÉE, USP
60 mg / capsule / gélule
100 capsules / gélules

Pfizer

INHIBITEUR DES RÉCEPTEURS BÊTA-ADRÉNERGIQUES
POSOLOGIE – ADULTE : Pour le traitement d'entretien seulement; de 60 à 320 mg une fois par jour.
Voir la monographie pour obtenir les renseignements complets.
Monographie fournie sur demande.
Conserver entre 15 et 30 °C.
Craint la chaleur, la lumière et l'humidité.
Garder hors de la portée des enfants.

FPO

0 66063 34700 1

C

ANTIBIOTIQUE
Posologie habituelle – Adulte : La dose habituelle est de 333 mg toutes les 8 heures, ou selon les recommandations du médecin. Les concentrations sanguines maximales sont obtenues lorsqu'Eryc 333 mg est administré 2 heures avant ou après un repas.
Pharmacien : Remettre avec le feuillet de renseignements.
Renseignements thérapeutiques fournis sur demande.
Conserver à une température ambiante stable (15 – 30 °C). Craint la lumière et l'humidité.

℞   DIN 00873454

LOT
EXP.

ERYC ®/MD
ERYTHROMYCIN DELAYED RELEASE CAPSULES USP
CAPSULES D'ÉRYTHROMYCINE À LIBÉRATION RETARDÉE, USP
Encapsulated enteric-coated pellets
Granules entérosolubles en capsules
333 mg/capsule
100 capsules

Pfizer

ANTIBIOTIC
Usual Adult Dose: The usual dose is 333 mg every 8 hours, or as directed by a physician. Maximum blood levels are obtained when Eryc 333 mg is given 2 hours before or after a meal.
Pharmacist: Dispense with Consumer Information leaflet.
Prescribing Information available on request.
Store at controlled room temperature (15 – 30°C).
Protect from light and moisture.

®/M.D. de Warner-Lambert Company LLC
Pfizer Canada Inc., Licensee / licencié
Kirkland (Québec) H9J 2M5
http://www.pfizer.ca; 1-800-463-6001
F00000077761-L2   26780-05-5   5010J33/3

Space for Pharmacode

D

Figure 11-9 A, Apo-Diltiaz controlled delivery capsules. **B,** Janumet modified-release tablets. **C,** Inderal extended-release capsules. **D,** ERYC delayed-release and enteric-coated capsules.

Bar-Code Symbols

Bar-code symbols appear on most medication labels as thin and heavy lines arranged in a group. Bar codes are particularly important at institutions where bar coding is used as part of the medication distribution system. Note the bar codes on the labels in Figures 11-2 *A*, 11-2 *B*, 11-6, and 11-9 *A–D*. Bar codes can also be used for stock reorder.

Route of Administration

The route of administration describes how a medication is to be administered. Examples of routes of administration are oral (PO), enteral (into the gastrointestinal tract through a tube), sublingual (SL), injection (intravenous [IV], intramuscular [IM], subcutaneous [SUBCUT]), optical, and topical. The route of administration may not be stated on labels for oral medications (see Figures 11-9, *A* to *D*). However, if a tablet or capsule is not to be swallowed, that information will be given. For example, the label for Nitrostat indicates that it is administered sublingually (under the tongue) (Figure 11-10). Unless specified otherwise, tablets, capsules, and caplets are intended for oral use. Any medication form intended for oral use should be administered orally.

Because certain tablets, capsules, and liquids are not always given orally, read the medication label carefully: any variation from oral administration is indicated on the label. Examples: sublingual tablets, otic suspension for use in ears, capsules that are placed in an inhaler and not swallowed. Liquid medications may be administered orally or by injection. Labels for liquid medications will indicate the route (e.g., "intravenous," "intramuscular," or "subcutaneous"). See Figures 11-11 to 11-13.

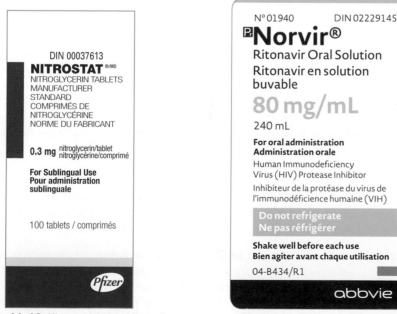

Figure 11-10 Nitrostat label (sublingual). **Figure 11-11** Norvir label (oral).

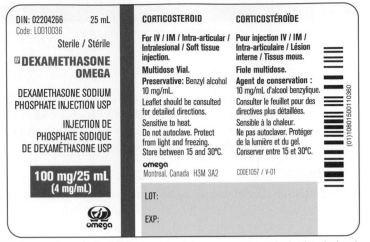

Figure 11-12 Dexamethasone label (intramuscular, intravenous, intra-articular, intralesional, or soft tissue).

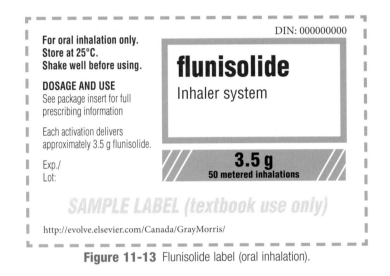

Figure 11-13 Flunisolide label (oral inhalation).

Total Volume

The labels of solutions for injection or oral liquids state the total volume as well as dosage strength. Total volume refers to the total fluid volume of a medication contained in a bottle, a vial, or an ampule.

There have been documented medication errors due to the misinterpretation of dosage strength and total volume. Health Canada and ISMP Canada (2015) recommend that the dosage strength per total volume be the prominent expression on single and multidose injectable product labels, followed in close proximity by the dosage strength per millilitre enclosed in parentheses (pp. 38–39). Note that the Zantac label shown in Figure 11-14 indicates that 40 mL is the vial size (total volume), the dosage strength per total volume of the vial is 1 g per 40 mL, and the dosage strength is 25 mg per mL.

Total Amount in Container

For solid forms of medication, such as tablets or capsules, the total amount is the total number of tablets or capsules in the container. The dosage strength is also indicated on the label of solid forms of medication.

Examples: In Figure 11-4, the total amount in the Isentress container is 60 tablets, whereas the dosage strength is 400 mg per tablet. In Figure 11-9, *A*, the total amount in the diltiazem container is 100 controlled-delivery capsules, whereas the dosage strength is 180 mg per controlled-delivery capsule. In Figure 11-14, the total volume of Ranitidine is 2 mL, whereas the solution

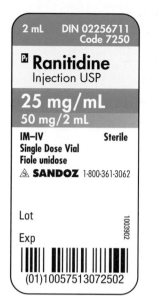

Figure 11-14 Ranitidine label (injectable).

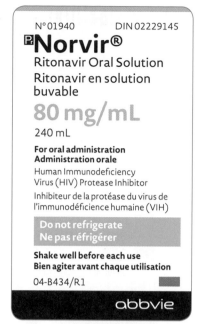

Figure 11-15 Norvir label (oral solution).

or liquid dosage strength is 50 mg per 2 mL (25 mg per mL). In Figure 11-15, the total volume of Norvir is 240 mL, whereas the solution or liquid dosage strength is 80 mg per mL.

> **(!) SAFETY ALERT!**
>
> It is important to recognize the difference between the amount per millilitre and the total volume to avoid confusion and errors. Do not confuse total volume or total amount in container with dosage strength. Confusing volume with dosage strength can cause a serious medication error.

Directions for Mixing or Reconstituting a Medication

When medication comes in a powdered form, the directions for how to mix or reconstitute it and with what solution are found on the label or package insert. The directions for reconstitution should be followed exactly as stated on the label for accuracy in administration. Note the directions on the label in Figure 11-16 for cefotaxime. In Figure 11-17, the directions for mixing fluconazole are shown on the side of the label. Reconstitution of solutions is discussed further in Chapter 17.

Precautions

Medications typically come with precautions (including warnings and alerts) that are related to safety, effectiveness, or administration. These precautions need to be followed. Storage alerts might also appear on the label and must be followed. Precautions may be printed on the label by the manufacturer or on a prescription medication label by the pharmacy that dispenses the medication. Always read precautions carefully and follow the instructions given precisely. Examples of precautions indicated on a label are "shake well," "protect from light," "may be habit forming." In Figure 11-17, the fluconazole label indicates a few precautions, including "For oral use only. Shake well before using." and "Protect from freezing." In Figure 11-18, the warning on the label for Lasix Special is "To be used under strict medical supervision in a hospital setting." Labels may also carry warnings for specific groups of patients. For example, a label may carry alerts for specific routes. For example, the Dilantin label warns that you should not give this medication parenterally (Figure 11-19).

Expiration Date

Medication labels contain information such as the expiration date (which may be indicated with the abbreviation *Exp*). The expiration date indicates the last date on which a

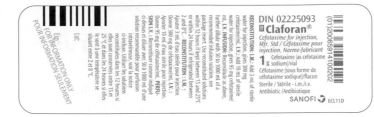

Figure 11-16 Cefotaxime label.

Figure 11-17 Fluconazole label.

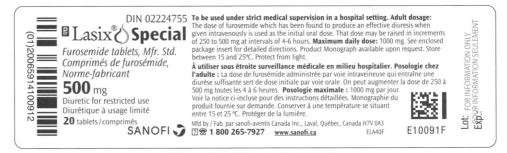

Figure 11-18 Lasix Special label.

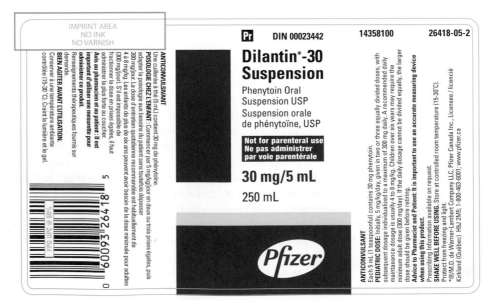

Figure 11-19 Dilantin label.

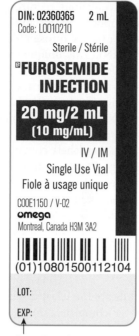

Location of expiry date.

Figure 11-20 Furosemide label.

medication should be used. Typically, the date appears as the month/year. This information can be found on the back or side of a label. Medications requiring reconstitution provide specific expiration instructions. In Figure 11-17, the fluconazole label reads "Discard unused portion." In the hospital setting, medications that have expired should be returned to the pharmacy. Note where the expiration date would be printed on the furosemide label in Figure 11-20. *Note:* The expiration date must always be checked on each medication, and the expiration date is always present on the actual prescription. The labels shown in this text may not all have expiration dates because they are used solely for educational purposes.

> **! SAFETY ALERT!**
>
> Remember to always read the expiration date. After the expiration date, the medication may lose its potency or cause adverse or different effects from those intended. Discard expired medications according to your organization's policy. For some medications, such as narcotics, disposal must be witnessed. Never give expired medications to a patient! Patients must be educated in *all* aspects of medication administration, so teach them to check medications for expiration dates and to discard medications that have expired properly. Teach patients that they can take unused or expired medications to any pharmacy in Canada. In some communities, the local police force also offers take-back programs so that people can easily and safely dispose of expired or unused medications. Encourage patients not to flush medications down the toilet or sink.

Additional Information

A medication label also includes the following information:
- **Storage directions.** This section of the medication label provides information as to how a medication should be stored to prevent the medication from losing its potency or effectiveness. Usually, information is given on the label relating to temperature for storing the medication. Note the storage direction on the famciclovir label (see Figure 11-2, *B*) and the Lupron label (see Figure 11-3). When medications come in a powdered form and must be reconstituted, the label usually indicates how long the medication is effective once it has been reconstituted. Note the storage direction for the reconstituted solution on the cefotaxime label (see Figure 11-16) and the fluconazole label (see Figure 11-17).

- **Lot numbers.** Food and Drug Regulations require that all medication packages be identified by a lot number. This number is important in the event that medications have to be recalled. Note the lot number on the furosemide label (see Figure 11-20).
- **Drug identification number (DIN).** This unique eight-digit number is assigned by Health Canada to a medication before it is marketed in Canada. A DIN is used to identify all medication products sold in a dosage form and is located on the label of prescription and over-the-counter medication products that have been evaluated and authorized for sale in Canada. Note the DIN on the cefotaxime label (see Figure 11-16): DIN 02225093.
- **Manufacturer's name.** All medication labels contain the name of the company that manufactured the medication (e.g., Pfizer, Apotex, GlaxoSmithKline). Omega is the manufacturer's name on the furosemide label in Figure 11-20. This information can be valuable if you have questions about the medication.
- **Abbreviations such as USP (United States Pharmacopoeia).** USP is an official national list of approved medications. Special guidelines are given to the manufacturer related to use and placement of these initials on medication labels. On the Zofran label in Figure 11-5, note that "USP" follows "Oral Solution." Also note the placement of USP on the Zantac label (see Figure 11-14).

Some medication labels may indicate the usual dosage on the label, while others may state to read the package insert for complete information. The "usual dosage" is how much medication is given in a single dose or in a 24-hour period. See Figure 11-2, *B* (famciclovir), which refers readers to the package insert for information on the usual dosage, and Figure 11-17 (fluconazole), which states the usual dosage for adults and children on the label.

The amount of information found on a medication label varies; however, some information is consistent on all labels (name of medication, dosage, amount in the package, manufacturer's name, expiration date, lot number).

Medication Labels for Combination Medications

Some medication labels may indicate that a medication contains two or more medications. Combination medications are sometimes ordered by the number of tablets, capsules, or millilitres to be given rather than by the dosage strength. Combination medications such as Janumet, which comes in several strengths, cannot be ordered without a specific dosage; the number of tablets alone is insufficient to fill the order. **Janumet must include the dosage!**

Example: Janumet, which is the trade name for an antihyperglycemic drug, is a combination of sitagliptin and metformin hydrochloride. In Figure 11-21, below the generic name shows the numbers 50 mg/500 mg. The first number specifies the amount of sitagliptin (50 mg) and the second number specifies

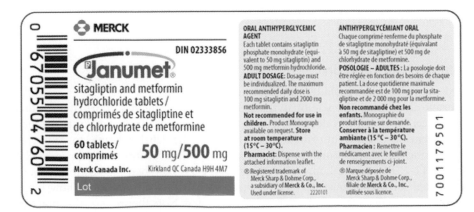

Figure 11-21 Janumet 50-500 label. The dosage strength of sitagliptin is 50 mg and that of metformin hydrochloride is 500 mg.

the amount of metformin hydrochloride (500 mg). This information is also indicated in fine print on the label. See sample labels for Janumet with different dosage strengths in Figures 11-22 and 11-23.

Example: Trimethoprim and sulfamethoxazole, an antibacterial that is also manufactured under the trade name Bactrim, is a combination of trimethoprim and sulfamethoxazole. In Figure 11-24, the trimethoprim and sulfamethoxazole label indicates that each tablet contains 80 mg of trimethoprim and

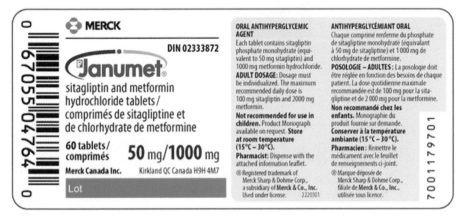

Figure 11-22 Janumet 50-1000 label. The dosage strength of sitagliptin is 50 mg and that of metformin hydrochloride is 1000 mg.

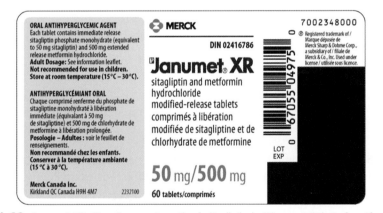

Figure 11-23 Janumet XR. The dosage strength of sitagliptin is 50 mg and that of metformin hydrochloride is 500 mg. *XR*, modified release.

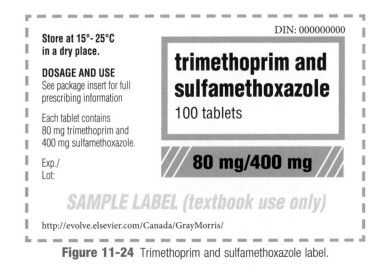

Figure 11-24 Trimethoprim and sulfamethoxazole label.

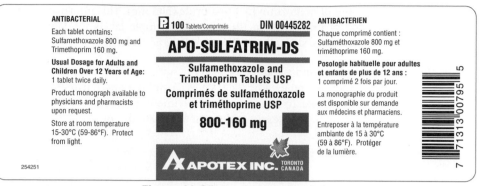

Figure 11-25 Apo-Sulfatrim-DS label.

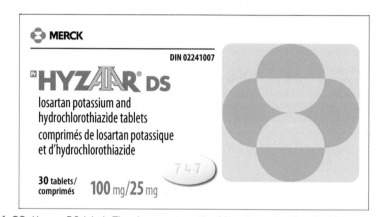

Figure 11-26 Hyzaar DS label. The dosage strength of losartan potassium is 100 mg with 25 mg of hydrochlorothiazide.

400 mg of sulfamethoxazole. In Figure 11-25, the Apo-Sulfatrim-DS label indicates that each tablet contains 160 mg of trimethoprim and 800 mg of sulfamethoxazole.

Remember that extra initials or abbreviations after a medication name identify additional medication in the preparation or a special action. For example, in Figure 11-25, Apo-Sulfatrim-DS DS is a double-strength tablet.

Example: Hyzaar DS is a combination of losartan potassium and hydrochlorothiazide (Figure 11-26).

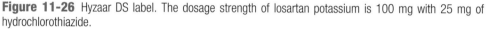

> **⚠ SAFETY ALERT!**
>
> The numbers beside a combination medication name (e.g., 10-100) identify the dosage strengths of each medication in the preparation. The initials that appear after a medication name (e.g., DS) identify additional medication in the preparation or a special action. Read labels carefully to validate that you have the correct medication and dosage for combination medications.

Although tablets and capsules that contain more than one medication are often ordered by the brand name and number of tablets to be given (e.g., Septra DS 1 tab PO BID), the health care provider may order this medication by another route, for example, IV. With the IV order, the nurse calculates the dosage to be given based on the strength of the trimethoprim. The nurse would learn such information by using appropriate resources, such as a drug reference, a pharmacist, a hospital formulary, and available information technology.

It is important to remember that some medications may not indicate their strength but are ordered by the number of tablets (e.g., multivitamin tablet 1 PO daily, Bactrim DS 1

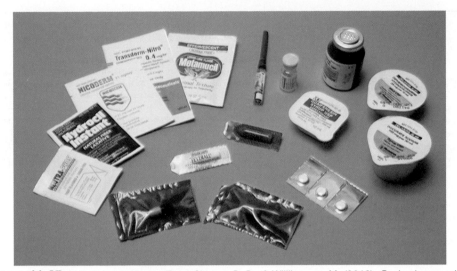

Figure 11-27 Unit-dose packages. (From Clayton, B. D., & Willihnganz, M. (2013). *Basic pharmacology for nurses* (16th ed.). St. Louis: Mosby.)

tablet PO BID, Percocet 1 tablet PO q4h prn). This is because these medications are available in one strength only. Some medications that contain a combination of medications in one strength only are also commonly ordered without indicating their strength.

Unit-Dose Packaging

Most medications administered in the hospital setting are available in unit dose. The pharmacy provides a 24-hour supply of each medication that can be dispensed in unit doses for patients. Unit-dose medications come to the unit in separately wrapped packages that include an individualized dose for a specific patient. The label on each package states the medication's generic name, trade name (if one exists), manufacturer, lot number, and expiration date. The strength is indicated on the medication label. The nurse must read the label on unit-dose packages and keep in mind that sometimes even this system may require calculation before medication administration. The pharmacy in some institutions also provides the unit with a supply of medications available in multidose containers. These medications may be in unit-dose packaging but are used a great deal by the patients on the unit. Examples are Tylenol and aspirin. Such medications may also be dispensed in bottles: for example, 100 tablets of aspirin 325 mg. Figure 11-27 shows examples of unit-dose packaging.

Most hospital units have a combination of unit-dose and multidose medications. Multidose packaging contains more than one dose of a medication. These medications may be part of the floor stock. Tablets, capsules, powders, and liquid medications may be supplied in stock bottles for dispensing. Parenteral medications in liquid form or in powdered form that requires reconstitution may come in multidose vials.

Medication Information

To decrease errors and manage the risks of medications and adverse effects, Health Canada mandates the format in which medication information is provided on prescription package inserts. The categories of information to be included in prescription package inserts include the highlights of prescribing information, boxed warnings, recent major changes, indications and usage, and adverse reactions. The adverse reactions section must include the following statement: "To report SUSPECTED ADVERSE REACTIONS, contact [Manufacturer] at [phone # and email address] or Health Canada at 1-866-225-0709 or http://www.healthcanada.gc.ca/medeffect." See Figure 11-28 for an excerpt from the prescribing information for the medication aspirin.

Over-the-Counter Labels

Over-the-counter (OTC) medicine is medication that a patient can purchase without a prescription. Health Canada requires that OTC labels include medication facts (the name

TARO-WARFARIN
Warfarin Sodium Tablets, USP
Anticoagulant

INFORMATION TO THE PATIENT

Please read this leaflet before you start taking TARO-WARFARIN (warfarin sodium) Tablets. Each time you renew your prescription, read the leaflet that comes with your medicine, just in case any information has changed. Remember, this leaflet does not take the place of talking to your health care provider (such as your doctor, nurse, or pharmacist). You and your health care provider should discuss TARO-WARFARIN Tablets when you start taking your medication and at regular checkups.

1. What are TARO-WARFARIN Tablets?
- TARO-WARFARIN is an anticoagulant drug. "Anti" means against and "coagulant" refers to blood clotting. An anticoagulant helps reduce clots from forming in the blood.
- TARO-WARFARIN is a narrow therapeutic index drug, which means that there is a narrow margin between too much and too little of the drug. Too much drug may cause you to bleed more. Too little drug may let a harmful clot form.

2. How do TARO-WARFARIN Tablets work?
- TARO-WARFARIN Tablets partially block the re-use of vitamin K in your liver. Vitamin K is needed to make clotting factors that help the blood to clot and prevent bleeding. Vitamin K is found naturally in foods such as leafy, green vegetables and certain vegetable oils.
- TARO-WARFARIN Tablets begin to reduce blood clotting within 24 hours after taking the drug. The full effect may take 72 to 96 hours to occur. The anti-clotting effects of a single dose of TARO-WARFARIN Tablets last 2 to 5 days, but it is important for you to take your dose everyday.

3. What is the most important information I should know when taking TARO-WARFARIN Tablets?
- Like all prescription drugs, TARO-WARFARIN Tablets may cause side effects. The most common side effect of TARO-WARFARIN Tablets is bleeding, which may be serious. However, the risk of serious bleeding is low when the effect of TARO-WARFARIN Tablets is within a range that is right for your specific medical condition. Notify your health care provider right away of any unusual bleeding or if signs or symptoms of bleeding occur (see Question 5).
- Do not take TARO-WARFARIN Tablets during pregnancy. Use effective measures to avoid pregnancy while taking TARO-WARFARIN Tablets.
- The dose of TARO-WARFARIN Tablets may be different for each patient. For example, older patients (age 60 years of age or older) appear to have a greater-than-expected response to TARO-WARFARIN Tablets so that as patient age increases, a lower dose of TARO-WARFARIN Tablets may be needed. Your health care provider will decide what dose is best for you. This dose may change from time to time.
- To decide on the dosage of TARO-WARFARIN Tablets you need, your health care provider will take a small amount of your blood to find out your prothrombin time, protime, or PT, for short. Protimes are often recorded as an INR (International Normalized Ratio), a standard way of reporting protimes.
- PT/INR tests are very important. They help your health care provider see how fast your blood is clotting and whether your dosage of TARO-WARFARIN Tablets should change.
- When you start taking TARO-WARFARIN Tablets, you may have PT/INR tests every day for a few days, then perhaps one time every week. These PT/INR tests and regular visits to a health care provider are very important for the success of therapy with TARO-WARFARIN Tablets. PT/INR tests will be needed at periodic intervals (such as one time per month) throughout your course of therapy to keep your PT/INR in the best range for your medical condition. Discuss with your health care provider the range that is right for you.
- Eat a normal balanced diet maintaining a consistent level of green leafy vegetables that contain high amounts of Vitamin K since the amount of vitamin K in your daily diet may affect TARO-WARFARIN Tablet therapy.
- Report any illness, such as throwing up (vomiting), loose or runny stools (diarrhea), an infection or fever to your health care provider.
- Tell anyone giving you medical or dental care that you are taking TARO-WARFARIN Tablets.
- Carry identification stating that you are taking TARO-WARFARIN Tablets.

4. How should I take TARO-WARFARIN Tablets?
- Take TARO-WARFARIN Tablets exactly the way your health care provider tells you and take it at the same time every day. You can take TARO-WARFARIN Tablets either with food or on an empty stomach. Your dosage may change from time to time depending on your response to TARO-WARFARIN Tablets.
- If you miss a dose of TARO-WARFARIN Tablets, notify your health care provider right away.

Take the dose as soon as possible on the same day, but do not take a double dose of TARO-WARFARIN Tablets the next day to make up for a missed dose.

5. What are the possible side effects of TARO-WARFARIN Tablets?
Your health care provider can tell you about possible side effects of TARO-WARFARIN Tablets, which include bleeding and allergic reactions. Please contact your health care provider right away if you experience signs or symptoms of bleeding or allergic reactions.

To lower the risk of bleeding, your PT/INR should be kept within a range that is right for you. Signs or symptoms of bleeding include:
- headache, dizziness, or weakness
- bleeding from shaving or other cuts that does not stop
- nosebleeds
- bleeding of gums when brushing your teeth
- throwing up blood
- unusual bruising (black-and-blue marks on your skin) for unknown reasons
- dark brown urine
- red or black color in your stool
- more bleeding than usual when you get your menstrual period or unexpected bleeding from the vagina
- unusual pain or swelling

Serious, but rare, side effects of TARO-WARFARIN Tablets include skin necrosis (death of skin tissue) and "purple toes syndrome", either of which may require removal of unhealthy tissue and/or amputation of the affected area. Talk with your health care provider for further information on these side effects.

Hypersensitivity/allergic reactions are reported infrequently. Signs or symptoms of these reactions may range from mild reactions (rash, itching, hives) to more severe reactions (trouble breathing, throat tightening or constriction, facial swelling, swollen lips or tongue, sudden low blood pressure).

6. What should I avoid while taking TARO-WARFARIN Tablets?
- Do not start, stop, or change any medicine except on the advice of your health care provider. TARO-WARFARIN Tablets interact with many different drugs, including aspirin and aspirin-containing ointments and skin creams. Tell your health care provider about any prescription and non-prescription (over-the-counter) drugs that you are taking including occasional use of headache medications.
- Do not make drastic changes in your diet, such as eating large amounts of green, leafy vegetables. The amount of vitamin K in your daily diet may affect therapy with TARO-WARFARIN Tablets.
- Do not attempt to change your weight by dieting, without first checking with your health care provider.
- Avoid alcohol consumption.
- Do not participate in any activity or sport that may result in serious injury.
- Avoid cutting yourself.

7. What do TARO-WARFARIN Tablets look like?
TARO-WARFARIN Tablets are available in many strengths, and each strength has a unique tablet color:

Tablet Strength	Tablet Color
1.0 mg	Pink
2.0 mg	Lavender
2.5 mg	Green
3.0 mg	Tan
4.0 mg	Blue
5.0 mg	Peach
6.0 mg	Teal
7.5 mg	Yellow
10.0 mg	White

Each round, single-scored tablet is imprinted on one side with the word "WARFARIN" and the numeric strength of the tablet. The other side of the tablet is imprinted with the name "TARO".

Be sure to check that the tablet shows "WARFARIN" and the right numeric strength before you take it.

For further information, please contact Taro Pharmaceuticals Inc. at 1-800-268-1975.

PK-3352-1

Figure 11-28 Prescribing information for Taro-Warfarin. (Copyright Taro Pharmaceuticals Inc. All Rights Reserved.)

**TO ORDER ADDITIONAL TARO-WARFARIN
PATIENT INFORMATION
LEAFLETS TO BE
DISPENSED WITH TARO-WAR-FARIN
PRESCRIPTIONS**

Call Taro Customer Service at:

1-800-268-1975 Ext 427

Order item PK-3352-1

**FOR MORE INFORMATION ON
TARO-WARFARIN
OR ANY OF TARO'S PRODUCTS
VISIT THE
TARO WEBSITE AT:**

www.taro.ca

Figure 11-28, cont'd

of the medication and its purpose), uses of the medication, warnings, and directions on how to take the medication. The format of an OTC label is simpler than the format of prescription medication labels.

Let's examine some sample medication labels to review and identify some of the important information on labels.

1. In Figure 11-29, note the following:

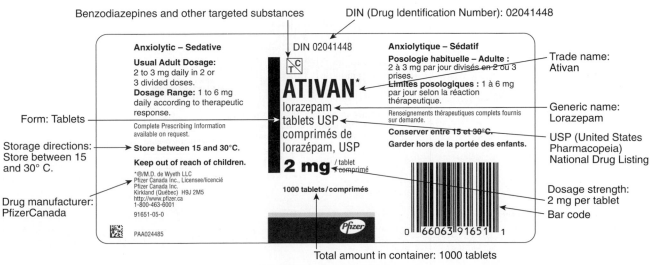

Figure 11-29 Ativan label.

2. In Figure 11-30, note the following:

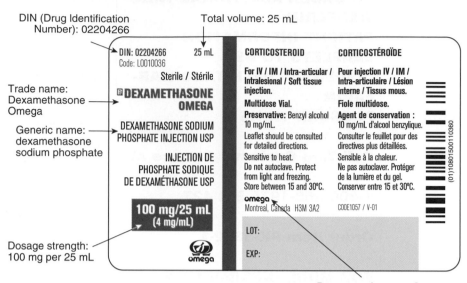

Figure 11-30 Dexamethasone label. Injection is the route; injectable liquid is the form.

3. In Figure 11-31, note the following:

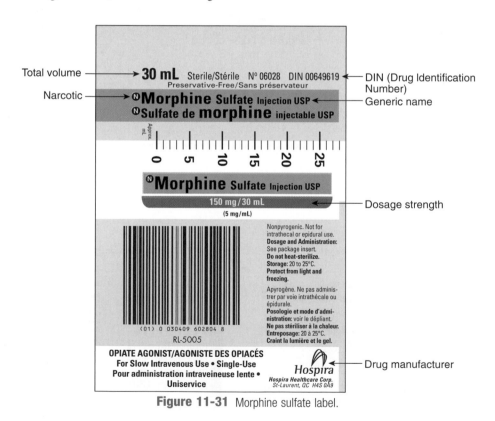

Figure 11-31 Morphine sulfate label.

4. In Figure 11-32, note the following:

Directions for mixing   Total name   Generic name

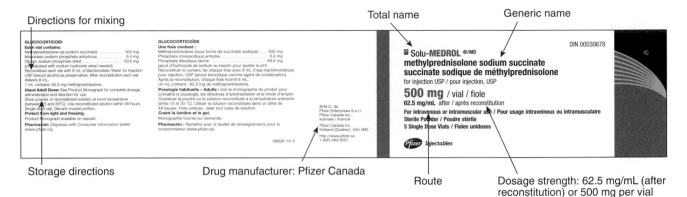

Storage directions   Drug manufacturer: Pfizer Canada   Route   Dosage strength: 62.5 mg/mL (after reconstitution) or 500 mg per vial

Figure 11-32 Solu-MEDROL label. Form is powder; it must be diluted for use.

5. In Figure 11-33, note the following:

Trade name

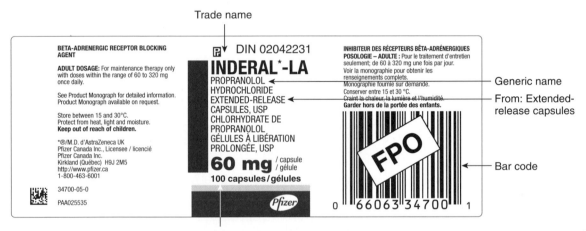

Generic name

From: Extended-release capsules

Bar code

Total amount in container: 100 capsules

Figure 11-33 Inderal-LA label.

6. In Figure 11-34, note the following:

Population medication used for

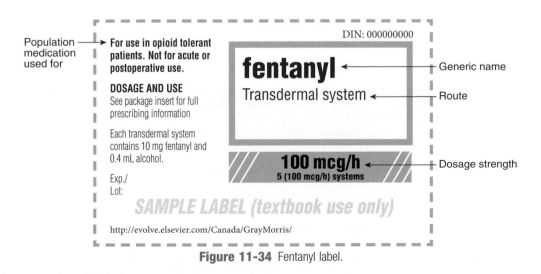

Generic name

Route

Dosage strength

Figure 11-34 Fentanyl label.

7. In Figure 11-35, note the following:

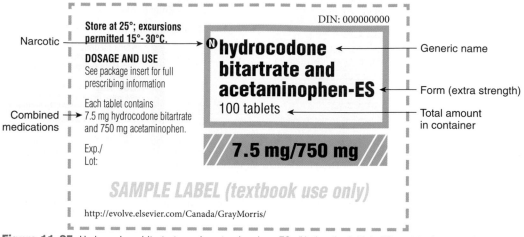

Figure 11-35 Hydrocodone bitartrate and acetaminophen-ES. (Notice the initials ES next to the generic name to indicate a special form.)

8. In Figure 11-36, note the following:

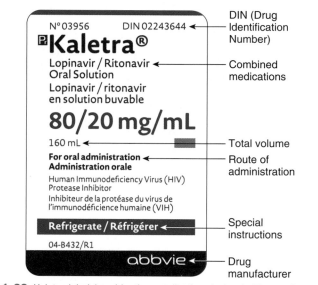

Figure 11-36 Kaletra label (combination medication: lopinavir 80 mg, ritonavir 20 mg).

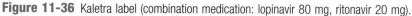

> ### POINTS TO REMEMBER
> - Read medication labels three times.
> - Identify directions for mixing when indicated.
> - Read labels carefully and do not confuse medication names; they are often deceptively similar. When in doubt, check appropriate resources, such as a drug reference or a pharmacist. Always cross-check medication names to avoid administering the wrong medication.
> - Read the label on combination medications carefully to ascertain whether you are administering the correct medication dosage.
> - Be aware that extra initials after a medication name may identify additional medication in the preparation or a special action.
> - Read labels carefully to identify trade and generic names, dosage strength, form, total amount in container or total volume, and route of administration.
> - Do not confuse special forms such as SR and XL with USP, the abbreviation for the official national list of approved medications.

- Read and follow directions relating to storage.
- Carefully read alerts on medication labels.
- Do not administer expired medications.
- When writing dosages, use *per* instead of a slash mark (/) because the slash mark can be misread or mistaken for the number *1*.
- Remember: administering the incorrect form of a medication is a medication error.

PRACTICE **PROBLEMS**

Read the labels and provide the information requested.

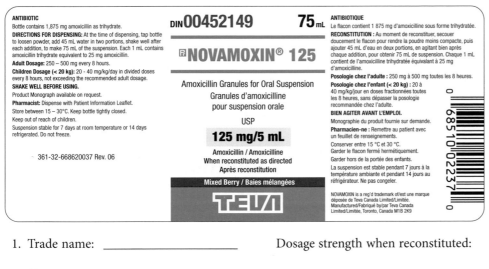

ANTIBIOTIC

Bottle contains 1,875 mg amoxicillin as trihydrate.

DIRECTIONS FOR DISPENSING: At the time of dispensing, tap bottle to loosen powder, add 45 mL water in two portions, shake well after each addition, to make 75 mL of the suspension. Each 1 mL contains amoxicillin trihydrate equivalent to 25 mg amoxicillin.

Adult Dosage: 250 – 500 mg every 8 hours.

Children Dosage (< 20 kg): 20 - 40 mg/kg/day in divided doses every 8 hours, not exceeding the recommended adult dosage.

SHAKE WELL BEFORE USING.

Product Monograph available on request.

Pharmacist: Dispense with Patient Information Leaflet.

Store between 15 – 30°C. Keep bottle tightly closed.

Keep out of reach of children.

Suspension stable for 7 days at room temperature or 14 days refrigerated. Do not freeze.

361-32-668620037 Rev. 06

DIN 00452149 **75 mL**

℞ NOVAMOXIN® 125

Amoxicillin Granules for Oral Suspension
Granules d'amoxicilline
pour suspension orale

USP

125 mg/5 mL

Amoxicillin / Amoxicilline
When reconstituted as directed
Après reconstitution

Mixed Berry / Baies mélangées

TEVA

ANTIBIOTIQUE

Le flacon contient 1 875 mg d'amoxicilline sous forme trihydratée.

RECONSTITUTION : Au moment de reconstituer, secouer doucement le flacon pour rendre la poudre moins compacte, puis ajouter 45 mL d'eau en deux portions, en agitant bien après chaque addition, pour obtenir 75 mL de suspension. Chaque 1 mL contient de l'amoxicilline trihydratée équivalant à 25 mg d'amoxicilline.

Posologie chez l'adulte : 250 mg à 500 mg toutes les 8 heures.

Posologie chez l'enfant (< 20 kg) : 20 à 40 mg/kg/jour en doses fractionnées toutes les 8 heures, sans dépasser la posologie recommandée chez l'adulte.

BIEN AGITER AVANT L'EMPLOI.

Monographie du produit fournie sur demande.

Pharmacien-ne : Remettre au patient avec un feuillet de renseignements.

Conserver entre 15 °C et 30 °C.
Garder le flacon fermé hermétiquement.
Garder hors de la portée des enfants.

La suspension est stable pendant 7 jours à la température ambiante et pendant 14 jours au réfrigérateur. Ne pas congeler.

NOVAMOXIN is a reg'd trademark of/est une marque déposée de Teva Canada Limited/Limitée.
Manufactured/Fabriqué by/par Teva Canada Limited/Limitée, Toronto, Canada M1B 2K9

1. Trade name: _____   Dosage strength when reconstituted:

   Generic name: _____   _____

   Form: _____   Total volume when mixed:

   _____

1 mL   DIN 00742813
Code 3000

℞ Hydroxyzine

Hydrochloride Injection USP

50 mg/mL

Sterile

IM only/IM seulement

⚠ SANDOZ 1-800-361-3062

Lot

Exp

1003827

(01)10057513030007

2. Trade name: _____   Dosage strength: _____

   Generic name: _____   Total volume: _____

   Form: _____

ANTIEPILEPTIC

Each tablet contains 270 mg divalproex sodium equivalent to 250 mg valproic acid.

Usual Dosage:
Epilepsy (Adults and Children): The recommended initial dose for children and adults is 15 mg/kg/day, increasing at one-week intervals by 5-10 mg/kg/day, to a maximum recommended dose of 60 mg/kg/day. If the total daily dose is 250 mg or greater, it should be given in a divided regimen.

Acute Mania (Adults): The recommended initial dose for adults is 250 mg 3 times a day. The dose should be increased as rapidly as possible to achieve the lowest therapeutic dose, to a maximum recommended dose of 60 mg/kg/day.

Swallow tablets whole.

PHARMACIST: PLEASE DISPENSE WITH THE PATIENT INFORMATION LEAFLET PROVIDED.

Product monograph available to physicians and pharmacists upon request.

Store at controlled room temperature 15-30°C (59-86°F) in tight, light-resistant containers.

330587

℞ 100 Tablets/Comprimés   DIN 02239699

APO-DIVALPROEX

Divalproex Sodium Enteric-Coated Tablets
Comprimés entéro-solubles de divalproex de sodium

Norme Apotex Standard

250 mg

ΑX APOTEX INC. TORONTO CANADA

ANTIÉPILEPTIQUE

Chaque comprimé contient 270 mg de divalproex de sodium équivalent à 250 mg d'acide valproïque.

POSOLOGIE HABITUELLE:
Épilepsie (adultes et enfants): La dose d'attaque recommandé chez les enfants et les adultes est de 15 mg/kg/jour, augmentant de 5-10 mg/kg/jour à des intervalles d'une semaine, jusqu'à la dose maximale recommandée de 60 mg/kg/jour. Si la dose quotidienne totale est d'au moins 250 mg, elle doit être administrée en prises fractionnées.

Manie aiguë (adultes): La posologie initiale recommandée chez les adultes est de 250 mg 3 fois/jour. La dose doit être augmentée aussi rapidement que possible de façon à atteindre la dose thérapeutique la plus faible, jusqu'à la dose maximale recommandée de 60 mg/kg/jour.

Avaler le comprimé entier.

PHARMACIEN: VEUILLEZ REMETTRE AVEC LE FEUILLET D'INFORMATION ÉTABLI À L'INTENTION DU PATIENT.

La monographie du produit est disponible sur demande aux médecins et pharmaciens.

Entreposer à la température ambiante contrôlée de 15 à 30°C (59 à 86°F) dans des flacons hermétiquement fermés et résistants à la lumière.

APOTEX INC. TORONTO CANADA M9L 1T9

3. Trade name: _____   Dosage strength: _____

   Generic name: _____   Total amount in container: _____

   DIN: _____

Store at 25°C; excursions permitted to 15°- 30°C.

DOSAGE AND USE
See package insert for full prescribing information

Each tablet contains 400 mg imatinib free base.

Exp./
Lot:

DIN: 000000000

imatinib mesylate
30 tablets

400 mg

SAMPLE LABEL (textbook use only)

http://evolve.elsevier.com/Canada/GrayMorris/

4. Generic name: _____   Total amount in container: _____

   Dosage strength: _____   Storage: _____

ANTICOAGULANT

Each tablet contains 5 mg warfarin sodium (crystalline).

Usual Adult Dosage: initially, 2 to 5 mg per day with dosage adjustments based on the results of INR and/or PT ratio determinations.

Product monograph available to physicians and pharmacists upon request.

Store at room temperature 15-30°C. Protect from light.

Replace cap tightly.

Pharmacists: Please dispense with the Patient Information Leaflet.

℞ 100 Tablets/Comprimés   DIN 02242928

APO-WARFARIN

Warfarin Sodium Tablets USP
Comprimés de warfarine sodique USP

5 mg

ΑX APOTEX INC. TORONTO CANADA

ANTICOAGULANT

Chaque comprimé contient 5 mg de warfarine sodique en forme cristallisée.

Posologie adulte usuelle: initier avec 2 à 5 mg par jour puis ajuster la dose au besoin selon les résultats des rapports de TP ou INR.

La monographie du produit est disponible sur demande aux médecins et pharmaciens.

Entreposer à la température ambiante de 15 à 30°C. **Protéger de la lumière.**

Reboucher hermétiquement.

Pharmacien: Remettre ce produit accompagné du feuillet de renseignements destinés au patient.

227552

5. Trade name: _____   Form: _____

   Dosage strength: _____   DIN: _____

   Total amount in container: _____

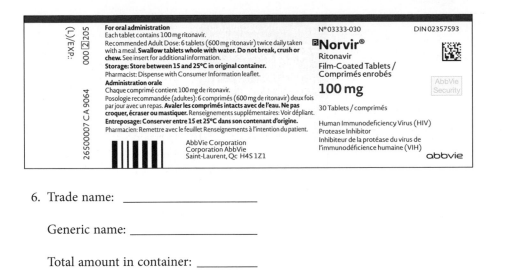

6. Trade name: _____

   Generic name: _____

   Total amount in container: _____

   Can this medication be crushed? _____

Answers on page 200.

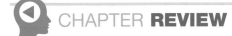 CHAPTER **REVIEW**

Read the labels and provide the information requested.

> Store at 25°C.
>
> DIN: 000000000
>
> **paricalcitol**
> 30 capsules
>
> **DOSAGE AND USE**
> See package insert for full
> prescribing information
>
> Each capsule contains
> 2 mcg paricalcitol.
>
> Exp./
> Lot:
>
> **2 mcg**
>
> *SAMPLE LABEL (textbook use only)*
>
> http://evolve.elsevier.com/Canada/GrayMorris/

1. Generic name: _____   Form: _____

   Total amount in container: _____   Dosage strength: _____

2 mL DIN 02048264
Code 2370

℞**Digoxin**
Injection C.S.D.

0.25 mg/mL

0.5 mg/2 mL

IV–IM **Sterile**

⚠ **SANDOZ** 1-800-361-3062

Lot

Exp

1004106

(01)10057513023702

2. Trade name: _____   Form: _____

   Generic name: _____   Dosage strength: _____

   DIN: _____

Store at 25°C.

DOSAGE AND USE
See package insert for full
prescribing information

Each tablet contains
10 mg tadalafil.

Exp./
Lot:

DIN: 000000000

tadalafil

30 tablets

10 mg

SAMPLE LABEL (textbook use only)

http://evolve.elsevier.com/Canada/GrayMorris/

3. Generic name: _____   Dosage strength: _____

   Storage: _____   Total amount in container: _____

   Form: _____

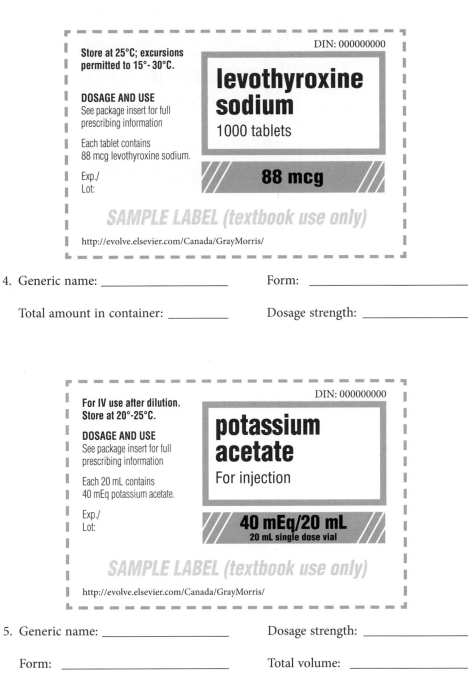

Store at 25°C; excursions permitted to 15°- 30°C.

DOSAGE AND USE
See package insert for full prescribing information

Each tablet contains 88 mcg levothyroxine sodium.

Exp./
Lot:

DIN: 000000000

levothyroxine sodium

1000 tablets

88 mcg

SAMPLE LABEL (textbook use only)

http://evolve.elsevier.com/Canada/GrayMorris/

4. Generic name: _____   Form: _____

   Total amount in container: _____   Dosage strength: _____

For IV use after dilution. Store at 20°-25°C.

DOSAGE AND USE
See package insert for full prescribing information

Each 20 mL contains 40 mEq potassium acetate.

Exp./
Lot:

DIN: 000000000

potassium acetate

For injection

40 mEq/20 mL
20 mL single dose vial

SAMPLE LABEL (textbook use only)

http://evolve.elsevier.com/Canada/GrayMorris/

5. Generic name: _____   Dosage strength: _____

   Form: _____   Total volume: _____

Keep refrigerated 2°-8°C.
ALERT: Find out about medications that should NOT be taken with saquinavir.

DOSAGE AND USE
See package insert for full prescribing information

Each capsule contains 200 mg saquinavir.

Exp./
Lot:

DIN: 000000000

saquinavir
180 soft gelatin capsules

200 mg

SAMPLE LABEL (textbook use only)

http://evolve.elsevier.com/Canada/GrayMorris/

6. Generic name: _____   Form: _____

   Usual dosage: _____   Dosage strength: _____

   Alert: _____   Total amount in container: _____

For IV infusion only. Inject 20 mL sterile water into vial. Shake vial until a clear solution is achieved and use within 12 hours.

DOSAGE AND USE
See package insert for full prescribing information

Each mL contains 1000 mg acyclovir.

Exp./
Lot:

DIN: 000000000

acyclovir
For injection

1000 mg

SAMPLE LABEL (textbook use only)

http://evolve.elsevier.com/Canada/GrayMorris/

7. Generic name: _____   Dosage strength after reconstitution:

   Form: _____   _____

   Directions for mixing: _____   Directions for use: _____

30 mL Sterile/Stérile N° 06028 DIN 00649619
Preservative-Free/Sans préservateur
ℕ**Morphine** Sulfate Injection USP
ℕ**Sulfate de morphine** injectable USP

Approx. mL

0 5 10 15 20 25

ℕ**Morphine** Sulfate Injection USP

150 mg / 30 mL
(5 mg/mL)

(01) 0 030409 602804 8
RL-5005

Nonpyrogenic. Not for intrathecal or epidural use.
Dosage and Administration: See package insert.
Do not heat-sterilize.
Storage: 20 to 25°C.
Protect from light and freezing.

Apyrogène. Ne pas administrer par voie intrathécale ou épidurale.
Posologie et mode d'administration: voir le dépliant.
Ne pas stériliser à la chaleur.
Entreposage: 20 à 25°C.
Craint la lumière et le gel.

OPIATE AGONIST/AGONISTE DES OPIACÉS
For Slow Intravenous Use • Single-Use
Pour administration intraveineuse lente •
Uniservice

Hospira
Hospira Healthcare Corp.
St-Laurent, QC H4S 0A9

8. Generic name: _____   Special notation: _____

   DIN: _____   Form: _____

   Total volume: _____   Dosage strength: _____

Store at or below 25°C.

DIN: 000000000

DOSAGE AND USE
See package insert for full prescribing information

Each sustained release capsule contains 25 mg topiramate.

Exp./
Lot:

topiramate
Sprinkle capsules

60 capsules

25 mg

SAMPLE LABEL (textbook use only)

http://evolve.elsevier.com/Canada/GrayMorris/

9. Generic name: _____   Form: _____

   Total amount in container: _____   Dosage strength: _____

DIN: 02360365   4 mL
Code: L0010211
                              Sterile / Stérile

℗FUROSEMIDE
INJECTION
              IV / IM

40 mg/4 mL
(10 mg/mL)
omega

DIURETIC
Single Use Vial
Leaflet on request.
Store between 15-30°C.
Protect from light.

DIURÉTIQUE
Fiole à usage unique.
Feuillet sur demande.
Conserver entre 15-30°C.
Protéger de la lumière.

LOT:

EXP:

C00E1151/V-01

omega
Montreal, Canada H3M 3A2

(01)10801500112111

10. Generic name: _____   Form: _____

     Dosage strength: _____   Total volume: _____

ANTIBACTERIAL AGENT
Each tablet contains ciprofloxacin
hydrochloride equivalent to 250 mg
of ciprofloxacin.
Usual Adult Dosage: depending on
severity of infection.
Urinary Tract: 250 mg or 500 mg
twice daily.
**Lower Respiratory Tract, Skin and
Soft Tissue, Bone and Joint:**
500 mg or 750 mg twice daily.
Infectious Diarrhea: 500 mg twice
daily.
Should not be used in prepubertal
patients.
Product monograph available to
physicians and pharmacists upon
request.
Store at controlled room temperature
15-30°C (59-86°F).

338723

℗ 100 Tablets/Comprimés   DIN 02229521

APO-CIPROFLOX

Ciprofloxacin Tablets USP
Comprimés de ciprofloxacine USP

250 mg

Ⓐ **APOTEX INC.** TORONTO CANADA

ANTIBACTÉRIEN
Chaque comprimé renferme de chlorhydrate
de ciprofloxacine équivalant à 250 mg de
ciprofloxacine.
Posologie habituelle pour adultes:
selon la gravité des infections.
Voies urinaires: 250 ou 500 mg deux
fois par jour.
**Voies respiratoires inférieures, peau,
tissus mous, os et articulations:**
500 mg ou 750 mg deux fois par jour.
Diarrhée infectieuse: 500 mg deux
fois par jour.
Ne pas administrer chez les personnes
prépubertaires.
La monographie du produit est
disponible sur demande aux médecins
et pharmaciens.
Entreposer à la température ambiante
contrôlée de 15 à 30°C (59 à 86°F).

APOTEX INC.
TORONTO
CANADA
M9L 1T9

7 71313 05159 0

11. Trade name: _____   Form: _____

     Generic name: _____   Dosage strength: _____

     Total amount in container: _____

Store at 25°C; excursions
permitted to 15°-30°C.
30 mL.

DOSAGE AND USE
See package insert for full
prescribing information

Each 10 mL contains
2 mg granisetron.

Exp./
Lot:

DIN: 000000000

granisetron
hydrochloride
For oral suspension

2 mg per 10 mL

SAMPLE LABEL (textbook use only)

http://evolve.elsevier.com/Canada/GrayMorris/

12. Generic name: _____   Dosage strength: _____

     Form: _____   Total volume: _____

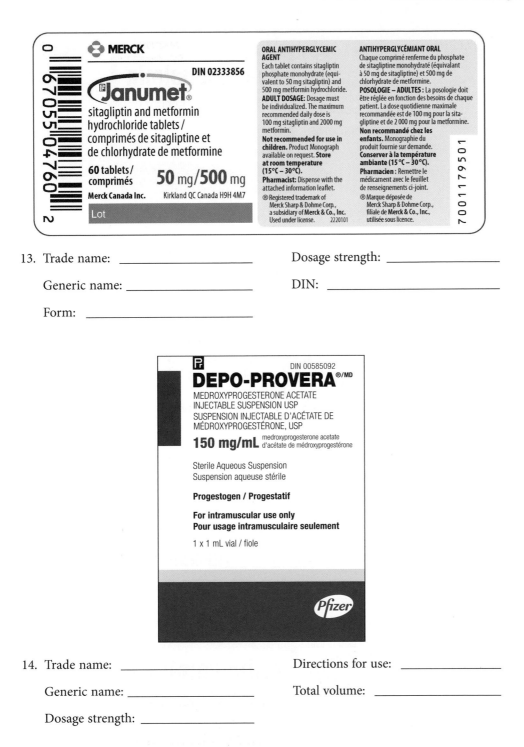

MERCK

DIN 02333856

Janumet®

sitagliptin and metformin
hydrochloride tablets /
comprimés de sitagliptine et
de chlorhydrate de metformine

60 tablets /
comprimés   **50** mg/**500** mg

Merck Canada Inc.   Kirkland QC Canada H9H 4M7

Lot

ORAL ANTIHYPERGLYCEMIC
AGENT
Each tablet contains sitagliptin
phosphate monohydrate (equivalent to 50 mg sitagliptin) and
500 mg metformin hydrochloride.
ADULT DOSAGE: Dosage must
be individualized. The maximum
recommended daily dose is
100 mg sitagliptin and 2000 mg
metformin.
Not recommended for use in
children. Product Monograph
available on request. **Store**
at room temperature
(15°C – 30°C).
Pharmacist: Dispense with the
attached information leaflet.
® Registered trademark of
Merck Sharp & Dohme Corp.,
a subsidiary of **Merck & Co., Inc.**
Used under license.   2220101

ANTIHYPERGLYCÉMIANT ORAL
Chaque comprimé renferme du phosphate
de sitagliptine monohydraté (équivalant
à 50 mg de sitagliptine) et 500 mg de
chlorhydrate de metformine.
POSOLOGIE – ADULTES : La posologie doit
être réglée en fonction des besoins de chaque
patient. La dose quotidienne maximale
recommandée est de 100 mg pour la sitagliptine et de 2 000 mg pour la metformine.
Non recommandé chez les
enfants. Monographie du
produit fournie sur demande.
Conserver à la température
ambiante (15°C – 30°C).
Pharmacien : Remettre le
médicament avec le feuillet
de renseignements ci-joint.
® Marque déposée de
Merck Sharp & Dohme Corp.,
filiale de **Merck & Co., Inc.,**
utilisée sous licence.

7001179501

13. Trade name: _____   Dosage strength: _____

    Generic name: _____   DIN: _____

    Form: _____

DIN 00585092

DEPO-PROVERA®/MD

MEDROXYPROGESTERONE ACETATE
INJECTABLE SUSPENSION USP
SUSPENSION INJECTABLE D'ACÉTATE DE
MÉDROXYPROGESTÉRONE, USP

150 mg/mL medroxyprogesterone acetate
d'acétate de médroxyprogestérone

Sterile Aqueous Suspension
Suspension aqueuse stérile

Progestogen / Progestatif

For intramuscular use only
Pour usage intramusculaire seulement

1 x 1 mL vial / fiole

Pfizer

14. Trade name: _____   Directions for use: _____

    Generic name: _____   Total volume: _____

    Dosage strength: _____

Suggested use: As a dietary supplement.

DOSAGE AND USE
See package insert for full prescribing information

Each tablet contains 2500 mcg cyanocobalmin.

Exp./
Lot:

DIN: 000000000

cyanocobalmin
90 sublingual tablets

2500 mcg

SAMPLE LABEL (textbook use only)

http://evolve.elsevier.com/Canada/GrayMorris/

15. Total amount in container: _____   Dosage strength: _____

   Form: _____   Suggested use: _____

3 mL   DIN 02242325
   Code 1282
Pr Amiodarone HCl
Injection Sandoz Standard
50 mg/mL 150 mg/3 mL
   Sterile
IV infusion only
Perfusion IV seulement
⚠ **SANDOZ**

**Single Use Vial.
Must be diluted.**

**Fiole à usage unique.
Doit être dilué.**

Sandoz Canada Inc.
1-800-361-3062

1003977

(01)10057513012829

Lot   Exp

16. Generic name: _____   Dosage strength: _____

   Form: _____   Total volume: _____

Directions for use: _____

**For IM, SC, or slow IV use.
Warning:** May be habit forming. Store at 15°-30°C.

DOSAGE AND USE
See package insert for full prescribing information

Each mL contains 2 mg hydromorphone hydrochloride.

Exp./
Lot:

DIN: 000000000

hydromorphone hydrochloride
For injection

2 mg/mL
20 mL multiple dose vial

SAMPLE LABEL (textbook use only)

http://evolve.elsevier.com/Canada/GrayMorris/

17. Generic name: _____   Dosage strength: _____

   Directions for use: _____   Total volume: _____

   Form: _____   Warning: _____

MERCK

ZOCOR®

DIN 00884359

simvastatin tablets, Merck Std.
comprimés de simvastatine,
norme de Merck

28 tablets / comprimés

40 mg

(side panel) 28 tablets comprimés ZOCOR® MERCK 40 mg

18. Trade name: _____   Dosage strength: _____

    Generic name: _____   DIN: _____

DIN 02138018

ᴺDemerol®

*Meperidine Hydrochloride
Tablets, Mfr. Std. / Comprimés
de chlorhydrate de mépéridine,
Norme-fabricant*

50 mg

Narcotic Analgesic /
Analgésique narcotique

100 tablets /comprimés

SANOFI

ED131A-C

Each tablet contains 50 mg meperidine hydrochloride.
Usual adult dose: 1 to 3 tablets as directed by a physician.
Store at 15-30°C. Detailed prescribing information available
upon request or at www.sanofi.ca. **Security seal over bottle
and cap.** — Chaque comprimé renferme 50 mg de
chlorhydrate de mépéridine. **Dose habituelle pour adultes :**
1 à 3 comprimés tel que prescrit par un médecin. Conserver
entre 15 et 30 °C. Renseignements posologiques détaillés
disponibles sur demande ou à l'adresse www.sanofi.ca.
Sceau de sécurité sur le flacon et le bouchon.

Manufactured by / Fabriqué
par sanofi-aventis Canada Inc.,
Laval, Québec, Canada H7V 0A3
☎ **1 800 265-7927**

50091682C

Pull here
Tirez ici

(side panel) Espace réservé pour lot et date de péremption

19. Generic name: _____   Dosage strength: _____

    Form: _____   Total amount in container: _____

OPIOID ANALGESIC

Each tablet contains 200 mg morphine sulfate.
Adult Dosage: Usual initial dose is 30 mg every 12 hours. Very elderly or
debilitated, 15 mg every 12 hours. Patients already taking oral morphine,
divide total daily dosage into two 12 hour doses. The 200 mg tablet may
be broken in half. Do not chew or crush the whole or half-tablets. Swallow
intact. Keep this product and all medicine out of the reach of children.
Pharmacist: Dispense with Patient Information Leaflet. Product
Monograph available on request. Store 15 – 30°C. Protect from light.
361-32-771960033T Rev. 01

DIN 02302802   **50** TABLETS COMPRIMÉS

ᴺTEVA

MORPHINE SR

200 mg

Morphine Sulfate
Sustained Release Tablets
Comprimés à libération
prolongée de sulfate de
morphine
Norme Teva Standard

TEVA

ANALGÉSIQUE OPIACÉ

Un comprimé renferme 200 mg de sulfate de morphine.
Posologie chez l'adulte : La dose de départ habituelle est de
30 mg toutes les 12 heures. Pour les personnes très âgées ou
affaiblies, 15 mg toutes les 12 heures. Pour les patients qui
prennent déjà de la morphine par voie orale, il faut diviser la
posologie quotidienne totale en deux doses égales,
administrées à 12 heures d'intervalle. Le comprimé de 200 mg
peut être coupé en deux. Les comprimés ou demi-comprimés
doivent être avalés entiers ; il ne faut pas les croquer ni les
écraser. Comme tout médicament, ranger ce produit hors de la
portée des enfants. **Pharmacien-ne :** Remettre au patient un
feuillet de renseignements. Monographie du produit fournie sur
demande. Conserver entre 15° – 30 °C, à l'abri de la lumière.
TEVA est une marque déposée de
TEVA Pharmaceutical Industries Ltd. used under license by / utilisée sous
licence par TEVA Canada Limited/ Limitée, Toronto, Canada M1B 2K9

20. Trade name: _____   Total amount in container: _____

    Generic name: _____   Dosage strength: _____

    Form: _____

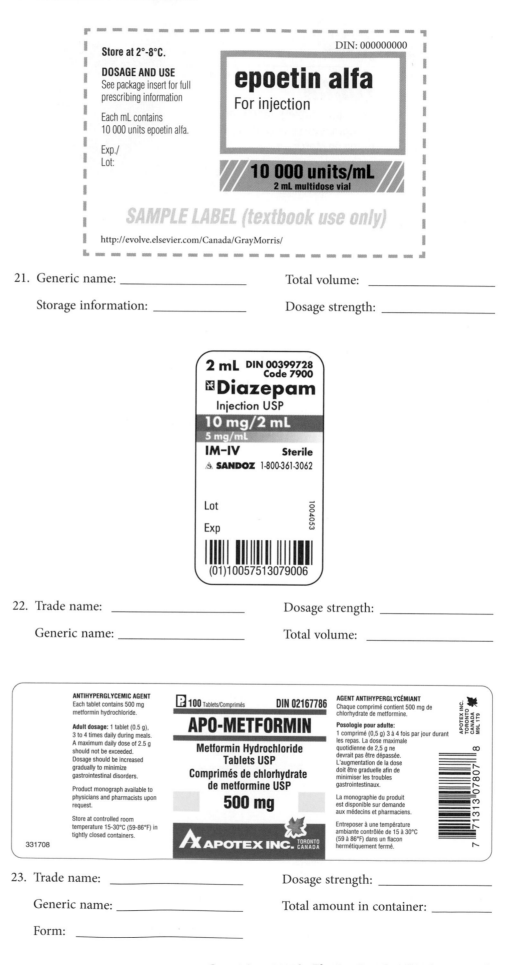

DIN: 000000000

Store at 2°-8°C.

DOSAGE AND USE
See package insert for full
prescribing information

Each mL contains
10 000 units epoetin alfa.

Exp./
Lot:

epoetin alfa
For injection

10 000 units/mL
2 mL multidose vial

SAMPLE LABEL (textbook use only)

http://evolve.elsevier.com/Canada/GrayMorris/

21. Generic name: _____   Total volume: _____

    Storage information: _____   Dosage strength: _____

2 mL DIN 00399728
Code 7900
℞ **Diazepam**
Injection USP
10 mg/2 mL
5 mg/mL
IM-IV   **Sterile**
⚠ **SANDOZ** 1-800-361-3062

Lot   1004053

Exp

(01)10057513079006

22. Trade name: _____   Dosage strength: _____

    Generic name: _____   Total volume: _____

ANTIHYPERGLYCEMIC AGENT
Each tablet contains 500 mg
metformin hydrochloride.

Adult dosage: 1 tablet (0.5 g),
3 to 4 times daily during meals.
A maximum daily dose of 2.5 g
should not be exceeded.
Dosage should be increased
gradually to minimize
gastrointestinal disorders.

Product monograph available to
physicians and pharmacists upon
request.

Store at controlled room
temperature 15-30°C (59-86°F) in
tightly closed containers.

331708

℞ **100** Tablets/Comprimés   DIN 02167786

APO-METFORMIN

Metformin Hydrochloride
Tablets USP
Comprimés de chlorhydrate
de metformine USP
500 mg

Ⓧ APOTEX INC. TORONTO CANADA

AGENT ANTIHYPERGLYCÉMIANT
Chaque comprimé contient 500 mg de
chlorhydrate de metformine.

Posologie pour adulte:
1 comprimé (0,5 g) 3 à 4 fois par jour durant
les repas. La dose maximale
quotidienne de 2,5 g ne
devrait pas être dépassée.
L'augmentation de la dose
doit être graduelle afin de
minimiser les troubles
gastrointestinaux.

La monographie du produit
est disponible sur demande
aux médecins et pharmaciens.

Entreposer à une température
ambiante contrôlée de 15 à 30°C
(59 à 86°F) dans un flacon
hermétiquement fermé.

APOTEX INC.
TORONTO
CANADA
M9L 1T9

7 71313 07807 8

23. Trade name: _____   Dosage strength: _____

    Generic name: _____   Total amount in container: _____

    Form: _____

CENTRAL NERVOUS SYSTEM STIMULANT

Each tablet contains 5 mg methylphenidate hydrochloride.

Adult Dosage: 20 - 30 mg/day in divided doses 2 or 3 times/day. Some patients may require 40 - 60 mg/day. Others, 10 - 15 mg/day.

Children 6 years and over: Initially 5 - 10 mg 3 times/day. Increase weekly by 5 - 10 mg/day. Individualize dosage up to 60 mg/day maximum.

PHARMACIST: PLEASE DISPENSE WITH THE PATIENT INFORMATION LEAFLET.

Prescribing information available to physicians and pharmacists upon request.

230381   Protect from heat (store between 15 and 30°C) and humidity.

100 Tablets/Comprimés   **DIN 02273950**

APO-METHYLPHENIDATE

Methylphenidate Hydrochloride Tablets USP
Comprimés de chlorhydrate de méthylphénidate USP

5 mg

APOTEX INC. TORONTO CANADA

STIMULANT DU SYSTÈME NERVEUX CENTRAL

Chaque comprimé contient 5 mg de chlorhydrate de méthylphénidate.

Posologie adulte: 20 à 30 mg/jour en doses fractionnées 2 ou 3 fois/jour. Certains patients peuvent avoir besoin de 40 à 60 mg/jour, tandis que d'autres n'ont besoin que de 10 à 15 mg/jour.

Enfants 6 ans et plus: Dose initiale: 5 à 10 mg 3 fois/jour. Augmenter chaque semaine, de 5 à 10 mg/jour. La posologie devrait être ajustée aux besoins individuels et ne devrait pas dépasser 60 mg/jour.

PHARMACIEN: VEUILLEZ REMETTRE AVEC LE FEUILLET D'INFORMATION ÉTABLI À L'INTENTION DU PATIENT.

Renseignements posologiques est disponible sur demande aux médecins et pharmaciens.

Protéger de la chaleur (conserver entre 15 et 30°C) et de l'humidité.

7 71313 16990 5

24. Generic name: _____   Dosage strength: _____

Instructions to pharmacist: _____

Store at 20°-25°C.

DOSAGE AND USE
See package insert for full prescribing information

Each tablet contains 200 mg amoxicillin and clavulanate potassium.

Exp./
Lot:

DIN: 000000000

amoxicillin and clavulanate potassium
20 chewable tablets

200 mg/28.5 mg

SAMPLE LABEL (textbook use only)

http://evolve.elsevier.com/Canada/GrayMorris/

25. Generic name: _____   Form: _____

Dosage strength: _____   Total amount in container: _____

For IM or IV use.
Store at controlled room temperature 15°-30°C.

DOSAGE AND USE
See package insert for full prescribing information

Each 5 mL contains 250 mcg fentanyl citrate.

Exp./
Lot:

DIN: 000000000

fentanyl citrate
For injection

250 mcg/5 mL
10 x 5 mL dosette ampuls

SAMPLE LABEL (textbook use only)

http://evolve.elsevier.com/Canada/GrayMorris/

26. Generic name: _____   Form: _____

Dosage strength: _____   Directions for use: _____

Sterile/Stérile **DIN 02319039**

Cefepime
for/pour injection
House Standard / Norme - maison

2.0 g

2.0 g per vial / par fiole
Single Use Vial / Fiole unidose
ANTIBIOTIC / ANTIBIOTIQUE
For IV use / Pour usage IV

Dose should be individualized.
Dosage and Administration: See outer carton and package insert. **RECONSTITUTION: I.V. / I.V. INFUSION:** See outer carton and package insert. **Store powder at 15-30°C or at 2-8°C. Protect from light.** Discard unused portion. Each single use vial contains 2 g cefepime (as cefepime HCl) and 1450 mg L-arginine.
La dose doit être adaptée à chaque patient.
Posologie et mode d'administration: Lire l'emballage et la notice ci-incluse. **RECONSTITUTION: I.V. / PERFUSION I.V.:** Lire l'emballage et la notice ci-incluse. **Conserver la poudre à 15 à 30°C ou à 2 à 8°C. Protéger de la lumière.** Jeter toute portion inutilisée. Une fiole unidose contient 2 g de céfépime (comme chlorhydrate de céfépime) et 1450 mg L-arginine.
Dist. by / dist. par: Apotex Inc.,Toronto, Canada

948006079

M.L. No. 763 TN/DRUGS/763
(01)0(07)7131319104

27. Generic name: _____   Dosage strength: _____

    Form: _____   Directions for use: _____

LAXATIVE
Each mL contains lactulose 667 mg and less than 147 mg galactose, less than 80 mg of lactose and less than 80 mg of the other sugars (epilactose and fructose). Non medicinal ingredients: D&C Yellow #10, FD&C Yellow #6 and purified water.
USUAL ADULT DOSE: 1 to 4 tablespoonfuls (15 to 60 mL) daily as required.
WARNINGS: Do not take for more than one week, unless your physician has ordered a special schedule for you. Overuse or extended use may cause dependence for bowel function. Should not be taken within 2 hours of another medicine because the desired effect of the other medication may be reduced. Should not be used in the presence of abdominal pain, nausea, fever or vomiting.
CAUTIONS: Persons who are diabetic should only use lactulose solution on the advice of a physician. Lactulose solution should not be used, except on the advice of a physician, by women who are pregnant or who may become pregnant.
CONTRAINDICATION: Should not be used by persons who require a low galactose diet.
Before taking this product, please tell your healthcare provider if you have allergies to the milk components, galactose or lactose and/or any ingredient(s) listed in the product.
Prescribing information available to physicians and pharmacists upon request.
Store at room temperature 15-30°C (59-86°F). Protect from freezing.
Product may develop some darkening or cloudy appearance, but not loss of therapeutic effect.
Safety seal under the cap.

500 mL   DIN 02242814

APO-LACTULOSE

Lactulose Solution USP
Solution de lactulose USP
Laxative/Laxatif

667 mg/mL

APOTEX INC. TORONTO CANADA

LAXATIF
Chaque mL contient 667 mg de lactulose et moins de 147 mg de galactose, moins de 80 mg de lactose et moins de 80 mg des autres sucres comme ingrédients inertes (epilactose et fructose).
Les ingrédients non médicinaux: colorant D&C jaune #10, colorant FD&C jaune #6 et eau purifiée.
POSOLOGIE HABITUELLE POUR ADULTES:
1 à 4 cuillerées à table (15 à 60 mL) par jour, selon le besoin.
MISES EN GARDE: Ne pas prendre au-delà d'une semaine, sauf sur recommandation d'un médecin. Le surdosage ou l'usage prolongé peut causer la dépendance de la fonction intestinale.
Ne devrait pas être pris en dedans de 2 heures avec un autre médicament, sinon l'effet de l'autre médicament pourrait être diminué. Ne doit pas être utilisé s'il y a douleurs abdominales, nausées, fièvre ou vomissements.
ATTENTION: Doit être pris seulement sur l'avis d'un médecin par les diabétiques. Ne doit pas être pris, sauf sur l'avis d'un médecin, par les femmes qui sont enceintes ou qui peuvent le devenir.
CONTRE-INDICATION:
Ne doit pas être pris par des personnes qui doivent suivre un régime à faible teneur en galactose.
Avant d'utiliser ce produit, consultez votre professionnel de la santé si vous êtes allergique aux composants du lait, galactose ou lactose ou à l'un des autres ingrédients.
Renseignements thérapeutiques disponible sur demande aux médecins et pharmaciens.
Entreposer à la température ambiante de 15 à 30°C (de 59 à 86°F). Protéger de la congélation.
Le produit peut prendre une apparence foncée ou brouillée, mais cela n'affecte pas son effect thérapeutique.
Sceau sécuritaire sous le bouchon.

APOTEX INC.
TORONTO
CANADA
M9L 1T9

373798

28. Total volume: _____   Form: _____

    Storage: _____   Dosage strength: _____

ANTIANGINAL AND ANTIHYPERTENSIVE
Adult Dosage: dosage must be individualized.
Chronic Stable Angina: Initial dose: 120 to 180 mg once daily. Dose range is 120 mg - 360 mg once daily.
Mild to Moderate Hypertension: Initial dose: 180 mg or 240 mg once daily. Dose range is 120 mg - 360 mg once daily.
– Maximum daily dose: 360 mg.
– Safe use in children not yet established.
Product monograph available to physicians and pharmacists upon request.
Store at room temperature 15-30°C.

234303

100 Capsules   **DIN 02230998**

APO-DILTIAZ CD

Diltiazem Hydrochloride
Controlled Delivery Capsules
Capsules à libération contrôlée de
Chlorhydrate de Diltiazem
Norme Apotex Standard

180 mg

APOTEX INC. TORONTO CANADA

ANTIANGINEUX ET ANTIHYPERTENSEUR
Posologie adulte: la posologie doit être individualisée.
Angine chronique stable: Dose initiale: 120 mg à 180 mg une fois par jour. La dose se situe entre 120 mg et 360 mg par jour en une prise.
Hypertension légère à modérée:
Dose initiale: 180 mg ou 240 mg une fois par jour. La dose se situe entre 120 mg et 360 mg par jour en une prise.
– Posologie quotidienne maximale: 360 mg.
– Innocuité chez l'enfant pas encore établie.
La monographie du produit est disponible sur demande aux médecins et pharmaciens.
Entreposer à la température ambiante de 15 à 30°C.

29. Trade name: _____   Dosage strength: _____

    Generic name: _____   Total amount in container: _____

    Form: _____

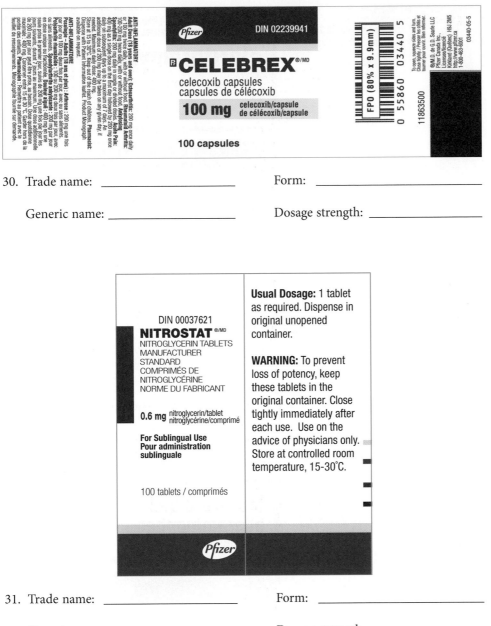

30. Trade name: _____   Form: _____

    Generic name: _____   Dosage strength: _____

31. Trade name: _____   Form: _____

    Generic name: _____   Dosage strength: _____

    Storage information: _____

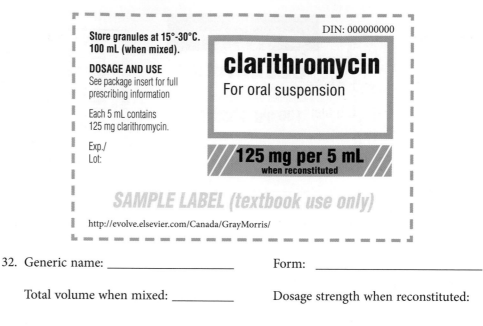

32. Generic name: _____   Form: _____

    Total volume when mixed: _____   Dosage strength when reconstituted:

    _____

Read the combination medication labels and answer the associated questions.

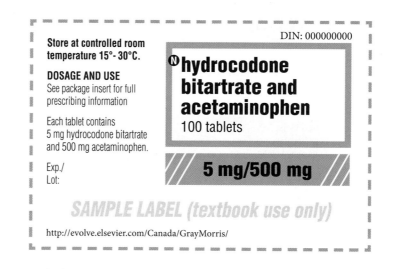

33. The route of administration for this medication would be _____.

34. This medication contains _____ mg of hydrocodone bitartrate and _____ mg of acetaminophen.

35. The total amount in the container is _____.

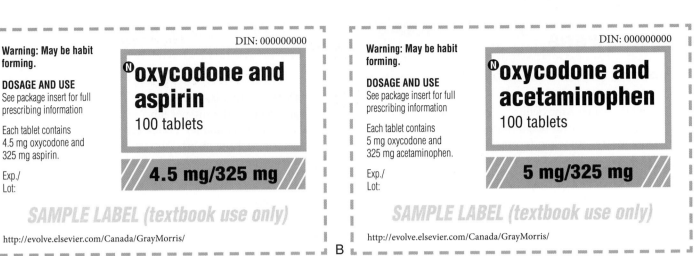

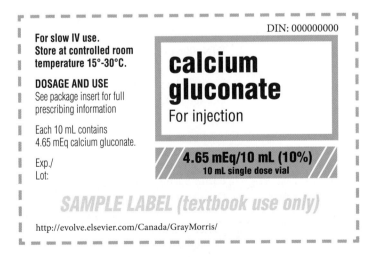

36. The prescriber ordered oxycodone and acetaminophen 1 tab PO q4h prn for pain. The nurse would use which of the medications (A or B) to administer the dosage?

_____

37. The difference between the medications oxycodone and aspirin and oxycodone and acetaminophen is that oxycodone and aspirin contains _____ of oxycodone hydrochloride and _____ of aspirin.

Oxycodone and acetaminophen contains _____ of oxycodone hydrochloride and _____ of acetaminophen.

38. If a patient is allergic to aspirin, which medication should the patient not be given?

_____

39. The dosage strength of this medication expressed as a percentage is

_____.

40. The dosage strength of this medication in mEq per mL is _____.

Answers on pages 200–202.

evolve

For additional practice problems, refer to the Safety in Medication Administration section of the Drug Calculations Companion, Version 5 on Evolve.

✳ ANSWERS

Answers to Practice Problems

1. Trade name: Novamoxin
   Generic name: Amoxicillin
   Form: Powder; oral suspension when reconstituted
   Dosage strength when reconstituted: 25 mg per mL
   Total volume when mixed: 75 mL

2. Generic name: Hydroxyzine hydrochloride
   Form: Injectable liquid
   Dosage strength: 50 mg per mL
   Total volume: 1 mL

3. Trade name: Apo-Divalproex
   Generic name: Divalproex sodium
   DIN: 02239699
   Dosage strength: 250 mg per tablet
   Total amount in container: 100 tablets

4. Generic name: Imatinib mesylate
   Dosage strength: 400 mg per tab
   Total amount in container: 30 tablets
   Storage: See package insert. Store at 25°C excursions permitted to 15°C to 30°C.

5. Trade name: Apo-Warfarin
   Form: Tablets
   Dosage strength: 5 mg per tablet
   DIN: 02242928
   Total amount in container: 100 tablets

6. Trade name: Norvir
   Generic name: Ritonavir
   Total amount in container: 30 tablets
   Can this medication be crushed? No. The label indicates tablets should be swallowed whole and not chewed, broken, or crushed.

Answers to Chapter Review

1. Generic name: Paricalcitol
   Total amount in container: 30 capsules
   Form: Capsules
   Dosage strength: 2 mcg (micrograms) per capsule

2. Generic name: Digoxin
   DIN: 02048264
   Form: Injectable liquid
   Dosage strength: 0.5 mg per 2 mL

3. Generic name: Tadalafil
   Storage: Store at 25°C
   Form: Tablets
   Dosage strength: 10 mg per tablet
   Total amount in container: 30 tablets

4. Generic name: Levothyroxine sodium
   Total amount in container: 1 000 tablets
   Form: Tablets
   Dosage strength: 88 mcg per tablet; 0.088 mg per tablet

5. Generic name: Potassium acetate
   Form: Injectable liquid
   Dosage strength: 40 mEq per 20 mL; 2 mEq per mL
   Total volume: 20 mL

6. Generic name: Saquinavir
   Usual dosage: See accompanying package insert
   Alert: Find out about medicines that should not be taken with saquinavir
   Form: Capsules; soft gelatin capsules
   Dosage strength: 200 mg per soft gelatin capsule
   Total amount in container: 180 soft gelatin capsules

7. Generic name: Acyclovir
   Form: Powder; injectable liquid once reconstituted
   Directions for mixing: Inject 20 mL sterile water for injection into vial, shake vial until a clear solution is achieved and use within 12 hours.
   Dosage strength after reconstitution: 1 000 mg per 20 mL
   Directions for use: For IV infusion only

8. Generic name: Morphine sulfate
   DIN: 00649619
   Total volume: 30 mL
   Form: Injectable liquid
   Dosage strength: 5 mg per mL
   Special notation: Narcotic

9. Generic name: Topiramate
   Total amount in container: 60 sprinkle capsules
   Form: Sprinkle capsules
   Dosage strength: 25 mg per sprinkle capsule

10. Generic name: Furosemide
    Dosage strength: 40 mg per 4 mL; 10 mg per mL
    Form: Injectable liquid
    Total volume: 4 mL

11. Trade name: Apo-Ciproflox
    Generic name: Ciprofloxacin
    Total amount in container: 100 tablets
    Form: Tablets
    Dosage strength: 250 mg per tablet

12. Generic name: Granisetron HCl
    Form: Oral suspension
    Dosage strength: 2 mg per 10 mL
    Total volume: 30 mL

13. Trade name: Janumet
    Generic name: Sitagliptin/metformin HCl
    Form: Tablets
    Dosage strength: 50 mg per tablet of sitagliptin and 500 mg per tablet of metformin HCl
    DIN: 02333856

14. Trade name: Depo-Provera
    Generic name: Medroxyprogesterone acetate
    Dosage strength: 150 mg per mL
    Directions for use: For intramuscular use only
    Total volume: 1 mL

15. Total amount in container: 90 sublingual tablets
    Form: Sublingual tablets
    Dosage strength: 2 500 mcg per sublingual tablet
    Suggested use: As a dietary supplement

16. Generic name: Amiodarone HCl
    Form: Injectable liquid
    Directions for use: For IV infusion only
    Dosage strength: 150 mg per 3 mL
    Total volume: 3 mL

17. Generic name: Hydromorphone hydrochloride
    Directions for use: For IM, SC (SUBCUT), or slow IV use
    Form: Injectable liquid
    Dosage strength: 2 mg per mL
    Total volume: 20 mL
    Warning: May be habit forming

18. Trade name: Zocor
    Generic name: Simvastatin
    Dosage strength: 40 mg per tablet
    DIN: 00884359

19. Generic name: Meperidine hydrochloride
    Form: Tablets
    Dosage strength: 50 mg per tablet
    Total amount in container: 100 tablets

20. Trade name: Teva Morphine SR
    Generic name: Morphine sulphate
    Form: Sustained-release tablets
    Total amount in container: 50 tablets
    Directions for use: Do not chew or crush the whole or half-tablets. Swallow intact.
    Dosage strength: 200 mg per sustained-release tablet

21. Generic name: Epoetin alfa
    Storage information: Store at 2°C to 8°C
    Total volume: 2 mL
    Dosage strength: 10 000 units per mL; 20 000 units per 2 mL

22. Generic name: Diazepam
    Dosage strength: 5 mg per mL
    Total volume: 2 mL

23. Trade name: APO-Metformin
    Generic name: Metformin hydrochloride
    Form: Tablets
    Dosage strength: 500 mg
    Total amount in container: 100 tablets

24. Generic name: Methylphenidate hydrochloride
    Instructions to pharmacist: Please dispense with the patient information leaflet.
    Dosage strength: 5 mg per tablet

25. Generic name: Amoxicillin and clavulanate potassium
    Dosage strength: 200 mg amoxicillin per chewable tablet and 28.5 mg clavulanate potassium per chewable tablet
    Form: Chewable tablets
    Total amount in container: 20 chewable tablets

26. Generic name: Fentanyl citrate
    Dosage strength: 250 mcg per 5 mL; 50 mcg per mL; 0.05 mg per mL
    Form: Injectable liquid
    Directions for use: For intravenous or intramuscular use

27. Generic name: Cefepime
    Form: Powder
    Dosage strength: 2 g per vial
    Directions for use: For IV use

28. Total volume: 500 mL
    Storage: Store at controlled room temperature 15° to 30°C (59° to 86°F). Do not freeze.
    Form: Oral solution
    Dosage strength: 667 mg per mL

29. Trade name: Apo-Diltiaz CD
    Generic name: Diltiazem hydrochloride
    Form: Controlled-delivery capsules
    Dosage strength: 180 mg per controlled-delivery capsule
    Total amount in container: 100 controlled-delivery capsules

30. Trade name: Celebrex
Generic name: Celecoxib
Form: Capsules
Dosage strength: 100 mg per capsule

31. Trade name: Nitrostat
Generic name: Nitroglycerin
Storage information: Store at controlled room
temperature 15°C to 30°C
Form: Tablets
Dosage strength: 0.6 mg per tablet

32. Generic name: Clarithromycin
Total volume when mixed: 100 mL
Form: Granules; oral suspension when reconstituted
Dosage strength when reconstituted: 125 mg per 5 mL

33. by mouth, PO

34. 5 mg of hydrocodone bitartrate and 500 mg of
acetaminophen

35. 100 tablets

36. B (oxycodone and acetaminophen)

37. 4.5 mg of oxycodone hydrochloride; 325 mg of
aspirin; 5 mg of oxycodone hydrochloride; and
325 mg of acetaminophen.

38. Oxycodone and aspirin

39. 10%

40. 0.465 mEq per mL

CHAPTER 12

Dosage Calculation Using the Ratio and Proportion Method

Objectives

After reviewing this chapter, you should be able to:

1. Understand how to use ratio and proportion to solve a given dosage calculation problem
2. Solve simple calculation problems using the ratio and proportion method

Several methods are used for calculating dosages. The most common are the *ratio and proportion method*, the *formula method* (Chapter 13), and the *dimensional analysis method* (Chapter 14). Students can choose the method they find easiest and most logical to use. This chapter discusses how to use ratio and proportion to calculate dosages. If necessary, review Chapter 3, on ratio and proportion.

Using Ratio and Proportion to Calculate Dosages

When you know three of the four values of a proportion, you can solve the proportion to determine the unknown quantity. In dosage calculation, it is often necessary to find only one unknown quantity. As you recall from Chapter 3, the proportion can be set up stating the terms using colons (ratio format) or as a fraction. Recall too that a proportion is an equation of two ratios of equal value. Before solving for the unknown quantity, it is essential to be competent in setting up the ratio and proportion correctly.

> **⚠ SAFETY ALERT!**
> If you set up the ratio and proportion incorrectly, you could calculate the dose incorrectly and administer the wrong dose, which could have serious consequences for the patient.

Suppose that you have a medication with a dosage strength of 50 mg per mL, and the prescriber orders a dose of 25 milligrams (mg). Ratio and proportion can be used to determine how many millilitres (mL) to administer. Remember to include the units of measurement when writing a ratio and proportion to avoid errors.

When setting up the ratio and proportion using the fraction format to calculate dosages, the known ratio is what you have available (what is on hand) or the information on the medication label. It is stated first (placed on the left side of the proportion). The desired dosage, or what is ordered to be administered, is the unknown (placed on the right side). Therefore, the ratio and proportion would be stated as follows.

Example:
$$\frac{50\,\text{mg}}{1\,\text{mL}} = \frac{25\,\text{mg}}{x\,\text{mL}}$$
$$\text{(known)} \quad \text{(unknown)}$$

When writing the ratio and proportion using ratio format, the known ratio—what you have available or the information on the medication label—is stated first, and the unknown ratio is stated second.

Example:
$$50 \, mg : 1 \, mL = 25 \, mg : x \, mL$$
$$\text{(known)} \qquad \text{(unknown)}$$

Solution: To solve for x, use the principles of ratio and proportion presented in Chapter 3.

$$\frac{50 \, mg}{1 \, mL} = \frac{25 \, mg}{x \, mL}$$
$$\text{(known)} \quad \text{(unknown)}$$

$$\frac{50x}{50} = \frac{25}{50}$$

$$x = 0.5 \, mL$$

Remember: the known is stated as the first fraction, and the unknown as the second. When using fraction format, solve by cross-multiplication.

or

$$50 \, mg : 1 \, mL = 25 \, mg : x \, mL$$
$$\text{(known)} \qquad \text{(unknown)}$$

$$50x = \text{product of extremes}$$
$$25 = \text{product of means}$$
$$50x = 25 \text{ is the equation}$$
$$\frac{50x}{50} = \frac{25}{50} \qquad \text{(Divide both sides by 50, the number in front of } x.\text{)}$$

$$x = 0.5 \, mL$$

! SAFETY ALERT!

Remember: when using ratio and proportion, write the units of measurement in the same sequence (in the examples, $\frac{mg}{mL} = \frac{mg}{mL}$ or mg:mL = mg:mL). Labelling all terms with their unit of measurement, including x, is also essential. These pointers are crucial to preventing calculation errors.

Example: Order: 40 mg PO of a medication.

Available: 20 mg tablets. How many tablets will the nurse administer?

Solution:
$$\frac{20 \, mg}{1 \, tab} = \frac{40 \, mg}{x \, tab}$$
$$\text{(known)} \quad \text{(unknown)}$$

$$\frac{20x}{20} = \frac{40}{20}$$
$$x = 2 \, tabs$$

or

$$20 \, mg : 1 \, tab = 40 \, mg : x \, tab$$
$$\text{(known)} \qquad \text{(unknown)}$$

$$\frac{20x}{20} = \frac{40}{20}$$
$$x = 2 \, tabs$$

Example: Order: Cefadroxil 1 g PO.

Available: 500 mg capsules. How many capsules will the nurse administer?

Solution: Notice that the dosage ordered is in a different unit from what is available. Proceed first by converting the units of measurement so they are the same. After making the conversion, set up the problem and calculate the dosage to be given. As shown in Chapter 6, ratio and proportion can be used for conversion.

Grams are converted to milligrams by using the conversion factor 1 000 mg = 1 g. After making the conversion of 1 g to 1 000 mg, the ratio is stated as follows:

$$\frac{500\ \text{mg}}{1\ \text{capsules}} = \frac{1000\ \text{mg}}{x\ \text{capsules}} \quad or \quad 500\ \text{mg} : 1\ \text{capsule} = 1000\ \text{mg} : x\ \text{capsules}$$

(known)   (unknown)   (known)   (unknown)

$$x = 2\ \text{caps} \qquad\qquad\qquad x = 2\ \text{caps}$$

An alternative method of solving might be to convert milligrams to grams. In this method, 500 mg would be converted to grams by using the same conversion factor: 1 000 mg = 1 g. However, decimals are common when units of measurement are changed from smaller to larger in the metric system: 500 mg = 0.5 g. Even though converting the milligrams to grams would produce the same final answer, *conversions that result in decimals are often the source of calculation errors.* Therefore, if possible, avoid conversions that require their use. As a rule, it is best to convert to the unit of measurement stated on the medication label. Doing so consistently can prevent confusion. As with the other examples, this proportion could be stated as a fraction as well.

For the purpose of learning to calculate dosages by using ratio and proportion, this chapter emphasizes the mathematics used to calculate the answer. Determining whether an answer is logical is essential and necessary in the calculation of medication. An answer *must make sense.* Determining whether an answer is logical will be discussed further in later chapters covering the calculation of dosages by various routes.

POINTS TO REMEMBER

When using the ratio and proportion method to calculate dosages:

- Make sure all units are in the same system of measurement before calculating. If they are not, a conversion will be necessary before calculating the dosage.
- When conversion of units is required, convert what is ordered to the unit of measurement stated on the medication available. Alternatively, convert the unit of measurement of the medication available to the unit of measurement in which the medication is ordered. Be consistent in how you make conversions. *Note:* Typically, the medication ordered is converted to the same unit of measurement of the medication available.
- When stating ratios, state the known ratio first. The known ratio is what is available or on hand or the information obtained from the medication label.
- State the unknown ratio second. The unknown ratio is the desired dosage, or what the prescriber has ordered.
- Write the units of measurement in the same sequence.

Example: $mg : mL = mg : mL$ *or* $= \dfrac{mg}{mL} = \dfrac{mg}{mL}$

- Label all terms of the ratios in the proportion with their unit of measurement, including *x.*
- Before calculating the dosage, make a mental estimate of the approximate and reasonable answer.
- Label the value you obtain for *x* (e.g., mL, tabs). Double-check the label for *x* by referring back to the label of *x* in the original ratio and proportion; it should be the same.
- Note that a proportion can be written in ratio format or fraction format.
- Double-check all calculations.
- Be consistent in how ratios are stated and conversions are done.
- Remember: an error in the setup of the ratio and proportion can cause an error in calculation.

PRACTICE **PROBLEMS**

Calculate the following dosages and indicate whether you need less than 1 tablet or more than 1 tablet. If necessary, review Chapter 3.

1. A patient is to receive 0.2 mg of a medication. The tablets available are 0.4 mg.

   How many tablets should the nurse administer? _____

2. A patient is to receive 1.25 mg of a medication. The tablets available are 0.625 mg.

   How many tablets should the nurse administer? _____

3. A patient is to receive 7.5 mg of a medication. The tablets available are 15 mg.

   How many tablets should the nurse administer? _____

4. A patient is to receive 10 mg of a medication. The tablets available are 20 mg.

   How many tablets should the nurse administer? _____

5. A patient is to receive 100 mg of a medication. The tablets available are 50 mg.

   How many tablets should the nurse administer? _____

Solve the following problems using ratio and proportion. Label answers correctly: tabs, capsules, or mL. Answers expressed in millilitres should be rounded to the nearest tenth where indicated. (*IM,* intramuscular; *IV,* intravenous; *mcg,* microgram; *mmol,* millimole; *PO,* orally; *SUBCUT,* subcutaneous.)

6. Order: 7.5 mg PO of a medication.

   Available: Tablets labelled 5 mg _____

7. Order: 45 mg PO of a medication.

   Available: Tablets labelled 30 mg _____

8. Order: 90 mg PO of a medication.

   Available: Capsules labelled 100 mg _____

9. Order: 0.25 mg IM of a medication.

   Available: 0.5 mg per mL _____

10. Order: 100 mg PO of a liquid medication.

    Available: 125 mg per 5 mL _____

11. Order: 20 mmol IV of a medication.

    Available: 40 mmol per 10 mL _____

12. Order: 5 000 units SUBCUT of a medication.

    Available: 10 000 units per mL _____

13. Order: 50 mg IM of a medication.

    Available: 80 mg per 2 mL _____

14. Order: 0.5 g PO of an antibiotic.

    Available: Capsules labelled 250 mg _____

15. Order: 400 mg PO of a liquid medication.

    Available: 125 mg per 5 mL _____

16. Order: 50 mg IM of a medication.

    Available: 80 mg per mL _____

17. Order: 60 mg IM of a medication.

    Available: 30 mg per mL _____

18. Order: 15 mg of a medication.

    Available: Tablets labelled 5 mg _____

19. Order: 0.24 g PO of a liquid medication.

    Available: 80 mg per 7.5 mL _____

20. Order: 20 g PO of a liquid medication.

    Available: 10 g per 15 mL _____

21. Order: 0.125 mg IM of a medication.

    Available: 0.5 mg per 2 mL _____

22. Order: 0.75 mg IM of a medication.

    Available: 0.25 mg per mL _____

23. Order: 375 mg PO of a liquid medication.

    Available: 125 mg per 5 mL _____

24. Order: 10 000 units SUBCUT of a medication.

    Available: 7 500 units per mL _____

25. Order: 0.45 mg PO of a medication.

    Available: Tablets labelled 0.3 mg _____

26. Order: 20 mg IM of a medication.

    Available: 25 mg per 1.5 mL _____

27. Order: 150 mg IV of a medication.

    Available: 80 mg per mL _____

28. Order: 2 mg IM of a medication.

    Available: 1.5 mg per 0.5 mL _____

29. Order: 500 mcg IV of a medication.

    Available: 750 mcg per 3 mL _____

30. Order: 0.15 mg IM of a medication.

    Available: 0.2 mg per 1.5 mL _____

31. Order: 1 100 units SUBCUT of a medication.

    Available: 1 000 units per 1.5 mL _____

32. Order: 0.6 g IV of a medication.

    Available: 1 g per 3.6 mL _____

33. Order: 3 g IV of a medication.

    Available: 1.5 g per mL _____

34. Order: 35 mg IM of a medication.

    Available: 40 mg per 2.5 mL _____

35. Order: 0.3 mg SUBCUT of a medication.

    Available: 1 000 mcg per 2 mL _____

36. Order: 200 mg IM of a medication.

    Available: 0.5 g per 2 mL _____

37. Order: 10 mmol IV of a medication.

    Available: 20 mmol per 10 mL _____

38. Order: 165 mg IV of a medication.

    Available: 55 mg per 1.1 mL _____

39. Order: 35 mg SUBCUT of a medication.

    Available: 45 mg per 1.2 mL _____

40. Order: 700 mg IM of a medication.

    Available: 1 000 mg per 2.3 mL _____

Use the ratio and proportion method to solve for the unknown quantity.

41. If 15 mL of solution contains 75 mg of medication, how many mg of medication are in 60 mL of solution? _____

42. A patient must take three tablets per day for 28 days. How many tablets should the pharmacy supply to fill this order? _____

43. A health care provider is instructed to administer 700 mL of a solution every 8 hours. How many hours will be needed to administer 2 100 mL?

_____

44. Two tablets contain a total of 6.25 mg of a medication. How many mg of medication are in 10 tablets? _____

45. If 80 mg of medication is in 480 mL of solution, how many mL of solution contain 60 mg of medication? _____

46. A patient is prescribed ondansetron hydrochloride (Apo-Ondansetron) 3 mg IV for post-operative nausea and vomiting. The medication is available in 2 mg per mL. How many mL should the nurse administer? _____

47. The nurse is to administer one dose of Hepatitis A & B Junior vaccine to a 15-year-old patient as a result of non-immune status. The vaccine is available in a single-dose pre-filled syringe of 10 mcg per 0.5 mL. How many mL should the nurse administer?

_____

48. The physician increased a patient's daily lansoprazole from 30 mg to 60 mg. The medication is available in 30-mg tablets and the patient already received one tablet this morning. How many additional tablets should the nurse administer to the patient during the day to fulfill the new daily dose?_____

Answers on pages 232–235.

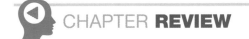 CHAPTER **REVIEW**

Part I

Calculate the number of tablets or capsules necessary to provide the dosage ordered using the labels or the information provided. Label answers correctly: tabs, capsules, mL.

1. Order: Phenobarbital 15 mg PO TID.

   Available: Phenobarbital tablets labelled 15 mg _____

2. Order: Apo-Divalproex 500 mg PO q12h.

Available:

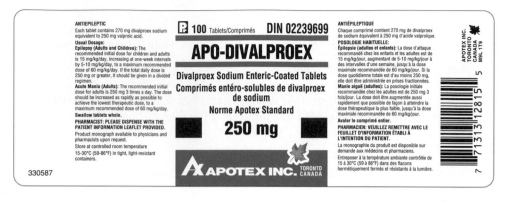

3. Order: Apo-Dipyridamole 50 mg PO QID.

Available:

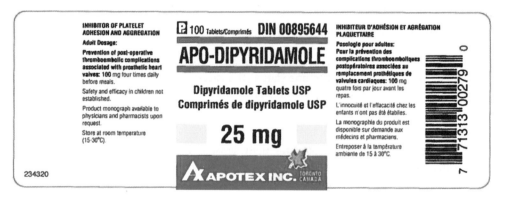

4. Order: Phenobarbital 60 mg PO at bedtime.

Available: Phenobarbital scored tablets (can be broken in half) labelled 30 mg

5. Order: Baclofen 20 mg PO TID.

Available: Baclofen scored tablets (can be broken in half) labelled 10 mg

6. Order: Isosorbide dinitrate 80 mg PO q12h.

   Available:

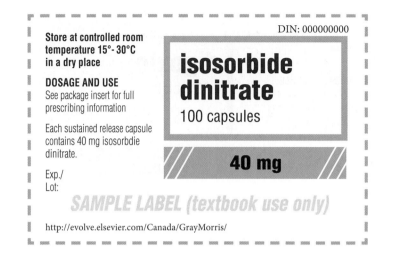

Store at controlled room
temperature 15°- 30°C
in a dry place

DOSAGE AND USE
See package insert for full
prescribing information

Each sustained release capsule
contains 40 mg isosorbdie
dinitrate.

Exp./
Lot:

DIN: 000000000

**isosorbide
dinitrate**
100 capsules

40 mg

SAMPLE LABEL (textbook use only)

http://evolve.elsevier.com/Canada/GrayMorris/

_____

7. Order: Dexamethasone 4 mg PO q6h.

   Available: Dexamethasone tablets labelled 2 mg   _____

8. Order: Diabeta 5 mg PO daily.

   Available:

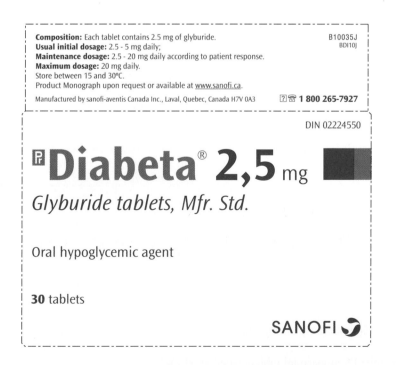

Composition: Each tablet contains 2.5 mg of glyburide.
Usual initial dosage: 2.5 - 5 mg daily;
Maintenance dosage: 2.5 - 20 mg daily according to patient response.
Maximum dosage: 20 mg daily.
Store between 15 and 30°C.
Product Monograph upon request or available at www.sanofi.ca.
Manufactured by sanofi-aventis Canada Inc., Laval, Quebec, Canada H7V 0A3

B10035J
BDI10J

☎ **1 800 265-7927**

DIN 02224550

Pr **Diabeta**® **2,5** mg
Glyburide tablets, Mfr. Std.

Oral hypoglycemic agent

30 tablets

SANOFI 🌀

_____

9. Order: Digoxin 125 mcg PO daily.

   Available: Digoxin scored tablets (can be broken in half)

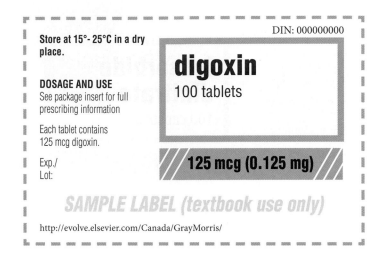

Store at 15°- 25°C in a dry place.

DOSAGE AND USE
See package insert for full prescribing information

Each tablet contains 125 mcg digoxin.

Exp./
Lot:

DIN: 000000000

digoxin
100 tablets

125 mcg (0.125 mg)

SAMPLE LABEL (textbook use only)

http://evolve.elsevier.com/Canada/GrayMorris/

_____

10. Order: Eltroxin 0.05 mg PO daily.

    Available: Eltroxin tablets labelled 50 mcg (0.05 mg) _____

11. Order: Clorazepate dipotassium 30 mg PO at bedtime.

    Available:

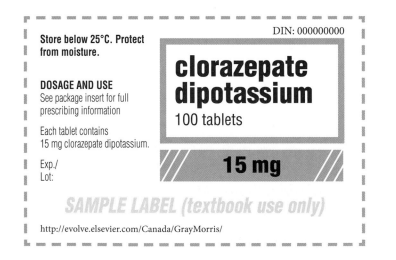

Store below 25°C. Protect from moisture.

DOSAGE AND USE
See package insert for full prescribing information

Each tablet contains 15 mg clorazepate dipotassium.

Exp./
Lot:

DIN: 000000000

clorazepate dipotassium
100 tablets

15 mg

SAMPLE LABEL (textbook use only)

http://evolve.elsevier.com/Canada/GrayMorris/

_____

12. Order: Phenobarbital 60 mg PO at bedtime.

    Available: Phenobarbital tablets labelled 60 mg _____

13. Order: Dimenhydrinate 100 mg PO q4h prn for nausea.

Available:

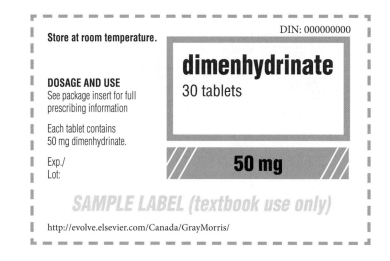

14. Order: Cephalexin 0.5 g PO QID.

Available:

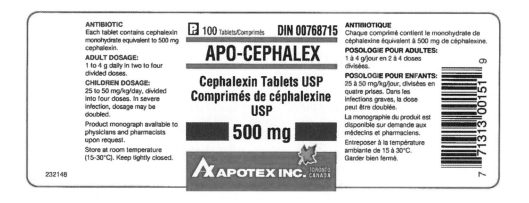

15. Order: Cogentin 2 mg PO BID.

Available: Cogentin tablets labelled 1 mg   _____

16. Order: Amoxicillin and clavulanate potassium 400 mg/57 mg PO q8h.

Available:

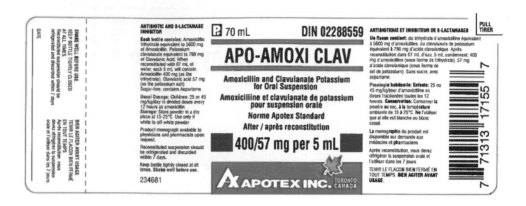

_____

17. Order: Zovirax 400 mg PO BID for 7 days.

Available: Zovirax capsules labelled 200 mg _____

18. Order: Rifampin 0.6 g PO daily.

Available:

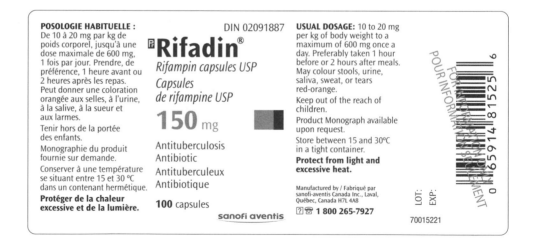

_____

19. Order: Carafate 1 000 mg PO BID.

Available: Carafate tablets labelled 1 g _____

20. Order: Cardizem 240 mg PO daily.

Available: Cardizem tablets labelled 120 mg _____

21. Order: Xanax 0.5 mg PO BID.

    Available: Scored tablets (can be broken in half)

    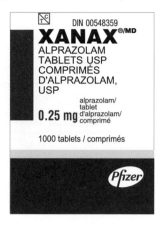

    _____

22. Order: Apo-Sulfatrim-DS 1 tab PO daily 3 times per week (Mon, Wed, Fri).

    Available:

    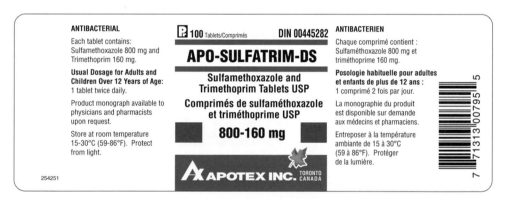

    _____

23. Order: Janumet 50/500 2 tablets PO daily.

    Available:

    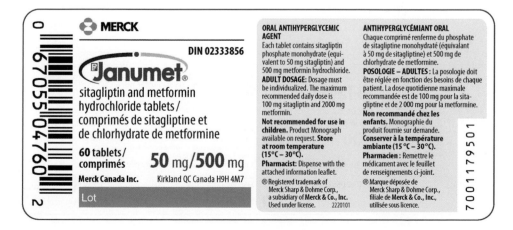

    _____

24. Order: Retrovir 0.2 g PO TID.

    Available: Retrovir capsules labelled 100 mg _____

25. Order: GlucoNorm 1 mg PO BID.

    Available:

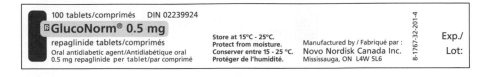

    _____

26. Order: Risperidone 1 mg PO BID.

    Available:

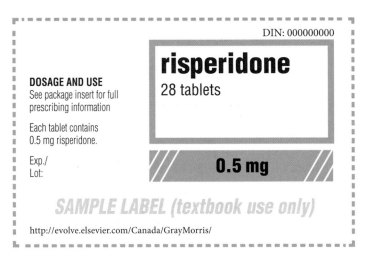

    _____

27. Order: Flagyl 0.5 g PO q8h.

    Available:

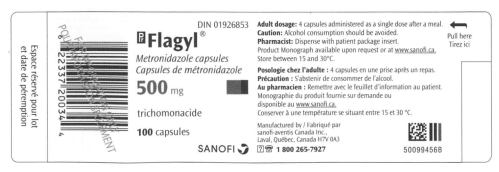

    _____

28. Order: Lopressor 100 mg PO BID.

    Available: Lopressor tablets labelled 50 mg   _____

29. Order: Furosemide 60 mg PO daily.

    Available:

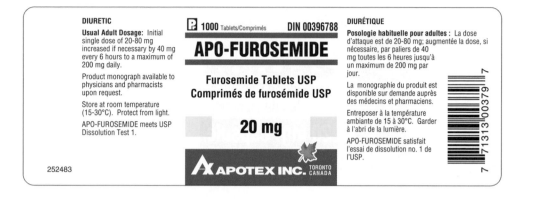

_____

30. Order: Motrin 0.6 g PO q6h prn for pain.

    Available: Motrin tablets labelled 300 mg   _____

31. Order: Potassium chloride extended-release tablets 30 mEq PO daily.

    Available:

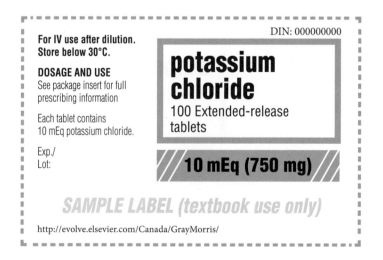

_____

32. Order: Mevacor 20 mg PO daily at 6:00 PM.

    Available: Mevacor tablets labelled 10 mg   _____

33. Order: Effexor 75 mg PO BID.

    Available: Effexor scored tablets (can be
    broken in half) labelled 37.5 mg   _____

34. Order: Nembutal 100 mg PO at bedtime.

    Available: Nembutal capsules labelled 50 mg _____

35. Order: Zeldox 40 mg PO BID.

    Available:

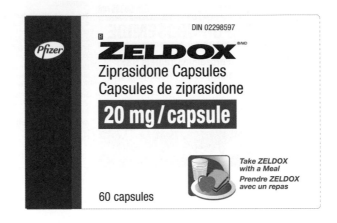

_____

36. Order: Ethosuximide 750 mg PO BID.

    Available:

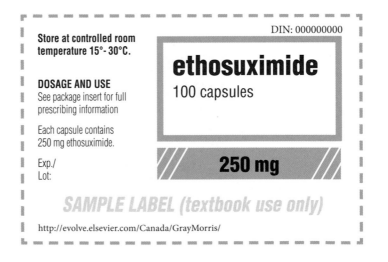

_____

37. Order: Prasugrel 10 mg PO daily.

    Available:

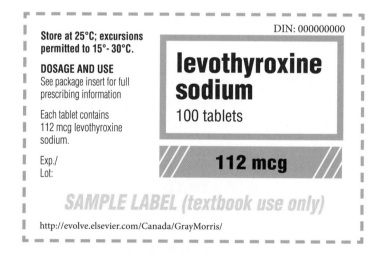

Store at 25°C; excursions permitted to 15°-30°C

DOSAGE AND USE
See package insert for full prescribing information

Each tablet contains 5 mg prasugrel.

Exp./
Lot:

DIN: 000000000

prasugrel
7 tablets

5 mg

SAMPLE LABEL (textbook use only)

http://evolve.elsevier.com/Canada/GrayMorris/

_____

38. Order: Levothyroxine sodium 0.112 mg PO daily.

    Available: Scored tablets (can be broken in half)

Store at 25°C; excursions permitted to 15°- 30°C.

DOSAGE AND USE
See package insert for full prescribing information

Each tablet contains 112 mcg levothyroxine sodium.

Exp./
Lot:

DIN: 000000000

levothyroxine sodium
100 tablets

112 mcg

SAMPLE LABEL (textbook use only)

http://evolve.elsevier.com/Canada/GrayMorris/

_____

39. Order: Apo-Digoxin 0.125 mg PO daily.

    Available: Apo-Digoxin scored tablets (can be broken in half) labelled 250 mcg (0.25 mg)   _____

40. Order: Apo-Raloxifene 0.06 g PO daily.

Available:

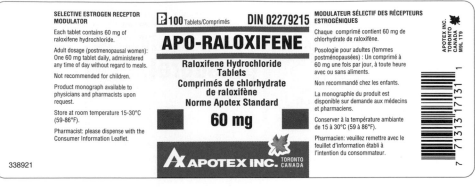

Answers on pages 235–236.

Part II

Calculate the volume necessary (in millilitres) to provide the dosage ordered using the labels or the information provided. Express your answers as a decimal fraction to the nearest tenth where indicated.

41. Order: Dilantin 100 mg by gastrostomy tube TID.

    Available: Dilantin 125 mg per 5 mL

    _____

42. Order: Benadryl 50 mg PO at bedtime.

    Available: Benadryl elixir 12.5 mg per 5 mL

    _____

43. Order: Gentamicin 50 mg IM q8h.

    Available:

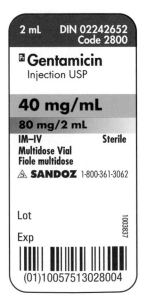

44. Order: Apo-Cefprozil 500 mg PO q12h.

   Available:

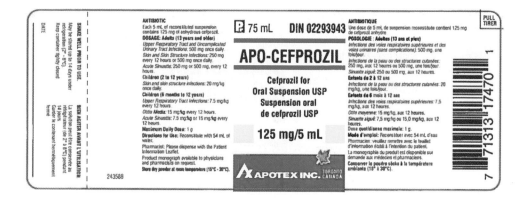

   _____

45. Order: Meperidine hydrochloride 50 mg IM q4h prn for pain.

   Available: Meperidine hydrochloride 75 mg per mL   _____

46. Order: Gentamicin 90 mg IV q8h.

   Available: Gentamicin 40 mg per mL   _____

47. Order: Morphine 15 mg SUBCUT q4h prn for pain.

   Available: Morphine labelled 15 mg per mL   _____

48. Order: Cyanocobalamin 1 000 mcg IM once monthly.

   Available:

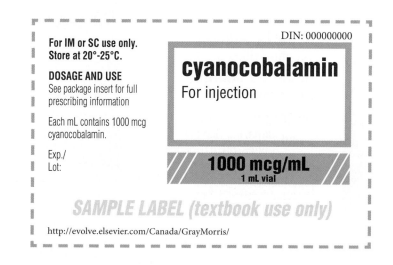

   _____

49. Order: Morphine 10 mg SUBCUT stat. (Express answer in hundredths.)

   Available: Morphine 15 mg per mL   _____

50. Order: Potassium chloride 20 mEq PO daily.

   Available:

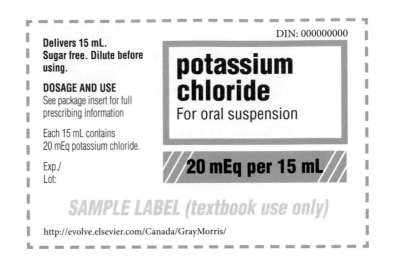

Delivers 15 mL.
Sugar free. Dilute before using.

DOSAGE AND USE
See package insert for full prescribing information

Each 15 mL contains 20 mEq potassium chloride.

Exp./
Lot:

DIN: 000000000

potassium chloride
For oral suspension

20 mEq per 15 mL

SAMPLE LABEL (textbook use only)

http://evolve.elsevier.com/Canada/GrayMorris/

_____

51. Order: Nystatin oral suspension 100 000 units swish and swallow q6h.

   Available: Nystatin oral suspension labelled 100 000 units per mL

_____

52. Order: Heparin 5 000 units SUBCUT daily.

   Available:

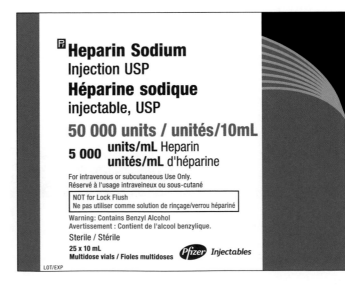

Ⓟ Heparin Sodium
Injection USP
Héparine sodique
injectable, USP

50 000 units / unités/10mL
5 000 units/mL Heparin
unités/mL d'héparine

For intravenous or subcutaneous Use Only.
Réservé à l'usage intraveineux ou sous-cutané

NOT for Lock Flush
Ne pas utiliser comme solution de rinçage/verrou hépariné

Warning: Contains Benzyl Alcohol
Avertissement : Contient de l'alcool benzylique.
Sterile / Stérile
25 x 10 mL
Multidose vials / Fioles multidoses   *Pfizer* Injectables

LOT/EXP

_____

53. Order: Atropine 0.2 mg SUBCUT stat.

    Available:

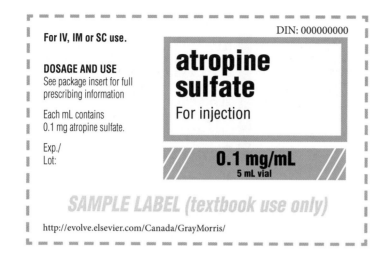

54. Order: Amoxicillin 500 mg PO q6h for 7 days.

    Available:

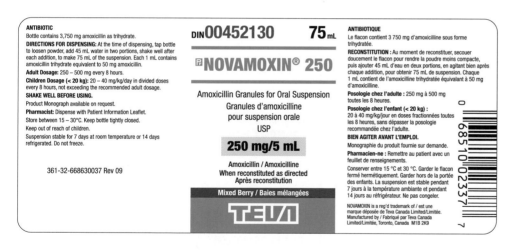

55. Order: Heparin 7500 units SUBCUT daily. (Express answer in hundredths.)

    Available: Heparin 10 000 units per mL   _____

56. Order: Methylprednisolone 70 mg IV daily.

    Available: Methylprednisolone labelled 40 mg per mL   _____

57. Order: Lorazepam 2 mg q4h prn for agitation.

    Available:

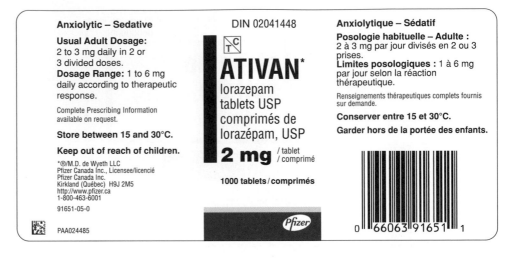

_____

58. Order: Hydroxyzine hydrochloride 25 mg IM on call to operating room (OR).

    Available:

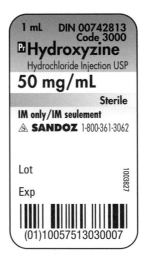

_____

59. Order: Phenobarbital (luminal) 90 mg IM stat.

    Available: Luminal 130 mg per mL

_____

60. Order: Octreotide Acetate 200 mcg SUBCUT q12h.

    Available:

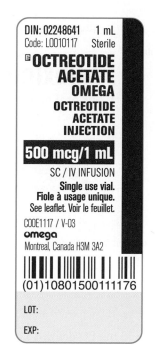

_____

61. Order: Ranitidine 150 mg IV daily.

    Available:

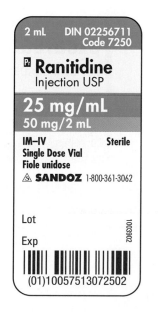

_____

62. Order: Amoxicillin 0.5 g PO q8h.

    Available:

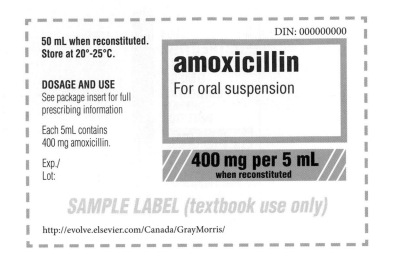

    _____

63. Order: Thorazine concentrate 75 mg PO daily.

    Available: Thorazine concentrate labelled 100 mg per mL _____

64. Order: Oxcarbazephine 300 mg PO BID.

    Available:

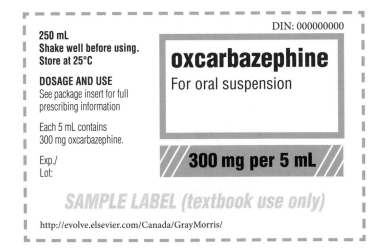

    _____

65. Order: Epivir 0.3 g PO BID.

    Available: Epivir oral solution labelled 10 mg per mL _____

66. Order: Ciprofloxacin 750 mg PO q12h.

    Available:

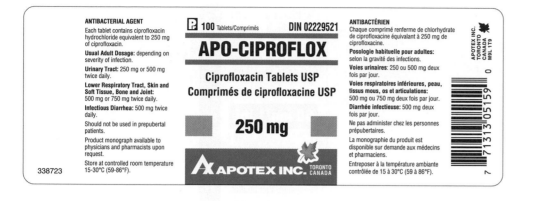

_____

67. Order: Prozac 40 mg PO daily.

    Available: Prozac oral solution labelled 20 mg per 5 mL _____

68. Order: Depo-Provera 0.4 g IM at bedtime once a week on Thursday.

    Available:

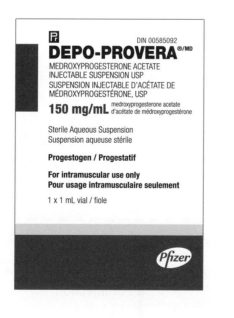

_____

69. Order: Diphenhydramine 35 mg IM q6h prn for itching.

   Available:

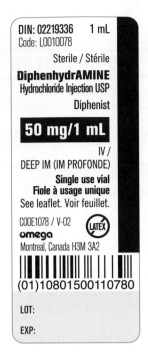

70. Order: Lactulose 30 g PO TID.

   Available: Lactulose oral solution labelled 10 g per 15 mL   _____

71. Order: Mellaril 40 mg PO BID.

   Available: Mellaril concentrate 30 mg per mL   _____

72. Order: Prochlorperazine 7 mg IM q4h prn for vomiting.

   Available:

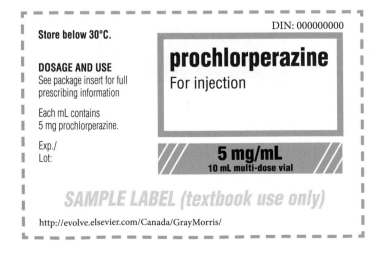

73. Order: Cefaclor 0.5 g PO q8h.

    Available:

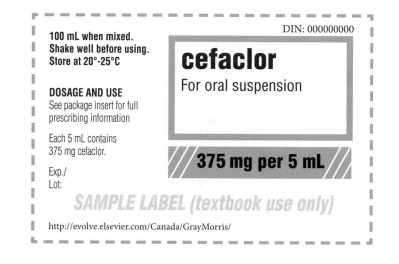

74. Order: Dilantin suspension 200 mg per nasogastric tube daily.

    Available:

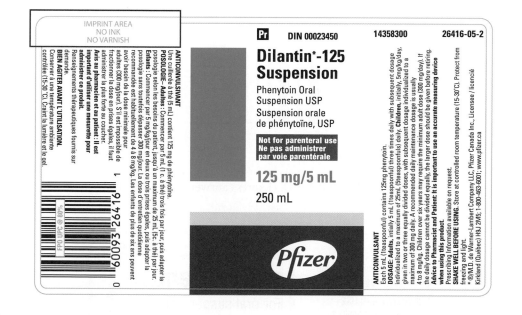

75. Order: Celestone 7 mg IM stat.

    Available: Celestone labelled 6 mg per mL

76. Order: Thiamine hydrochloride 75 mg IM daily.

Available:

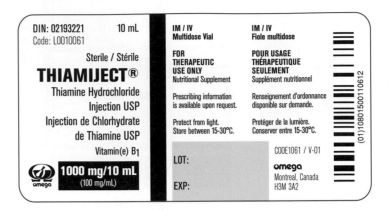

_____

77. Order: Epinephrine 0.25 mg IV stat.

Available:

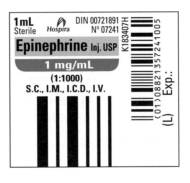

_____

78. Order: Alprazolam 0.25 mg PO BID. (Express answer in hundredths.)

Available:

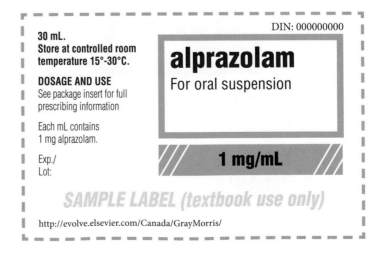

_____

79. Order: Cefpodoxime proxetil 100 mg PO q12h for 10 days.

    Available:

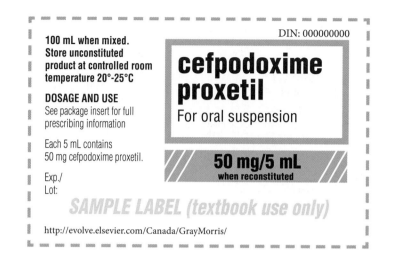

80. Order: Zithromax oral suspension 500 mg PO for 1 dose stat then 250 mg daily for 3 days. Determine the amount to administer for the stat dose.

    Available:

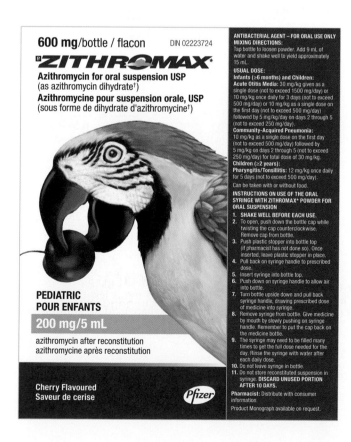

evolve

For additional practice problems, refer to the Methods of Calculating Dosages section of the Drug Calculations Companion, Version 5 on Evolve.

Answers on page 236.

✷ ANSWERS

Answers to Practice Problems

1. Less than 1 tab

2. More than 1 tab

3. Less than 1 tab

4. Less than 1 tab

5. More than 1 tab

6.
$$\frac{5\,mg}{1\,tab} = \frac{7.5\,mg}{x\,tab}$$

$$\frac{5x}{5} = \frac{7.5}{5}$$

or

$$5\,mg : 1\,tab = 7.5\,mg : x\,tab$$

$$\frac{5x}{5} = \frac{7.5}{5}$$

$$x = \frac{7.5}{5}$$

$x = 1.5$ tabs or $1\frac{1}{2}$ tabs. 5 mg is less than 7.5 mg; therefore, you will need more than 1 tab to administer the dosage.

7.
$$\frac{30\,mg}{1\,tab} = \frac{45\,mg}{x\,tab}$$

$$\frac{30x}{30} = \frac{45}{30}$$

$$x = \frac{45}{30}$$

or

$$30\,mg : 1\,tab = 45\,mg : x\,tab$$

$$\frac{30x}{30} = \frac{45}{30}$$

$$x = \frac{45}{30}$$

$x = 1.5$ tabs or $1\frac{1}{2}$ tabs. 45 mg is greater than 30; therefore, you will need more than 1 tab to administer the dosage.

8.
$$\frac{100\,mg}{1\,cap} = \frac{90\,mg}{x\,capsule}$$

$$\frac{100x}{100} = \frac{90}{100}$$

$$x = \frac{90}{100}$$

or

$$100\,mg : 1\,capsule = 90\,mg : x\,capsule$$

$$\frac{100x}{100} = \frac{90}{100}$$

$$x = \frac{90}{100}$$

$x = 1$ capsule. It would be impossible to administer 0.9 of a capsule. A 10% margin of difference is allowed between what is ordered and what is administered. When this 10% safety margin is used, no more than 110 mg and no less than 90 mg may be given.

The prescriber ordered (90 mg). The capsules available are 100 mg. Capsules are not divisible. Administering 1 capsule is within the 10% margin of difference allowed.

9.
$$\frac{0.5\,mg}{1\,mL} = \frac{0.25\,mg}{x\,mL}$$

$$\frac{0.5x}{0.5} = \frac{0.25}{0.5}$$

$$x = \frac{0.25}{0.5}$$

or

$$0.5\,mg : 1\,mL = 0.25\,mg : x\,mL$$

$$\frac{0.5x}{0.5} = \frac{0.25}{0.5}$$

$$x = \frac{0.25}{0.5}$$

$x = 0.5$ mL, 0.25 mg is less than 0.5 mg; therefore, you will need less than 1 mL to administer the dosage.

10.
$$\frac{125 \text{ mg}}{5 \text{ mL}} = \frac{100 \text{ mg}}{x \text{ mL}}$$

$$\frac{125x}{125} = \frac{500}{125}$$

$$x = \frac{500}{125}$$

or

$$125 \text{ mg} : 5 \text{ mL} = 100 \text{ mg} : x \text{ mL}$$

$$\frac{125x}{125} = \frac{500}{125}$$

$$x = \frac{500}{125}$$

$x = 4$ mL. 100 mg is less than 125 mg; therefore, you will need less than 5 mL to administer the dosage.

11.
$$\frac{40 \text{ mmol}}{10 \text{ mL}} = \frac{20 \text{ mmol}}{x \text{ mL}}$$

$$\frac{40x}{40} = \frac{200}{40}$$

$$40 \text{ mmol} : 10 \text{ mL} = 20 \text{ mmol} : x \text{ mL}$$

$$\frac{40x}{40} = \frac{200}{40}$$

$$x = \frac{200}{40}$$

$x = 5$ mL. 20 mmol is less than 40 mmol; therefore, you will need less than 10 mL to administer the dosage.

12.
$$\frac{10000 \text{ units}}{1 \text{ mL}} = \frac{5000 \text{ units}}{x \text{ mL}}$$

$$\frac{10000x}{10000} = \frac{5000}{10000}$$

$$x = \frac{5000}{10000}$$

or

$$10000 \text{ units} : 1 \text{ mL} = 5000 \text{ units} : x \text{ mL}$$

$$\frac{10000x}{10000} = \frac{5000}{10000}$$

$$x = \frac{5000}{10000}$$

$x = 0.5$ mL, 10 000 units is greater than 5 000 units; therefore, you will need less than 1 mL to administer the dosage.

13.
$$\frac{80 \text{ mg}}{2 \text{ mL}} = \frac{50 \text{ mg}}{x \text{ mL}}$$

$$\frac{80x}{80} = \frac{100}{80}$$

$$x = \frac{100}{80}$$

or

$$80 \text{ mg} : 2 \text{ mL} = 50 \text{ mg} : x \text{ mL}$$

$$\frac{80x}{80} = \frac{100}{80}$$

$$x = \frac{100}{80}$$

$x = 1.25 = 1.3$ mL. 50 mg is less than 80 mg; therefore, you will need less than 2 mL to administer the dosage.

14. Conversion factor: $1\,000$ mg = 1 g (0.5 g = 500 mg)

$$\frac{250 \text{ mg}}{1 \text{ capsules}} = \frac{500 \text{ mg}}{x \text{ capsules}}$$

$$\frac{250x}{250} = \frac{500}{250}$$

or

$$250 \text{ mg} : 1 \text{ capsule} = 500 \text{ mg} : x \text{ capsule}$$

$$\frac{250x}{250} = \frac{500}{250}$$

$$x = \frac{500}{250}$$

$x = 2$ capsules. 500 mg is greater than 250 mg; therefore, you will need more than 1 capsule to administer the dosage.

15.
$$\frac{125 \text{ mg}}{5 \text{ mL}} = \frac{400 \text{ mg}}{x \text{ mL}}$$

$$\frac{125x}{125} = \frac{2000}{125}$$

$$x = \frac{2000}{125}$$

or

$$125 \text{ mg} : 5 \text{ mL} = 400 \text{ mg} : x \text{ mL}$$

$$\frac{125x}{125} = \frac{2000}{125}$$

$$x = \frac{2000}{125}$$

$x = 16$ mL. 400 mg is greater than 125 mg; therefore, you will need more than 5 mL to administer the dosage.

16.

$$\frac{80 \text{ mg}}{1 \text{ mL}} = \frac{50 \text{ mg}}{x \text{ mL}}$$

$$\frac{80x}{80} = \frac{50}{80}$$

$$x = \frac{50}{80}$$

or

$$80 \text{ mg} : 1 \text{ mL} = 50 \text{ mg} : x \text{ mL}$$

$$\frac{80x}{80} = \frac{50}{80}$$

$$x = \frac{50}{80}$$

$x = 0.62 = 0.6$ mL. 50 mg is less than 80 mg; therefore, you will need less than 1 mL to administer the dosage.

17.

$$\frac{30 \text{ mg}}{1 \text{ mL}} = \frac{60 \text{ mg}}{x \text{ mL}}$$

$$\frac{30x}{30} = \frac{60}{30}$$

$$x = \frac{60}{30}$$

or

$$30 \text{ mg} : 1 \text{ mL} = 60 \text{ mg} : x \text{ mL}$$

$$\frac{30x}{30} = \frac{60}{30}$$

$$x = \frac{60}{30}$$

$x = 2$ mL. 30 mg is less than 60 mg; therefore, you will need more than 1 mL to administer the dosage.

18.

$$\frac{5 \text{ mg}}{1 \text{ tab}} = \frac{15 \text{ mg}}{x \text{ tab}}$$

$$\frac{5x}{5} = \frac{15}{5}$$

or

$$5 \text{ mg} : 1 \text{ tab} = 15 \text{ mg} : x \text{ tab}$$

$$\frac{5x}{5} = \frac{15}{5}$$

$$x = \frac{15}{5}$$

$x = 3$ tabs. 15 mg is greater than 5 mg; therefore, you will need more than 1 tab to administer the dosage.

19. Conversion factor: 1 000 mg = 1 g (0.24 g = 240 mg)

$$\frac{80 \text{ mg}}{7.5 \text{ mL}} = \frac{240 \text{ mg}}{x \text{ mL}}$$

$$\frac{80x}{80} = \frac{1800}{80}$$

$$x = \frac{1800}{80}$$

or

$$80 \text{ mg} : 7.5 \text{ mL} = 240 \text{ mg} : x \text{ mL}$$

$$\frac{80x}{80} = \frac{1800}{80}$$

$$x = \frac{1800}{80}$$

$x = 22.5$ mL. 240 mg is greater than 80 mg; therefore, you would need more than 7.5 mL to administer the dosage.

20.

$$\frac{10 \text{ g}}{15 \text{ mL}} = \frac{20 \text{ g}}{x \text{ mL}}$$

$$\frac{10x}{10} = \frac{300}{10}$$

$$x = \frac{300}{10}$$

or

$$10 \text{ g} : 15 \text{ mL} = 20 \text{ g} : x \text{ mL}$$

$$\frac{10x}{10} = \frac{300}{10}$$

$$x = \frac{300}{10}$$

$x = 30$ mL. 20 g is greater than 10 g; therefore, you would need more than 15 mL to administer the dosage.

21.

$$\frac{0.5 \text{ mg}}{2 \text{ mL}} = \frac{0.125 \text{ mg}}{x \text{ mL}}$$

$$\frac{0.5x}{0.5} = \frac{0.25}{0.5}$$

or

$$0.5 \text{ mg} : 2 \text{ mL} = 0.125 \text{ mg} : x \text{ mL}$$

$$\frac{0.5x}{0.5} = \frac{0.25}{0.5}$$

$$x = \frac{0.25}{0.5}$$

$x = 0.5$ mL, 0.125 mg is less than 0.5 mg; therefore, you will need less than 2 mL to administer the dosage.

22.
$$\frac{0.25 \text{ mg}}{1 \text{ mL}} = \frac{0.75 \text{ mg}}{x \text{ mL}}$$

$$\frac{0.25x}{0.25} = \frac{0.75}{0.25}$$

or

$$0.25 \text{ mg} : 1 \text{ mL} = 0.75 \text{ mg} : x \text{ mL}$$

$$\frac{0.25x}{0.25} = \frac{0.75}{0.25}$$

$$x = \frac{0.75}{0.25}$$

$x = 3$ mL. 0.75 mg is greater than 0.25 mg; therefore, you will need more than 1 mL to administer the dosage.

23.
$$\frac{125 \text{ mg}}{5 \text{ mL}} = \frac{375 \text{ mg}}{x \text{ mL}}$$

$$\frac{125x}{125} = \frac{375 \times 5}{125}$$

or

$$125 \text{ mg} : 5 \text{ mL} = 375 \text{ mg} : x \text{ mL}$$

$$\frac{125x}{125} = \frac{375 \times 5}{125}$$

$$x = \frac{1875}{125}$$

$x = 15$ mL. 375 mg is greater than 125 mg; therefore, you will need more than 5 mL to administer the dosage.

24.
$$\frac{7500 \text{ units}}{1 \text{ mL}} = \frac{10000 \text{ units}}{x \text{ mL}}$$

$$\frac{7500x}{7500} = \frac{10000}{7500}$$

or

$$7500 \text{ units} : 1 \text{ mL} = 10000 \text{ units} : x \text{ mL}$$

$$\frac{7500x}{7500} = \frac{10000}{7500}$$

$$x = \frac{10000}{7500}$$

$x = 1.33 = 1.3$ mL. 10 000 units is greater than 7 500 units; therefore, you will need more than 1 mL to administer the dosage.

25.
$$\frac{0.3 \text{ mg}}{1 \text{ tab}} = \frac{0.45 \text{ mg}}{x \text{ tab}}$$

$$\frac{0.3x}{0.3} = \frac{0.45}{0.3}$$

or

$$0.3 \text{ mg} : 1 \text{ tab} = 0.45 \text{ mg} : x \text{ tab}$$

$$\frac{0.3x}{0.3} = \frac{0.45}{0.3}$$

$$x = \frac{0.45}{0.3}$$

$x = 1.5$ tabs or $1\frac{1}{2}$ tabs. 0.45 mg is greater than 0.3 mg; therefore, you will need more than 1 tab to administer the dosage.

✎ **NOTE**

For questions 26–45 and Chapter Review Parts I and II, only answers are shown. If needed, review the setup of problems in Practice Problems 6–25.

26. 1.2 mL	31. 1.7 mL	36. 0.8 mL	41. 300 mg	46. 1.5 mL
27. 1.9 mL	32. 2.2 mL	37. 5 mL	42. 84 tabs	47. 0.5 mL
28. 0.7 mL	33. 2 mL	38. 3.3 mL	43. 24 hours	48. 1 tab
29. 2 mL	34. 2.2 mL	39. 0.9 mL	44. 31.25 mg	
30. 1.1 mL	35. 0.6 mL	40. 1.6 mL	45. 360 mL	

Answers to Chapter Review Part I

1. 1 tab	6. 2 sustained-release (SR) capsules	10. 1 tab	15. 2 tabs	20. 2 tabs
2. 2 tabs		11. 2 tabs	16. 5 mL	21. 2 tabs
3. 2 tabs		12. 1 tab	17. 2 capsules	22. 1 tab (DS)
4. 2 tabs	7. 2 tabs	13. 2 tabs	18. 4 capsules	23. 2 tabs
5. 2 tabs	8. 2 tabs	14. 1 tab	19. 1 tab	24. 2 capsules
	9. 1 tab			

25. 2 tabs	29. 3 tabs	33. 2 tabs	37. 2 tabs
26. 2 tabs	30. 2 tabs	34. 2 capsules	38. 1 tab
27. 1 cap	31. 3 tabs	35. 2 capsules	39. $\frac{1}{2}$ tab *or* 0.5 tab
28. 2 tabs	32. 2 tabs	36. 3 capsules	40. 1 tab

Answers to Chapter Review Part II

41. 4 mL	49. 0.67 mL	57. 1 tab	65. 30 mL	73. 6.7 mL
42. 20 mL	50. 15 mL	58. 0.5 mL	66. 3 tabs	74. 8 mL
43. 1.3 mL	51. 1 mL	59. 0.7 mL	67. 10 mL	75. 1.2 mL
44. 20 mL	52. 1 mL	60. 0.4 mL	68. 2.7 mL	76. 0.8 mL
45. 0.7 mL	53. 2 mL	61. 6 mL	69. 0.7 mL	77. 0.3 mL
46. 2.3 mL	54. 10 mL	62. 6.3 mL	70. 45 mL	78. 0.25 mL
47. 1 mL	55. 0.75 mL	63. 0.8 mL	71. 1.3 mL	79. 10 mL
48. 1 mL	56. 1.8 mL	64. 5 mL	72. 1.4 mL	80. 12.5 mL

CHAPTER 13

Dosage Calculation Using the Formula Method

Objectives

After reviewing this chapter, you should be able to:

1. Identify the information to place in the formula for dosage calculation

2. Calculate dosages using the formula $\dfrac{D}{H} \times Q = x$

3. Calculate the number of tablets, capsules, or caplets to administer using the formula method

4. Calculate the volume of medication in solution to administer using the formula method

This chapter shows how to use the *formula method* to calculate the amount of medication to administer. The formula method involves identifying the components of the formula in the problem, placing that information into the formula, and calculating the dosage.

Total reliance on a formula without thinking and asking yourself whether an answer is reasonable can result in errors in calculation and an administration error.

When using a formula, always use it consistently and in its entirety to avoid calculation errors. Always ask, "Is the answer obtained reasonable?"

As Cohen (2010) notes, dosages of more than two or three tablets, capsules, or vials are unusual. Anything exceeding that amount should be a red flag to you, even if the answer is obtained from the use of a formula. Use formulas to validate the dosage you think is reasonable, not the reverse. **Think** before you calculate. Always estimate **before** applying a formula. Thinking first will allow you to detect errors and alert you to try again and question the results you obtained.

> ! **SAFETY ALERT!**
>
> **Avoid Dosage Calculation Errors**
>
> Do not rely solely on formulas when calculating dosages to be administered. Use critical thinking skills such as considering what the answer should be, reasoning, problem solving, and finding rational justification for your answer. Formulas should be used as tools for validating the dosage you THINK should be given.

Formula for Calculating Dosages

The formula presented in this chapter can be used when calculating dosages in the same system of measurement. When the desired dosage and the dosage on hand are in different systems, convert them to the same system before using the formula, using one of the methods learned for conversion in Chapter 6. It is important to learn and memorize the following formula and its components:

$$\frac{D}{H} \times Q = x$$

Let's examine what each initial in the formula means.

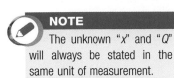

D = The **desired dosage**, or what the prescriber has ordered, including the units of measurement (mg, g, mL, etc.).

H = The dosage strength available; what you **have** on **hand** or written on the medication label, including the unit of measurement (mg, g, mL, etc.).

Q = The **quantity** or volume in the unit of measurement that contains the dosage that is available. For example, "Q" is labelled accordingly as tablet, capsule, millilitre, litre, and so on.

x = The **unknown**, which is the dosage to be administered.

Always insert the quantity value for "**Q**" into the formula, even though when solving problems that involve solid forms of medication (tablets, capsules, etc.), "**Q**" is always 1. Doing so will prevent errors when calculating dosages of medications in solution (oral liquids or injectables) in which the solution quantity can be more or less than 1 (e.g., per 10 mL). When solving problems for medications in solution, the quantity value for "**Q**" varies and must always be included.

The dosage strength indicated on the labels of medications in solution may state the quantity of medication per 1 millilitre of solution (e.g., 25 mg per mL) or per multiple millilitres of solution (e.g., 80 mg per 2 mL, 125 mg per 5 mL). Some liquid medications may also express the quantity in amounts less than a millilitre (e.g., 2 mg per 0.5 mL).

When setting up the formula, notice that "**D**," which is the desired dosage, is in the numerator, and "**H**," which is the dosage strength you have available, is placed in the denominator of the fraction.

All factors in the formula, including "*x*," must be labelled with their unit of measurement to ensure accuracy.

! **SAFETY ALERT!**

Omitting the amount for "**Q**" can lead to an error in dosage calculation. Labelling all factors in the formula with their unit of measurement, including "*x*," is a safeguard against errors in calculation. **Before** you calculate the dosage using the formula, always make a mental estimate of the approximate and reasonable answer.

Applying the Formula

Now that we have reviewed the factors in the formula, let's review the steps in the formula method (Box 13-1) before beginning to calculate dosages using the formula.

BOX 13-1 Steps in Calculating Dosages Using the Formula Method

1. Memorize the formula, or verify the formula from a resource.
2. Make sure that all measures are in the same system and unit of measurement; if not, a conversion must be done *before* calculating the dosage.
3. Place the information from the problem into the formula in the correct position, with all factors in the formula labelled correctly, including "*x*."
4. Think logically, and consider what an approximate and reasonable amount to administer would be.
5. Calculate your answer using the formula $\dfrac{D}{H} \times Q = x$.
6. Label all answers: tabs, capsules, mL, etc.

Let's look at sample problems illustrating the use of the formula.

Example: Order: 0.375 mg PO of a medication.

Available: Tablets labelled 0.25 mg

Solution: The desired dosage is 0.375 mg; the dosage strength available is 0.25 mg per tablet. No conversion is necessary. What is desired is in the same system and unit of measurement as what you have on hand.

✔ FORMULA SETUP

$$\frac{D}{H} \times Q = x$$

The desired dosage (D) is 0.375 mg. You have on hand (H) 0.25 mg per (Q) 1 tablet. The label on x is tablet. Notice that the label on x is always the same as the label on Q.

$$\frac{(D)\,0.375\,\text{mg}}{(H)\,0.25\,\text{mg}} \times (Q)\,1\,\text{tab} = x\,\text{tab}$$

$$x = \frac{0.375}{0.25} \times 1$$

$$x = \frac{0.375}{0.25}$$

$$x = 1.5 = 1\frac{1}{2}\,\text{tabs}$$

Therefore, x = 1.5 tabs, or $1\frac{1}{2}$ tabs. (Because 0.375 mg is greater than 0.25 mg, you will need more than 1 tab to administer 0.375 mg.) *Note:* Although 1.5 tabs is the same as $1\frac{1}{2}$ tabs, for administration purposes, it would be best to state it as $1\frac{1}{2}$ tabs.

Example: Order: 7 000 units IM of a medication.

Available: 10 000 units in 2 mL

Solution: $$\frac{(D)\,7\,000\,\text{units}}{(H)\,10\,000\,\text{units}} \times (Q)\,2\,\text{mL} = x\,\text{mL}$$

$$x = \frac{7\,000}{10\,000} \times 2$$

$$x = \frac{14}{10}$$

$$x = 1.4\,\text{mL}$$

! SAFETY ALERT!

Omitting Q here could result in an error. A liquid form of medication is involved. Q must be included because the amount varies and is not always per 1 mL.

RULE

Dealing with Different Systems or Units of Measurement

Whenever the desired dosage and what is on hand are in different systems or units of measurement, follow these steps:

1. Choose the appropriate conversion factor.
2. Convert the desired dosage to the same system and unit of measurement as what is available by using one of the methods presented in Chapter 6.
3. Use the formula $\frac{D}{H} \times Q = x$ to calculate the dosage to administer.

The metric system is the principal system used in the measurement of medications. When converting is required before calculating a dosage, convert units to their metric equivalent when possible to decrease the chance of a calculation error.

Example: Order: 0.1 mg PO of a medication daily.

Available: Tablets labelled 50 mcg

Solution: Convert 0.1 mg to mcg. The conversion factor to use is 1 mg = 1 000 mcg. Therefore, 0.1 mg = 100 mcg

Now that the desired dosage and the dosage on hand are in the same system and unit of measurement, use the formula presented to calculate the dosage to administer.

$$\frac{(D)\,100\text{ mcg}}{(H)\,50\text{ mcg}} \times (Q)\,1\text{ tab} = x\text{ tab}$$

$$x = \frac{100}{50} \times 1$$

$$x = \frac{100}{50}$$

$$x = 2\text{ tabs}$$

Therefore, $x = 2$ tabs. (Because 100 mcg is greater than 50 mcg, you will need more than 1 tab to administer the desired dosage.)

Example: Order: 0.2 g PO of a liquid medication.

Available: 125 mg per 5 mL

Solution: Convert 0.2 g to mg. The conversion factor to use is 1 000 mg = 1 g. Therefore, 0.2 g = 200 mg.

Now that the desired dosage and the dosage on hand are in the same system and unit of measurement, use the formula presented to calculate the dosage to administer.

$$\frac{(D)\,200\text{ mg}}{(H)\,125\text{ mg}} \times (Q)\,5\text{ mL} = x\text{ mL}$$

$$x = \frac{200 \times 5}{125}$$

$$x = \frac{1\,000}{125}$$

$$x = 8\text{ mL}$$

Therefore, $x = 8$ mL (Because 200 mg is greater than 125 mg, you will need more than 5 mL to administer the desired dosage.)

Example: Order: 10 mg subcutaneous of a medication.

Available: 30 mg per mL (Express the answer to the nearest tenth.)

Solution: No conversion is required; the dosage ordered is in the same system and unit of measurement as the dosage strength available.

$$\frac{(D)\,10\,mg}{(H)\,30\,mg} \times (Q)\,1\,mL = x\,mL$$

$$x = \frac{10}{30} \times 1$$

$$x = \frac{10}{30}$$

$$x = \frac{1}{3} = 0.33 = 0.3\,mL$$

Therefore, $x = 0.33 = 0.3$ mL rounded to the nearest tenth. (Because 30 mg is greater than 10 mg, you will need less than 1 mL to administer the desired dosage.)

NOTE

As you will learn in Chapter 16, stating the answer as $\frac{1}{3}$ mL (fraction) would be incorrect. A millilitre is a metric measurement and is expressed as a decimal number.

CRITICAL THINKING

Always think critically, even when using a formula. It is an essential step in estimating what is reasonable and logical in terms of a dosage. Critical thinking will help prevent errors in calculation caused by setting up the problem incorrectly or careless math and will remind you to double-check your calculation and identify any error.

Remember to memorize the formula presented and follow the steps sequentially. Check **FIRST** to see if a conversion is required; if so, convert so that the desired dosage and the dosage on hand are in the same system and unit of measurement, set up factors in the formula, **THINK** critically as to a reasonable answer, and calculate the dosage using the formula to validate the dosage you anticipated was reasonable.

SAFETY ALERT!

Always double-check your math. Errors can be made in simple calculations because of lack of caution. Always ask yourself whether the answer you have obtained is reasonable and correct.

POINTS TO REMEMBER

When using the formula method to calculate dosages:

- Use the formula $\frac{D}{H} \times Q = x$ to calculate the dosage to administer.
- Note that the Q is always 1 for solid forms of medication (tablets, capsules, etc.) but varies when medications are in liquid form. Do not omit "Q" even when it is 1.
- Before the dosage to be given is calculated, ensure that the desired dosage is in the same system and unit of measurement as the dosage strength available or a conversion is necessary.
- Set up the factors in the formula labelled with the units of measurement, including "*x*."
- Think about what a reasonable answer would be.
- Calculate the dosage to administer using the formula to validate your answer as to what was reasonable.
- Label all answers correctly: tabs, capsules, mL, etc.
- Remember: the use of a formula does not eliminate the need to think critically.
- Always systematically follow these steps: **convert** if necessary, set up the factors in the formula, **THINK** about what a reasonable answer would be, **calculate** the dosage to administer using the formula.
- Double-check all your math, and think about whether the answer obtained is logical.

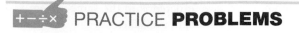 PRACTICE **PROBLEMS**

Calculate the following dosages using the formula method. Label all answers correctly: tabs or capsules.

1. Order: 0.4 mg PO of a medication.

   Available: Tablets labelled 0.2 mg _____

2. Order: 0.75 g PO of a medication.

   Available: Capsules labelled 250 mg _____

3. Order: 90 mg PO of a medication.

   Available: Tablets labelled 60 mg _____

4. Order: 7.5 mg PO of a medication.

   Available: Tablets labelled 2.5 mg _____

5. Order: 0.05 mg PO of a medication.

   Available: Tablets labelled 25 mcg _____

6. Order: 0.4 mg PO of a medication.

   Available: Tablets labelled 200 mcg _____

7. Order: 1 000 mg PO of a medication.

   Available: Tablets labelled 500 mg _____

8. Order: 0.6 g PO of a medication.

   Available: Capsules labelled 600 mg _____

9. Order: 1.25 mg PO of a medication.

   Available: Tablets labelled 625 mcg _____

Calculate the following dosages in millilitres; round your answer to the nearest tenth where indicated. Label all answers in mL.

10. Order: 10 mg SUBCUT of a medication.

    Available: 15 mg per mL _____

11. Order: 400 mg PO of an oral solution.

    Available: Oral solution labelled 200 mg per 5 mL _____

12. Order: 15 mmol PO of an oral solution.

    Available: Oral solution labelled 20 mmol per 10 mL _____

13. Order: 125 mg PO of an oral solution.

    Available: Oral solution labelled 250 mg per 5 mL _____

14. Order: 0.025 mg PO of an oral solution.

    Available: Oral solution labelled 0.05 mg per 5 mL _____

15. Order: 375 mg PO of an oral solution.

    Available: Oral solution labelled 125 mg per 5 mL _____

16. A patient who is 10 years old is receiving cephalexin (Keflex) 100 mg suspension PO QID. The medication is labelled 125 mg per 5 mL. How many mL should the nurse administer? _____

17. A patient is prescribed amoxicillin 500 mg PO q8h for an upper respiratory tract infection. The medication is available in a suspension of 125 mg per 5 mL. How many mL should the patient receive at the 1400 dose? _____

18. A patient received dimenhydrinate (Gravol) 25 mg IV for post-op nausea and vomiting. The Gravol is available in 50 mg per mL vials. How many mL should the nurse administer? _____

19. A physician ordered ciprofloxacin (Cipro) 0.4 g IV for a patient who had a colon resection done yesterday. Cipro is available in single-dose vials of 400 mg per 40 mL. How many mL should the patient receive with each dose? _____

20. A nurse is preparing to administer octreotide (Sandostatin) 200 mcg SUBCUT to a patient. The medication is available in 500 mcg per mL. How many mL should the patient receive? _____

Answers on pages 260–262.

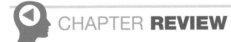 CHAPTER **REVIEW**

Calculate the following dosages using the label or the information provided. Label answers correctly: tabs, capsules, caplets, or mL. Answers expressed in millilitres should be rounded to the nearest tenth where indicated.

1. Order: Phenobarbital 30 mg PO TID.

    Available: Phenobarbital tablets labelled 30 mg _____

2. Order: Crixivan 0.8 g PO q8h.

Available:

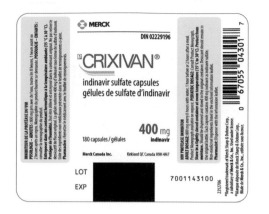

_____

3. Order: Piroxicam 20 mg PO daily.

Available:

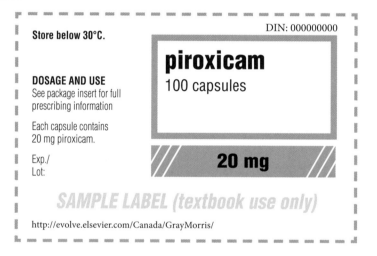

_____

4. Order: Hydrochlorothiazide 50 mg PO BID.

Available:

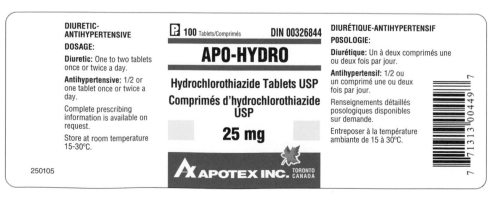

_____

5. Order: Acetaminophen 650 mg PO q4h prn for pain.

   Available:

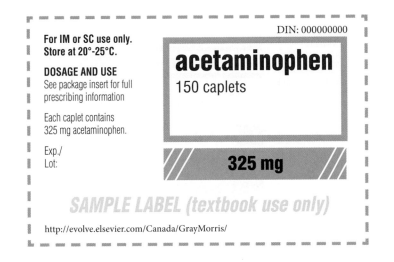

_____

6. Order: Digoxin 0.375 mg PO daily.

   Available: Digoxin scored tablets (can be broken in half) labelled 250 mcg (0.25 mg)

_____

7. Order: Flagyl 0.5 g PO BID for 1 week.

   Available: Flagyl tablets labelled 500 mg   _____

8. Order: Seconal 100 mg PO at bedtime.

   Available: Seconal capsules labelled 100 mg   _____

9. Order: Verapamil hydrochloride SR 240 mg PO daily.

   Available:

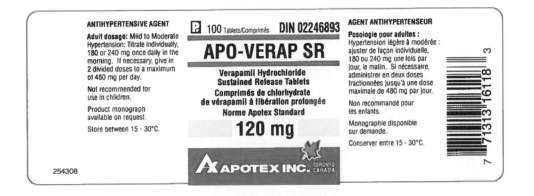

_____

10. Order: Ibuprofen 0.8 g PO q8h prn for pain.

    Available:

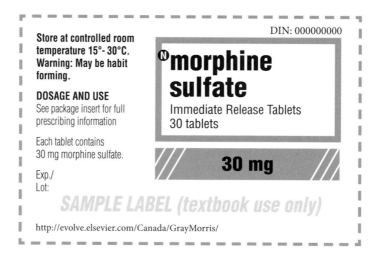

11. Order: Morphine (immediate release tablets) 30 mg PO q4h prn for pain.

    Available: Morphine scored tablets (can be broken in half)

Store at controlled room temperature 15°- 30°C. Warning: May be habit forming.

DOSAGE AND USE
See package insert for full prescribing information

Each tablet contains 30 mg morphine sulfate.

Exp./
Lot:

DIN: 000000000

(N) **morphine sulfate**

Immediate Release Tablets
30 tablets

30 mg

SAMPLE LABEL (textbook use only)

http://evolve.elsevier.com/Canada/GrayMorris/

12. Order: Cephradine 0.5 g PO q6h.

    Available: Cephradine capsules labelled 250 mg

13. Order: Benztropine mesylate 0.5 mg PO at bedtime.

    Available:

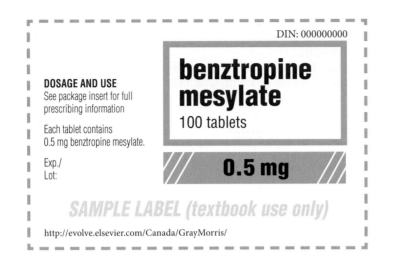

    _____

14. Order: Chlordiazepoxide hydrochloride 50 mg PO q4h prn for 24 hours for acute alcohol withdrawal.

    Available:

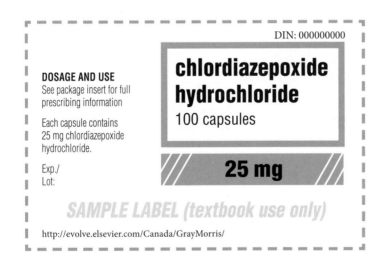

    _____

15. Order: Dilantin (extended capsules) 60 mg PO BID.

    Available: Dilantin (extended capsules) labelled 30 mg   _____

16. Order: Meperidine hydrochloride 50 mg IM q4h prn for pain.

    Available: Meperidine hydrochloride labelled 75 mg per mL   _____

17. Order: Methylprednisolone sodium succinate 80 mg IV daily.

    Available:

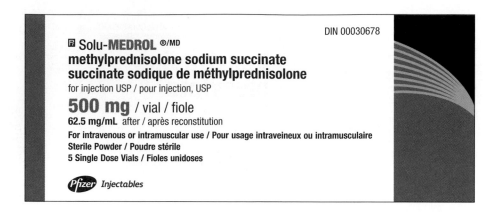

18. Order: Diltiazem 20 mg IV stat.

    Available:

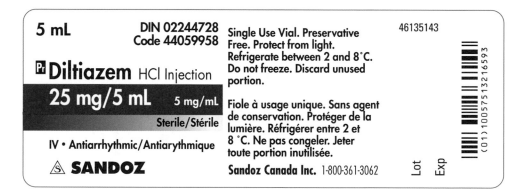

19. Order: Amoxicillin 300 mg PO q8h.

    Available: Amoxicillin oral suspension labelled 125 mg per 5 mL

20. Order: Amoxicillin 0.5 g by nasogastric tube q6h.

    Available:

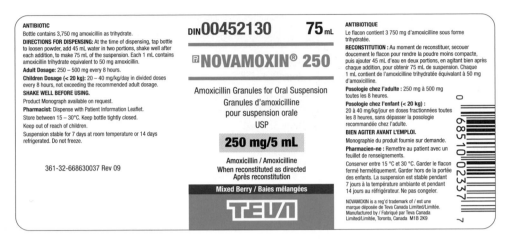

    _____

21. Order: Phenobarbital elixir 45 mg PO BID.

    Available: Phenobarbital elixir labelled 20 mg per 5 mL   _____

22. Order: Heparin 3 000 units SUBCUT BID.

    Available:

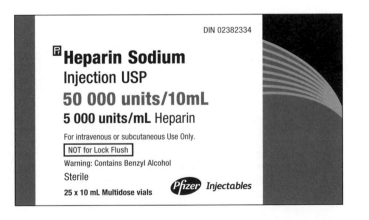

    _____

23. Order: Penicillin G 600 000 units IM q12h.

    Available: Penicillin G labelled 300 000 units per mL   _____

24. Order: Gentamicin 70 mg IV q8h.

    Available:

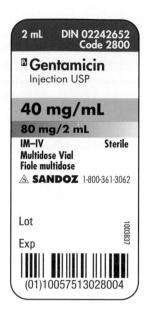

    _____

25. Order: Potassium chloride 20 mmol IV in 1 000 mL 0.9% normal saline.

    Available:

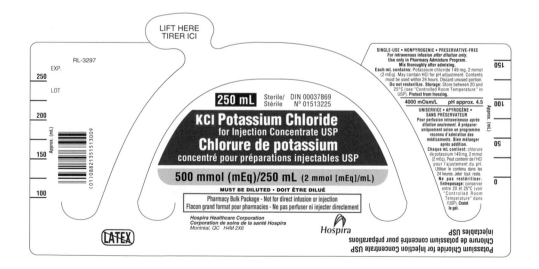

    _____

26. Order: Folic acid 1 000 mcg IM daily for 10 days.

    Available: Folic acid labelled 5 000 mcg per mL   _____

27. Order: Vistaril 100 mg IM stat.

    Available: Vistaril labelled 50 mg per mL   _____

28. Order: Morphine sulphate 6 mg SUBCUT q4h prn for pain.

    Available:

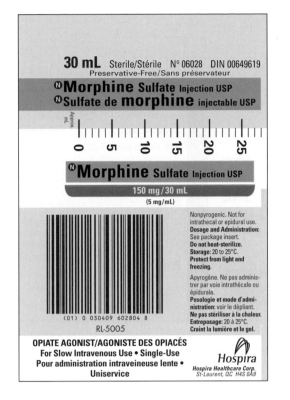

_____

29. Order: Atropine 0.3 mg IM stat.

    Available: Atropine labelled 0.4 mg per mL   _____

30. Order: Stadol 1 mg IM q4h prn for pain.

    Available: Stadol labelled 2 mg per mL   _____

31. Order: Ativan 1 mg IM stat.

    Available: Ativan labelled 4 mg per mL   _____

32. Order: Lincomycin 0.5 g IM q12h.

    Available:

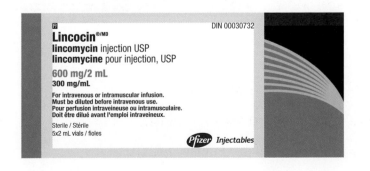

_____

33. Order: Robinul 0.4 mg IM stat on call to operating room (OR).

    Available: Robinul labelled 0.2 mg per mL   _____

34. Order: Aminophylline 80 mg IV q6h.

    Available:

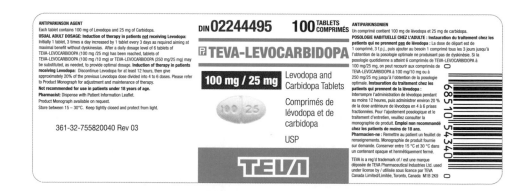

35. Order: Lithium citrate oral solution 300 mg PO TID.

    Available: Lithium citrate labelled 300 mg per 5 mL   _____

36. Order: Teva-Levocarbidopa 100-25 PO QID.

    Available:

37. Order: Gemfibrozil 0.6 g PO BID 30 minutes before meals.

    Available:

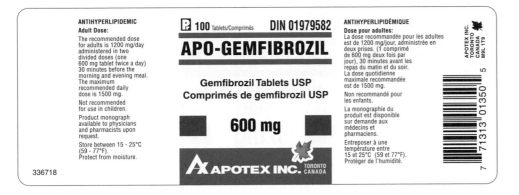

38. Order: Fenofibrate 108 mg PO daily.

    Available:

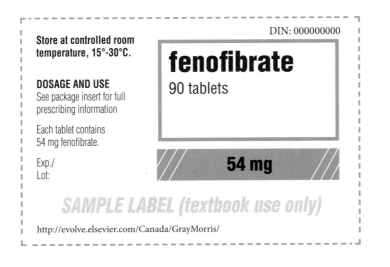

39. Order: Potassium chloride 10 mmol IV in 1 000 mL D5W (dextrose 5% solution).

    Available: Potassium chloride 20 mL vial labelled 40 mmol (2 mmol per mL)

40. Order: Prednisone 7.5 mg PO BID.

Available:

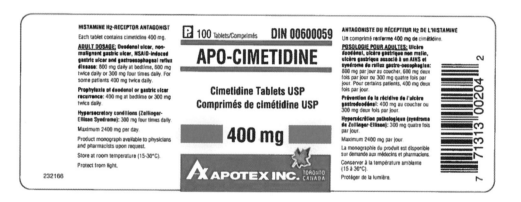

41. Order: Cimetidine 800 mg PO at bedtime.

Available:

42. Order: Depo-Provera 650 mg IM once a week (on Mondays).

Available: Depo-Provera labelled 400 mg per mL _____

43. Order: Ranitidine 0.4 g IV BID.

Available:

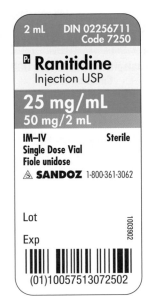

_____

44. Order: Leucovorin calcium 0.1 g IVPB q12h.

Available:

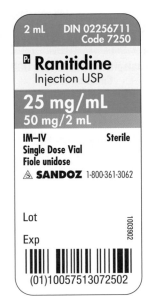

_____

45. Order: Cipro 1.5 g PO q12h.

Available: Cipro tablets labelled 750 mg   _____

46. Order: Enalapril maleate 5 mg PO daily.

    Available:

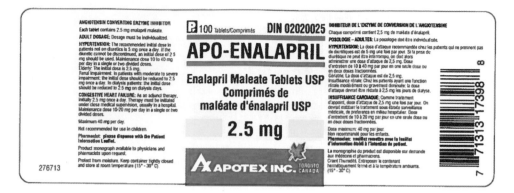

47. Order: Clozapine 50 mg PO BID.

    Available:

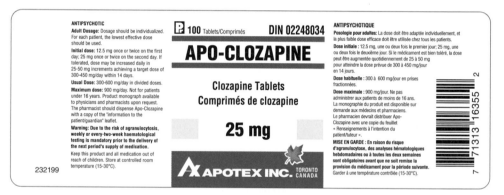

48. Order: Azithromycin 450 mg PO QID for 5 days.

    Available:

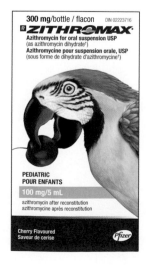

49. Order: Benadryl 30 mg PO TID.

Available: Oral solution labelled 12.5 mg per 5 mL   _____

50. Order: Primidone 125 mg PO daily.

Available: Oral solution labelled 250 mg per 5 mL   _____

51. Order: Metformin hydrochloride 750 mg PO BID with meals.

Available:

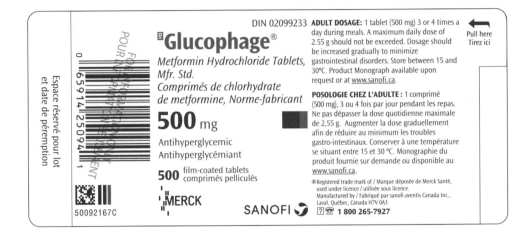

_____

52. Order: Inderal 120 mg PO BID.

Available:

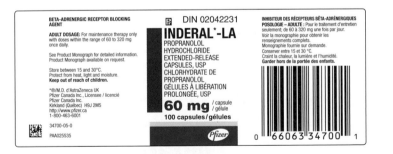

_____

53. Order: Furosemide 30 mg PO every day at 9 AM.

    Available: Lasix scored tablets (can be broken in half)

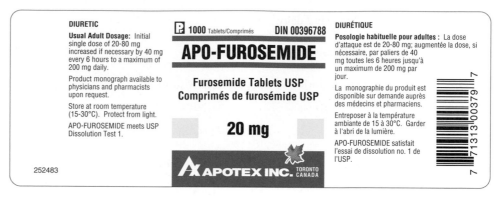

54. Order: Janumet 50 mg/1 000 mg PO BID.

    Available:

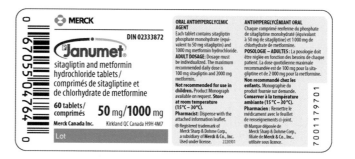

55. Order: Bexarotene 150 mg PO daily ac.

    Available:

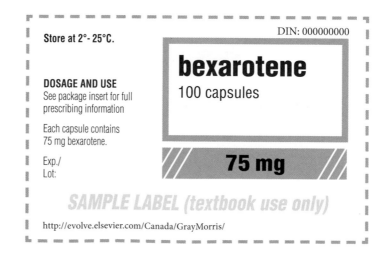

56. Order: Glyburide 7.5 mg PO daily with breakfast.

    Available: Glyburide tablets labelled 2.5 mg   _____

57. Order: Clarithromycin 0.5 g PO q12h for 10 days.

    Available:

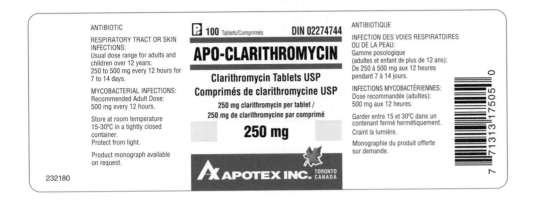

    _____

58. Order: Donepezil 5 mg PO every day at bedtime.

    Available:

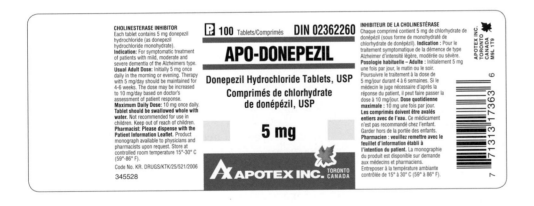

    _____

59. Order: Lasix 8 mg IM stat.

    Available: Lasix solution labelled 20 mg per 2 mL   _____

60. Order: Metoprolol SR 0.2 g PO daily.

Available:

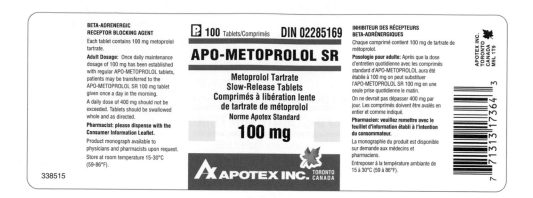

Answers on page 262.

✳ ANSWERS

Answers to Practice Problems

1. $\dfrac{0.4 \text{ mg}}{0.2 \text{ mg}} \times 1 \text{ tab} = x \text{ tab}$

   $x = \dfrac{0.4}{0.2}$

   $x = 2$ tabs. 0.4 mg is greater than 0.2 mg; therefore, you will need more than 1 tab to administer the dosage.

2. Conversion factor: 1 000 mg = 1 g (0.75 g = 750 mg)

   $\dfrac{750 \text{ mg}}{250 \text{ mg}} \times 1 \text{ capsule} = x \text{ capsule}$

   $x = \dfrac{750}{250}$

   $x = 3$ capsules. 750 mg is greater than 250 mg; therefore, you will need more than 1 capsule to administer the dosage.

3. $\dfrac{90 \text{ mg}}{60 \text{ mg}} \times 1 \text{ tab} = x \text{ tab}$

   $x = \dfrac{90}{60}$

   $x = 1.5$ or $1\dfrac{1}{2}$ tabs. 90 mg is greater than 60 mg; therefore, you will need more than 1 tab to administer the dosage.

4. $\dfrac{7.5 \text{ mg}}{2.5 \text{ mg}} \times 1 \text{ tab} = x \text{ tab}$

   $x = \dfrac{7.5}{2.5}$

   $x = 3$ tabs. 7.5 mg is greater than 2.5 mg; therefore, you will need more than 1 tab to administer the dosage.

---

evolve

For additional practice problems, refer to the Methods of Calculating Dosages section of the Drug Calculations Companion, Version 5 on Evolve.

5. Conversion factor: 1 000 mcg = 1 mg
(0.05 mg = 50 mcg)

$$\frac{50\,mcg}{25\,mcg} \times 1\,tab = x\,tab$$

$$x = \frac{50}{25}$$

x = 2 tabs. 50 mcg is greater than 25 mcg; therefore, you will need more than 1 tab to administer the dosage.

6. Conversion factor: 1 000 mcg = 1 mg
(0.4 mg = 400 mcg)

$$\frac{400\,mcg}{200\,mcg} \times 1\,tab = x\,tab$$

$$x = \frac{400}{200}$$

x = 2 tabs. 400 mcg is greater than 200 mcg; therefore, you will need more than 1 tab to administer the dosage.

7. $\frac{1\,000\,mg}{500\,mg} \times 1\,tab = x\,tab$

$$x = \frac{1\,000}{500}$$

x = 2 tabs. 1 000 mg is greater than 500 mg; therefore, you will need more than 1 tab to administer the dosage.

8. Conversion factor: 1 000 mg = 1 g (0.6 g = 600 mg)

$$\frac{600\,mg}{600\,mg} \times 1\,capsule = x\,capsule$$

$$x = \frac{600}{600}$$

x = 1 capsule. 0.6 g = 600 mg and 600 mg capsules are available; therefore, give 1 capsule to administer the dosage.

9. Conversion factor: 1 000 mcg = 1 mg
(1.25 mg = 1 250 mcg)

$$\frac{1\,250\,mcg}{625\,mcg} \times 1\,tab = x\,tab$$

$$x = \frac{1\,250}{625}$$

x = 2 tabs. 1 250 mcg is greater than 625 mcg; therefore, you will need more than 1 tab to administer the dosage.

10. $\frac{10\,mg}{15\,mg} \times 1\,mL = x\,mL$

$$x = \frac{10}{15}$$

x = 0.66 = 0.7 mL. 10 mg is less than 15 mg; therefore, you will need less than 1 mL to administer the dosage.

11. $\frac{400\,mg}{200\,mg} \times 5\,mL = x\,mL$

$$x = \frac{2\,000}{200}$$

x = 10 mL. 400 mg is greater than 200 mg; therefore, you will need more than 5 mL to administer the dosage.

12. $\frac{15\,mmol}{20\,mmol} \times 10\,mL = x\,mL$

$$x = \frac{150}{20}$$

x = 7.5 mL. 15 mmol is less than 20 mmol; therefore, you will need less than 10 mL to administer the dosage.

13. $\frac{125\,mg}{250\,mg} \times 5\,mL = x\,mL$

$$x = \frac{625}{250}$$

x = 2.5 mL. 125 mg is less than 250 mg; therefore, you will need less than 5 mL to administer the dosage.

14. $\frac{0.025\,mg}{0.05\,mg} \times 5\,mL = x\,mL$

$$x = \frac{0.125}{0.05}$$

x = 2.5 mL. 0.025 mg is less than 0.05 mg; therefore, you will need less than 5 mL to administer the dosage.

15. $\frac{375\,mg}{125\,mg} \times 5\,mL = x\,mL$

$$x = \frac{1\,875}{125}$$

x = 15 mL. 375 mg is greater than 125 mg; therefore, you will need more than 5 mL to administer the dosage.

16. $\dfrac{100\,\text{mg}}{125\,\text{mg}} \times 5\,\text{mL} = x\,\text{mL}$

$x = \dfrac{500}{125} = 4\,\text{mL}$

17. $x = \dfrac{500\,\text{mg}}{125\,\text{mg}} \times 5\,\text{mL} = x\,\text{mL}$

$x = \dfrac{2\,500}{125} = 20\,\text{mL}$

18. $x = \dfrac{25\,\text{mg}}{50\,\text{mg}} \times 1\,\text{mL} = x\,\text{mL}$

$x = \dfrac{25}{50} = 0.5\,\text{mL}$

19. $\quad 0.4\,\text{g} \times 1\,000 = 400\,\text{mg}$

$\dfrac{400\,\text{mg}}{400\,\text{mg}} \times 40\,\text{mL} = x\,\text{mL}$

$x = \dfrac{16\,000}{400} = 40\,\text{mL}$

20. $\dfrac{200\,\text{mcg}}{500\,\text{mcg}} \times 1\,\text{mL} = x\,\text{mL}$

$x = \dfrac{200}{500} = 0.4\,\text{mL}$

Answers to Chapter Review

NOTE

For Chapter Review problems, only answers are shown. If needed, review the setup of problems in Practice Problems 1–15.

1. 1 tab

2. 2 capsules

3. 1 capsule

4. 2 tabs

5. 2 caplets

6. $1\frac{1}{2}$ tabs *or* 1.5 tabs

7. 1 tab

8. 1 capsule

9. 2 tablets

10. 2 tabs

11. 1 tab

12. 2 capsules

13. 1 tab

14. 2 capsules

15. 2 capsules (extended)

16. 0.7 mL

17. 1.3 mL

18. 4 mL

19. 12 mL

20. 10 mL

21. 11.3 mL

22. 0.6 mL

23. 2 mL

24. 1.8 mL

25. 10 mL

26. 0.2 mL

27. 2 mL

28. 1.2 mL

29. 0.8 mL

30. 0.5 mL

31. 0.3 mL

32. 1.7 mL

33. 2 mL

34. 3.2 mL

35. 5 mL

36. 1 tab

37. 1 tab

38. 2 tabs

39. 5 mL

40. 1.5 tabs

41. 2 tabs

42. 1.6 mL

43. 16 mL

44. 10 mL

45. 2 tabs

46. 2 tabs

47. 2 tabs

48. 22.5 mL

49. 12 mL

50. 2.5 mL

51. 1.5 tab

52. 2 caps

53. $1\frac{1}{2}$ tabs *or* 1.5 tabs

54. 1 tab

55. 2 capsules

56. 3 tabs

57. 2 tabs *or* 2 film tabs

58. 1 tab

59. 0.8 mL

60. 2 tabs (slow release)

CHAPTER 14

Dosage Calculation Using the Dimensional Analysis Method

Objectives

After reviewing this chapter, you should be able to:

1. Define dimensional analysis
2. Implement unit cancellation in dimensional analysis
3. Perform conversions using dimensional analysis
4. Calculate dosages using the dimensional analysis method

In this chapter, you will learn how to use the *dimensional analysis* as a method for calculating dosages. Dimensional analysis was introduced in Chapter 6 as a method for converting measurements within the same system or between systems. You may prefer the dimensional analysis method to the ratio and proportion method or the formula method. When using dimensional analysis, no memorization of a formula is required, and one equation is used even if a conversion is required. However, memorization of the common equivalents is a **must.**

Dimensional analysis is a simple technique with a fancy name for the process of manipulating units to get the desired unit. By manipulating units, you are able to eliminate or cancel unwanted units. Dimensional analysis is considered a common-sense approach and, as already stated, it eliminates the need to memorize a formula and uses only one equation. Once the concepts related to dimensional analysis are mastered, it can be used to calculate dosages.

Dimensional analysis is also referred to as the *factor-label method* or the *unit factor method.* Dimensional analysis can be viewed as a problem-solving method. It can be used for all calculations you may encounter once you become comfortable with the process. This chapter provides examples of how this method can be used to calculate dosages.

Although some may find the formal name *dimensional analysis* intimidating, this method is quite simple once you have worked a few problems. This method will be applied to a variety of dosage calculations as we proceed through this text. Remember, as stated in the discussion of calculation methods in Chapter 12, it is important that you choose a method of calculation you are comfortable with and use it consistently.

Understanding the Basics of Dimensional Analysis

Let's begin by looking at how dimensional analysis can be used to make a conversion before we look at its use in calculating dosages. In previous chapters, you learned about *conversion factors:* for example, 1 g = 1 000 mg, 1 kg = 1 000 g. When we begin using dimensional analysis for dosage calculations, you will quickly see how it allows multiple factors to be

263

entered in one equation. This method is particularly useful when a medication is ordered in one unit of measurement but is available in another. Although multiple factors can be placed in a dimensional analysis equation, you can decide to do the conversion before you set up the equation using one of the methods learned in earlier chapters, or you can use dimensional analysis to perform the conversion before calculating the dosage.

Performing Conversions Using Dimensional Analysis

The conversion factors you learned are written in fraction format when dimensional analysis is used to perform conversions. For example, the conversion factor 1 kg = 1 000 g is written as follows:

$$\frac{1\,kg}{1\,000\,g} \quad or \quad \frac{1\,000\,g}{1\,kg}$$

NOTE
You have not changed the value of the unit: you have simply rewritten the conversion factor in a fraction format.

Now let's look at how to use dimensional analysis to convert units of measurement. An equivalent (conversion factor) will give you two fractions:

NOTE
How the fraction is written depends on the unit you want to cancel or eliminate to get the desired unit.

Examples:

$$2.2\,lb = 1\,kg = \frac{2.2\,lb}{1\,kg} \quad or \quad \frac{1\,kg}{2.2\,lb}$$

$$1\,000\,mcg = 1\,mg = \frac{1\,000\,mcg}{1\,mg} \quad or \quad \frac{1\,mg}{1\,000\,mcg}$$

Which fraction to use depends on the desired unit you are converting to. Choose the fraction that has the desired unit in the numerator.

To Make Conversions Using Dimensional Analysis

1. Identify the desired unit you are converting to.
2. Identify the equivalent needed.
3. Write the conversion factor in fraction format, keeping the desired unit in the numerator of the fraction. This is written first in the equation, followed by a multiplication sign (×). (Notice that the unit in the numerator is the same as the unit you desire.)
4. Label all factors in the equation, and label the desired unit x.
5. Identify the unwanted or undesired units, and cancel them. Reduce to lowest terms if possible.
6. If all the labels except the answer label (the desired unit) are not eliminated, recheck the equation.
7. Perform the necessary mathematical operations to solve for the unknown x.

(!) SAFETY ALERT!
Stating the conversion factor incorrectly will not allow you to cancel undesired units. Knowing when the equation is set up correctly is an important part of dimensional analysis.

Let's look at sample problems illustrating the use of dimensional analysis.

Example 1: 1.5 g = _____ mg

✓ PROBLEM SETUP

1. The desired unit is mg.
2. Conversion factor: 1 g = 1 000 mg
3. Write the conversion factor in fraction format, keeping milligrams (mg) in the numerator to allow you to cancel the unwanted unit, grams (g). Write the conversion factor first in the equation, followed by a multiplication sign (×). (Notice the unit in the numerator of the first fraction is the same as the desired unit.)
4. Label all factors in the equation.

5. Identify unwanted or undesired units (grams, in this case), and cancel them.
6. Perform the necessary mathematical operations to solve for the unknown x.

Solution:

$$x \text{ mg} = \frac{1\,000 \text{ mg}}{1 \cancel{g}} \times 1.5 \cancel{g}$$

or

$$x \text{ mg} = \frac{1\,000 \text{ mg}}{1 \cancel{g}} \times \frac{1.5 \cancel{g}}{1}$$

$$1\,000 \text{ mg} \times 1.5 = 1\,500 \text{ mg}$$

$$x = 1\,500 \text{ mg}$$

The problem in Example 1 could also be solved by decimal movement. It is shown in this format to illustrate dimensional analysis.

> **RULE**
>
> Placing a 1 under a value does not alter the value of the number. What you desire or are looking for is labelled x.

Example 2: 110 lb = _____ kg

✓ PROBLEM SETUP

1. The desired unit is kg.
2. Conversion factor: 2.2 lb = 1 kg
3. Proceed with the rest of the steps to set up and solve the problem.

Solution:

$$x \text{ kg} = \frac{1 \text{ kg}}{2.2 \cancel{lb}} \times 110 \cancel{lb}$$

or

$$x \text{ kg} = \frac{1 \text{ kg}}{2.2 \cancel{lb}} \times \frac{110 \cancel{lb}}{1}$$

$$x = \frac{110}{2.2}$$

$$x = 50 \text{ kg}$$

> **RULE**
>
> All factors entered in the equation must always include the quantity and unit of measurement. State all answers following the rules of the system. When there is more than one equivalent for a unit of measurement, use the conversion factor used most often.

 PRACTICE **PROBLEMS**

Set up the following problems using dimensional analysis; cancel the units. Do not solve.

1. $8\frac{1}{2}$ tsp = _____ mL   4. 2 tbsp = _____ mL

2. 15 mg = _____ g   5. 0.007 g = _____ mg

3. 400 mcg = _____ mg   6. 0.5 L = _____ mL

7. 529 mg = _____ g   9. 46.4 kg = _____ lb

8. 1 600 mL = _____ L   10. 5 cm = _____ in

Answers on page 282.

> ⚙ **POINTS TO REMEMBER**
> - Identify the desired unit, and label it *x*.
> - State the equivalent (conversion factor) in fraction format with the desired unit in the numerator.
> - Label all factors in the equation, including "*x*."
> - State the conversion factor first in the equation, followed by a multiplication sign (×).
> - Remember the rules relating to conversion (see Chapter 6).
> - Cancel the undesired units.

Dosage Calculation Using Dimensional Analysis

As stated previously, dimensional analysis can be used to calculate dosages with a single equation. A single equation can also be used to calculate the dosage when the desired dosage is in units that differ from what is available. When using dimensional analysis to calculate dosages, it is important to extract the essential information needed from the problem. See Box 14-1.

In earlier chapters relating to calculating dosages, you learned how to read medication labels. Remember: dosages are always expressed in relation to the form or unit of measurement that contains them.

Examples: 100 mg per tab, 500 mg per capsule, 40 mg per 2 mL.

When dimensional analysis is used to calculate dosages, the preceding examples become crucial factors in the equation and are entered as a fraction with a numerator and a denominator.

BOX 14-1   Steps in Calculating Dosages Using Dimensional Analysis

1. Identify the desired unit in the calculation. With solid forms of medication, the unit will be tab, capsule, or caplet. For parenteral and oral liquid medications, the unit will be mL. Think about what a reasonable dosage would be before you calculate.
2. On the left side of the equation, place *x* with the name or appropriate abbreviation of what you desire or are looking for (e.g., tab, capsule, caplet, mL).
3. On the right side of the equation, place the available dosage strength in a fraction format. Ensure that the abbreviation or unit of measurement matches the desired unit in the numerator.
4. Enter the additional factors from the problem, usually the dosage ordered, to the right of the available dosage strength. Set up this information as a fraction and match the unit of measurement in the numerator with the unit of measurement in the denominator of the preceding fraction.
5. Cancel the like units of measurement on the right side of the equation. The remaining unit of measurement should match the unit of measurement on the left side of the equation and be the desired unit. Reduce to lowest terms if possible.
6. Solve for the unknown *x*.

Let's look at examples using these steps.

Example 1:   Order: Furosemide 40 mg PO daily.

Available: Tablets labelled 20 mg

1. The desired unit is tab. Think about what a reasonable dosage would be before you calculate.

2. On the left side of the equation, place x with the name or abbreviation of the desired unit.

$$x \text{ tab} =$$

3. On the right side of the equation, place the available information from the problem in fraction format, with the unit of measurement matching the desired unit in the numerator. (In this problem, each tab contains 20 mg.)

$$x \text{ tab} = \frac{1 \text{ tab}}{20 \text{ mg}}$$

4. Enter the additional factors from the problem—the dosage ordered—to the right of the available dosage strength. Match the unit in the numerator with the unit in the preceding denominator (in this problem, the dosage ordered is 40 mg). Placing a 1 under a numerator does not change its value.

Amount to Available Dosage
administer   dosage   ordered
   ↓   ↓   ↓

$$x \text{ tab} = \frac{1 \text{ tab}}{20 \text{ mg}} \times \frac{40 \text{ mg}}{1}$$

5. Cancel the like units of measurement on the right side of the equation. The remaining unit of measurement should match the unit on the left side of equation: the desired unit.
6. Proceed with the necessary mathematical operations to solve for the unknown x. Notice that after cancellation of units (mg), the desired unit of measurement to be administered remains (tab, in this problem).

$$x \text{ tab} = \frac{1 \text{ tab}}{20 \text{ mg}} \times \frac{40 \text{ mg}}{1}$$

$$x = \frac{1 \times 40}{20}$$

$$x = \frac{40}{20}$$

$$x = 2 \text{ tabs}$$

Now let's look at an example with parenteral medications. Follow the same steps used in Example 1.

Example 2: Order: Gentamicin 55 mg IM q8h.

Available: Gentamicin 80 mg per 2 mL (round to the nearest tenth)

1. The desired unit is mL. Think about what a reasonable dosage would be before you calculate.
2. On the left side of the equation, place x with the name or abbreviation of the desired unit.

$$x \text{ mL} =$$

3. On the right side of the equation, place the available information from the problem in fraction format, with the unit of measurement matching the desired unit in the numerator.

$$x \text{ mL} = \frac{2 \text{ mL}}{80 \text{ mg}}$$

4. Enter the additional factors from the problem—the dosage ordered—to the right of the available dosage strength. Match the unit in the numerator with the unit in the preceding denominator (in this problem, the dosage ordered is 55 mg).

$$\underset{\substack{\text{Amount to}\\\text{administer}\\\downarrow}}{x\,\text{mL}} = \underset{\substack{\text{Available}\\\text{dosage}\\\downarrow}}{\frac{2\,\text{mL}}{80\,\text{mg}}} \times \underset{\substack{\text{Dosage}\\\text{ordered}\\\downarrow}}{\frac{55\,\text{mg}}{1}}$$

5. Cancel the like units of measurement on the right side of the equation. The remaining unit of measurement should match the unit on the left side of the equation: the desired unit.
6. Solve for the unknown x.

$$x\,\text{mL} = \frac{2\,\text{mL}}{80\,\cancel{\text{mg}}} \times \frac{55\,\cancel{\text{mg}}}{1}$$

$$x = \frac{2 \times 55}{80}$$

$$x = \frac{110}{80} = 1.37$$

$$x = 1.37\,\text{mL}$$

As previously mentioned, dimensional analysis can be used when a medication is ordered in one unit of measurement but available in another, which necessitates a conversion. However, the same steps are followed as previously shown.

- An additional fraction is entered into the equation as the second fraction. This fraction is the conversion factor needed. The numerator must match the unit of measurement of the previous denominator.
- The last fraction is the dosage ordered. This is written so that the numerator of the fraction matches the unit of measurement in the denominator of the fraction immediately before.

Let's look at an example:

Example 3: Order: Ampicillin 0.5 g IM q6h.

Available: Ampicillin labelled 250 mg per mL

1. The desired unit is mL. Think about what a reasonable dosage would be before you calculate.
2. On the left side of the equation, place x with the name or abbreviation of the desired unit.

$$x\,\text{mL} =$$

3. On the right side of the equation, place the available information from the problem in a fraction format, with the unit of measurement matching the desired unit in the numerator.

$$x\,\text{mL} = \frac{1\,\text{mL}}{250\,\text{mg}}$$

4. The order is for 0.5 g, and the medication is available in 250 mg. Therefore, a conversion is needed. From previous chapters, we know 1 g = 1 000 mg; this conversion factor is placed next, in the form of a fraction (the unit in the numerator of this fraction must match the unit in the denominator of the immediately preceding fraction).

$$x \text{ mL} = \frac{1 \text{ mL}}{250 \text{ mg}} \times \frac{1\,000 \text{ mg}}{1 \text{ g}}$$

5. Next, place the dosage ordered in the equation. The unit in the numerator will match the unit in the preceding denominator (in this problem, the dosage ordered is 0.5 g).

$$x \text{ mL} = \underset{\downarrow}{\underset{\text{dosage}}{\underset{\text{Available}}{}}} \quad \underset{\downarrow}{\underset{\text{factor}}{\underset{\text{Conversion}}{}}} \quad \underset{\downarrow}{\underset{\text{ordered}}{\underset{\text{Dosage}}{}}}$$

$$x \text{ mL} = \frac{1 \text{ mL}}{250 \text{ mg}} \times \frac{1\,000 \text{ mg}}{1 \text{ g}} \times \frac{0.5 \text{ g}}{1}$$

6. Cancel the like units of measurement on the right side of the equation. The remaining unit of measurement should match the unit on the left side of equation: the desired unit. Notice that mg and g cancel, leaving the desired unit, mL.

$$x \text{ mL} = \frac{1 \text{ mL}}{250 \text{ m\!\!\!/g}} \times \frac{1\,000 \text{ m\!\!\!/g}}{1 \text{ \!\!\!/g}} \times \frac{0.5 \text{ \!\!\!/g}}{1}$$

$$x = \frac{1\,000 \times 0.5}{250}$$

$$x = \frac{500}{250}$$

$$x = 2 \text{ mL}$$

SAFETY ALERT!

Incorrect placement of units of measurement in the equation will not allow cancellation of units and can result in an error in calculation. Dimensional analysis does not eliminate thinking about what a reasonable answer should be.

POINTS TO REMEMBER

When using dimensional analysis to calculate dosages:

- Identify the unit of medication you want to administer; for example, tab, capsule, caplet, mL. The desired unit is written **FIRST** to the left of the equation followed by an equal sign (=).
- Always **THINK** about what a reasonable amount to administer would be before you calculate.
- Note that the unit of measurement in the numerator on the left of the equal sign should be the same unit of measurement in the numerator of the **first fraction** on the right side of the equation.
- If a conversion is necessary, place the conversion factor on the right side of the equation, as the second fraction.
- Place the dosage ordered at the end of the equation, as the final fraction.
- Cancel the like units of measurement. When all the cancellations have been made, only the desired unit should remain (e.g., tab, capsule, mL).
- Include the quantity and unit of measurement in all factors entered into the equation.
- Keep in mind that incorrect placement of units of measurement will not allow you to cancel units and can result in an incorrect answer.
- Note that critical thinking and reasoning are essential even with dimensional analysis.

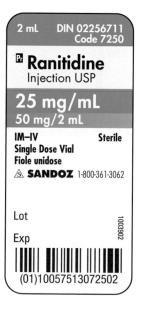

PRACTICE **PROBLEMS**

Set up the following problems using dimensional analysis. Do not solve.

11. Order: 0.3 g of a liquid medication.

    Available: 0.4 g per 1.5 mL _____

12. Order: 15 mg of a liquid medication.

    Available: 15 mg per mL _____

13. Order: Ampicillin 1 g PO stat.

    Available: Ampicillin capsules labelled 500 mg _____

14. Order: Cefaclor 250 mg PO TID.

    Available: Cefaclor oral suspension labelled 125 mg per 5 mL _____

15. Order: Ranitidine 150 mg IV daily.

    Available:

| 2 mL | DIN 02256711 |
| | Code 7250 |

℞ **Ranitidine**
Injection USP

25 mg/mL
50 mg/2 mL

IM–IV   Sterile
Single Dose Vial
Fiole unidose
⚠ **SANDOZ** 1-800-361-3062

Lot

Exp

(01)10057513072502

_____

16. Order: Methyldopa 0.5 g PO daily.

    Available:

    DIN: 000000000

    DOSAGE AND USE
    See package insert for full
    prescribing information

    Each tablet contains
    250 mg methyldopa.

    Exp./
    Lot:

    methyldopa
    100 tablets

    250 mg

    SAMPLE LABEL (textbook use only)

    http://evolve.elsevier.com/Canada/GrayMorris/

    _____

17. Order: Digoxin 0.125 mg PO daily.

    Available: Scored tablets (can be broken in half)   _____

    DIN: 000000000

    **Store at 25°C; excursions
    permitted to 15°- 30°C.**

    DOSAGE AND USE
    See package insert for full
    prescribing information

    Each tablet contains
    250 mcg digoxin.

    Exp./
    Lot:

    digoxin
    100 tablets

    250 mcg (0.25 mg)

    SAMPLE LABEL (textbook use only)

    http://evolve.elsevier.com/Canada/GrayMorris/

    _____

18. Order: Phenytoin 300 mg PO TID.

    Available: Phenytoin oral suspension labelled 125 mg per 5 mL

    _____

19. Order: Ciprofloxacin 0.5 g PO q12h.

    Available:

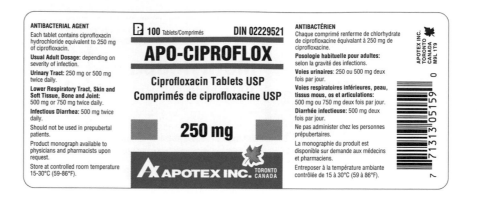

_____

20. Order: Clindamycin 0.3 g IV q6h.

    Available: Clindamycin labelled 150 mg per mL   _____

Answers on page 282.

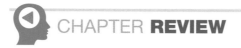 CHAPTER **REVIEW**

Calculate the following dosages using the dimensional analysis method. Use the labels or the information provided. Label answers correctly: tabs, capsules, or mL. Answers expressed in millilitres should be rounded to the nearest tenth where indicated.

1. Order: Meclizine hydrochloride 50 mg PO daily.

    Available:

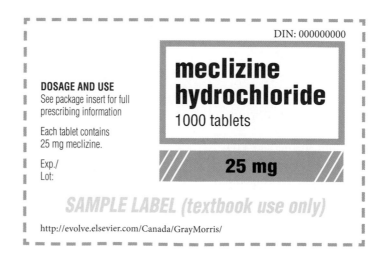

_____

2. Order: Potassium chloride 20 mmol in 1 L of D5W (dextrose 5% solution).

Available:

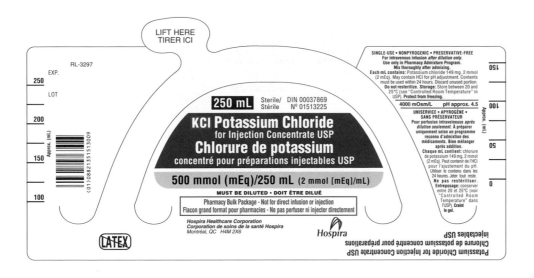

3. Order: Morphine sulphate 20 mg IM stat.

Available:

4. Order: Apo-Escalitopram 20 mg PO daily.

Available:

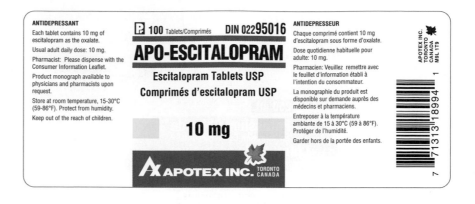

5. Order: Captopril 25 mg PO daily.

Available: Captopril tablets labelled 12.5 mg

6. Order: Thiamine 80 mg IM stat.

Available:

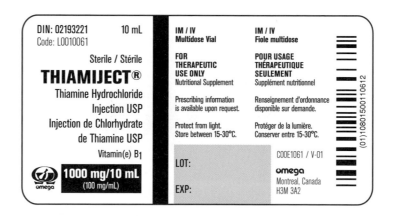

7. Order: Heparin 6 500 units SUBCUT q12h.

Available: Heparin 10 000 units per mL (Express answer in hundredths.)

8.　Order: Terbutaline 5 mg PO TID.

　　Available:

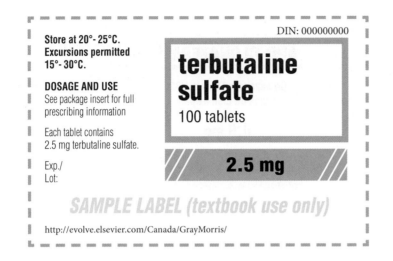

9.　Order: Labetalol 200 mg PO BID.

　　Available: Labetalol tablets labelled 100 mg　　　————————

10.　Order: Methylprednisolone 175 mg IV daily.

　　Available: Methylprednisolone labelled 500 mg per 8 mL　　————————

11.　Order: Pentoxifylline ER tablets 0.4 g PO TID.

　　Available: Pentoxifylline ER tablets 400 mg　　————————

12.　Order: Apo-Clarithromycin 0.5 g PO q12h for 7 days.

　　Available:

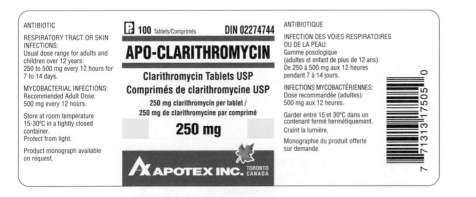

13. Order: Clonazepam 0.5 mg PO BID.

    Available:

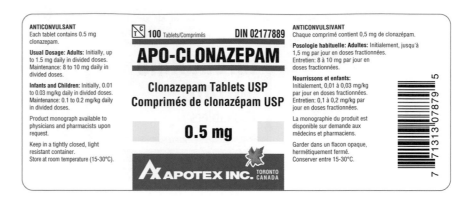

14. Order: Quinidine gluconate 200 mg IM q8h.

    Available: Quinidine gluconate labelled 80 mg per mL _____

15. Order: Protamine sulphate 25 mg IV stat.

    Available:

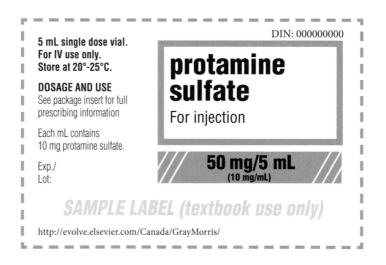

16. Order: Methotrexate 15 mg IM every week (on Monday).

    Available:

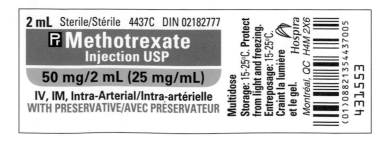

17. Order: Theophylline 0.4 g PO BID.

    Available:

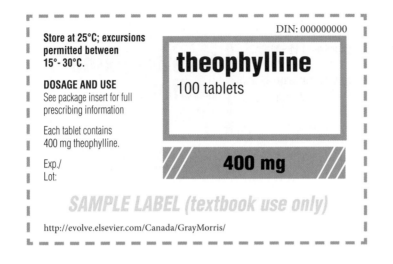

    _____

18. Order: Diphenhydramine 60 mg IM stat.

    Available: Diphenhydramine labelled 50 mg per mL _____

19. Order: Cefaclor 0.4 g PO q8h.

    Available:

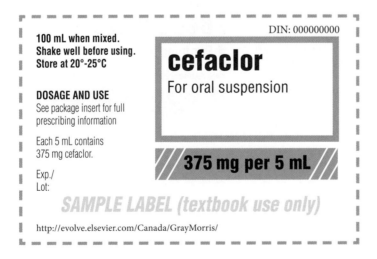

    _____

20. Order: Levothyroxine sodium 0.075 mg PO daily.

   Available: Scored tablets (can be broken in half)

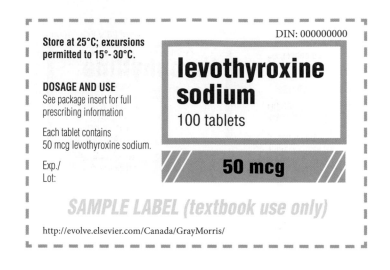

_____

21. Order: Haloperidol decanoate 0.25 g IM monthly.

   Available:

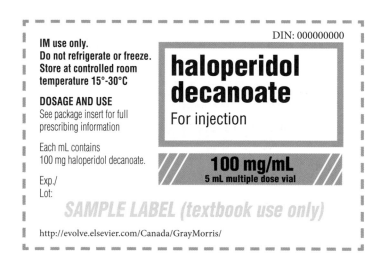

_____

22. Order: Dexamethasone 1.5 mg IV stat.

    Available:

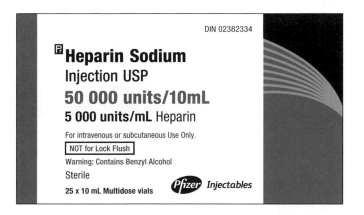

_____

23. Order: Heparin 5 000 units SUBCUT stat.

    Available:

Heparin Sodium
Injection USP
50 000 units/10mL
5 000 units/mL Heparin

For intravenous or subcutaneous Use Only.
NOT for Lock Flush
Warning: Contains Benzyl Alcohol
Sterile
25 x 10 mL Multidose vials   *Pfizer* Injectables

DIN 02382334

_____

24. Order: Strattera 0.1 g PO daily.

Available:

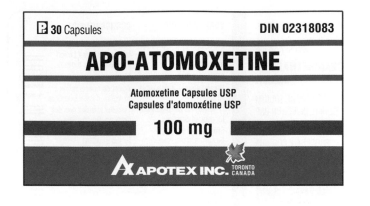

_____

25. Order: Erythromycin oral suspension 150 mg PO BID.

Available:

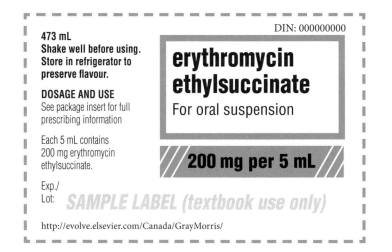

_____

26. Order: Darbepoetin alfa 0.02 mg SUBCUT once weekly.

    Available:

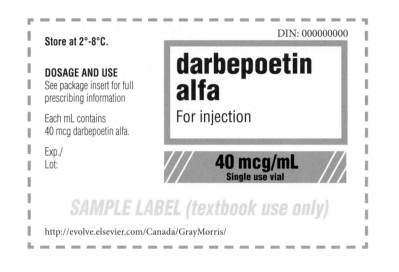

_____

For questions 27–34, set up the problem using dimensional analysis and make the conversion as indicated.

27. 79 lb = _____ kg (round to nearest tenth)

28. 5 mcg = _____ mg

29. 2 400 mL = _____ L

30. 8 in = _____ cm

31. 1.25 mcg = _____ mg

32. 240 mL = _____ oz

33. 1.75 mg = _____ mcg

34. 125 mL = _____ L

Answers on pages 283–285.

For additional practice problems, refer to the Methods of Calculating Dosages section of the Drug Calculations Companion, Version 5 on Evolve.

✳ ANSWERS

Answers to Practice Problems

NOTE

The following problems could be set up without placing 1 under a value; placing a 1 under the value as shown in the setup for Practice Problems 1–20 does not alter the value of the number.

1. $x \, \text{mL} = \dfrac{5 \, \text{mL}}{1 \, \text{tsp}} \times \dfrac{8\frac{1}{2} \, \text{tsp}}{1}$

2. $x \, \text{g} = \dfrac{1 \, \text{g}}{1000 \, \text{mg}} \times \dfrac{15 \, \text{mg}}{1}$

3. $x \, \text{mg} = \dfrac{1 \, \text{mg}}{1000 \, \text{mcg}} \times \dfrac{400 \, \text{mcg}}{1}$

4. $x \, \text{mL} = \dfrac{15 \, \text{mL}}{1 \, \text{tbsp}} \times \dfrac{2 \, \text{tbsp}}{1}$

5. $x \, \text{mg} = \dfrac{1000 \, \text{mg}}{1 \, \text{g}} \times \dfrac{0.007 \, \text{g}}{1}$

6. $x \, \text{mL} = \dfrac{1000 \, \text{mL}}{1 \, \text{L}} \times \dfrac{0.5 \, \text{L}}{1}$

7. $x \, \text{g} = \dfrac{1 \, \text{g}}{1000 \, \text{mg}} \times \dfrac{529 \, \text{mg}}{1}$

8. $x \, \text{L} = \dfrac{1 \, \text{L}}{1000 \, \text{mL}} \times \dfrac{1600 \, \text{mL}}{1}$

9. $x \, \text{lb} = \dfrac{2.2 \, \text{lb}}{1 \, \text{kg}} \times \dfrac{46.4 \, \text{kg}}{1}$

10. $x \, \text{in} = \dfrac{1 \, \text{in}}{2.5 \, \text{cm}} \times \dfrac{5 \, \text{cm}}{1}$

11. $x \, \text{mL} = \dfrac{1.5 \, \text{mL}}{0.4 \, \text{g}} \times \dfrac{0.3 \, \text{g}}{1}$

12. $x \, \text{mL} = \dfrac{1 \, \text{mL}}{15 \, \text{mg}} \times \dfrac{15 \, \text{mg}}{1}$

13. $x \, \text{capsule} = \dfrac{1 \, \text{capsule}}{500 \, \text{mg}} \times \dfrac{1000 \, \text{mg}}{1 \, \text{g}} \times \dfrac{1 \, \text{g}}{1}$

14. $x \, \text{mL} = \dfrac{5 \, \text{mL}}{125 \, \text{mg}} \times \dfrac{250 \, \text{mg}}{1}$

15. $x \, \text{mL} = \dfrac{1 \, \text{mL}}{25 \, \text{mg}} \times \dfrac{150 \, \text{mg}}{1}$

   or

   $x \, \text{mL} = \dfrac{2 \, \text{mL}}{50 \, \text{mg}} \times \dfrac{150 \, \text{mg}}{1}$

16. $x \, \text{tab} = \dfrac{1 \, \text{tab}}{250 \, \text{mg}} \times \dfrac{1000 \, \text{mg}}{1 \, \text{g}} \times \dfrac{0.5 \, \text{g}}{1}$

17. $x \, \text{tab} = \dfrac{1 \, \text{tab}}{0.25 \, \text{mg}} \times \dfrac{0.125 \, \text{mg}}{1}$

18. $x \, \text{mL} = \dfrac{5 \, \text{mL}}{125 \, \text{mg}} \times \dfrac{300 \, \text{mg}}{1}$

19. $x \, \text{tab} = \dfrac{1 \, \text{tab}}{250 \, \text{mg}} \times \dfrac{1000 \, \text{mg}}{1 \, \text{g}} \times \dfrac{0.5 \, \text{g}}{1}$

20. $x \, \text{mL} = \dfrac{1 \, \text{mL}}{150 \, \text{mg}} \times \dfrac{1000 \, \text{mg}}{1 \, \text{g}} \times \dfrac{0.3 \, \text{g}}{1}$

Answers to Chapter Review

1. $x \text{ tab} = \dfrac{1 \text{ tab}}{25 \text{ mg}} \times \dfrac{50 \text{ mg}}{1}$

$x = \dfrac{50}{25}$

$x = 2 \text{ tabs}$

2. $x \text{ mL} = \dfrac{15 \text{ mL}}{\underset{3}{30 \text{ mEq}}} \times \dfrac{\overset{2}{20 \text{ mEq}}}{1}$

$x = \dfrac{15 \times 2}{3}$

$x = \dfrac{30}{3}$

$x = 10 \text{ mL}$

3. $x \text{ mL} = \dfrac{1 \text{ mL}}{5 \text{ mg}} \times \dfrac{20 \text{ mg}}{1}$

$x = \dfrac{20}{5}$

$x = 4 \text{ mL}$

4. $x \text{ tab} = \dfrac{1 \text{ tab}}{10 \text{ mg}} \times \dfrac{20 \text{ mg}}{1}$

$x = \dfrac{20}{10}$

$x = 2 \text{ tabs}$

5. $x \text{ tab} = \dfrac{1 \text{ tab}}{12.5 \text{ mg}} \times \dfrac{25 \text{ mg}}{1}$

$x = \dfrac{25}{12.5}$

$x = 2 \text{ tabs}$

6. $x \text{ mL} = \dfrac{1 \text{ mL}}{100 \text{ mg}} \times \dfrac{80 \text{ mg}}{1}$

$x = \dfrac{80}{100}$

$x = 0.8 \text{ mL}$

7. $x \text{ mL} = \dfrac{1 \text{ mL}}{10\,000 \text{ units}} \times \dfrac{6\,500 \text{ units}}{1}$

$x = \dfrac{6\,500}{10\,000}$

$x = 0.65 \text{ mL}$

8. $x \text{ tab} = \dfrac{1 \text{ tab}}{2.5 \text{ mg}} \times \dfrac{5 \text{ mg}}{1}$

$x = \dfrac{5}{2.5}$

$x = 2 \text{ tabs}$

9. $x \text{ tab} = \dfrac{1 \text{ tab}}{100 \text{ mg}} \times \dfrac{200 \text{ mg}}{1}$

$x = \dfrac{200}{100}$

$x = 2 \text{ tabs}$

10. $x \text{ mL} = \dfrac{8 \text{ mL}}{500 \text{ mg}} \times \dfrac{175 \text{ mg}}{1}$

$x = \dfrac{8 \times 175}{500}$

$x = \dfrac{1\,400}{500}$

$x = 2.8 \text{ mL}$

11. $x \text{ tab} = \dfrac{1 \text{ tab}}{400 \text{ mg}} \times \dfrac{1\,000 \text{ mg}}{1 \text{ g}} \times \dfrac{0.4 \text{ g}}{1}$

$x = \dfrac{1\,000 \times 0.4}{400}$

$x = \dfrac{400}{400}$

$x = 1 \text{ tab (ER)}$

12. $x \text{ tab} = \dfrac{1 \text{ tab}}{\underset{1}{250 \text{ mg}}} \times \dfrac{\overset{4}{1\,000 \text{ mg}}}{1 \text{ g}} \times \dfrac{0.5 \text{ g}}{1}$

$x = \dfrac{4 \times 0.5}{1}$

$x = \dfrac{2}{1}$

$x = 2 \text{ tab}$

13. $x \text{ tab} = \dfrac{1 \text{ tab}}{0.5 \text{ mg}} \times \dfrac{0.5 \text{ mg}}{1}$

$x = \dfrac{0.5}{0.5}$

$x = 1 \text{ tab}$

14. $x \text{ mL} = \dfrac{1 \text{ mL}}{80 \text{ mg}} \times \dfrac{200 \text{ mg}}{1}$

$x = \dfrac{200}{80}$

$x = 2.5 \text{ mL}$

15. $x \text{ mL} = \dfrac{1 \text{ mL}}{10 \text{ mg}} \times \dfrac{25 \text{ mg}}{1}$

$x = \dfrac{25}{10}$

$x = 2.5 \text{ mL}$

or

$x \text{ mL} = \dfrac{5 \text{ mL}}{50 \text{ mg}} \times \dfrac{25 \text{ mg}}{1}$

$x = \dfrac{5 \times 25}{50}$

$x = \dfrac{125}{50}$

$x = 2.5 \text{ mL}$

16. $x \text{ mL} = \dfrac{1 \text{ mL}}{25 \text{ mg}} \times \dfrac{15 \text{ mg}}{1}$

$x = \dfrac{15}{25}$

$x = 0.6 \text{ mL}$

or

$x \text{ mL} = \dfrac{10 \text{ mL}}{250 \text{ mg}} \times \dfrac{15 \text{ mg}}{1}$

$x = \dfrac{10 \times 15}{250}$

$x = \dfrac{150}{250}$

$x = 0.6 \text{ mL}$

17. $x \text{ tab} = \dfrac{1 \text{ tab}}{400 \text{ mg}} \times \dfrac{1000 \text{ mg}}{1 \text{ g}} \times \dfrac{0.4 \text{ g}}{1}$

$x = \dfrac{1000 \times 0.4}{400}$

$x = \dfrac{400}{400}$

$x = 1 \text{ tab}$

18. $x \text{ mL} = \dfrac{1 \text{ mL}}{50 \text{ mg}} \times \dfrac{60 \text{ mg}}{1}$

$x = \dfrac{60}{50}$

$x = 1.2 \text{ mL}$

19. $x \text{ mL} = \dfrac{5 \text{ mL}}{375 \text{ mg}} \times \dfrac{1000 \text{ mg}}{1 \text{ g}} \times \dfrac{0.4 \text{ g}}{1}$

$x = \dfrac{5000 \times 0.4}{375}$

$x = \dfrac{2000}{375}$

$x = 5.33 \text{ mL} = 5.3 \text{ mL (to the nearest tenth)}$

20. $x \text{ tab} = \dfrac{1 \text{ tab}}{0.05 \text{ mg}} \times \dfrac{0.075 \text{ mg}}{1}$

$x = \dfrac{0.075}{0.05}$

$x = 1.5 \text{ tabs or } 1\frac{1}{2} \text{ tabs (``} 1\frac{1}{2} \text{ tabs'' preferred for administrative purposes)}$

21. $x \text{ mL} = \dfrac{1 \text{ mL}}{100 \text{ mg}} \times \dfrac{1000 \text{ mg}}{1 \text{ g}} \times \dfrac{0.25 \text{ g}}{1}$

$x = \dfrac{1000 \times 0.25}{100}$

$x = \dfrac{250}{100}$

$x = 2.5 \text{ mL}$

22. $x \text{ mL} = \dfrac{1 \text{ mL}}{4 \text{ mg}} \times \dfrac{1.5 \text{ mg}}{1}$

$x = \dfrac{1.5}{4}$

$x = 0.37 \text{ mL} = 0.4 \text{ mL (to the nearest tenth)}$

23. $x \text{ mL} = \dfrac{1 \text{ mL}}{5000 \text{ units}} \times \dfrac{5000 \text{ units}}{1}$

$x = \dfrac{5000}{5000}$

$x = 1 \text{ mL}$

24. $x \text{ capsule} = \dfrac{1 \text{ capsule}}{100 \text{ mg}} \times \dfrac{1\,000 \text{ mg}}{1 \text{ g}} \times \dfrac{0.1 \text{ g}}{1}$

$x = \dfrac{1\,000 \times 0.1}{100}$

$x = \dfrac{100}{100}$

$x = 1 \text{ capsule}$

25. $x \text{ mL} = \dfrac{5 \text{ mL}}{200 \text{ mg}} \times \dfrac{150 \text{ mg}}{1}$

$x = \dfrac{5 \times 150}{200}$

$x = \dfrac{750}{200}$

$x = 3.75 \text{ mL} = 3.8 \text{ mL} \text{ (to the nearest tenth)}$

26. $x \text{ mL} = \dfrac{1 \text{ mL}}{40 \text{ mcg}} \times \dfrac{1\,000 \text{ mcg}}{1} \times \dfrac{0.02 \text{ mg}}{1}$

$x = \dfrac{1\,000 \times 0.02}{40}$

$x = \dfrac{20}{40}$

$x = 0.5 \text{ mL}$

27. $x \text{ kg} = \dfrac{1 \text{ kg}}{2.2 \text{ lb}} \times \dfrac{79 \text{ lb}}{1}$

$x = \dfrac{79}{2.2}$

$x = 35.9 \text{ kg} \text{ (to the nearest tenth)}$

28. $x \text{ mg} = \dfrac{1 \text{ mg}}{1\,000 \text{ mcg}} \times \dfrac{5 \text{ mcg}}{1}$

$x = \dfrac{5}{1\,000}$

$x = 0.005 \text{ mg}$

29. $x \text{ L} = \dfrac{1 \text{ L}}{1\,000 \text{ mL}} \times \dfrac{2\,400 \text{ mL}}{1}$

$x = \dfrac{2\,400}{1\,000}$

$x = 2.4 \text{ L}$

30. $x \text{ cm} = \dfrac{2.5 \text{ cm}}{1 \text{ in}} \times \dfrac{8 \text{ in}}{1}$

$x = \dfrac{2.5 \times 8}{1}$

$x = 20 \text{ cm}$

31. $x \text{ mg} = \dfrac{1 \text{ mg}}{1\,000 \text{ mcg}} \times \dfrac{1.25 \text{ mcg}}{1}$

$x = \dfrac{1.25}{1\,000}$

$x = 0.00125 \text{ mg}$

32. $x \text{ oz} = \dfrac{1 \text{ oz}}{30 \text{ ml}} \times \dfrac{240 \text{ ml}}{1}$

$x = \dfrac{240}{30}$

$x = 8 \text{ oz}$

33. $x \text{ mcg} = \dfrac{1\,000 \text{ mcg}}{1 \text{ mg}} \times \dfrac{1.75 \text{ mg}}{1}$

$x = \dfrac{1\,000 \times 1.75}{1}$

$x = 1\,750 \text{ mcg}$

34. $x \text{ L} = \dfrac{1 \text{ L}}{1\,000 \text{ mL}} \times \dfrac{125 \text{ mL}}{1}$

$x = \dfrac{125}{1\,000}$

$x = 0.125 \text{ L}$

UNIT FOUR

Oral and Parenteral Dosage Forms and Insulin

Oral medications are the easiest, most economical, and most frequently used medications, but sometimes parenteral (through a route other than the gastrointestinal tract) dosage routes are necessary. Both oral and parenteral medications are available in liquid or powdered form. Medications that are available in powdered form must be reconstituted and administered in liquid form. In addition to oral and parenteral dosage forms, this unit examines the varying types of insulin.

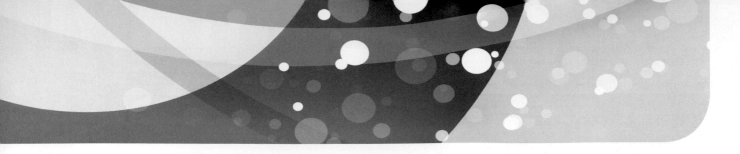

CHAPTER 15
Oral Medications

Objectives

After reviewing this chapter, you should be able to:

1. Identify the forms of oral medication
2. Identify the information on an oral medication label to be used in calculating dosages
3. Calculate dosages of solid and oral liquid medications using the ratio and proportion method, the formula method, or the dimensional analysis method
4. Apply the principles of tablet and liquid preparation to obtain a logical dosage

The easiest, most economical, and most commonly used method of medication administration is by mouth (PO). Medications for oral administration come in several forms including tablets (tab), capsules, and caplets. Medications for oral use also come as liquid preparations. The Practice Problems in this chapter will require careful reading of labels in order to safely and accurately calculate dosages to administer. To calculate dosages correctly, the nurse needs to understand the principles that apply to the administration of medications by this route.

In an effort to increase medication safety and reduce errors, patient safety organizations have recommended that all medications be available in unit-dose packaging. The Institute for Safe Medication Practices Canada (ISMP Canada) and the Canadian Patient Safety Institute (CPSI) recommend dispensing medication in the form in which it is to be administered to help prevent medication errors.

Calculations involving tablets and capsules and their preparation for administration are usually simple. Let's discuss the various forms of solid medication.

Forms of Solid Medication

Tablets

Tablets are the most common form of solid oral medications. Tablets are preparations of powdered medications that have been moulded into various sizes and shapes. Tablets come in a variety of dosage strengths. There are different types of tablets and shapes.

Caplets. A caplet is a tablet that has an elongated shape (oval) and is coated for ease of swallowing. Tylenol is available in caplet form.

Scored Tablets. Scored tablets are designed to administer a dosage that is less than what is available in a single tablet. In other words, scored tablets have indentations or markings that allow you to break the tablet into halves or quarters. The medication in scored tablets is evenly distributed throughout the tablet and allows the dose to be divided evenly when a scored tablet is broken. Only scored tablets should be broken because there is no way to determine the dosage being administered when a nonscored tablet is broken. Breaking a tablet that is unscored could lead to the administration of an inaccurate dosage if the tablet is not divided equally. The purpose of the groove or indentation is to provide a guide for breaking a whole tablet into a fractional part. Figure 15-1 shows an example of a scored tablet. Breaking a scored tablet to administer the dosage ordered is allowed but not optimal. Always check to see whether the tablet is available in another dosage strength before breaking a scored tablet. **Remember: use practices that put patient safety first.** It is safest and more accurate to administer the least number of whole, undivided tablets possible. Breaking tablets should be done only if tablets are scored and no other option exists to administer the dosage.

SAFETY ALERT!

Breaking an unscored tablet is risky and dangerous and can lead to the administration of an unintended dosage. Question and/or verify any calculation you perform that indicates administering a portion of a tablet that is unscored.

A pill or tablet cutter is readily available in most pharmacies and can be used to evenly cut tablets appropriately. Figure 15-2 shows a pill/tablet cutter. A drug reference should always be consulted before cutting a tablet. Many tablets come in a form that allows slow and steady release of the active drug. These forms cannot be cut, crushed, or chewed. Capsules and enteric-coated, timed-release, sustained-release, and controlled-release tablets cannot be cut. Nurses must use caution when instructing patients to cut tablets.

TIPS FOR CLINICAL PRACTICE

If the calculation of a medication dosage requires that a tablet be cut in half, divide the tablet along the scoring created by the manufacturer. If possible, use a pill or tablet cutter to divide a tablet in half to help ensure accuracy of a dose.

Enteric-Coated Tablets. Enteric-coated tablets have a special coating that protects them from the effects of gastric secretions and prevents them from dissolving in the stomach. They are dissolved and absorbed in the small intestine. The enteric coating also prevents the medication from becoming a source of irritation to the gastric mucosa, thereby

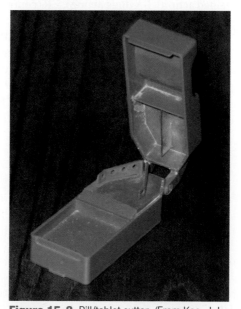

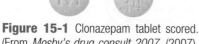

Figure 15-1 Clonazepam tablet scored. (From *Mosby's drug consult 2007*. (2007). St. Louis: Mosby.)

Figure 15-2 Pill/tablet cutter. (From Kee, J. L., & Marshall, S. M. (2013). *Clinical calculations: With applications to general and specialty areas* (7th ed.). St. Louis: Saunders.)

preventing gastrointestinal upset. Examples include enteric-coated aspirin and iron tablets, such as ferrous gluconate. Enteric-coated tablets should never be crushed, broken, or chewed because crushing, breaking, and chewing them destroys the special coating and defeats its purpose. They must be swallowed whole with their coating intact.

Sublingual Tablets. Sublingual tablets are designed to be placed under the tongue, where they dissolve in saliva and the medication is absorbed. Sublingual tablets should never be swallowed because doing so will prevent them from achieving their desired effect. Nitroglycerine tablets, which are used for the relief of acute chest pain, are usually administered sublingually.

Buccal Tablets. Buccal tablets are absorbed by the mucosa of the mouth. They are placed between the gums and cheek. Figure 15-3 shows placement of sublingual and buccal tablets. Tablets for buccal and sublingual administration should never be swallowed.

Layered Tablets. Some tablets contain different layers or have cores that separate different medications that may be incompatible with one another; thus, incompatible ingredients may be separated and released at different times as the tablet passes through the gastrointestinal tract (Figure 15-4).

Medications in a layered form have become available in which one or more medications can be released immediately from the coating, whereas the same or other medications can be released on a sustained basis from the tablet core. An example of this kind of medication is zolpidem (Ambien CR). Ambien CR is formulated in a two-layer tablet. The first layer of the tablet dissolves quickly to help in falling asleep, and the second layer dissolves slowly overnight to help the person stay asleep.

Film Tabs. A film tab is a tablet sealed with a film. The special coating helps to protect the stomach. Examples of medications that come as film tabs are clarithromycin and erythromycin.

Disintegrating Tablets. Orally disintegrating tablets dissolve rapidly, usually within seconds of being placed on the tongue. They are used for their rapid onset of action, such as in the treatment of migraine headaches. They are also used for patients who have difficulty swallowing. Clonazepam (Clonapam), which is an anticonvulsant, is an example of an orally disintegrating tablet.

Chewable Tablets. Chewable tablets are designed to be chewed and must be chewed to be effective. Examples of medications that come in chewable form are amoxicillin and clavulanate potassium tablets as well as calcium supplement tablets.

Timed-Release and Extended-Release Tablets. Look for abbreviations such as SA (sustained action), LA (long acting), CR (controlled release), DR (delayed release), ER (extended release), or XL (extended release). Medication from these types of tablets is not released immediately but over a period of time at specific intervals. These types of preparations should not be crushed, chewed, or broken; they should be swallowed whole. If a timed-release or extended-release tablet is crushed, chewed, or broken, all of the medication will be administered at one time and absorbed rapidly. Examples are nifedipine (Apo-Nifed), verapamil (Apo-Verap), and theophylline (Phyllocotin).

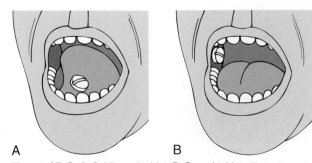

Figure 15-3 A, Sublingual tablet. **B,** Buccal tablet. (From Clayton, B. D., & Willihnganz, M. (2013). *Basic pharmacology for nurses* (16th ed.). St. Louis: 2013, Mosby.)

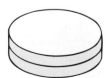

Figure 15-4 Layered tablet. (From Clayton, B. D., & Willihnganz, M. (2013). *Basic pharmacology for nurses* (16th ed.). St. Louis: 2013, Mosby.)

Capsules

A capsule is a form of medication that contains a powder, liquid, or oil enclosed in a hard or soft gelatin. Capsules come in a variety of colours, sizes, and dosages. Some capsules have special shapes and colourings to identify which company produced them. Capsules are also available in timed-release and sustained-release forms that work over a period of time.

Capsules should always be administered whole to achieve the desired result (e.g., sustained release capsules). Sustained-release and timed-release capsules should not be divided or crushed. Always consult an appropriate drug reference or a pharmacist when in doubt as to whether to open a capsule. Examples of medications that come in capsule form are ampicillin, tetracycline, and docusate sodium.

Spansules are special capsules that contain granules of medications. Spansules may be opened and mixed in soft food; however, the granules cannot be crushed or dissolved. The granules delay the release of the medication.

Sprinkle capsules are also available for oral administration. Sprinkle capsules can be swallowed whole or opened and sprinkled on a food such as applesauce. Topiramate (Topamax) and divalproex sodium (Apo-Divalproex) are examples of medication that comes in sprinkle capsules.

> **① SAFETY ALERT!**
>
> Not all medications can be crushed. Medications such as timed-release or extended-release tablets and capsules have special coatings to prevent the medication from being absorbed too quickly. Altering medications that should be administered whole may change the action of the medication and possibly cause unintended effects. Always consult a drug reference or a pharmacist before crushing a medication or opening a capsule to ensure that a medication can be safely administered to avoid harm to the patient.

Although there are other forms of solid preparations for oral administration—such as lozenges and troches—tablets, capsules, and pulvules (proprietary capsules containing a dosage of a medication in powdered form) are the most common forms of solids that require calculation that the nurse will encounter. Figure 15-5 shows types of solid oral medications.

Medications may sometimes be ordered for administration enterally—into the gastrointestinal tract by a specially placed tube. For example, medication can be administered via a gastrostomy tube (GT) inserted directly through the abdomen into the stomach after a percutaneous endoscopic gastrostomy (PEG). Medications administered by a tube will have to be crushed and dissolved in a small amount of warm water. Determine whether an alternative form of the medication exists if it cannot be crushed, such as oral liquid form. Check with the prescriber as to whether the medication can be ordered in an alternative form.

Availability of the Same Medication in Different Forms and Dosages

Sometimes the same medication comes in different forms and dosages. For example, as noted earlier, nitroglycerine (anti-anginal) is available in sublingual tablets. However, it is

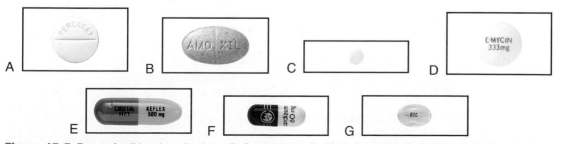

Figure 15-5 Types of solid oral medications. **A,** Scored tablet. **B,** Chewable tablet. **C,** Sublingual. **D,** Timed-release tablet. **E,** Capsule. **F,** Timed-release capsule. **G,** Gelatin capsule.

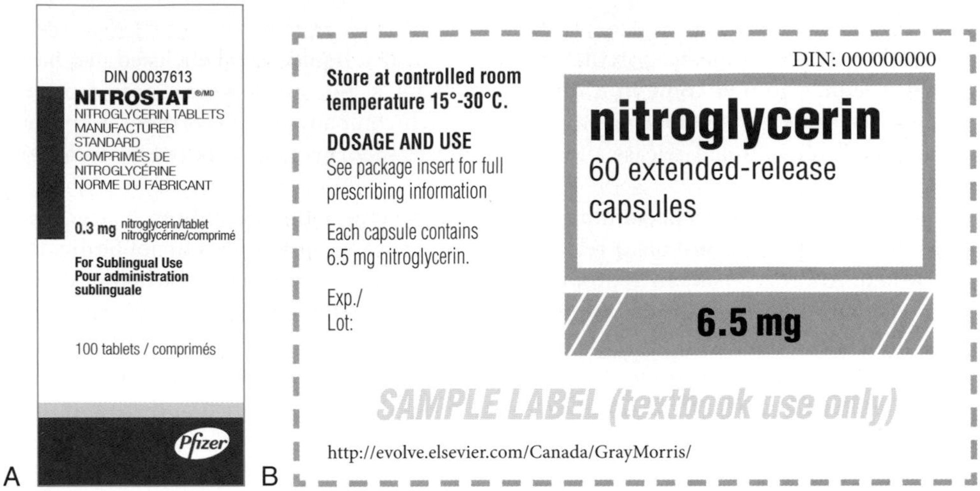

Figure 15-6 A, Nitrostat 0.3 mg sublingual tablets. **B,** Nitroglycerine 6.5 mg extended-release capsules.

> **NOTE**
> Nitroglycerine spray is now available in 0.4 mg per metered dose. It is administered sublingually or sprayed on the tongue for quick onset.

> **NOTE**
> The allowance for a 10% variation between what is ordered and what is administered is often applied to adults but not necessarily to children.

also available in extended-release capsules and a spray as well as in different dosages. See Figure 15-6 with sample labels for two forms of nitroglycerine.

In an emergency situation, the sublingual tablet would be administered for immediate effect. Sublingual tablets and extended-release capsules or tablets must be administered whole.

Calculating Dosages of Tablets and Capsules

When administering medications, you will have to calculate the number of tablets or capsules needed to administer the dosage ordered. To help determine if your calculated dosage is sensible, accurate, and safe, remember the points that follow.

> **POINTS TO REMEMBER**
> - Do not divide tablets that are unscored. Unscored tablets are administered in whole amounts only. If a patient has difficulty swallowing a tablet, check to see if a liquid preparation of the same medication is available. Never crush or open a timed-release tablet or capsule or empty its contents into a liquid or food; doing so may cause the release of all the medication at once. Seek advice from a pharmacist if unsure.
> - Know that pulvules are proprietary capsules containing a dose of a medication in powdered form. For example, the popular antidepressant fluoxetine (Prozac) comes in pulvule form (proprietary capsules are owned by a corporation under a trademark or patent).
> - Be aware that tablets and capsules may be available in different strengths for administration, and you may have a choice when giving a dosage. For example, let's say that 75 mg of a medication is ordered. You determine that the medication is available in tablet or capsule form in 10 mg, 25 mg, or 50 mg. When deciding the best combination of tablets or capsules to give, choose the strength that would allow the least number of tablets or capsules to be administered without breaking a tablet, if possible, because breaking is found to result in variations in dosage. In the example given, the best combination for administering 75 mg is one 50-mg tablet or capsule and one 25-mg tablet or capsule.
> - Note that only scored tablets are intended to be divided. It is safest and most accurate not to divide tablets and to give the fewest number of whole (undivided) tablets possible.
> - Keep in mind that the maximum number of tablets or capsules given to a patient to achieve a single dose is usually three. The minimum tablet is usually one half $(\frac{1}{2})$. Recheck your calculation if a single dose does not seem logical. It is not best practice to administer more than three or less than one-half tablet. However, for some human immunodeficiency virus (HIV) medications in tablet

or capsule form, the patient may have to take more than three to achieve the desired dosage. For example, if a patient has been prescribed ritonavir 400 mg PO q12h (available 100 mg per tab), then a single dose is four tablets. Although many HIV medications come in liquid form, many patients prefer to take tablets or capsules.
- When using the ratio and proportion, the formula method, or the dimensional analysis method to calculate tablet and capsule dosages, remember that each tablet or capsule contains a certain weight of the medication. The weight indicated on the label is per tablet or per capsule. This is particularly important when you are reading a medication label on a bottle or single unit-dose package.
- Always consult a drug reference or a pharmacist when in doubt as to whether a capsule may be opened or pierced or whether a tablet can be crushed.

Here are some sample problems that illustrate how to calculate the number of tablets or capsules to administer.

Example 1: Order: Digoxin 0.375 mg PO daily.

Available: Digoxin scored tablets labelled 0.25 mg

✔ PROBLEM SETUP

1. Note that no conversion is necessary; the ordered and available medication are in the same system and unit of measurement:
Order: 0.375 mg
Available: 0.25 mg
2. Think: Tablets are scored and 0.375 mg is greater than 0.25 mg. Therefore, more than 1 tab is needed to administer the correct dosage.
3. Calculate the dosage to administer using the ratio and proportion method, the formula method, or the dimensional analysis method.

✔ Solution Using Ratio and Proportion

$$0.25 \, mg : 1 \, tab = 0.375 \, mg : x \, tab$$
$$\text{(known)} \qquad \text{(unknown)}$$
$$\text{(what is available)} \quad \text{(what is ordered)}$$
$$\frac{0.25x}{0.25} = \frac{0.375}{0.25}$$
$$x = \frac{0.375}{0.25}$$

Therefore, $x = 1.5$ tabs or $1\frac{1}{2}$ tabs. (It is best to state it as $1\frac{1}{2}$ tabs for administration purposes.)

✔ Solution Using the Formula Method

$$\frac{\text{(D)} \, 0.375 \, mg}{\text{(H)} \, 0.25 \, mg} \times \text{(Q)} \, 1 \, tab = x \, tab$$
$$x = \frac{0.375}{0.25}$$
$$x = 1.5 = 1\frac{1}{2} \, tabs$$

NOTE

You can administer $1\frac{1}{2}$ tabs because the tablets are scored. The ratio and proportion method could have been written in fraction format as well. (If necessary, review Chapter 3 on ratio and proportion.)

✔ Solution Using Dimensional Analysis

$$x \text{ tab} = \frac{1 \text{ tab}}{0.25 \text{ mg}} \times \frac{0.375 \text{ mg}}{1}$$

$$x = \frac{0.375}{0.25}$$

$$x = 1\frac{1}{2} \text{ tabs}$$

Example 2: Order: Ampicillin 0.5 g PO q6h.

Available: Ampicillin capsules labelled 250 mg per capsule

1. Order: 0.5 g
   Available: 250-mg capsules
2. After making the necessary conversion, think about what is a reasonable amount to administer.
3. Calculate the dosage to administer using the ratio and proportion method, the formula method, or the dimensional analysis method.
4. Label your final answer (tabs, capsules).

> **NOTE**
> A conversion is necessary. The dosage ordered and the available dosage strength are in the same system of measurement (metric), but the units are different: grams (g) and milligrams (mg). Before calculating the dosage to be administered, the dosage ordered and the available dosage strength must be in the same units.

✔ PROBLEM SETUP

1. Note that conversion from grams to milligrams is necessary. Conversion factor:
   1 000 mg = 1 g

$$1\,000 \text{ mg} : 1 \text{ g} = x \text{ mg} : 0.5 \text{ g}$$

$$x = 1\,000 \times 0.5$$

$$x = 500 \text{ mg}$$

Therefore, 0.5 g is equal to 500 mg. Converting the grams to milligrams eliminated a decimal, which is often the source of calculation errors. Converting milligrams to grams would necessitate a decimal. Whenever possible, conversions that result in a decimal should be avoided to decrease the chance of calculation errors. Remember, a ratio and proportion could also be stated as a fraction. If necessary, review Chapter 3. Because the measurements in this problem are metric, conversion can also be undertaken by moving the decimal the desired number of places (0.5 g = 0.500 = 500 mg).

2. After making the conversion, calculate the dosage to administer using the ratio and proportion method, the formula method, or the dimensional analysis method. In this problem, we will use the answer obtained from converting what was ordered to what is available (0.5 g = 500 mg). Remember that if dimensional analysis is used, you need only one equation; even if conversion is required, you can choose to do the conversion first and then set up the problem in dimensional analysis.

> **NOTE**
> Two capsules is a logical answer. Capsules are administered in whole amounts; they cannot be divided. Using the value obtained from converting milligrams to grams in this problem would also net a final answer of 2 capsules.

✔ Solution Using Ratio and Proportion

$$250 \text{ mg} : 1 \text{ capsule} = 500 \text{ mg} : x \text{ capsule}$$

$$\frac{250x}{250} = \frac{500}{250}$$

$$x = \frac{500}{250}$$

$$x = 2 \text{ capsules}$$

✔ Solution Using the Formula Method

$$\frac{\text{(D)}\, 500\,\text{mg}}{\text{(H)}\, 250\,\text{mg}} \times \text{(Q)}\, 1\,\text{capsule} = x\,\text{capsule}$$

$$x = \frac{500}{250}$$

$$x = 2\,\text{capsules}$$

✔ Solution Using Dimensional Analysis

$$x\,\text{capsule} = \frac{1\,\text{capsule}}{250\,\cancel{\text{mg}}} \times \frac{1\,000\,\cancel{\text{mg}}}{1\,\cancel{\text{g}}} \times \frac{0.5\,\cancel{\text{g}}}{1}$$

$$x = \frac{1\,000 \times 0.5}{250}$$

$$x = \frac{500}{250}$$

$$x = 2\,\text{capsules}$$

Setup if conversion is done first, using dimensional analysis:

$$x\,\text{mg} = \frac{1\,000\,\text{mg}}{1\,\cancel{\text{g}}} \times 0.5\,\cancel{\text{g}}$$

$$x = \frac{1\,000 \times 0.5}{1}$$

$$x = \frac{500}{1}$$

$$x = 500\,\text{mg}$$

Setup to calculate dosage using dimensional analysis after the conversion is made:

$$x\,\text{capsule} = \frac{1\,\text{capsule}}{250\,\cancel{\text{mg}}} \times \frac{500\,\cancel{\text{mg}}}{1}$$

$$x = \frac{500}{250}$$

$$x = 2\,\text{capsules}$$

Note: It is easier to set up the problem by using one equation that will allow you to convert what was ordered to the available strength and calculate the dosage required.

Example 3: Order: Thorazine 100 mg PO TID.

Available: Thorazine tablets labelled 25 mg and 50 mg

✔ PROBLEM SETUP

1. Note that no conversion is necessary.
2. Think: 100 mg is greater than the 25-mg and 50-mg tablets available. Therefore, more than 1 tablet is needed to administer the dosage. The patient should always be given the strength of tablets or capsules that would require the least number to be taken.

3. In this problem, be aware that if you select the 50-mg tablets, the patient would be administered 2 tablets. Using 25-mg tablets would require that the patient be administered 4 tabs.

✔ **Solution Using Ratio and Proportion**

$$50\,mg : 1\,tab = 100\,mg : x\,tab$$

$$\frac{50x}{50} = \frac{100}{50}$$

$$x = 2\,tabs\,(50\,mg\,each)$$

✔ **Solution Using the Formula Method**

$$\frac{(D)\,100\,mg}{(H)\,50\,mg} \times Q\,(1\,tab) = x\,tab$$

$$x = \frac{100}{50}$$

$$x = 2\,tabs\,(50\,mg\,each)$$

✔ **Solution Using Dimensional Analysis**

$$x\,tab = \frac{1\,tab}{50\,mg} \times \frac{100\,mg}{1}$$

$$x = \frac{100}{50}$$

$$x = 2\,tabs\,(50\,mg\,each)$$

Example 3 could have been calculated without the use of ratio and proportion, dimensional analysis, or a formula. This is common when problems provide more than one dosage strength. In the case where a conversion is required, you would perform the conversion and choose the appropriate dosage strength to administer the least number of tablets or capsules. Add the dosage strengths chosen to ensure that the result is equivalent to what was ordered.

Variation of Tablet and Capsule Problems

At times, you must calculate the total number of tablets or capsules needed for a dosage. This requires knowing the dose and the frequency. Numerous scenarios could arise, but for the purpose of illustration, let's look at two examples. In both cases, the patient is going out of town on vacation and needs to determine whether it is necessary to refill the prescription before leaving.

Example: A patient has an order for Valium 10 mg PO QID (four times a day) and has 5-mg tablets. The patient is leaving town for 7 days and asks how many tablets to bring.

Solution: To obtain a dose of 10 mg, the patient requires two 5-mg tablets. Therefore, eight 5-mg tablets are necessary to administer the dosage QID.
    Number of tablets needed per day (8) × Number of days needed for (7) = Total number of tablets needed

$$8 \times 7 = 56$$

Example: A patient is instructed to take 30 mg PO of a medication stat (immediately) as an initial dose and 20 mg TID (three times a day) thereafter. The medication is available in 10-mg tablets. The patient is leaving town for 3 days and asks how many tablets to bring.

Solution: To obtain the stat dose of 30 mg, the patient will require three 10-mg tablets. To obtain the 20-mg dosage TID, the patient will require six 10-mg tablets.

Number of tablets needed per day (6) × Number of days needed for (3) = Total number of tablets needed

$$6 \times 3 = 18 + 3 \text{ (stat dose)} = 21 \text{ tablets}$$

Determining the Dosage to Be Given Each Time

Example: A patient is to receive 1 g of a medication PO daily. The medication should be given in four equally divided doses. How many milligrams should the patient receive each time the medication is administered?

Solution: $$\frac{\text{Total daily allowance}}{\text{Number of doses per day}} = \text{Dosage to be administered}$$

$$\frac{1\,g\,(1\,000\,mg)}{4} = 250 \text{ mg each time the medication is administered}$$

POINTS TO REMEMBER

When calculating dosages of solid medication:

- Before calculating a dosage, be sure that the dosage ordered and the available dosage strength are in the same system and unit of measurement. When a conversion is required, it is usually best to convert the dosage ordered to the available dosage strength.
- Regardless of the calculation method used, think critically about what is a reasonable amount to administer. Think and question any dosage that seems unreasonable.
- State dosages as you are actually going to administer them. Example: 0.5 tab = $\frac{1}{2}$ tab.
- Do not break tablets that are unscored.
- Keep in mind that it is safer to administer the least number of whole tablets possible without scoring.
- Read labels carefully and choose the correct medication to administer to match the order and dosage amount.
- When there is a choice of tablets or capsules in varying strengths, choose the strength that allows administration of the least number of tablets or capsules.
- Consult a drug reference or a pharmacist when in doubt about a dosage to be administered.

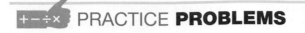

PRACTICE **PROBLEMS**

Calculate the correct number of tablets or capsules to be administered in the following problems using the labels or the information provided. Use any of the methods presented to calculate the dosage. Label your answers correctly: tabs, capsules.

1. Order: Levothyroxine sodium 0.025 mg PO daily.

   Available: Scored tablets (can be broken in half)

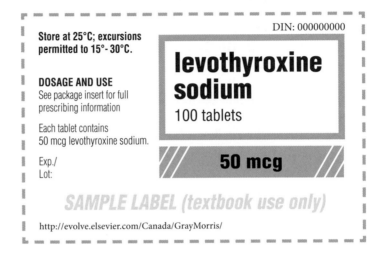

2. Order: Warfarin Sodium 7.5 mg PO at bedtime.

   Available: Scored tablets (can be broken in half)

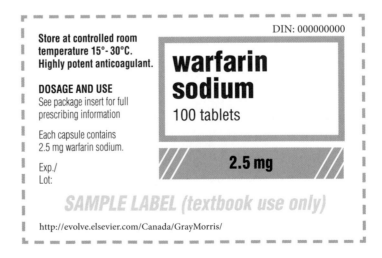

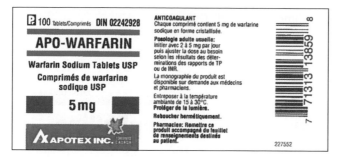

What is the appropriate strength of tablet to use?   _____

3. Order: Digoxin 0.125 mg PO daily.

   Available: Scored tablets (can be broken in half)

Store at 15°- 25°C in a dry place.

DIN: 000000000

DOSAGE AND USE
See package insert for full prescribing information

Each tablet contains 125 mcg digoxin.

Exp./
Lot:

digoxin
100 tablets

/// **125 mcg (0.125 mg)** ///

SAMPLE LABEL (textbook use only)

http://evolve.elsevier.com/Canada/GrayMorris/

Store at 15°- 30°C in a dry place.

DIN: 000000000

DOSAGE AND USE
See package insert for full prescribing information

Each tablet contains 500 mcg digoxin.

Exp./
Lot:

digoxin
100 tablets

/// **500 mcg (0.5 mg)** ///

SAMPLE LABEL (textbook use only)

http://evolve.elsevier.com/Canada/GrayMorris/

   a. What is the appropriate strength of tablet to use?   _____

   b. What will you administer?   _____

4. Order: Ampicillin 1 g PO q6h.

   Available: Ampicillin capsules labelled 500 mg and 250 mg

   a. What is the appropriate strength of capsule to use?   _____

   b. How many capsules are needed for each dose?   _____

   c. What is the total number of capsules needed if the medication is ordered for 7 days?   _____

5. Order: Cellcept 750 mg PO BID.

   Available: Cellcept capsules labelled 250 mg   _____

6. Order: Theophylline 0.4 g PO daily.

Available:

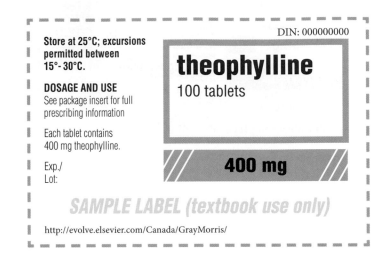

7. Order: Carbamazepine 200 mg PO TID.

Available:

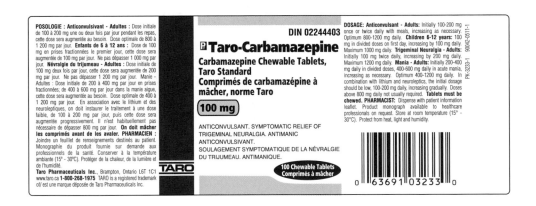

How many tablets will you administer for each dose? _____

8. Order: Phenobarbital 90 mg PO at bedtime.

Available: Phenobarbital 15-mg tabs and 30-mg tabs

a. What is the appropriate strength of tablet to administer? _____

b. How many tablets of which strength will you administer? _____

9. Order: Abacavir sulfate 0.6 g PO daily.

    Available:

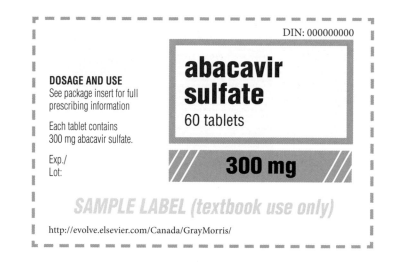

10. Order: Chlorpromazine 100 mg PO TID.

    Available:

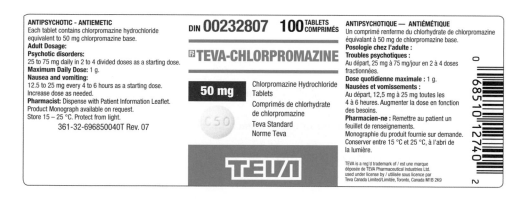

    How many tablets are needed for 3 days? _____

11. Order: Verapamil 120 mg PO TID. Hold for systolic blood pressure less than 100, heart rate less than 55.

    Available: Verapamil scored tablets labelled 80 mg and 40 mg

    How many tablets of which strength will you administer? _____

12. Order: Divalproex sodium 1 g PO daily.

    Available:

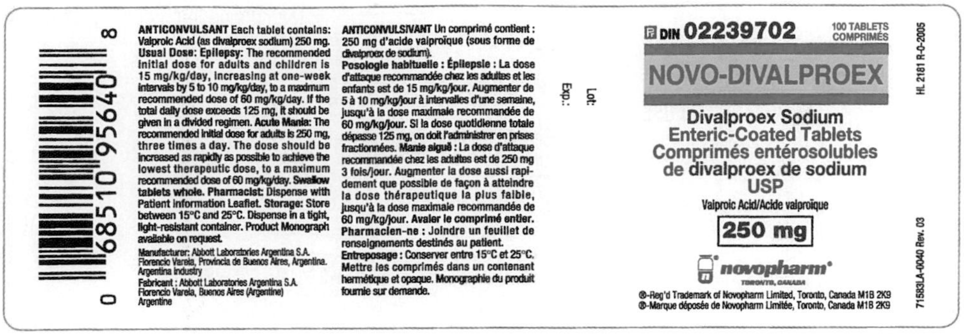

____

13. Order: Dexamethasone 6 mg PO daily.

    Available: Dexamethasone scored tablets labelled 0.5 mg, 4 mg, and 6 mg

    How many tablets of which strength will you administer? ______________

14. Order: Torsemide 20 mg PO daily.

    Available: Torsemide tablets labelled 10 mg ______________

15. Order: Cimetidine (Tagamet) 400 mg PO BID.

    Available: Cimetidine tablets labelled 200 mg

    How many tablets will you administer for each dose? ______________

16. Order: Indomethacin 150 mg PO BID.

    Available:

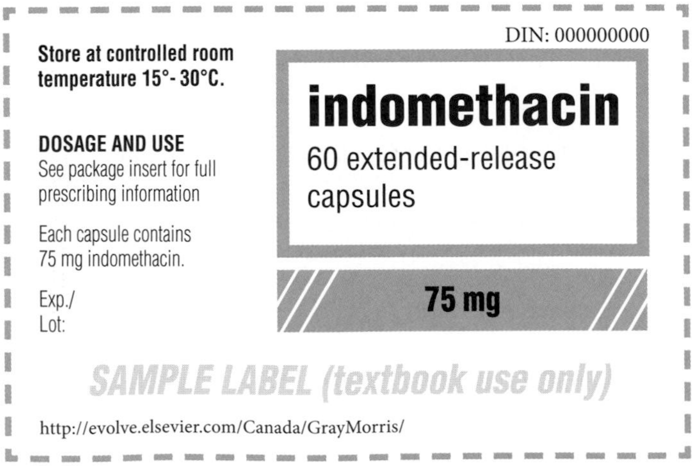

    How many capsules will you administer for each dose? ______________

17. Order: Sulfasalazine 1 g PO q6h.

Available:

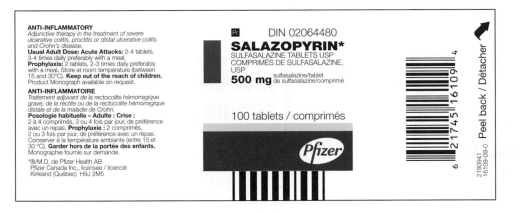

How many tablets will you administer for each dose?   _____

18. Order: Duloxetine hydrochloride (delayed-release capsules) 60 mg PO daily.

Available:

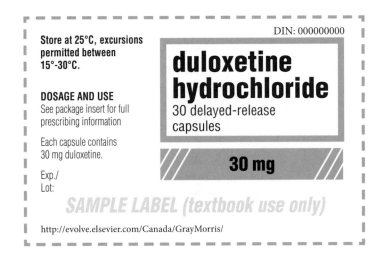

How many capsules will you administer for each dose?   _____

19. Order: Levothyroxine sodium 75 mcg PO daily.

    Available: Scored tablets (can be broken in half)

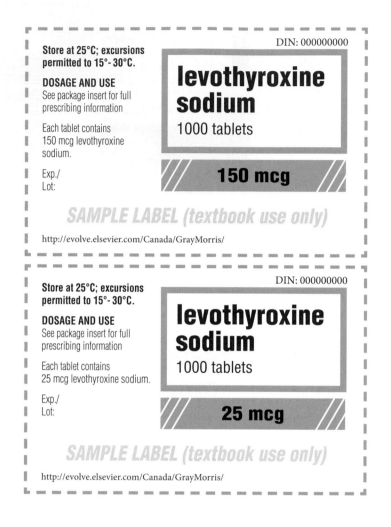

(Top label)

Store at 25°C; excursions permitted to 15°- 30°C.

DOSAGE AND USE
See package insert for full prescribing information

Each tablet contains 150 mcg levothyroxine sodium.

Exp./
Lot:

DIN: 000000000

levothyroxine sodium
1000 tablets

150 mcg

SAMPLE LABEL (textbook use only)

http://evolve.elsevier.com/Canada/GrayMorris/

(Bottom label)

Store at 25°C; excursions permitted to 15°- 30°C.

DOSAGE AND USE
See package insert for full prescribing information

Each tablet contains 25 mcg levothyroxine sodium.

Exp./
Lot:

DIN: 000000000

levothyroxine sodium
1000 tablets

25 mcg

SAMPLE LABEL (textbook use only)

http://evolve.elsevier.com/Canada/GrayMorris/

How many tablets of which strength will you administer? _____

20. Order: Captopril 25 mg PO q8h.

    Available:

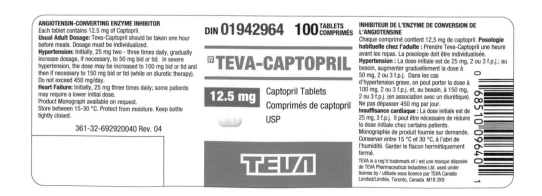

ANGIOTENSIN-CONVERTING ENZYME INHIBITOR
Each tablet contains 12.5 mg of Captopril.
Usual Adult Dosage: Teva-Captopril should be taken one hour before meals. Dosage must be individualized.
Hypertension: Initially, 25 mg two - three times daily, gradually increase dosage, if necessary, to 50 mg bid or tid. In severe hypertension, the dose may be increased to 100 mg bid or tid and then if necessary to 150 mg bid or tid (while on diuretic therapy). Do not exceed 450 mg/day.
Heart Failure: Initially, 25 mg three times daily; some patients may require a lower initial dose.
Product Monograph available on request.
Store between 15-30 °C. Protect from moisture. Keep bottle tightly closed.

361-32-692920040 Rev. 04

DIN **01942964** **100** TABLETS COMPRIMÉS

℞**TEVA-CAPTOPRIL**

12.5 mg Captopril Tablets
Comprimés de captopril
USP

TEVA

INHIBITEUR DE L'ENZYME DE CONVERSION DE L'ANGIOTENSINE
Chaque comprimé contient 12,5 mg de captopril. **Posologie habituelle chez l'adulte :** Prendre Teva-Captopril une heure avant les repas. La posologie doit être individualisée.
Hypertension : La dose initiale est de 25 mg, 2 ou 3 f.p.j.; au besoin, augmenter graduellement la dose à 50 mg, 2 ou 3 f.p.j. Dans les cas d'hypertension grave, on peut porter la dose à 100 mg, 2 ou 3 f.p.j. et, au besoin, à 150 mg, 2 ou 3 f.p.j. (en association avec un diurétique). Ne pas dépasser 450 mg par jour.
Insuffisance cardiaque : La dose initiale est de 25 mg, 3 f.p.j. Il peut être nécessaire de réduire la dose initiale chez certains patients.
Monographie de produit fournie sur demande. Conserver entre 15 °C et 30 °C, à l'abri de l'humidité. Garder le flacon hermétiquement fermé.
TEVA is a reg'd trademark of / est une marque déposée de TEVA Pharmaceutical Industries Ltd. used under license by / utilisée sous licence par TEVA Canada Limited/Limitée, Toronto, Canada M1B 2K9

21. Order: Amoxicillin and clavulanate potassium 400 mg/57 mg PO q8h (dosage based on amoxicillin).

Available:

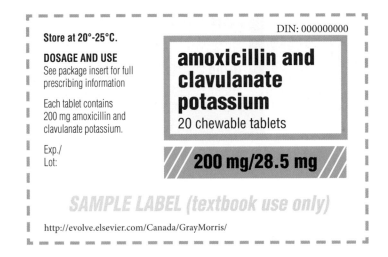

Store at 20°-25°C.

DOSAGE AND USE
See package insert for full prescribing information

Each tablet contains 200 mg amoxicillin and clavulanate potassium.

Exp./
Lot:

DIN: 000000000

amoxicillin and clavulanate potassium
20 chewable tablets

200 mg/28.5 mg

SAMPLE LABEL (textbook use only)

http://evolve.elsevier.com/Canada/GrayMorris/

_____

22. Order: Aspirin 650 mg PO q4h prn for pain.

Available: Aspirin tablets labelled 325 mg   _____

23. Order: Dilantin (extended release) capsules 0.2 g PO TID.

Available: Dilantin (extended release) capsules labelled 100 mg   _____

24. Order: Ibuprofen 800 mg PO q6h prn for pain.

Available:

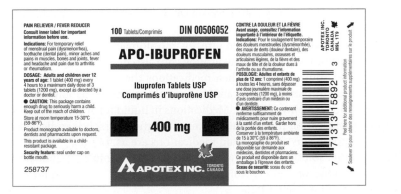

PAIN RELIEVER / FEVER REDUCER
Consult inner label for important information before use.
Indications: For temporary relief of menstrual pain (dysmenorrhea), toothache (dental pain), minor aches and pains in muscles, bones and joints, fever and headache and pain due to arthritis or rheumatism.
DOSAGE: Adults and children over 12 years of age: 1 tablet (400 mg) every 4 hours to a maximum daily dose of 3 tablets (1200 mg), except as directed by a doctor or dentist.
● **CAUTION:** This package contains enough drug to seriously harm a child. Keep out of the reach of children.
Store at room temperature 15-30°C (59-86°F).
Product monograph available to doctors, dentists and pharmacists upon request.
This product is available in a child-resistant package.
Security feature: seal under cap on bottle mouth.

258737

100 Tablets/Comprimés   DIN 00506052

APO-IBUPROFEN

Ibuprofen Tablets USP
Comprimés d'ibuprofène USP

400 mg

APOTEX INC. TORONTO CANADA

CONTRE LA DOULEUR ET LA FIÈVRE
Avant usage, consultez l'information importante à l'intérieur de l'étiquette.
Indications: Pour le soulagement temporaire des douleurs menstruelles (dysménorrhée), des maux de dents (douleur dentaire), des douleurs musculaires, osseuses et articulaires légères, de la fièvre et des maux de tête et de la douleur dues à l'arthrite ou au rhumatisme.
POSOLOGIE: Adultes et enfants de plus de 12 ans: 1 comprimé (400 mg) à toutes les 4 heures, sans dépasser une dose journalière maximale de 3 comprimés (1200 mg), à moins d'avis contraire d'un médecin ou d'un dentiste.
● **AVERTISSEMENT:** Ce contenant renferme suffisamment de médicaments pour nuire gravement à la santé d'un enfant. Garder hors de la portée des enfants. Conserver à la température ambiante de 15 à 30°C (59 à 86°F). La monographie du produit est disponible sur demande aux médecins, dentistes et pharmaciens. Ce produit est disponible dans un emballage à l'épreuve des enfants. **Sceau de sécurité:** sceau du col sous le bouchon.

APOTEX INC. TORONTO CANADA M9L 1T9

_____

25. Order: Minoxidil 0.03 g PO daily.

    Available:

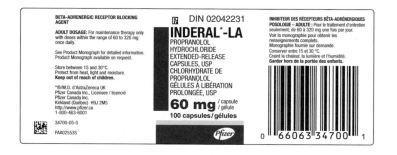

26. Order: Inderal-LA 120 mg PO daily.

    Available:

Answers on pages 341–343.

Calculating Dosages of Oral Liquids

Medications are also available in liquid form for oral administration. Oral liquid medications are desirable to use for patients who have dysphagia (difficulty swallowing) or who are receiving medications through various types of tubes such as nasogastric (tube in nose to stomach), gastrostomy (tube placed directly into stomach), or jejunostomy (tube placed directly into intestine). Oral liquid medications are also desired for use in young children, infants, and older adult patients. When medications that cannot be crushed are ordered for administration to patients who cannot ingest them, the availability of the medication in liquid form should be investigated. Medications in liquid form contain a specific amount or weight of a medication in a given amount of solution, which is indicated on the label. The most common forms of oral liquid medications are as follows:

- **Elixir**—Alcohol solution that is sweet and aromatic. Example: Phenobarbital elixir.
- **Suspension**—One or more medications finely divided into a liquid such as water. Example: Penicillin suspension.
- **Syrup**—Medication dissolved in concentrated solution of sugar and water. Example: Docusate sodium (Colace).

Oral liquid medications also come as tinctures, emulsions, and extract preparations for oral use. Although oral liquids may be administered by means other than by mouth (e.g., nasogastric tube, gastrostomy), they should **never** be given by any other route, such as the intravenous (IV) route or by injection.

When calculating dosages of oral liquids, the methods presented in Chapters 12 to 14 can be used. For oral liquids, you must calculate the volume or amount of liquid that

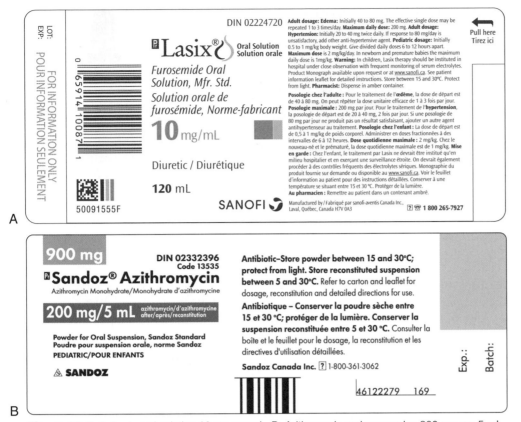

Figure 15-7 A, Lasix oral solution 10 mg per mL. **B,** Azithromycin oral suspension 200 mg per 5 mL.

contains the prescribed dosage of the medication. This information is usually indicated on the medication label and can be expressed per millilitre: for example, 25 mg per mL, 10 mg per mL (Figure 15-7, *A*). The amount may also be expressed in terms of multiple millilitres of solution, such as 80 mg per 2 mL, 200 mg per 5 mL (Figure 15-7, *B*).

Oral liquids can be measured in small amounts of volume, and a greater range of dosages can be ordered for administration. When calculating oral liquids, the stock, or what you have available, is in liquid form; therefore, the label (unit) on your answer will always be expressed in liquid measurements such as millilitres.

Measuring Oral Liquids

Oral liquid medications can be measured in several ways:
- **A medicine cup,** which is a plastic cup calibrated in metric and household measurements, can be used. Pour the liquid medication at eye level and read at the meniscus (a curvature made by the solution) while the cup is on a flat surface (Figure 15-8). Always pour liquid medications with the label facing you to avoid covering the label with your hand or obscuring label information if the medication drips down the side of the container.
- **A calibrated dropper** is also used for measuring oral liquid medication (Figure 15-9).

> ! **SAFETY ALERT!**
> **A calibrated dropper should be used ONLY for the medication for which it is intended; droppers are not interchangeable.** Drop size varies from one dropper to another.

If a dropper comes with a medication, it can only be used for that medication. Some medicine droppers are calibrated in millilitres or by actual dosage. Patients who are being

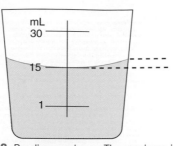

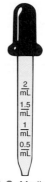

Figure 15-8 Reading meniscus. The meniscus is caused by the surface tension of the solution against the walls of the container. The surface tension causes the formation of a concave or hollowed curvature on the surface of the solution. Read the level at the lowest point of the concave. (From Clayton, B. D., & Willihnganz, M. (2013). *Basic pharmacology for nurses* (16th ed.). St. Louis: Mosby.)

Figure 15-9 Medicine dropper. (Modified from Clayton, B. D., & Willihnganz, M. (2013). *Basic pharmacology for nurses* (16th ed.). St. Louis: Mosby.)

discharged and taking oral liquid medications at home should be instructed to use only the dropper or other measuring device that comes with the particular medication.

- **An oral syringe** may also be used to measure and administer oral liquid medication. The medication is poured in a medicine cup and drawn up in the oral syringe (which has no needle). This tool is often used when the amount desired cannot be measured accurately in a cup. For example, 6.3 mL cannot be measured accurately in a standard medicine cup; however, the medication may be drawn up in an oral syringe and then squirted into a cup or administered orally. Solutions can be measured by using a specially calibrated oral syringe to ensure accurate and safe dosages (Figure 15-10). Oral syringes are not sterile, are often available in colours, and have an off-centre (eccentric) tip. These features make it easy to distinguish them from hypodermic syringes. Only use oral syringes with oral medications. Figure 15-11 shows how to fill an oral syringe from a medicine cup.

Some oral liquid medications come in premeasured containers that allow the patient to drink right out of the container, eliminating the need to transfer it to a medicine cup.

Before we proceed to calculate oral liquid medications, let's review some helpful pointers.

1. The label on the medication container must be read carefully to determine the dosage strength in the volume of solution because it varies.

> **! SAFETY ALERT!**
>
> Do not confuse dosage strength with total volume. Read labels carefully. Confusing dosage strength with total volume can result in errors when performing calculations and lead to the administration of an unintended dose.

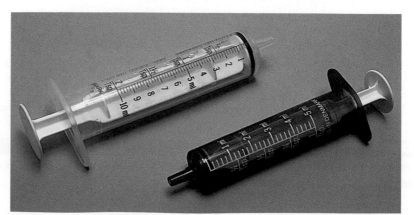

Figure 15-10 Oral syringes. (Courtesy Chuck Dresner. From Clayton, B. D., & Willihnganz, M. (2013). *Basic pharmacology for nurses* (16th ed.). St. Louis: Mosby.)

Figure 15-11 Filling a syringe directly from a medicine cup. (Modified from Clayton, B. D., & Willihnganz, M. (2013). *Basic pharmacology for nurses* (16th ed.). St. Louis: Mosby.)

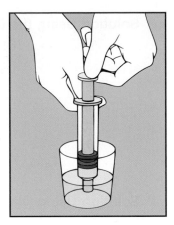

For example, the label on a medication may indicate a total volume of 100 mL, but the dosage strength may be 125 mg per 5 mL. It must be noted that dosage strength can be written on solutions in several ways to indicate the same thing. For example, 125 mg per 5 mL may be written as 125 mg/5 mL or 125 mg = 5 mL. Other examples of dosage strength are 20 mg per mL, 20 mg/mL, 200 mg/5 mL, and 200 mg per 5 mL.

SAFETY ALERT!

Although dosage strengths may be written on solution labels in different ways—for example, 40 mg per 2 mL or 40 mg/2 mL—ISMP Canada recommends that the slash mark (/) not be used to separate doses. The slash mark has been mistaken for the number *1*. Use *per* rather than the slash mark to separate doses.

2. Answers are labelled with liquid measurements. Example: mL.
3. The same methods (ratio and proportion, the formula method, or dimensional analysis) and steps used to calculate dosages of solid forms of medication are used to calculate oral liquid dosages.

Now let's look at some sample problems that illustrate how to calculate the amount of oral liquids to administer.

Example 1: Order: Phenytoin 200 mg PO TID.

Available: Phenytoin suspension labelled 125 mg per 5 mL

✔ PROBLEM SETUP

1. Note that no conversion is necessary.
2. Think: What would be a logical answer? Looking at the information in Example 1, you can assume that the answer will be more than 5 mL.
3. Calculate the dosage to administer using the ratio and proportion method, the formula method, or the dimensional analysis method.
4. Label the final answer with the correct unit of measurement. In this case, the unit is millilitres. Remember: the answer has no meaning if written without the appropriate unit of measurement.

✔ Solution Using Ratio and Proportion

$$125 \, \text{mg} : 5 \, \text{mL} = 200 \, \text{mg} : x \, \text{mL}$$

$$\text{(known)} \qquad \text{(unknown)}$$

$$125x = 200 \times 5$$

$$\frac{125x}{125} = \frac{1\,000}{125}$$

$$x = \frac{1\,000}{125}$$

$$x = 8 \, \text{mL}$$

NOTE

When possible, the numbers may be reduced to lowest terms to make them smaller and easier to deal with.

✔ Solution Using the Formula Method

$$\frac{(D)\,200\,mg}{(H)\,125\,mg} \times (Q)\,5\,mL = x\,mL$$

$$x = \frac{200}{125} \times 5$$

$$x = \frac{1\,000}{125}$$

$$x = 8\,mL$$

✔ Solution Using Dimensional Analysis

$$x\,mL = \frac{5\,mL}{125\,\cancel{mg}} \times \frac{200\,\cancel{mg}}{1}$$

$$x = \frac{1\,000}{125}$$

$$x = 8\,mL$$

Example 2: Order: Lactulose 30 g PO TID.

Available: Lactulose labelled 10 g per 15 mL

✔ Solution Using Ratio and Proportion

$$10\,g:15\,mL = 30\,g:x\,mL$$

$$\frac{10x}{10} = \frac{450}{10}$$

$$x = \frac{450}{10}$$

$$x = 45\,mL$$

✔ Solution Using the Formula Method

$$\frac{(D)\,30\,g}{(H)\,10\,g} \times (Q)\,15\,mL = x\,mL$$

$$x = \frac{30 \times 15}{10}$$

$$x = \frac{450}{10}$$

$$x = 45\,mL$$

✔ Solution Using Dimensional Analysis

$$x\,mL = \frac{15\,mL}{10\,\cancel{g}} \times \frac{30\,\cancel{g}}{1}$$

$$x = \frac{450}{10}$$

$$x = 45\,mL$$

Example 3: Order: Cefdinir 0.3 g PO q12h.

Available: Cefdinir oral suspension labelled 125 mg per 5 mL

Note: Convert grams to milligrams. 1 000 mg = 1 g.

NOTE

A conversion is necessary before calculating the dosage. What the prescriber has ordered is different from what is available.

Any of the methods presented for converting can be used. Because the measurements are metric in this problem, the other method that can be used is to move the decimal point the desired number of places (0.3 g = 0.300 = 300 mg).

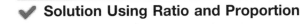

✔ Solution Using Ratio and Proportion

$$125 \text{ mg} : 5 \text{ mL} = 300 \text{ mg} : x \text{ mL}$$

$$\frac{125x}{125} = \frac{300 \times 5}{125}$$

$$x = \frac{1\,500}{125}$$

$$x = 12 \text{ mL}$$

✔ Solution Using the Formula Method

NOTE

Some medication orders state the specific amount to be given and therefore require no calculation. Examples: milk of magnesia 30 mL PO at bedtime; Robitussin 15 mL PO q4h prn; Fer-In-Sol 0.2 mL PO daily.

$$\frac{(D) \, 300 \text{ mg}}{(H) \, 125 \text{ mg}} \times (Q) \, 5 \text{ mL} = x \text{ mL}$$

$$x = \frac{300 \times 5}{125}$$

$$x = \frac{1\,500}{125}$$

$$x = 12 \text{ mL}$$

✔ Solution Using Dimensional Analysis

$$x \text{ mL} = \frac{5 \text{ mL}}{125 \text{ mg}} \times \frac{1\,000 \text{ mg}}{1 \text{ g}} \times \frac{0.3 \text{ g}}{1}$$

$$x = \frac{5\,000 \times 0.3}{125}$$

$$x = \frac{1\,500}{125}$$

$$x = 12 \text{ mL}$$

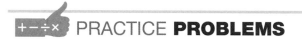

POINTS TO **REMEMBER**

When calculating dosages of oral liquids:

- Use the same methods and steps used to calculate dosages of solid medication (tabs, capsules).
- Regardless of the calculation method used, think critically about what is a reasonable amount. Think and question any dosage that seems unreasonable.
- Read labels carefully on medication containers; identify the dosage strength contained in a certain amount of solution.
- Be aware that dosage strength on solutions can be written several ways. Do not confuse it with total volume (total amount in container). Use "per" to separate dosages when writing.
- For accurate measurement, pour oral solutions at eye level on a flat surface and read the measurement at eye level.
- Always pour away from the label to keep hands from covering it and spills from obscuring it.
- Know that administering accurate dosages of liquid medications may require the use of calibrated droppers or oral syringes. Oral syringes are designed for oral use; they are not sterile.
- Use a calibrated measuring device only for the medication it is intended for.

PRACTICE **PROBLEMS**

Calculate the following dosages of oral liquids in millilitres using the labels or the information provided. Do not forget to label your answer. Round answers to the nearest tenth where indicated.

27. Order: Docusate sodium syrup 100 mg by jejunostomy tube TID.

    Available: Docusate sodium syrup 50 mg per 15 mL   _____

28. Order: Clarithromycin 100 mg PO q12h.

    Available:

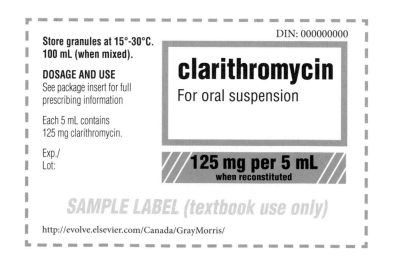

Store granules at 15°-30°C.
100 mL (when mixed).

DIN: 000000000

DOSAGE AND USE
See package insert for full
prescribing information

Each 5 mL contains
125 mg clarithromycin.

Exp./
Lot:

clarithromycin
For oral suspension

125 mg per 5 mL
when reconstituted

SAMPLE LABEL (textbook use only)

http://evolve.elsevier.com/Canada/GrayMorris/

_____

29. Order: Potassium chloride 40 mEq PO daily.

    Available:

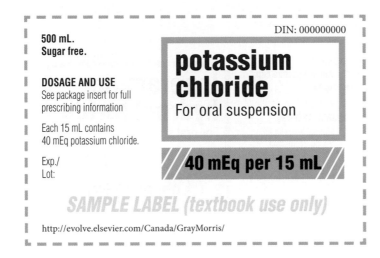

    500 mL.
    Sugar free.

    DOSAGE AND USE
    See package insert for full
    prescribing information

    Each 15 mL contains
    40 mEq potassium chloride.

    Exp./
    Lot:

    DIN: 000000000

    potassium
    chloride
    For oral suspension

    40 mEq per 15 mL

    SAMPLE LABEL (textbook use only)

    http://evolve.elsevier.com/Canada/GrayMorris/

    _____

30. Order: Theophylline elixir 120 mg PO BID.

    Available: Theophylline elixir 80 mg per 15 mL   _____

31. Order: Erythromycin oral suspension 250 mg PO q6h.

    Available: Erythromycin oral suspension labelled 200 mg per 5 mL

    _____

32. Order: Phenytoin 100 mg PO TID.

    Available: Phenytoin oral suspension 125 mg per 5 mL   _____

33. Order: Digoxin 125 mcg PO daily.

    Available:

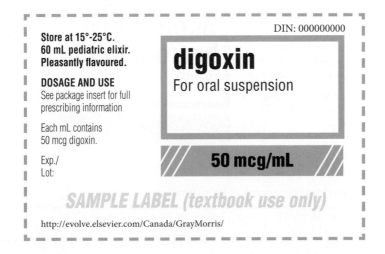

    Store at 15°-25°C.
    60 mL pediatric elixir.
    Pleasantly flavoured.

    DOSAGE AND USE
    See package insert for full
    prescribing information

    Each mL contains
    50 mcg digoxin.

    Exp./
    Lot:

    DIN: 000000000

    digoxin
    For oral suspension

    50 mcg/mL

    SAMPLE LABEL (textbook use only)

    http://evolve.elsevier.com/Canada/GrayMorris/

    _____

34. Order: Loperamide hydrochloride 4 mg PO as initial dose and then 2 mg after each loose stool.

   Available:

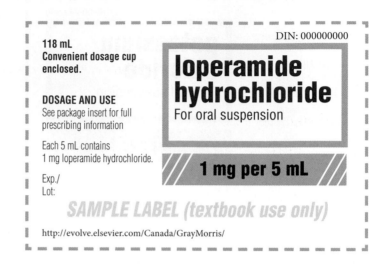

118 mL
Convenient dosage cup enclosed.

DOSAGE AND USE
See package insert for full prescribing information

Each 5 mL contains
1 mg loperamide hydrochloride.

Exp./
Lot:

DIN: 000000000

loperamide hydrochloride
For oral suspension

1 mg per 5 mL

SAMPLE LABEL (textbook use only)

http://evolve.elsevier.com/Canada/GrayMorris/

   How many mL will you administer for the initial dose? _____

35. Order: Amoxicillin 0.5 g PO q6h.

   Available: Amoxicillin oral suspension labelled 125 mg per 5 mL

   _____

36. Order: Phenobarbital 60 mg PO at bedtime.

   Available: Phenobarbital elixir 20 mg per 5 mL   _____

37. Order: Thioridazine hydrochloride 150 mg PO BID.

   Available:

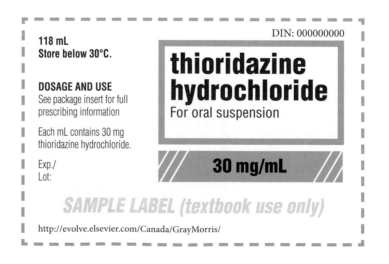

118 mL
Store below 30°C.

DOSAGE AND USE
See package insert for full prescribing information

Each mL contains 30 mg thioridazine hydrochloride.

Exp./
Lot:

DIN: 000000000

thioridazine hydrochloride
For oral suspension

30 mg/mL

SAMPLE LABEL (textbook use only)

http://evolve.elsevier.com/Canada/GrayMorris/

   _____

38. Order: Diphenhydramine HCl 25 mg PO BID prn for agitation.

    Available: Diphenhydramine hydrochloride elixir 12.5 mg per 5 mL

    _____

39. Order: Lithium carbonate 600 mg PO at bedtime.

    Available: Lithium citrate syrup. Each 5 mL contains lithium carbonate 300 mg. Each unit-dose container contains 5 mL

    a. How many mL are needed to administer the dosage? _____

    b. How many containers of the medication will you need to administer the dosage? _____

40. Order: Haldol 10 mg PO BID.

    Available: Haldol concentrate labelled 2 mg per mL _____

41. Order: Erythromycin ethylsuccinate oral suspension (E.E.S.) 0.5 g by gastrostomy tube q6h.

    Available:

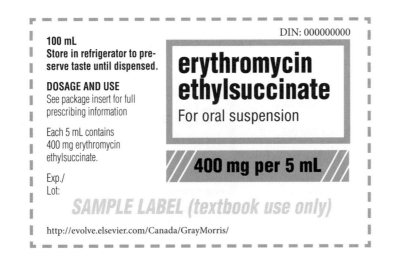

100 mL
Store in refrigerator to pre-serve taste until dispensed.

DOSAGE AND USE
See package insert for full prescribing information

Each 5 mL contains 400 mg erythromycin ethylsuccinate.

Exp./
Lot:

DIN: 000000000

erythromycin ethylsuccinate
For oral suspension

400 mg per 5 mL

SAMPLE LABEL (textbook use only)

http://evolve.elsevier.com/Canada/GrayMorris/

    _____

42. Order: Penicillin V potassium 500 000 units PO QID.

Available:

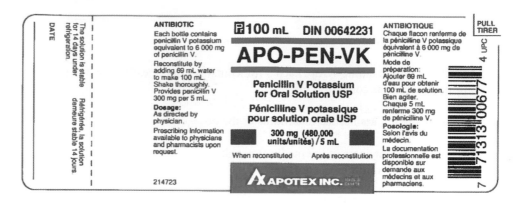

43. Order: Cephalexin 1 g by nasogastric tube q6h.

Available: Cephalexin oral suspension 125 mg per 5 mL   _____

44. Order: Valproic acid 500 mg PO daily.

Available:

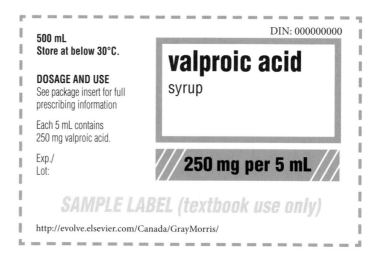

45. Order: Acetaminophen 650 mg by nasogastric tube q4h prn for temperature higher than 38.5°C.

Available:

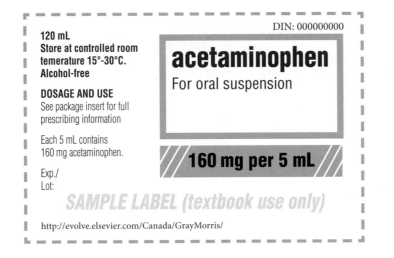

46. Order: Cimetidine 400 mg PO q6h.

Available: Cimetidine oral liquid labelled 300 mg per 5 mL

47. Order: Lamivudine 150 mg PO BID.

Available:

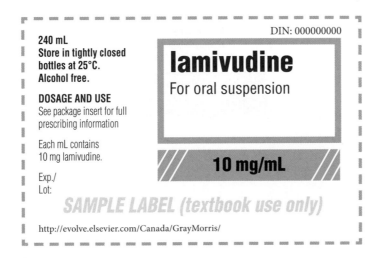

48. Order: Zidovudine 0.3 g PO BID.

Available:

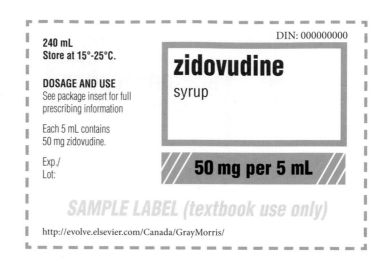

49. Order: Amoxicillin 375 mg PO q8h.

Available:

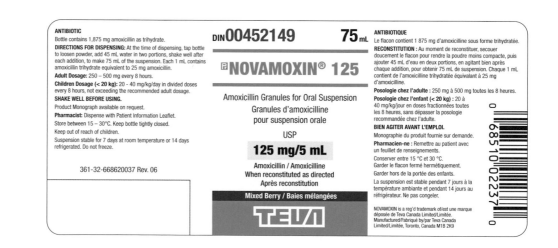

50. Order: Norvir 600 mg PO BID.

Available:

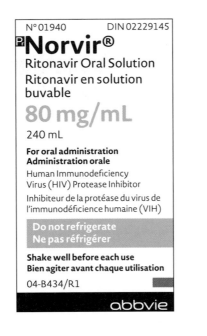

51. Order: Amoxicillin and clavulanate potassium 0.25 g PO q8h (ordered according to the dose of amoxicillin).

Available:

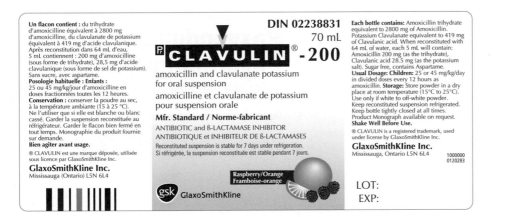

52. Order: Fluoxetine hydrochloride 30 mg PO daily in AM.

    Available:

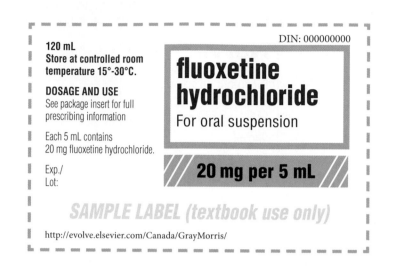

53. Order: Ranitidine 150 mg BID by nasogastric tube.

    Available: Ranitidine syrup labelled 15 mg per mL

    _____

54. Order: Oxycodone hydrochloride 30 mg PO q12h prn for pain.

    Available:

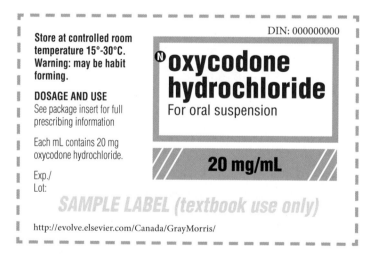

Answers on pages 344–346.

CLINICAL **REASONING**

1. **Scenario:** Order: Digoxin 0.75 mg PO daily. In preparing to administer medications, you find 0.125 mg tabs (scored) in the medication drawer for the patient.

   a. Based on the tablets available, how many would you have to administer? _____

   b. What action should you take? _____

   c. What is the rationale for your action? _____

2. **Scenario:** Order: Fluconazole 150 mg PO daily. The pharmacy sends two 100-mg unscored tabs.

   a. What action should you take to administer the dosage ordered? _____

   b. What is the rationale for your action? _____

3. **Scenario:** Order: Oxycodone and acetaminophen 2 tabs PO q4h prn for pain for a patient who is allergic to aspirin. The nurse administers Oxycodone and aspirin 2 tabs.

Warning: May be habit forming.

DOSAGE AND USE
See package insert for full prescribing information

Each tablet contains 4.5 mg oxycodone and 325 mg aspirin.

Exp./
Lot:

DIN: 000000000

ᴺoxycodone and aspirin
100 tablets

4.5 mg/325 mg

SAMPLE LABEL (textbook use only)

http://evolve.elsevier.com/Canada/GrayMorris/

Warning: May be habit forming.

DOSAGE AND USE
See package insert for full prescribing information

Each tablet contains 5 mg oxycodone and 325 mg acetaminophen.

Exp./
Lot:

DIN: 000000000

ᴺoxycodone and acetaminophen
100 tablets

5 mg/325 mg

SAMPLE LABEL (textbook use only)

http://evolve.elsevier.com/Canada/GrayMorris/

---

   a. What patient right was violated? _____

   b. What contributed to the error? _____

   c. What is the potential outcome of the error? _____

   d. What preventive measures could have been taken to prevent the error? _____

Answers on page 347.

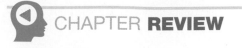

CHAPTER **REVIEW**

Calculate the following dosages using the labels or the information provided. Express volume answers in millilitres; round answers to the nearest tenth as indicated. Remember to label answers: tab, capsules, mL.

1. Order: Acetaminophen 975 mg PO q6h prn for earache.

    Available:

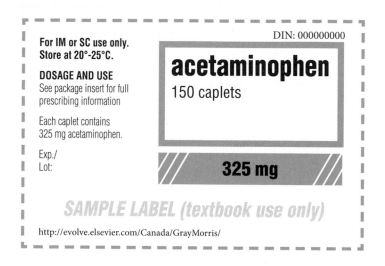

2. Order: Linezolid 400 mg PO q12h.

    Available:

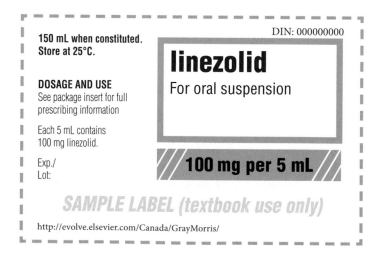

3. Order: Metoprolol tartrate 100 mg PO BID. Hold for blood pressure less than 100/60.

   Available:

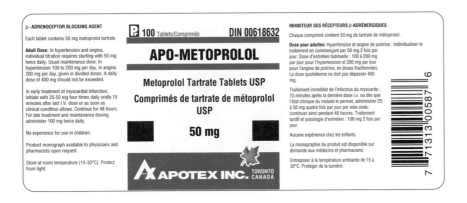

4. Order: Carvedilol 18.75 mg PO BID.

   Available:

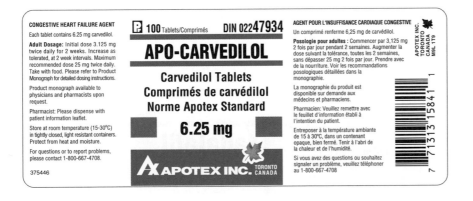

5. Order: Janumet 50 mg/500 mg PO BID.

   Available:

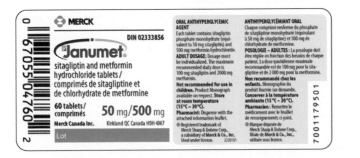

6. Order: Zithromax 250 mg PO daily for 3 days.

Available:

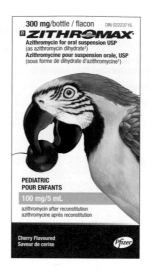

7. Order: Tadalafil 20 mg PO 1 h before sexual activity for a patient with erectile dysfunction.

Available:

_____

8. Order: Lorazepam 1 mg PO q4h prn for agitation.

Available: Lorazepam tablets labelled 0.5 mg   _____

9. Order: Lopressor 25 mg per nasogastric tube BID.

Available: Lopressor scored tablets labelled 50 mg   _____

10. Order: Spironolactone and hydrochlorothiazide 100 mg PO daily.

    Available:

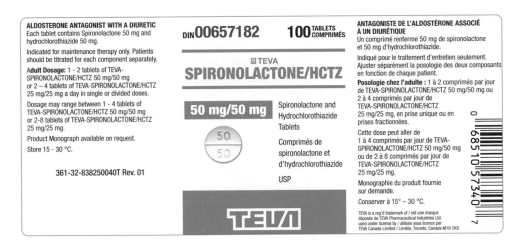

11. Order: Digoxin 0.1 mg PO daily.

    Available:

12. Order: Amoxicillin 0.475 g PO q6h.

Available:

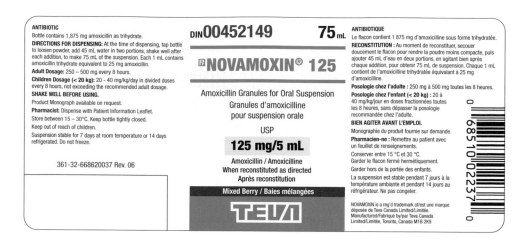

ANTIBIOTIC
Bottle contains 1,875 mg amoxicillin as trihydrate.
DIRECTIONS FOR DISPENSING: At the time of dispensing, tap bottle to loosen powder, add 45 mL water in two portions, shake well after each addition, to make 75 mL of the suspension. Each 1 mL contains amoxicillin trihydrate equivalent to 25 mg amoxicillin.
Adult Dosage: 250 – 500 mg every 8 hours.
Children Dosage (< 20 kg): 20 - 40 mg/kg/day in divided doses every 8 hours, not exceeding the recommended adult dosage.
SHAKE WELL BEFORE USING.
Product Monograph available on request.
Pharmacist: Dispense with Patient Information Leaflet.
Store between 15 – 30°C. Keep bottle tightly closed.
Keep out of reach of children.
Suspension stable for 7 days at room temperature or 14 days refrigerated. Do not freeze.

361-32-668620037 Rev. 06

DIN**00452149**   **75** mL

℗**NOVAMOXIN®** 125

Amoxicillin Granules for Oral Suspension
Granules d'amoxicilline
pour suspension orale

USP

125 mg/5 mL

Amoxicillin / Amoxicilline
When reconstituted as directed
Après reconstitution

Mixed Berry / Baies mélangées

TEVA

ANTIBIOTIQUE
Le flacon contient 1 875 mg d'amoxicilline sous forme trihydratée.
RECONSTITUTION : Au moment de reconstituer, secouer doucement le flacon pour rendre la poudre moins compacte, puis ajouter 45 mL d'eau en deux portions, en agitant bien après chaque addition, pour obtenir 75 mL de suspension. Chaque 1 mL contient de l'amoxicilline trihydratée équivalant à 25 mg d'amoxicilline.
Posologie chez l'adulte : 250 mg à 500 mg toutes les 8 heures.
Posologie chez l'enfant (< 20 kg) : 20 à 40 mg/kg/jour en doses fractionnées toutes les 8 heures, sans dépasser la posologie recommandée chez l'adulte.
BIEN AGITER AVANT L'EMPLOI.
Monographie du produit fournie sur demande.
Pharmacien-ne : Remettre au patient avec un feuillet de renseignements.
Conserver entre 15 °C et 30 °C.
Garder le flacon fermé hermétiquement.
Garder hors de la portée des enfants.
La suspension est stable pendant 7 jours à la température ambiante et pendant 14 jours au réfrigérateur. Ne pas congeler.
NOVAMOXIN is a reg'd trademark of/est une marque déposée de Teva Canada Limited/Limitée.
Manufactured/Fabriqué by/par Teva Canada Limitée/Limited, Toronto, Canada M1B 2K9

0 68510 02237 0

13. Order: Hydrochlorothiazide 12.5 mg PO daily. Hold for blood pressure less than 90/60.

Available: Scored tablets (can be broken in half)

DIURETIC-ANTIHYPERTENSIVE
DOSAGE:
Diuretic: One to two tablets once or twice a day.
Antihypertensive: 1/2 or one tablet once or twice a day.
Complete prescribing information is available on request.
Store at room temperature 15-30°C.

250105

℗ **100** Tablets/Comprimés   DIN 00326844

APO-HYDRO

Hydrochlorothiazide Tablets USP
Comprimés d'hydrochlorothiazide USP

25 mg

A APOTEX INC. TORONTO CANADA

DIURÉTIQUE-ANTIHYPERTENSIF
POSOLOGIE:
Diurétique: Un à deux comprimés une ou deux fois par jour.
Antihypertensif: 1/2 ou un comprimé une ou deux fois par jour.
Renseignements détaillés posologiques disponibles sur demande.
Entreposer à la température ambiante de 15 à 30°C.

7 71313 00449 7

14. Order: Acetaminophen 500 mg by nasogastric tube q4h prn for temperature higher than 38.5°C.

Available:

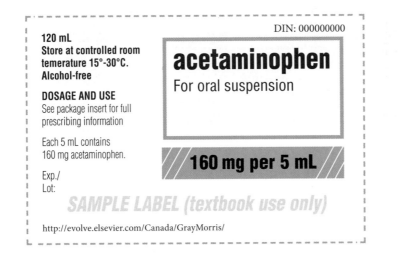

_____

15. Order: Escitalopram 20 mg PO daily in the PM.

Available: Escitalopram oral solution labelled 5 mg per 5 mL   _____

16. Order: Elixophyllin elixir 300 mg by nasogastric tube BID.

Available: Elixophyllin elixir labelled 160 mg per 15 mL   _____

17. Order: Xanax 0.75 mg PO TID.

Available:

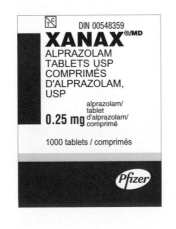

_____

18. Order: GlucoNorm 3 mg PO BID.

    Available:

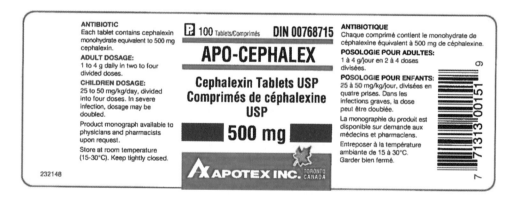

    Which dosage strength will be best to use?   _____

19. Order: Meclizine HCl (Antivert) 25 mg PO daily.

    Available: Meclizine HCl tablets labelled 12.5 mg   _____

20. Order: Cephalexin 0.5 g PO BID.

    Available:

ANTIBIOTIC
Each tablet contains cephalexin monohydrate equivalent to 500 mg cephalexin.
ADULT DOSAGE:
1 to 4 g daily in two to four divided doses.
CHILDREN DOSAGE:
25 to 50 mg/kg/day, divided into four doses. In severe infection, dosage may be doubled.
Product monograph available to physicians and pharmacists upon request.
Store at room temperature (15-30°C). Keep tightly closed.
232148

℞ 100 Tablets/Comprimés   DIN 00768715
APO-CEPHALEX
Cephalexin Tablets USP
Comprimés de céphalexine USP
500 mg
⚕APOTEX INC. TORONTO CANADA

ANTIBIOTIQUE
Chaque comprimé contient le monohydrate de céphalexine équivalent à 500 mg de céphalexine.
POSOLOGIE POUR ADULTES:
1 à 4 g/jour en 2 à 4 doses divisées.
POSOLOGIE POUR ENFANTS:
25 à 50 mg/kg/jour, divisées en quatre prises. Dans les infections graves, la dose peut être doublée.
La monographie du produit est disponible sur demande aux médecins et pharmaciens.
Entreposer à la température ambiante de 15 à 30°C. Garder bien fermé.

_____

21. Order: Clonidine 0.5 mg PO TID. Hold for blood pressure less than 100/60.

    Available: Clonidine tablets labelled 0.1 mg, 0.2 mg, 0.3 mg

    Which would be the best combination to administer to the patient?

    _____

22. Order: Nitrostat 0.3 mg sublingual (SL) stat.

     Available:

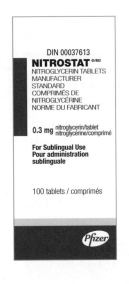

_____

23. Order: Procainamide hydrochloride extended release 1 g PO q12h.

     Available:

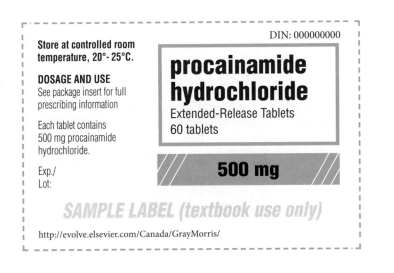

_____

24. Order: Lactulose 20 g by gastrostomy tube BID.

    Available:

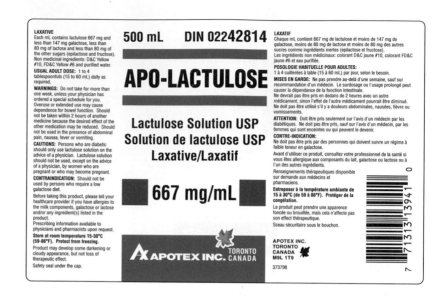

25. Order: Cephalexin 1 g PO q6h for 5 days.

    Available:

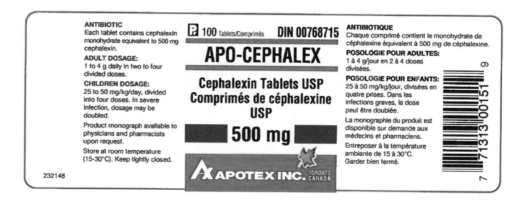

26. Order: Clozapine 50 mg PO daily.

    Available:

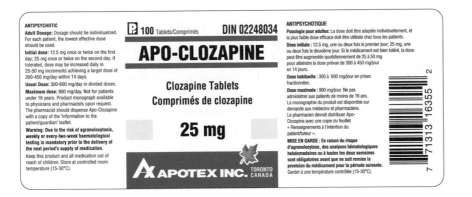

    a. How many tabs will you administer for each dose?   _____

    b. How many tabs will be needed for 7 days?   _____

27. Order: Lipitor 30 mg PO daily.

    Available:

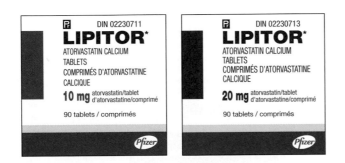

    What will you administer to the patient?   _____

28. Order: Cimetidine 0.8 g PO TID.

    Available:

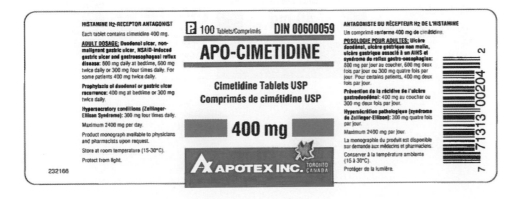

    _____

29. Order: Cefprozil 0.5 g PO q12h.

    Available:

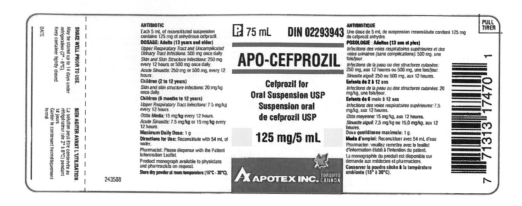

30. Order: Esomeprazole magnesium (delayed release) 40 mg PO daily for 4 weeks.

    Available:

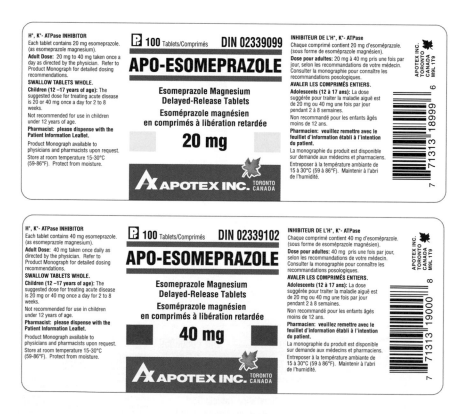

What will you administer to the patient?

31. Order: Cefprozil 235 mg PO q8h.

    Available:

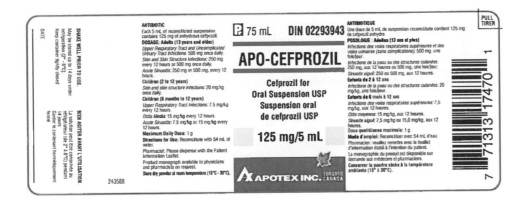

32. Order: Rosiglitazone maleate 8 mg PO daily.

    Available:

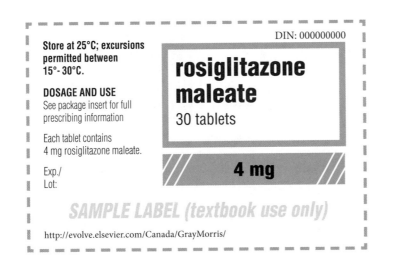

33. Order: Allopurinol 0.25 g PO daily.

   Available: Scored tablets (can be broken in half)

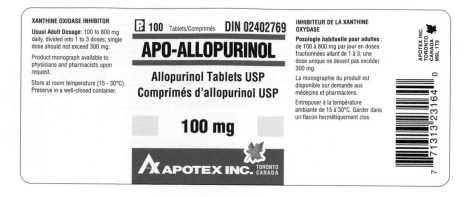

34. Order: Zeldox 120 mg PO BID.

   Available:

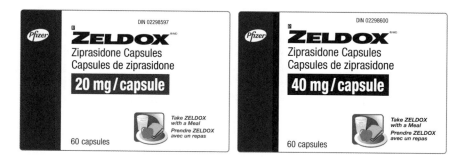

   What will you administer to the patient? _____

35. Order: Furosemide (Lasix) 100 mg by gastrostomy tube once a day.

   Available:

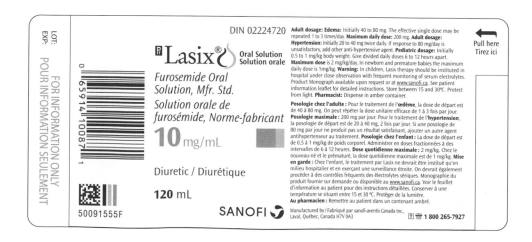

36. Order: Atomoxetine hydrochloride 0.1 g PO daily.

    Available:

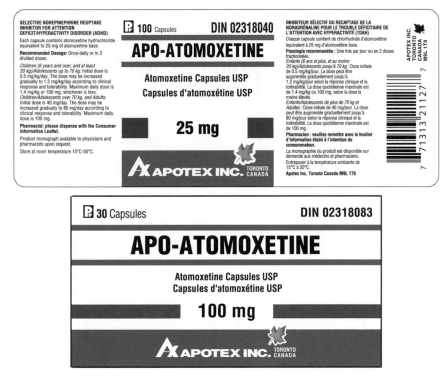

    Which dosage strength will you administer? _____

37. Order: Sildenafil citrate 50 mg PO $\frac{1}{2}$ hour before sexual activity for a patient with erectile dysfunction.

    Available:

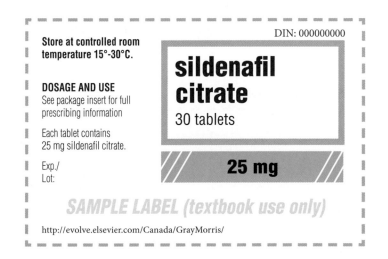

    _____

38. Order: Tranxene 30 mg PO BID.

    Available: Tranxene tablets labelled 15 mg _____

39. Order: Valproic acid 1 g PO daily.

    Available:

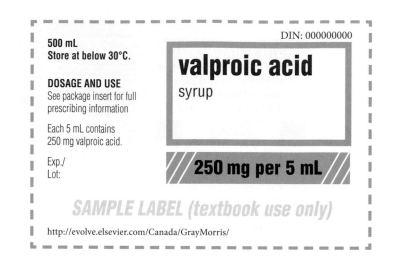

40. Order: Levothyroxine sodium 175 mcg PO daily.

    Available:

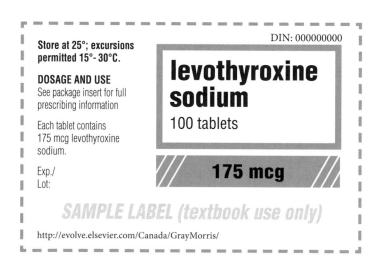

41. Order: Olanzapine 10 mg PO BID.

    Available:

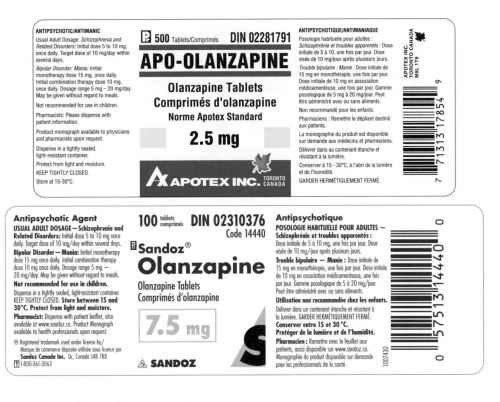

    What will you administer to the patient?   _____

42. Order: Bupropion hydrochloride 150 mg PO BID.

    Available:

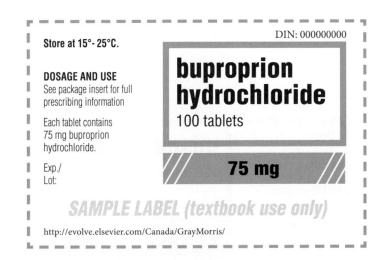

    _____

43. Order: Sertraline 100 mg PO daily.

    Available:

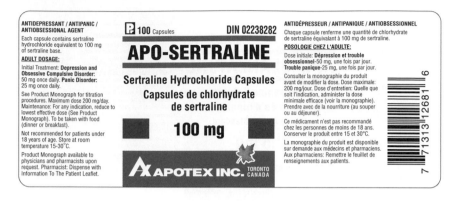

44. Order: Famciclovir 0.25 g PO TID for 5 days.

    Available:

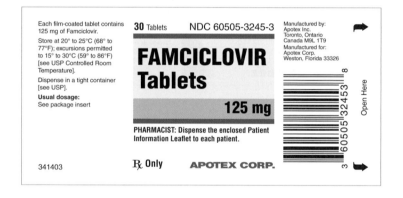

45. Order: Misoprostol 200 mcg PO QID.

    Available:

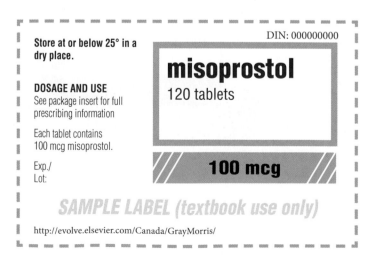

46. Order: Oxcarbazepine 0.6 g PO BID.

    Available:

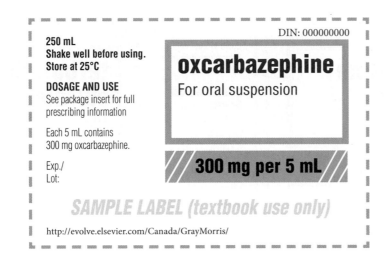

    _____

47. Order: Benadryl 100 mg PO at bedtime.

    Available: Benadryl capsules labelled 50 mg   _____

48. Order: Dilantin 60 mg PO BID.

    Available:

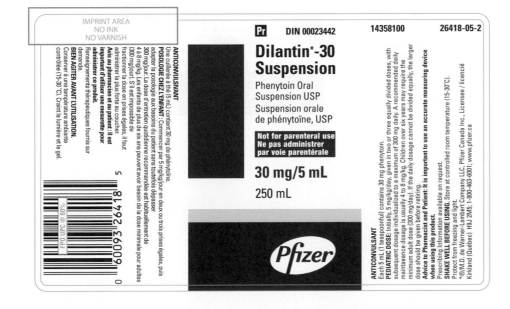

    _____

49. Order: Terbutaline sulphate 15 mg PO daily.

Available:

DIN: 000000000

Store at 20°-25°C.
Excursion permitted
15°-30°C.

DOSAGE AND USE
See package insert for full
prescribing information

Each tablet contains
5 mg terbutaline sulfate.

Exp./
Lot:

**terbutaline
sulfate**
100 tablets

5 mg

SAMPLE LABEL (textbook use only)

http://evolve.elsevier.com/Canada/GrayMorris/

DIN: 000000000

Store at 20°- 25°C.
Excursions permitted
15°- 30°C.

DOSAGE AND USE
See package insert for full
prescribing information

Each tablet contains
2.5 mg terbutaline sulfate.

Exp./
Lot:

**terbutaline
sulfate**
100 tablets

2.5 mg

SAMPLE LABEL (textbook use only)

http://evolve.elsevier.com/Canada/GrayMorris/

How many of which dosage strength will you administer? _____

50. Order: Erythromycin 0.666 g PO q6h.

Available:

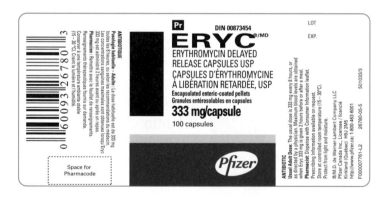

Answers on page 347.

evolve

For additional practice problems, refer to the Basic Calculations section of the Drug Calculations Companion,
Version 5 on Evolve.

✳ ANSWERS

Answers to Practice Problems

The answers to the Practice Problems include the rationale for the answer, where indicated. Where necessary, the method for calculating the dosage is shown as well.

> **✎ NOTE**
> Unless stated, no conversion is required to calculate the dosage. In problems that required a conversion before calculating the dosage, the problem setup shown illustrates the problem after appropriate conversions have been made.

1. $0.025 \text{ mg} = 25 \text{ mcg} (1\,000 \text{ mg} = 1 \text{ mg})$

   $$50 \text{ mcg} : 1 \text{ tab} = 25 \text{ mcg} : x \text{ tab}$$

   or

   $$\frac{25 \text{ mcg}}{50 \text{ mcg}} \times 1 \text{ tab} = x \text{ tab}$$

   Answer: 0.5 or $\frac{1}{2}$ tab. This is an acceptable answer because the tabs are scored. (For administration purposes, state as "$\frac{1}{2}$ tab.") Note that the problem could have been done without converting by using the dosage indicated on the label in mg. This setup would net the same answer:

   $$0.05 \text{ mg} : 1 \text{ tab} = 0.025 \text{ mg} : x \text{ tab}$$
   $$\frac{0.025 \text{ mg}}{0.05 \text{ mg}} \times 1 \text{ tab} = x \text{ tab}$$

2. It would be best to administer one of the 5-mg tabs and one of the 2.5-mg tabs

   $(5 \text{ mg} + 2.5 \text{ mg} = 7.5 \text{ mg}).$

3. a. 125-mcg tablet is the appropriate strength to use $(0.125 \text{ mg} = 125 \text{ mcg}).$
   b. 1 tab. Even though the tabs are scored, one half of 500 mcg would still be twice the desired dosage.

   $$125 \text{ mcg} : 1 \text{ tab} = 125 \text{ mcg} : x \text{ tab}$$

   or

   $$\frac{125 \text{ mcg}}{125 \text{ mcg}} \times 1 \text{ tab} = x \text{ tab}$$

   Answer: 1 tab

4. a. 500-mg capsules would be appropriate to use.
   b. 2 capsules (500 mg each). $1\,000 \text{ mg} = 1 \text{ g}$; therefore, 2 capsules of 500 mg each would be the least number of capsules. Using the 250-mg strength capsules would require 4 capsules.

   $$500 \text{ mg} : 1 \text{ capsule} = 1\,000 \text{ mg} : x \text{ capsule}$$
   $$\frac{1\,000 \text{ mg}}{500 \text{ mg}} \times 1 \text{ capsule} = x \text{ capsule}$$
   $$x = 2 \text{ capsules}$$

   c. 2 capsules q6h = 8 capsules. Multiplying the number of capsules needed by the number of days gives you the number of capsules required.

   $$8 \text{ (number of capsules per day)} \times 7 \text{ (number of days)} = 56 \text{ (total capsules needed)}$$

5. $$250 \text{ mg} : 1 \text{ capsule} = 750 \text{ mg} : x \text{ capsule}$$

   $$\frac{750 \text{ mg}}{250 \text{ mg}} \times 1 \text{ capsule} = x \text{ capsule}$$

   Answer: 3 capsules. The dosage ordered is more than the available strength; therefore, you will need more than 1 capsule to administer the dosage.

6. $0.4 \text{ g} = 400 \text{ mg} (1 \text{ g} = 1\,000 \text{ mg})$

   $$400 \text{ mg} : 1 \text{ tab} = 400 \text{ mg} : x \text{ tab}$$
   $$\frac{400 \text{ mg}}{400 \text{ mg}} \times 1 \text{ tab} = x \text{ tab}$$

   Answer: 1 tab. 1 tab, 400 mg, is equal to 0.4 g; therefore, only 1 tab is needed to administer the dosage.

7. $$100 \text{ mg} : 1 \text{ tab} = 200 \text{ mg} : x \text{ tab}$$

   or

   $$\frac{200 \text{ mg}}{100 \text{ mg}} \times 1 \text{ tab} = x \text{ tab}$$

   Answer: 2 tabs (chewable). The dosage ordered is more than the available strength; therefore, you will need more than 1 tab to administer the dosage.

8. a. 30-mg tablets

   b. Three 30-mg tablets. This strength will allow the patient to take 3 tabs to achieve the desired dosage, as opposed to six 15-mg tabs. This dosage is logical because the maximum number of tablets administered is generally three.

$$30 \, mg : 1 \, tab \, = \, 90 \, mg : x \, tab$$

   or

$$\frac{90 \, mg}{30 \, mg} \times 1 \, tab \, = \, x \, tab$$

   Answer: three 30-mg tabs

9. 0.6 g = 600 mg (1 g = 1 000 mg)

$$300 \, mg : 1 \, tab \, = \, 600 \, mg : x \, tab$$
$$\frac{600 \, mg}{300 \, mg} \times 1 \, tab \, = \, x \, tab$$

   Answer: 2 tabs. The dosage ordered is more than the available strength; therefore, you will need more than 1 tab to administer the dosage.

10. $$50 \, mg : 1 \, tab = 100 \, mg : x \, tab$$

   or

$$\frac{100 \, mg}{50 \, mg} \times 1 \, tab \, = \, x \, tab$$

   Answer: You need 2 tabs to administer 100 mg. 2 tabs TID (three times a day) = 6 tabs × 3 days = 18 tabs.

11. It would be best to administer one 80-mg tab and one 40-mg tab (80 + 40 = 120 mg). This would be the least number of tablets.

12. 1 g = 1 000 mg

$$250 \, mg : 1 \, tab \, = \, 1 \, 000 \, mg : x \, tab$$
$$\frac{1 \, 000 \, mg}{250 \, mg} \times 1 \, tab \, = \, x \, tab$$

   Answer: 4 tabs. The dosage ordered is more than the available strength; therefore, you will need more than 1 tab to administer the dosage.

13. Choose the 6-mg tab and give 1 tab, which allows the patient to swallow the least number of tabs without dividing tabs.

$$6 \, mg : 1 \, tab \, = \, 6 \, mg : x \, tab$$

   or

$$\frac{6 \, mg}{6 \, mg} \times 1 \, tab \, = \, x \, tab$$

   Answer: one 6-mg tab

14. $$10 \, mg : 1 \, tab = 20 \, mg : x \, tab$$

   or

$$\frac{20 \, mg}{10 \, mg} \times 1 \, tab \, = \, x \, tab$$

   Answer: 2 tabs. The dosage ordered is more than the available strength; therefore, you will need more than 1 tab to administer the dosage.

15. $$200 \, mg : 1 \, tab = 400 \, mg : x \, tab$$

   or

$$\frac{400 \, mg}{200 \, mg} \times 1 \, tab \, = \, x \, tab$$

   Answer: 2 tabs. The dosage ordered is more than the available strength; therefore, you will need more than 1 tab to administer the dosage.

16. $$75 \, mg : 1 \, capsule = 150 \, mg : x \, capsule$$

   or

$$\frac{150 \, mg}{75 \, mg} \times 1 \, capsule \, = \, x \, capsule$$

   Answer: 2 capsules (extended release). The dosage ordered is more than the available strength; therefore, you will need more than 1 capsule to administer the dosage.

17. Convert 1 g to 1 000 mg (1 000 mg = 1 g)

$$500 \text{ mg} : 1 \text{ tab} = 1\,000 \text{ mg} : x \text{ tab}$$

or

$$\frac{1\,000 \text{ mg}}{500 \text{ mg}} \times 1 \text{ tab} = x \text{ tab}$$

Answer: 2 tabs. The dosage ordered is more than the available strength; therefore, you will need more than 1 tab to administer the dosage.

18. $$30 \text{ mg} : 1 \text{ capsule} = 60 \text{ mg} : x \text{ capsule}$$

or

$$\frac{60 \text{ mg}}{30 \text{ mg}} \times 1 \text{ capsule} = x \text{ capsule}$$

Answer: 2 capsules (delayed release). The dosage ordered is more than the available strength; therefore, you will need more than 1 capsule to administer the dosage.

19. It would be best to administer three 25-mcg tablets. Although the tabs are scored, it is best to administer tabs whole rather than breaking them. Variation in dosage can occur if tablets are broken.

20. $$12.5 \text{ mg} : 1 \text{ tab} = 25 \text{ mg} : x \text{ tab}$$

or

$$\frac{25 \text{ mg}}{12.5 \text{ mg}} \times 1 \text{ tab} = x \text{ tab}$$

Answer: 2 tabs. The dosage ordered is more than the available strength; therefore, you will need more than 1 tab to administer the dosage.

21. $$200 \text{ mg} : 1 \text{ tab} = 400 \text{ mg} : x \text{ tab}$$

$$\frac{400 \text{ mg}}{200 \text{ mg}} \times 1 \text{ tab} = x \text{ tab}$$

Answer: 2 tabs (chewable). The dosage ordered is more than the available strength; therefore, you will need more than 1 tab to administer the dosage.

22. $$325 \text{ mg} : 1 \text{ tab} = 650 \text{ mg} : x \text{ tab}$$

or

$$\frac{650 \text{ mg}}{325 \text{ mg}} \times 1 \text{ tab} = x \text{ tab}$$

Answer: 2 tabs. The dosage ordered is more than the available strength; therefore, you will need more than 1 tab to administer the dosage.

23. Conversion is necessary. Conversion factor: 1 000 mg = 1 g. Therefore, 0.2 g = 200 mg.

$$100 \text{ mg} : 1 \text{ capsule} = 200 \text{ mg} : x \text{ capsule}$$

or

$$\frac{200 \text{ mg}}{100 \text{ mg}} \times 1 \text{ capsule} = x \text{ capsule}$$

Answer: 2 capsules (extended release). The dosage ordered is more than the available strength; therefore, you will need more than 1 capsule to administer the dosage.

24. $$400 \text{ mg} : 1 \text{ tab} = 800 \text{ mg} : x \text{ tab}$$

or

$$\frac{800 \text{ mg}}{400 \text{ mg}} \times 1 \text{ tab} = x \text{ tab}$$

Answer: 2 tabs. The dosage ordered is more than the available strength; therefore, you will need more than 1 tab to administer the dosage.

25. Conversion is necessary. Conversion factor: 1 000 mg = 1 g. Therefore, 0.03 g = 30 mg.

$$10 \text{ mg} : 1 \text{ tab} = 30 \text{ mg} : x \text{ tab}$$

or

$$\frac{30 \text{ mg}}{10 \text{ mg}} \times 1 \text{ tab} = x \text{ tab}$$

Answer: 3 tabs. The dosage ordered is more than the available strength; therefore, you will need more than 1 tab to administer the dosage. Generally, 3 tabs is the maximum number of tabs that should be given.

26. $$60 \text{ mg} : 1 \text{ capsule} = 120 \text{ mg} : x \text{ capsule}$$

$$\frac{120 \text{ mg}}{60 \text{ mg}} \times 1 \text{ capsule} = x \text{ capsule}$$

Answer: 2 capsules. The dosage ordered is more than the available strength; therefore, you will need more than 1 capsule to administer the dosage.

NOTE

The setup shown for problems that required conversion reflects the conversion of what the prescriber ordered to the available strength. Unless stated in problems 27–54, no conversion is required to calculate the dosage.

27.   50 mg : 15 mL = 100 mg : x mL

or

$$\frac{100\ mg}{50\ mg} \times 15\ mL = x\ mL$$

Answer: 30 mL. The dosage ordered is two times more than the available strength; therefore, you will need more than 15 mL to administer the dosage.

28.   125 mg : 5 mL = 100 mg : x mL

or

$$\frac{100\ mg}{125\ mg} \times 5\ mL = x\ mL$$

Answer: 4 mL. The dosage ordered is less than the available strength; therefore, you will need less than 5 mL to administer the dosage.

29.   40 mEq : 15 mL = 40 mEq : x mL

or

$$\frac{40\ mEq}{40\ mEq} \times 15\ mL = x\ mL$$

Answer: 15 mL. The dosage ordered is contained in 15 mL of the medication.

30.   80 mg : 15 mL = 120 mg : x mL

or

$$\frac{120\ mg}{80\ mg} \times 15\ mL = x\ mL$$

Answer: 22.5 mL. The dosage ordered is more than the available strength; therefore, you will need more than 15 mL to administer the dosage.

31.   200 mg : 5 mL = 250 mg : x mL

or

$$\frac{250\ mg}{200\ mg} \times 5\ mL = x\ mL$$

Answer: 6.3 mL. The dosage ordered is more than the available strength; therefore, you will need more than 5 mL to administer the dosage. The answer to the nearest tenth is 6.3 mL.

32.   125 mg : 5 mL = 100 mg : x mL

or

$$\frac{100\ mg}{125\ mg} \times 5\ mL = x\ mL$$

Answer: 4 mL. The amount ordered is less than the available strength; therefore, you will need less than 5 mL to administer the dosage.

33. Use the microgram equivalent to calculate the dosage.

50 mcg : 1 mL = 125 mcg : x mL

or

$$\frac{125\ mcg}{5\ mcg} \times 1\ mL = x\ mL$$

Answer: 2.5 mL (2.5 mL is metric and stated with a decimal). The dosage ordered is more than the available strength; therefore, you will need more than 1 mL to administer the dosage.

34.   1 mg : 5 mL = 4 mg : x mL

or

$$\frac{4\ mg}{1\ mg} \times 5\ mL = x\ mL$$

Answer: 20 mL. The dosage ordered is more than the available strength; therefore, you will need more than 5 mL to administer the dosage.

35. Conversion is required. Conversion factor: 1 000 mg = 1 g. Therefore, 0.5 g = 500 mg.

125 mg : 5 mL = 500 mg : x mL

or

$$\frac{500\ mg}{125\ mg} \times 5\ mL = x\ mL$$

Answer: 20 mL. The dosage ordered is four times more than the available strength; therefore, you will need more than 5 mL to administer the dosage.

36. 20 mg : 5 mL = 60 mg : x mL

$$\frac{20x}{20} = \frac{300}{20}$$

or

$$\frac{60 \, \text{mg}}{20 \, \text{mg}} \times 5 \, \text{mL} = x \, \text{mL}$$

Answer: 15 mL. The dosage ordered is more than the available strength; therefore, you will need more than 5 mL to administer the dosage.

37. 30 mg : 1 mL = 150 mg : x mL

or

$$\frac{150 \, \text{mg}}{30 \, \text{mg}} \times 1 \, \text{mL} = x \, \text{mL}$$

Answer: 5 mL. The dosage ordered is five times more than the available strength; therefore, you will need more than 1 mL to administer the dosage.

38. 12.5 mg : 5 mL = 25 mg : x mL

or

$$\frac{25 \, \text{mg}}{12.5 \, \text{mg}} \times 5 \, \text{mL} = x \, \text{mL}$$

Answer: 10 mL. The dosage ordered is two times more than the available strength; therefore, you will need more than 5 mL to administer the dosage.

39. The label indicates that 5 mL = 300 mg of the medication.

300 mg : 5 mL = 600 mg : x mL

or

$$\frac{600 \, \text{mg}}{300 \, \text{mg}} \times 5 \, \text{mL} = x \, \text{mL}$$

a. 10 mL. The dosage ordered is two times more than the available strength; therefore, you will need more than 5 mL to administer the dosage.
b. Two containers are needed. One container contains 300 mg.

40. 2 mg : 1 mL = 10 mg : x mL

or

$$\frac{10 \, \text{mg}}{2 \, \text{mg}} \times 1 \, \text{mL} = x \, \text{mL}$$

Answer: 5 mL. The dosage ordered is five times more than the available strength; therefore, you will need more than 1 mL to administer the dosage.

41. Conversion is required. Conversion factor: 1 000 mg = 1 g. Therefore, 0.5 g = 500 mg.

400 mg : 5 mL = 500 mg : x mL

$$\frac{500 \, \text{mg}}{400 \, \text{mg}} \times 5 \, \text{mL} = x \, \text{mL}$$

Answer: 6.25 = 6.3 mL. The dosage ordered is more than the available strength; therefore, you will need more than 5 mL to administer the dosage.

42. 480 000 units : 5 mL = 500 000 units : x mL

$$\frac{500 \, 000 \, \text{units}}{480 \, 000 \, \text{units}} \times 5 \, \text{mL} = x \, \text{mL}$$

Answer: x = 5.2 mL. The dosage ordered is more than the available strength; therefore, you will need more than 5 mL to administer the dosage.

43. Conversion is required. Conversion factor: 1 g = 1 000 mg.

125 mg : 5 mL = 1 000 mg : x mL

or

$$\frac{1 \, 000 \, \text{mg}}{125 \, \text{mg}} \times 5 \, \text{mL} = x \, \text{mL}$$

Answer: 40 mL. The dosage ordered is more than the available strength; therefore, you will need more than 5 mL to administer the dosage.

44. 250 mg : 5 mL = 500 mg : x mL

$$\frac{500 \, \text{mg}}{250 \, \text{mg}} \times 5 \, \text{mL} = x \, \text{mL}$$

Answer: 10 mL. The dosage ordered is more than the available strength; therefore, you will need more than 5 mL to administer the dosage.

45. $160 \text{ mg} : 5 \text{ mL} = 650 \text{ mg} : x \text{ mL}$

$$\frac{650 \text{ mg}}{160 \text{ mg}} \times 5 \text{ mL} = x \text{ mL}$$

Answer: 20.31 = 20.3 mL. The dosage ordered is four times more than the available strength; therefore, you will need more than 5 mL to administer the dosage.

46. $300 \text{ mg} : 5 \text{ mL} = 400 \text{ mg} : x \text{ mL}$

or

$$\frac{400 \text{ mg}}{300 \text{ mg}} \times 5 \text{ mL} = x \text{ mL}$$

Answer: 6.66 = 6.7 mL to the nearest tenth. The dosage ordered is more than the available strength; therefore, you will need more than 5 mL to administer the dosage.

47. $10 \text{ mg} : 1 \text{ mL} = 150 \text{ mg} : x \text{ mL}$

or

$$\frac{150 \text{ mg}}{10 \text{ mg}} \times 1 \text{ mL} = x \text{ mL}$$

Answer: 15 mL. The dosage ordered is more than the available strength; therefore, you will need more than 1 mL to administer the dosage.

48. Conversion is necessary. Conversion factor: 1 000 mg = 1 g. Therefore, 0.3 g = 300 mg.

$$50 \text{ mg} : 5 \text{ mL} = 300 \text{ mg} : x \text{ mL}$$

or

$$\frac{300 \text{ mg}}{50 \text{ mg}} \times 5 \text{ mL} = x \text{ mL}$$

Answer: 30 mL. The dosage ordered is more than the available strength; therefore, you will need more than 5 mL to administer the dosage.

49. $125 \text{ mg} : 5 \text{ mL} = 375 \text{ mg} : x \text{ mL}$

$$\frac{375 \text{ mg}}{125 \text{ mg}} \times 5 \text{ mL} = x \text{ mL}$$

Answer: 15 mL. The dosage ordered is three times more than the available strength; therefore, you will need more than 5 mL to administer the dosage.

50. $80 \text{ mg} : 1 \text{ mL} = 600 \text{ mg} : x \text{ mL}$

or

$$\frac{600 \text{ mg}}{80 \text{ mg}} \times 1 \text{ mL} = x \text{ mL}$$

Answer: 7.5 mL. The dosage ordered is more than the available strength; therefore, you will need more than 1 mL to administer the dosage.

51. Conversion is necessary. Conversion factor: 1 000 mg = 1 g. Therefore, 0.25 g = 250 mg.

$$200 \text{ mg} : 5 \text{ mL} = 250 \text{ mg} : x \text{ mL}$$
$$\frac{250 \text{ mg}}{200 \text{ mg}} \times 5 \text{ mL} = x \text{ mL}$$

Answer: 6.25 = 6.3 mL. The dosage ordered is more than the available strength; therefore, you will need more than 5 mL to administer the dosage.

52. $20 \text{ mg} : 5 \text{ mL} = 30 \text{ mg} : x \text{ mL}$

or

$$\frac{30 \text{ mg}}{20 \text{ mg}} \times 5 \text{ mL} = x \text{ mL}$$

Answer: 7.5 mL. The dosage ordered is more than the available strength; therefore, you will need more than 5 mL to administer the dosage.

53. $15 \text{ mg} : 1 \text{ mL} = 150 \text{ mg} : x \text{ mL}$

or

$$\frac{150 \text{ mg}}{15 \text{ mg}} \times 1 \text{ mL} = x \text{ mL}$$

Answer: 10 mL. The dosage ordered is 10 times more than the available strength; therefore, you will need more than 1 mL to administer the dosage.

54. $20 \text{ mg} : 1 \text{ mL} = 30 \text{ mg} : x \text{ mL}$

or

$$\frac{30 \text{ mg}}{20 \text{ mg}} \times 1 \text{ mL} = x \text{ mL}$$

Answer: 1.5 mL, the dosage ordered is more than the available strength; therefore, you will need more than 1 mL to administer the dosage.

Answers to Clinical Reasoning Questions

1. a. 6 tablets
   b. Question the order before administering. Double-check your calculation with another nurse. If the order is correct, check with the pharmacist regarding available dosage strengths for the medication. Check a reliable and reputable drug reference for the usual dosage and action of this medication.
   c. Any calculation that requires you to administer more than the maximum number of tablets or capsules, which is usually three, to achieve a single dose should be questioned and rechecked. An unusual number of tablets or capsules should alert the nurse to a possible error in prescribing, transcribing, or calculation.

2. a. After checking a reliable and reputable drug reference for the usual dosage, contact the pharmacist regarding the available dosage strengths for the medication.
   b. The dosage ordered would require that the tablets be broken to administer the dosage. The tablets are unscored and should not be broken. Unscored tablets will not break evenly, and there is no way to determine the dosage being administered. Breaking an unscored tablet could lead to the administration of an unintended dosage.

3. a. The right medication
   b. In preparing the medication, the nurse did not read the label carefully and administered Percodan, the wrong medication, which has a similar spelling to Percocet. By not reading the label carefully, the nurse did not notice that combination medications contain more than one medication; in this case, Percodan contains aspirin. Percocet contained Tylenol.
   c. A medication error occurred because the wrong medication was administered. The patient was allergic to aspirin and could have had a reaction from mild to a severe anaphylactic reaction (dyspnea, airway obstruction, shock, and in some cases death).
   d. The error could have been prevented by carefully reading the medication label three times while preparing the medication. The nurse must use caution when administering medications that look alike or that have similar spellings. Tablets or capsules that contain more than one medication must be read carefully. (Percocet contains acetaminophen [Tylenol] and Percodan contains aspirin.)

✏️ **NOTE**

For Chapter Review problems, only answers are shown. If needed, review the setup of problems in Practice Problems 1–54 if needed.

Answers to Chapter Review

1. 3 caps
2. 20 mL
3. 2 tabs
4. 3 tabs
5. 1 tab
6. 12.5 mL
7. 2 tabs
8. 2 tabs
9. $\frac{1}{2}$ tab
10. 2 tabs
11. 2 mL
12. 19 mL
13. $\frac{1}{2}$ tab
14. 15.6 mL
15. 20 mL
16. 28.1 mL
17. 3 tabs
18. One 2-mg tab and two 0.5-mg tabs
19. 2 tabs
20. 1 tab
21. One 0.3-mg tab and one 0.2-mg tab
22. 1 tab
23. 2 tabs (extended release)
24. 30 mL
25. 2 tablets
26. a. 2 tabs
    b. 14 tabs
27. One 10-mg tab and one 20-mg tab
28. 2 tabs
29. 20 mL
30. One 40-mg tablet
31. 9.4 mL
32. 2 tabs
33. $2\frac{1}{2}$ tabs
34. Three 40-mg capsules
35. 10 mL
36. 100-mg capsules
37. 2 tabs
38. 2 tabs
39. 20 mL
40. 1 tab
41. One 7.5-mg tab and one 2.5-mg tab
42. 2 tabs
43. 1 capsule
44. 2 tabs
45. 2 tabs
46. 10 mL
47. 2 capsules
48. 10 mL
49. Three 5-mg tabs
50. 2 caps (delayed release; enteric coated)

CHAPTER **16**
Parenteral Medications

Objectives

After reviewing this chapter, you should be able to:

1. Identify the various types of syringes used for parenteral administration
2. Read parenteral medication labels and identify dosage strengths
3. Read and measure dosages on syringes
4. Calculate dosages of parenteral medications already in solution
5. Identify the appropriate syringe to administer the dosage based on the dosage calculation

The term *parenteral* is used to indicate medications that are administered by any route other than through the gastrointestinal system. The term *parenteral* is commonly used to refer to the administration of medications by injection with the use of a needle and syringe into body tissue. In this text, use of *parenteral* means injection routes such as intramuscular (IM), subcutaneous (SUBCUT), intradermal (ID), and intravenous (IV):

- **IM**—Injection into a muscle; for example, Demerol is administered IM for pain.
- **SUBCUT**—Injection into subcutaneous tissue; for example, insulin is administered SUBCUT in the management of diabetes.
- **ID**—Injection administered under the skin; for example, tuberculin or mantoux skin test to assess for exposure to tuberculosis is administered ID.
- **IV**—Injection into a vein; medication can be administered directly (IV push) or it can be diluted in a larger volume of IV fluid and infused over a period of time (IV infusion). Antibiotics and other medications may be administered IV.

Medications administered by the parenteral route generally act more quickly than oral medications because they are absorbed more rapidly into the bloodstream. It is important to note that the absorption rates vary for medications administered by this route, and dosages can vary when the same medication is administered by different routes. For example, a medication administered IV will produce the desired effect more rapidly than the same medication administered IM. The parenteral route may be desired when rapid action of a medication is necessary for a patient who is unable to take a medication orally because of emesis (vomiting), has a nonfunctioning gastrointestinal (GI) tract, or is unconscious.

Medications for parenteral use are available as a sterile solution or liquid that can be absorbed and distributed without causing irritation to the tissues. Parenteral medications are also available in powdered form that must be diluted with a liquid or solvent (reconstituted) before it can be used. Reconstitution of medications in powdered form will be covered in Chapter 17.

Packaging of Parenteral Medications

Medications for parenteral use may be packaged in various forms, including ampules, vials, mix-o-vials, cartridges, and prefilled syringes.

- **Ampules.** An ampule is a sealed glass container designed to hold a single dose (for single use) of medication (Figure 16-1). It has a constricted neck that is designed to snap (break) open. The neck of the ampule may be scored or have a darkened line or ring around it to indicate where it should be snapped to withdraw the medication. The neck is snapped off by using a plastic protective sleeve, an alcohol wipe, or sterile gauze. A filter needle (a needle with a filter inside) should always be attached to the syringe to withdraw the medication from the ampule, the filter needle removed, and an appropriate needle used for administration. A filter needle prevents the withdrawal of glass or rubber particulate (Perry, Potter, & Elkin, 2012). The medication is withdrawn into the syringe by gently pulling back on the plunger, which creates a negative pressure and allows the medication to be pulled into the syringe.

- **Vials.** A vial is a plastic or glass container that has a rubber stopper or diaphragm on the top. The rubber stopper is covered with a metal lid or plastic cover to maintain sterility until the vial is used for the first time. Multidose vials contain more than one dose of the medication. Single-dose vials contain a single dose of medication. Many medications are prepared in a single dose to reduce the chance of error. Even if medication is in a single-dose vial, it should still be measured and not just drawn up. The medication in a vial may be in liquid (solution) form (as shown in Figure 16-2), or it may contain a powder that must be reconstituted before administration (as shown in Figure 16-3). Reconstitution is discussed further in Chapter 17.

    In contrast to the ampule, the vial is a closed system. Before a solution can be withdrawn from a vial, the same volume of air must be injected into the vial. For large volumes of solution to be withdrawn, a small volume of air is required to initiate the flow of medication.

> ### (i) TIPS FOR CLINICAL PRACTICE
>
> It is important to note that single-dose vials and ampules contain a little extra medication; it is important to carefully measure the amount of medication to be withdrawn.

- **Mix-o-vials.** Some medications come in a mix-o-vial (Figure 16-4). The mix-o-vial usually contains a single dose of a medication. It has two compartments separated by a rubber stopper. The top compartment contains the sterile liquid (diluent), and the bottom compartment contains the powdered medication. When pressure is applied to the top of the vial, the rubber stopper that separates the medication and liquid is released. This action allows the liquid and medication to be mixed, thereby dissolving the medication (Figure 16-5).

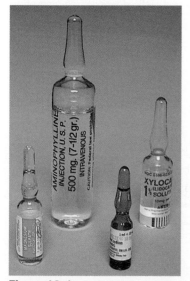

Figure 16-1 Medication in ampules. (From Perry, A. G., Potter, P. A., & Elkin, M. K. (2012). *Nursing interventions and clinical skills* (5th ed.). St. Louis: Mosby.)

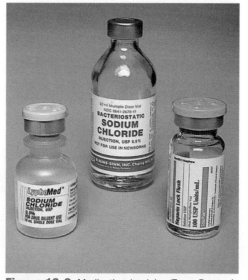

Figure 16-2 Medication in vials. (From Perry, A. G., Potter, P. A., & Elkin, M. K. (2012). *Nursing interventions and clinical skills* (5th ed.). St. Louis: Mosby.)

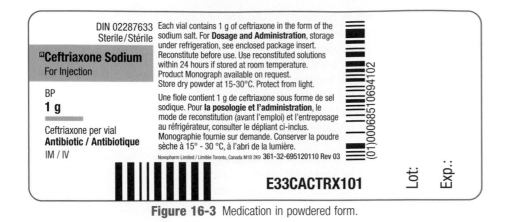

DIN 02287633
Sterile / Stérile

ᴼ**Ceftriaxone Sodium**
For Injection

BP
1 g

Ceftriaxone per vial
Antibiotic / Antibiotique
IM / IV

Each vial contains 1 g of ceftriaxone in the form of the sodium salt. For **Dosage and Administration**, storage under refrigeration, see enclosed package insert. Reconstitute before use. Use reconstituted solutions within 24 hours if stored at room temperature. Product Monograph available on request. Store dry powder at 15-30°C. Protect from light.

Une fiole contient 1 g de ceftriaxone sous forme de sel sodique. Pour **la posologie et l'administration**, le mode de reconstitution (avant l'emploi) et l'entreposage au réfrigérateur, consulter le dépliant ci-inclus. Monographie fournie sur demande. Conserver la poudre sèche à 15° - 30 °C, à l'abri de la lumière.

Novopharm Limited / Limitée Toronto, Canada M1B 2K9   361-32-695120110 Rev 03

(01)00066851069410 2

E33CACTRX101

Lot:

Exp.:

Figure 16-3 Medication in powdered form.

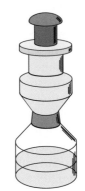

Figure 16-4 Mix-o-vial. (From Clayton, B. D., & Willihnganz, M. (2013). *Basic pharmacology for nurses* (16th ed.). St. Louis: Mosby.)

- **Cartridges.** Some medications are packaged in a prefilled glass or plastic container. The cartridge is clearly marked, indicating the amount of medication in it. Certain cartridges require a special holder called a *Tubex* or *Carpuject* to release the medication from the cartridge. The cartridge contains a single dose of medication. The white plastic portion on the end of the Carpuject (Figure 16-6, *A*) can also be removed, exposing a rubber stopper in which a needle can be inserted to remove calculated amounts.

  If the dosage to administer is less than the amount contained in the unit, discard the unused portion, if any.

- **Prefilled syringes (premeasured).** Some medications come prepared for administration in a prefilled syringe—with or without a needle attached. Prefilled syringes are single-dose syringes that contain a specific amount of medication and are designed to be used only once. The amount desired is calculated, the excess is disposed of (in the presence of another nurse when the medication is a narcotic), and the calculated dosage is administered. EpiPens (Figure 16-6, *B*) and Hepatitis B vaccines are examples of medications that come in a prefilled syringe.

⚠ SAFETY ALERT!

To safely administer the prescribed amount from a cartridge or a prefilled syringe, the amount of medication in excess of what is prescribed should be discarded before administration.

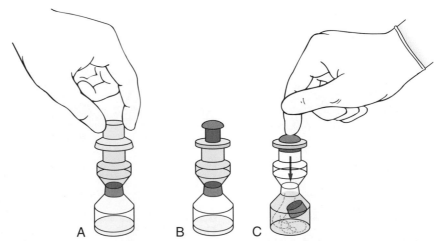

Figure 16-5 Mix-o-vial directions. **A,** Remove plastic lid protector. **B,** Powdered drug is in lower half; diluent is in upper half. **C,** Push firmly on the diaphragm-plunger. Downward pressure dislodges the divider between the two chambers. (Modified from Clayton, B. D., & Willihnganz, M. (2013). *Basic pharmacology for nurses* (16th ed.). St. Louis: Mosby.)

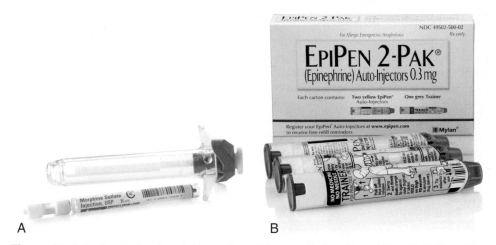

Figure 16-6 A, Carpuject syringe holder and needleless, prefilled sterile cartridge. **B,** EpiPen 2-Pak. (**A,** From Hospira, Inc., Lake Forest, IL. **B,** From Mylan Specialty L.P., Basking Ridge, NJ.)

Syringes

Syringes are available in various sizes with different capacities and calibration. Syringes are made of plastic or glass, but plastic syringes are more commonly used. They are disposable and designed for one-time use only. Syringes have three parts (Figure 16-7):

1. **The barrel:** The outer calibrated portion that holds the medication. It has calibration markings on the outer portion.
2. **The plunger:** The inner device that is moved backward to withdraw and measure the medication and is pushed to eject the medication from the syringe. The plunger fits into the barrel.
3. **The tip:** The end of the syringe that holds the needle. The tip can be plain (slip tip) or Luer-Lok (Figure 16-8).

Syringes are classified as Luer-Lok or non–Luer-Lok (have a slip tip). Both are disposable and designed for one-time use. Luer-Lok syringes require special needles that are twisted onto the tip and lock themselves in place, which prevents inadvertent removal of the needle. Non–Luer-Lok syringes require needles that slip onto the tip (Potter, Perry, Stockert, et al., 2013). The needle fits onto the tip of the syringe. Needles come in various lengths and diameters. The nurse chooses the needle according to the patient's size, the type of tissue being injected into, and the viscosity of the medication to be injected. Some syringes also come with a needle attached that cannot be detached from the syringe.

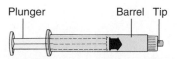

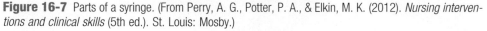

Figure 16-7 Parts of a syringe. (From Perry, A. G., Potter, P. A., & Elkin, M. K. (2012). *Nursing interventions and clinical skills* (5th ed.). St. Louis: Mosby.)

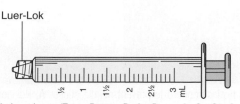

Figure 16-8 3-mL Luer-Lok syringe. (From Potter, P. A., Perry, A. G., Stockert, P., et al. (2013). *Fundamentals of nursing* (9th ed.). St. Louis: Mosby.)

Safety Needles and Needleless Syringes

It is important to note that needle-stick prevention has become increasingly important to avoid the transmission of blood-borne infections from contaminated needles. Consequently, special prevention techniques (e.g., no recapping of a needle after use) and special equipment (e.g., syringes with a sheath or guard that covers the needle after it is withdrawn from the skin) have been developed to decrease the chance of needle-stick injury (Figure 16-9). Another advancement in safety needle technology is the safety glide syringe, which contains a protective needle guard that can be activated by a single finger to cover and seal the needle after injection (Figure 16-10). Needleless syringe systems have also been designed to prevent needle sticks. They may be used to withdraw medication from a vial and to add medication to an IV for medication administration (Figure 16-11).

> **! SAFETY ALERT!**
>
> Protection from needle-stick injuries requires that needles never be recapped and always be correctly disposed of in special puncture-resistant containers.

Types of Syringes

The three types of syringes are hypodermic, tuberculin, and insulin.

Hypodermic Syringes. Hypodermic syringes come in a variety of sizes, from 0.5 to 60 millilitres (mL) and larger. Syringes are calibrated (or marked) in millilitres but hold varying capacities. Of the small-capacity syringes, the 3-mL syringe is used most often for the administration of medication doses that are more than 1 mL; however, hypodermic syringes are also available in larger sizes (10 mL, 20 mL, 50 mL, and larger). Figure 16-12 shows a 3-mL and a 1-mL syringe.

> **! SAFETY ALERT!**
>
> It is critical that the calibration (or scale) on a small hypodermic be read carefully. Misreading the calibration could lead to a medication error.

For small hypodermics, decimal numbers are used to express dosages (e.g., 1.2 mL, 0.3 mL). Notice that small hypodermics up to 3 mL in size also have fractions on them (see Figure 16-12, *A*). However, some syringes indicate 0.5 mL, 1.5 mL, etc., instead of fractions. The use of decimals on syringes correlates with the use of decimals in the metric system; therefore, a dosage should be stated in millilitres as a decimal.

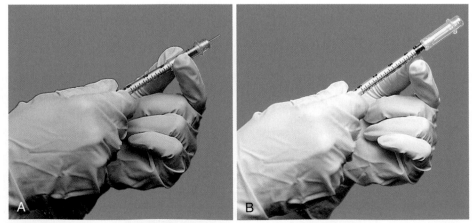

Figure 16-9 Needle with plastic guard to prevent needle sticks. **A,** Position of guard before injection. **B,** After injection the guard locks in place, covering the needle. (From Perry, A. G., Potter, P. A., & Elkin, M. K. (2012). *Nursing interventions and clinical skills* (5th ed.). St. Louis: Mosby.)

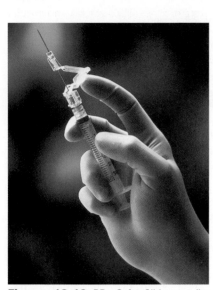

Figure 16-10 BD SafetyGlide needle. (Courtesy and © Becton, Dickinson, and Company, Franklin Lakes, NJ.)

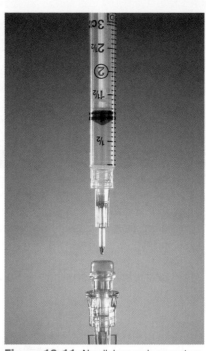

Figure 16-11 Needleless syringe system. (Courtesy and © Becton, Dickinson, and Company, Franklin Lakes, NJ.)

Notice in Figure 16-12, *A* (3-mL syringe) the side that indicates mL. There are 10 spaces between the largest markings. This spacing indicates that the syringe is marked in tenths of a millilitre. Each of the lines is 0.1 mL. The longer lines indicate half (0.5) and full millilitre measures.

In Figure 16-12, *B*, the 1-mL syringe is marked in hundredths (0.01) of a millilitre and tenths (0.1) of a millilitre. Each of the small lines is 0.01 mL, with the slightly longer lines equal to 0.05, 0.1, 0.15, 0.2, and so on.

When looking at the syringe shown in Figure 16-13, notice the rubber ring. When you are measuring medication and reading the medication withdrawn, the forward edge of the plunger head indicates the amount of medication withdrawn. Do not become confused by the second, bottom ring or by the raised section (middle) of the suction tip. The point where the rubber plunger edge makes contact with the barrel is the spot that should be lined up with the amount desired.

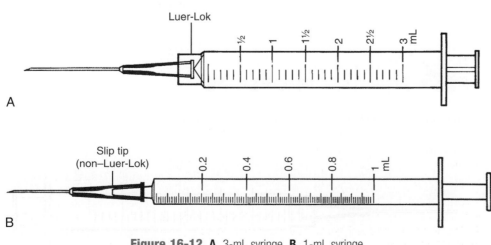

Figure 16-12 **A,** 3-mL syringe. **B,** 1-mL syringe.

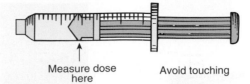

Measure dose here   Avoid touching

Figure 16-13 Reading measured amount of medication in a syringe. (From Potter, P. A., Perry, A. G., Stockert, P., et al. (2013). *Fundamentals of nursing* (9th ed.). St. Louis: Mosby.)

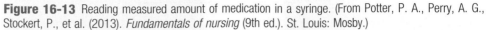

SAFETY ALERT!

Understanding the calibration on a syringe is critical to accurately measure a medication dose. The calibration on a syringe can differ depending on the size of the syringe. Check the calibration of the syringe you are using carefully. If medication is not accurately measured, an incorrect dosage can be administered, resulting in serious consequences to the patient.

Let's examine the syringes that follow to illustrate specific amounts in a syringe.

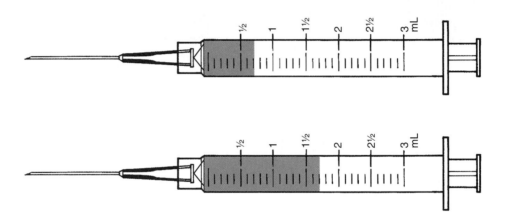

Because the small-capacity syringes are used most often to administer medications, it is very important to know how to read them to withdraw amounts accurately.

POINTS TO REMEMBER

- Small-capacity hypodermics are calibrated in millilitres; the 3-mL syringe is used most often to administer dosages that are between 1 mL and 3 mL. Dosages administered with them must correlate to the calibration.
- Syringes are labelled with the abbreviation mL, which is the measurement for volume.

+−÷× PRACTICE **PROBLEMS**

Shade in the indicated amounts on the syringes in millilitres.

1. 0.8 mL

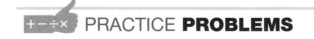

2. 1.2 mL

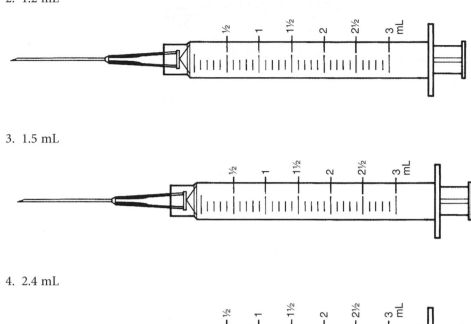

3. 1.5 mL

4. 2.4 mL

Indicate the number of millilitres shaded in on the following syringes.

5.

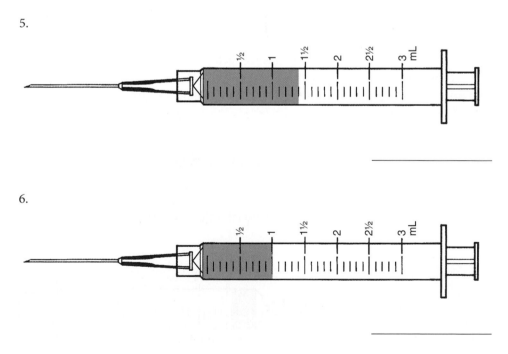

_____

6.

_____

7.

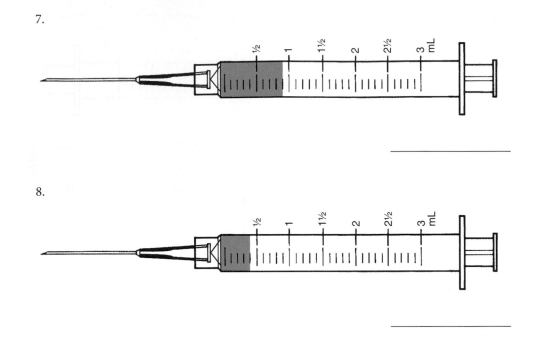

8.

Answers on pages 408–409.

Large Capacity Syringes. Large hypodermics (5, 6, 10, and 12 mL) are used when volumes that are more than 3 mL are desired. These syringes are used to measure whole numbers of millilitres as opposed to smaller units such as a tenth of a millilitre. Syringes that are 5, 6, 10, or 12 mL in size are calibrated in increments of fifths of a millilitre (0.2 mL), with the whole numbers indicated by long lines. Figure 16-14, *A,* shows 0.8 mL of medication measured in a 5-mL syringe, and Figure 16-14, *B,* shows 7.8 mL measured in a 10-mL syringe. Syringes that are 20 mL and larger are calibrated in whole millilitre increments and can have other measurements, such as ounces, on them.

Large hypodermics (5, 6, 10, 12 mL, and even higher) are commonly used to prepare medications for IV administration. These syringes are sometimes referred to as *intravenous syringes.*

> ### TIPS FOR CLINICAL PRACTICE
>
> The larger the syringe, the larger the calibration. Example: In 5-mL and 10-mL syringes, each shorter calibration measures two tenths of a millilitre (0.2 mL). To be safe, always examine the calibration of the syringes available and use the one best suited for the volume to be administered.

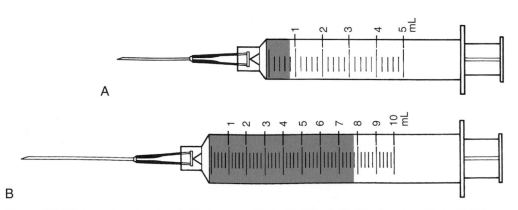

A

B

Figure 16-14 Large hypodermics. **A,** 5-mL syringe filled with 0.8 mL. **B,** 10-mL syringe filled with 7.8 mL.

PRACTICE **PROBLEMS**

Indicate the number of millilitres shaded in on the following syringes.

9.

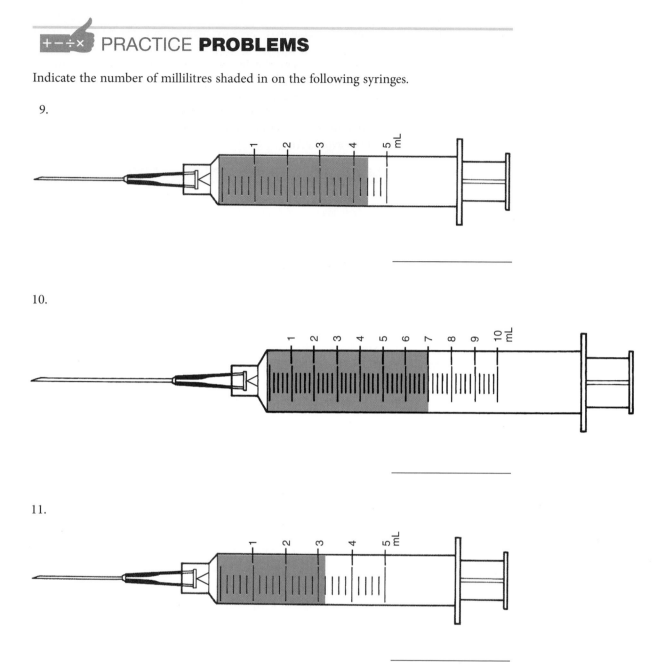

10.

11.

_____

Answers on page 409.

Tuberculin Syringes. A tuberculin syringe is a narrow syringe that has a capacity of 0.5 mL or 1 mL. The 1 mL size is used most often. The volume of a tuberculin syringe can be measured on the millilitre scale. The syringe is calibrated in hundredths (0.01 mL) and tenths (0.1 mL) of a millilitre. The markings on the syringe are closer together to indicate how small the calibration is (Figure 16-15).

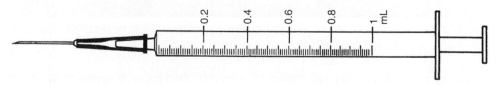

Figure 16-15 Tuberculin syringe. (From Potter, P. A., Perry, A. G., Stockert, P., et al. (2013). *Fundamentals of nursing* (9th ed.). St. Louis: Mosby.)

Tuberculin syringes are used to accurately measure medications given in very small volumes (e.g., heparin). This syringe is also often used in pediatrics and for diagnostic purposes (e.g., skin testing for tuberculosis). Vaccines are also administered using a tuberculin syringe. It is recommended that dosages less than 0.5 mL be measured with a tuberculin syringe to make certain that the correct dosage is administered to a patient. Dosages such as 0.42 mL and 0.37 mL can be measured accurately with a tuberculin syringe. Measuring the correct dosage with a tuberculin syringe requires extreme care. Read the markings on the syringe carefully to avoid error.

> **(!) SAFETY ALERT!**
> Be careful when measuring medications in a syringe. Being off by even a small amount on the syringe scale can be critical. The syringe you use to administer medication must provide the calibration you need to accurately measure the dose.

Insulin Syringes. Insulin syringes are used for the subcutaneous injection of insulin and are calibrated in units rather than millilitres. Insulin is measured in units and always ordered in units. Insulin syringes marked with "U-100" indicate that they are calibrated for administration of U-100 insulin only. The most common strength of insulin is 100 units per mL, which is referred to as "units 100" insulin and is abbreviated as "U-100."

> **(!) SAFETY ALERT!**
> The insulin syringe marked "U-100" is used for the administration of U-100 insulin only. "U-100" insulin indicates that the strength of insulin is 100 units per mL. Never measure other medications measured in units in an insulin syringe.

There are two types of insulin syringes: Lo-Dose U-100 and standard U-100 insulin syringes. Lo-Dose insulin syringes have 50- or 30-unit capacities. They should be used for small doses of insulin (50 units or less) because they more accurately measure these doses. **A 50-unit Lo-Dose insulin syringe** has a capacity of 50 units. It is calibrated in 1-unit increments up to 50 units per 0.5 mL (Figure 16-16, *B*).

A **30-unit Lo-Dose insulin syringe** has a capacity of 30 units. It is used to administer doses of less than 30 units. The 30-unit Lo-Dose insulin syringe is calibrated in 1-unit increments or 30 units per 0.3 mL. The 30-unit insulin syringe is commonly used in pediatrics (Figure 16-16, *C*).

The **standard U-100 insulin syringe** has a capacity of 100 units of insulin per millilitre. A single-scaled standard 100-unit insulin syringe is calibrated in 2-unit increments (Figure 16-16, *A*). To avoid error in measurement, an odd number of units (e.g., 27 units) should not be prepared with this type of syringe.

The standard U-100 insulin syringe is also available in a **dual-scale** version, which is calibrated in 2-unit increments. It has a scale with even-numbered 2-unit increments (2, 4, etc.) on one side and a scale with odd-numbered 2-unit increments (1, 3, etc.) on the other. The best way to use this type of syringe is to measure odd-numbered doses on the scale with the odd-numbered calibration and to measure even-numbered doses on the scale with the even-numbered calibration (Figure 16-17). For insulin, it is not necessary to use the methods of calculation presented because the insulin syringe is designed to measure insulin dosages. Reading insulin syringes and being attentive to their calibration is an essential skill for safety. Insulin dosages are discussed in more detail in Chapter 18.

> **(✎) NOTE**
> Insulin syringes do not have detachable needles. The needle, hub, and barrel are inseparable.

> **(!) SAFETY ALERT!**
> Insulin is a high-alert medication. All hospitals have a policy for insulin to be independently double-checked by another nurse before administration to a patient.

Before proceeding to the calculation of parenteral dosages, it is necessary to review parenteral labels. Understanding these labels and which information is essential are important in determining the correct dosage to administer.

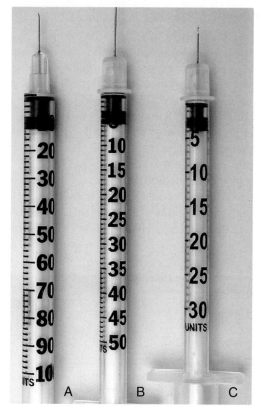

Figure 16-16 Insulin syringes. **A,** 1-mL size (100 units). **B,** Lo-Dose (50 units). **C,** Lo-Dose (30 units). (From Macklin, D., Chernecky, L., & Infortuna, H. (2011). *Math for clinical practice* (2nd ed.). St. Louis: Mosby.)

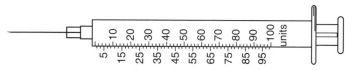

Figure 16-17 1-mL capacity insulin syringe (100 units) with dual-scale odd- and even-numbered calibration. (Courtesy and © Becton, Dickinson, and Company, Franklin Lakes, NJ.)

POINTS TO REMEMBER

- When parenteral medications are prepared for administration, it is important to use the correct syringe for accurate administration of the dosage.
- Medications are prepared and labelled with the dosage strength given per millilitre (mL). Small-capacity hypodermic syringes are marked in tenths of a millilitre (0.1 mL). The 3-mL size is used most often to administer medication volumes greater than 1 mL.
- Hypodermic syringes—5, 6, 10, and 12 mL—are marked in increments of 0.2 mL and 1 mL.
- Hypodermic syringes—20 mL and larger—are marked in 1-mL increments and may have other markings, such as ounces.
- Tuberculin syringes or 1-mL syringes are small syringes marked in tenths and hundredths of a millilitre. They are used to administer small dosages and are recommended for use with a dosage that is less than 0.5 mL.
- Insulin syringes marked with "U-100" are calibrated for administration of U-100 insulin only.
- Insulin is measured in units and should be administered only with an insulin syringe.
- The insulin syringe and the tuberculin syringe are different. Confusion of the two can cause a medication error.
- Dosages in millilitres should be expressed as decimals even when the syringe is marked with fractions.
- If the dosage of a medication cannot be accurately measured, it should not be administered.

Reading Parenteral Labels

The information on a parenteral label is similar to the information on an oral liquid label. A parenteral label contains the total volume of the container and the dosage strength (amount of medication in solution) expressed in millilitres. Table 16-1 presents sample dosage strengths written on labels and their interpretation. Read parenteral labels carefully to determine the dosage strength and volume. Let's examine some labels.

The ranitidine label in Figure 16-18 indicates that the total size of the vial is 2 mL and that the dosage strength is 25 milligrams (mg) per mL. The medroxyprogesterone (Depo-Provera) label in Figure 16-19 indicates that the total vial size is 5 mL and that the dosage strength is 50 mg per mL.

Dosage strengths for parenteral medications are commonly expressed as the amount of medication contained in a volume of solution (in millilitres). Parenteral labels can also express the dosage strength for medications in percentages, ratios, units, millimoles (mmol), or milliequivalents (mEq). Read labels carefully to identify the unit of measurement as well as the dosage strength.

TABLE 16-1 Sample Dosage Strengths	
Label	**Interpretation**
Diazepam 5 mg/mL	1 mL contains 5 mg of diazepam
Naloxone 0.4 mg/mL	1 mL contains 0.4 mg of naloxone
Digoxin 500 mcg/2 mL	2 mL contains 500 mcg of digoxin

Note: The slash (/) mark is used here to illustrate the expression of the dosage strength as written on labels. When expressing dosage strengths, do not use the slash mark. Use *per*. Note that "per mL" is recommended by the Institute for Safe Medication Practices Canada (ISMP Canada) because the slash mark has been mistaken for the number 1.

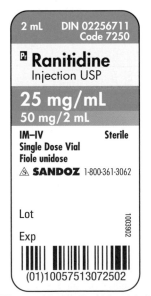

Figure 16-18 Ranitidine label.

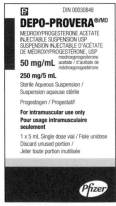

Figure 16-19 Depo-Provera label.

PRACTICE **PROBLEMS**

Use the labels provided to answer the questions.

12. Use the aminophylline label to answer the following questions:

   a. What is the total volume of the ampule? _____

   b. What is the dosage strength? _____

   c. If 250 mg was ordered, how many
      mL would need to be administered? _____

DIN: 00582662 10 mL Code: L0010021 Sterile / Stérile ℞ **AMINOPHYLLINE INJECTION USP** omega **250 mg/10 mL (25 mg/mL)**	**BRONCHODILATOR** **Slow IV injection** **Single Use Vial.** **Each mL contains:** 25 mg of Aminophylline (equivalent to 21.4 mg anhydrous Theophylline). Osmolarity of solution is 0.18 mOsmol/mL and pH between 8.6 and 9.0. Leaflet should be consulted for detailed directions. Protect from light. Store between 15 and 30°C. LOT: EXP:	**BRONCHODILATATEUR** **Injection IV lente** **Fiole à usage unique.** **Chaque mL contient** : 25 mg d'aminophylline (équivalent à 21,4 mg de théophylline anhydre). L'osmolarité de la solution est de 0,18 mOsmol/mL et son pH se situe entre 8,6 et 9,0. Consulter le feuillet pour des directives plus détaillées. Protéger de la lumière. Conserver entre 15 et 30°C. CODE 1021 / V-02 omega Montreal, Canada H3M 3A2 (01)10801500110216

13. Use the lorazepam label to answer the following questions:

   a. What is the total volume of the vial? _____

   b. What is the dosage strength? _____

   c. What is the route of administration? _____

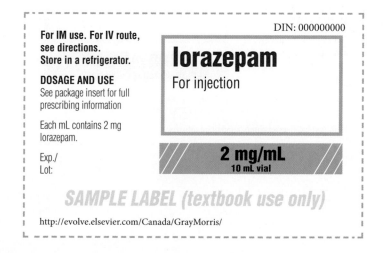

**For IM use. For IV route,
see directions.
Store in a refrigerator.**

DOSAGE AND USE
See package insert for full
prescribing information

Each mL contains 2 mg
lorazepam.

Exp./
Lot:

DIN: 000000000

lorazepam
For injection

2 mg/mL
10 mL vial

SAMPLE LABEL (textbook use only)

http://evolve.elsevier.com/Canada/GrayMorris/

14. Use the chlorpromazine hydrochloride label to answer the following questions:

   a. What is the total volume of the vial? _____

   b. What is the dosage strength? _____

   c. If 50 mg was ordered, how many mL would need to be administered? _____

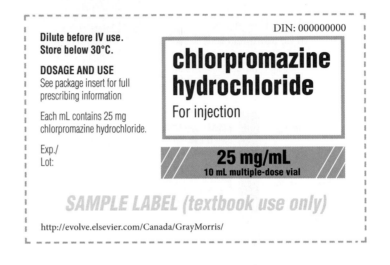

Dilute before IV use.
Store below 30°C.

DOSAGE AND USE
See package insert for full prescribing information

Each mL contains 25 mg chlorpromazine hydrochloride.

Exp./
Lot:

DIN: 000000000

chlorpromazine hydrochloride

For injection

25 mg/mL
10 mL multiple-dose vial

SAMPLE LABEL (textbook use only)

http://evolve.elsevier.com/Canada/GrayMorris/

15. Use the trimethobenzamide hydrochloride label to answer the following questions:

   a. What is the total volume of the vial? _____

   b. What is the dosage strength? _____

   c. If 50 mg was ordered, how many millilitres would need to be administered? _____

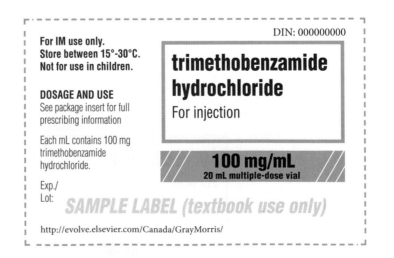

For IM use only.
Store between 15°-30°C.
Not for use in children.

DOSAGE AND USE
See package insert for full prescribing information

Each mL contains 100 mg trimethobenzamide hydrochloride.

Exp./
Lot:

DIN: 000000000

trimethobenzamide hydrochloride

For injection

100 mg/mL
20 mL multiple-dose vial

SAMPLE LABEL (textbook use only)

http://evolve.elsevier.com/Canada/GrayMorris/

16. Use the leuprolide acetate label to answer the following questions:

    a. What is the total volume of the vial? _____

    b. What is the dosage strength? _____

    c. What is the route of administration? _____

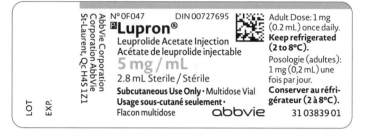

17. Use the hydromorphone label to answer the following questions:

    a. What is the total volume of the vial? _____

    b. What is the dosage strength? _____

    c. What does the scheduling symbol indicate
       for this medication type? _____

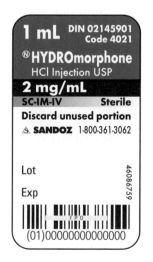

18. Use the Humira label to answer the following questions:

    a. What is the route of administration? _____

    b. What is the dosage strength? _____

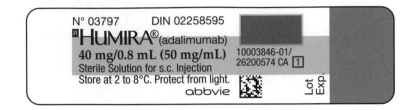

N° 03797   DIN 02258595
HUMIRA®(adalimumab)
40 mg/0.8 mL (50 mg/mL)
Sterile Solution for s.c. Injection
Store at 2 to 8°C. Protect from light.
abbvie
10003846-01/
26200574 CA [1]
Lot
Exp.

19. Use the furosemide label to answer the following questions:

    a. What is the total volume of the vial? _____

    b. What is the dosage strength? _____

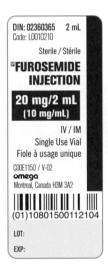

DIN: 02360365   2 mL
Code: L0010210
Sterile / Stérile
**FUROSEMIDE
INJECTION**
20 mg/2 mL
(10 mg/mL)
IV / IM
Single Use Vial
Fiole à usage unique
CODE1150 / V-02
omega
Montreal, Canada H3M 3A2
(01)10801500112104
LOT:
EXP:

20. Use the Diflucan label to answer the following questions:

    a. What is the dosage strength?   _____

    b. What is the route of administration?   _____

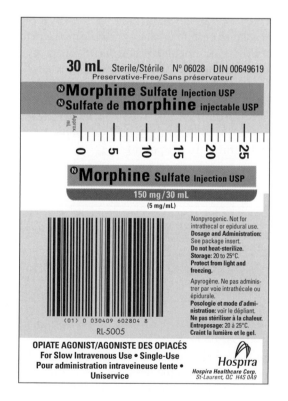

21. Use the morphine sulfate label to answer the following questions:

    a. What is the total volume of the ampule?   _____

    b. What is the dosage strength?   _____

22. Use the amiodarone label to answer the following questions:

  a. What is the total volume of the vial? _____

  b. What is the dosage strength? _____

  c. What is the route of administration? _____

3 mL DIN 02242325 Code 1282 **℞ Amiodarone** HCl Injection Sandoz Standard 50 mg/mL **150 mg/3 mL** *Sterile* IV infusion only Perfusion IV seulement ⚠ **SANDOZ**	Single Use Vial. Must be diluted. Fiole à usage unique. Doit être dilué. Sandoz Canada Inc. 1-800-361-3062 1003977 (01)10057513012829 Lot Exp

Answers on page 409.

Parenteral Medications Labelled in Percentage Strength

Medications that are labelled in percentage strength indicate the percentage of the solution and the total volume of the vial or ampule. Although percentage is used to indicate dosage strength on the label, an expression of the dosage strength in metric measurement is also included. For example, notice that the label for lidocaine 1% that follows also states that there are 10 mg per mL. As discussed in Chapter 4, a percentage solution is the number of grams (g) of solute (the medication) per 100 mL of diluent (the solution). In the lidocaine label shown, lidocaine 1% contains 1 g of medication per 100 mL of solution, 1 g per 100 mL = 1 000 mg per 100 mL = 10 mg per mL.

20 mL Vial Sterile/Stérile Nº 04276   DIN 00884154   **Lidocaine**   **Hydrochloride** Injection USP   **1%**   **200 mg/ 20 mL**   (10 mg/mL)   **For Infiltration and Nerve Block**   Multidose • With Preservative • Latex-Free   Not for Epidural or Caudal Use • Nonpyrogenic   **Each mL contains:** Lidocaine HCl 10 mg, methylparaben 1 mg (preservative), sodium chloride and water for injection. May contain HCl and/or NaOH (pH adjustment). **Storage:** 20 to 25°C. **Protect from freezing.**   Ne pas utiliser pour un blocage caudal ou épidural • Apyrogène   **Chaque mL contient:** chlorhydrate de lidocaïne 10 mg, méthylparabène 1 mg (préservateur), chlorure de sodium et eau pour préparations injectables. Peut contenir du HCl et/ou du NaOH (pour l'ajustement du pH). **Entreposage:** 20 à 25°C. **Craint le gel.**   RL-4383   *Montréal, QC H4M 2X6*   **Hospira**

Often no calculation is necessary when medications expressed in percentage strength are given. The prescriber usually states the number of millilitres to prepare or the number of ampules or vials to administer. For example, calcium gluconate 10% may be ordered as "Administer 1 vial of 10% calcium gluconate or 10 mL of 10% calcium gluconate" (see the label that follows).

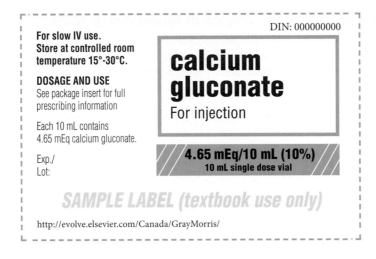

Parenteral Medications Labelled in Ratio Strength

A medication commonly expressed in terms of ratio strength is epinephrine. Medications that are labelled in ratio strength also include an expression of dosage strength in metric measurement (and are often ordered by number of millilitres). For example, notice that the label for epinephrine that follows states 1:1000 and indicates 1 mg per mL. Ratio strength solutions, as discussed in Chapter 3, express the number of grams of the medication per total millilitres of solution. Epinephrine 1:1000 contains 1 g of medication per 1000 mL solution, 1 g:1000 mL = 1000 mg:1000 mL = 1 mg:1 mL.

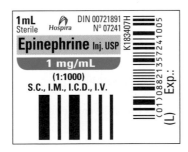

Parenteral Medications Labelled in Units

Some medications measured in units for parenteral administration are heparin, Pitocin, insulin, and penicillin (see the heparin and insulin labels that follow). Notice that labels for medications measured in units indicate the number of units per millilitre; for example, Apidra 100 units per mL, heparin 1000 units per mL. Units express the amount of medication present in 1 mL of solution, and they are specific to the medication used. Units measure a medication in terms of its action.

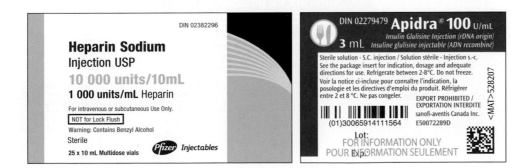

Parenteral Medications Labelled in Millimoles or Milliequivalents

Potassium and sodium bicarbonate are medications that are typically expressed in millimoles. Like units, millimoles are specific measurements that have no conversion to another system and are specific to the medication used. Millimoles are used to measure electrolytes (e.g., potassium) and the ionic activity of a medication. One millimole is equal to one thousandth ($\frac{1}{1000}$) of a gram-molecule. This definition is often used by a chemist or pharmacist.

As noted in Chapter 5, milliequivalents are also used to measure electrolytes and may still be seen on medication labels (but the preferred measurement for electrolytes in Canada is millimoles). (See the potassium chloride label that follows.)

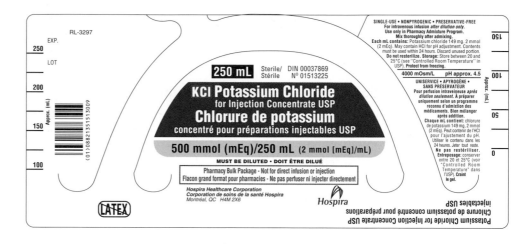

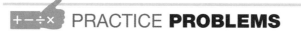 PRACTICE **PROBLEMS**

Use the labels provided to answer the questions.

23. Use the potassium chloride label to answer the following questions:

    a. What is the total volume of the vial?　　　　　　＿＿＿＿＿＿＿＿

    b. What is the dosage in mmol per mL?　　　　　　＿＿＿＿＿＿＿＿

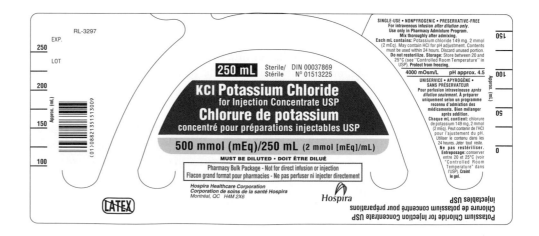

24. Use the sodium chloride label to answer the following questions:

    a. What is the total volume of the vial?   _____

    b. What is the dosage strength expressed in mmol per mL?   _____

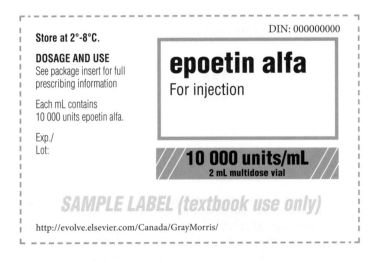

DIN: 00402230   30 mL
Code: L0010004

Sterile / Stérile

SODIUM CHLORIDE INJECTION USP 23.4%

CHLORURE DE SODIUM INJECTION USP 23,4 %

omega **120 mEq/30 mL**
       (4 mEq/mL)

CONCENTRATE / CONCENTRÉ

INTRAUTERINE / INTRAVENOUS, DILUTE BEFORE USE.

Single Use Vial
Discard unused portion.

Hypertonic Solution
120 mmol/30 mL (4 mmol/mL)
Osmolarity: 8 mOsmol/mL

Store between 15 and 30°C.

LOT:

EXP:

INTRA-UTÉRINE / INTRAVEINEUSE, DILUER AVANT USAGE.

Fiole à usage unique
Jeter toute partie inutilisée.

Solution hypertonique
120 mmol/30 mL (4 mmol/mL)
Osmolarité : 8 mOsmol/mL

Conserver entre 15 et 30°C.

C00E1004 / V-02   LATEX

omega
Montreal, Canada H3M 3E4

(01)10801500110049

25. Use the epoetin alfa label to answer the following questions:

    a. What is the total volume of the vial?   _____

    b. What is the dosage strength?   _____

DIN: 000000000

Store at 2°-8°C.

DOSAGE AND USE
See package insert for full prescribing information

Each mL contains 10 000 units epoetin alfa.

Exp./
Lot:

epoetin alfa
For injection

10 000 units/mL
2 mL multidose vial

SAMPLE LABEL (textbook use only)

http://evolve.elsevier.com/Canada/GrayMorris/

26. Use the insulin label to answer the following questions:

    a. What is the total volume of the vial? _____

    b. What is the dosage strength? _____

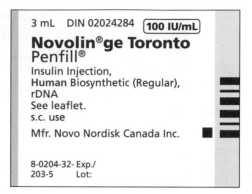

27. Use the oxytocin label to answer the following questions:

    a. What is the total volume of the vial? _____

    b. What is the dosage strength? _____

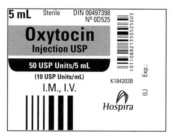

Answers on page 409.

> ## TIPS FOR CLINICAL PRACTICE
>
> Read the labels on parenteral medications carefully. Labels on parenteral medications include a variety of units to express dosage strengths. To calculate dosages to administer, it is important to know the strength of the medication in solution per millilitre. Confusing dosage strength with total volume can lead to a medication error.

Calculating Parenteral Dosages

As previously stated, parenteral dosages can be calculated by using the same rules and methods used to calculate oral dosages. The ratio and proportion method, the formula method, and the dimensional analysis method have been presented in earlier chapters. The following guidelines will help you calculate a dosage that is logical, reasonable, and accurate.

Guidelines for Calculating Parenteral Dosages

To calculate parenteral dosages, convert if necessary, **THINK,** and calculate using one of the methods presented (ratio and proportion, the formula method, or dimensional analysis).

When calculating and preparing an injectable dosage, keep the following in mind:

- The 3-mL syringe is calibrated in 0.1-mL increments. Round millilitres to the nearest tenth when measuring using a 3-mL syringe; **never round to a whole unit.** If a dosage calculation does not work out evenly to the tenths place, then carry division to the hundredths place (two decimal places) and round to the nearest tenth.

Example: 1.75 mL = 1.8 mL

- The 1-mL (tuberculin syringe) is calibrated in 0.01 mL increments. If the math calculation does not work out evenly to the hundredths place, then the division is carried to the thousandths place and rounded to the hundredths place.

Example: 0876 mL = 0.88 mL. It is recommended that dosages less than 0.5 mL be measured with a 1-mL syringe.

- Large syringes (5, 6, 10, and 12 mL) are calibrated in 0.2-mL increments. Dosages are also expressed to the nearest tenth.
- Dosages should be measured in millilitres, and the answer should be labelled accordingly.
- Insulin is measured and administered in units.

For injectable medications, there are guidelines on the amount of medication that can be administered in a single site. When the amount to administer exceeds the amount that can be administered in a single site, divide the amount into two injections. When administering medications by injection, the condition of the patient, the site selected, and the absorption and consistency of the medication must be considered. Depending on his or her condition, a patient may not be able to tolerate the maximum dosage volume.

> **⚠ SAFETY ALERT!**
>
> When the dosage for parenteral administration exceeds the guidelines of volume that can be administered in a single injection site, it should be questioned and the calculation double-checked. Perhaps a higher dosage strength is available, so check with the prescriber. A dosage that is larger than the maximum volume is rare and can cause harm to the patient.

Intramuscular

The maximum volume to administer in a single intramuscular site is as follows:

- Average-sized adult = 3 mL (for deltoid muscle, 1 mL)
- Children ages 6 to 12 years = 2 mL
- Children ages 0 to 5 years = 1 mL

It should be noted that IM injections are less common in the clinical setting than in the past.

Subcutaneous

The maximum volume to administer in a single subcutaneous site for an adult is 1 mL.

Intravenous

Injectable solutions that are added to an IV solution may have a volume of more than 5 mL.

> **ⓘ TIPS FOR CLINICAL PRACTICE**
>
> It is critical to choose the correct size syringe to ensure accurate measurement.

Calculating Injectable Medications According to the Syringe

Now that you have an understanding of syringes and guidelines, let's begin calculating dosages.

Regardless of what method you use to calculate, apply the following steps:

1. Check to make sure the desired dosage and dosage on hand are in the same system and unit of measurement.
2. Think critically about what the answer should logically be before you calculate.
3. Consider the type of syringe to use. **The cardinal rule should always be that any dosage given must be able to be measured accurately in the syringe you are using.**
4. Solve using the ratio and proportion method, the formula method, or the dimensional analysis method.

Let's look at some sample problems calculating parenteral dosages.

Example: Order: Gentamicin 75 mg IM q8h.

Available: Gentamicin labelled 40 mg per mL

Note: No conversion is necessary. Think: The dosage ordered is going to be more than 1 mL but less than 2 mL. Set up the problem and solve.

✔ Solution Using Ratio and Proportion

$$40 \, \text{mg} : 1 \, \text{mL} = 75 \, \text{mg} : x \, \text{mL}$$

$$\frac{40x}{40} = \frac{75}{40}$$

$$x = 1.87 = 1.9 \, \text{mL}$$

The answer here is rounded to the nearest tenth of a millilitre. Remember that you are using a small hypodermic syringe marked in tenths of a millilitre.

✔ Solution Using the Formula Method

$$\frac{(D) \, 75 \, \text{mg}}{(H) \, 40 \, \text{mg}} \times (Q) \, 1 \, \text{mL} = x \, \text{mL}$$

$$x = \frac{75}{40} \times 1$$

$$x = 1.87 = 1.9 \, \text{mL}$$

✔ Solution Using Dimensional Analysis

$$x \, \text{mL} = \frac{1 \, \text{mL}}{40 \, \cancel{\text{mg}}} \times \frac{75 \, \cancel{\text{mg}}}{1}$$

$$x = \frac{75}{40}$$

$$x = 1.87 = 1.9 \, \text{mL}$$

This syringe shows 1.9 mL drawn up:

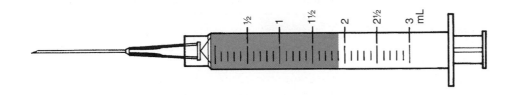

Example: Order: Ceftriaxone 0.25 g IM stat q12h.

Available: Ceftriaxone labelled 350 mg per 1 mL

In this problem, a conversion is necessary. Conversion factor: 1 000 mg = 1 g. Convert what is ordered to what is available: 0.25 g = 250 mg.
Think: The dosage you will need to give is less than 1 mL, and it is being given intramuscularly. Therefore, the dosage should fall within the range that is safe for IM administration. The solution, after making the necessary conversion, follows.

✔ Solution Using Ratio and Proportion

$$350 \text{ mg} : 1 \text{ mL} = 250 \text{ mg} : x \text{ mL}$$

$$\frac{350x}{350} = \frac{250}{350}$$

$$x = \frac{250}{350}$$

$$x = 0.71 = 0.7 \text{ mL}$$

✔ Solution Using the Formula Method

$$\frac{(D) 250 \text{ mg}}{(H) 350 \text{ mg}} \times (Q) 1 \text{ mL} = x \text{ mL}$$

$$x = \frac{250}{350} \times 1$$

$$x = 0.71 = 0.7 \text{ mL}$$

✔ Solution Using Dimensional Analysis

$$x \text{ mL} = \frac{1 \text{ ml}}{350 \text{ mg}} \times \frac{1\,000 \text{ mg}}{1 \text{ g}} \times \frac{0.25 \text{ g}}{1}$$

$$x = \frac{1\,000 \times 0.25}{350}$$

$$x = \frac{250}{350}$$

$$x = 0.71 = 0.7 \text{ mL}$$

This syringe shows 0.7 mL drawn up:

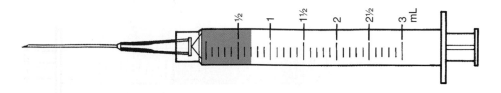

Example: Order: Glycopyrrolate 100 mcg IM stat.

Available: Glycopyrrolate 0.2 mg per 1 mL

✅ PROBLEM SETUP

1. Note that a conversion is necessary. Conversion factor: 1 000 micrograms (mcg) = 1 mg. To eliminate the decimal point, convert what is available to what is ordered. 0.2 mg = 200 mcg. If what is ordered were converted to what is available (100 mcg = 0.1 mg), you would get the same answer (the problem shown illustrates both the ratio and proportion and the formula methods).
2. Think: You will need less than 1 mL to administer the dosage.
3. Calculate the dosage to administer using the ratio and proportion method, the formula method, or the dimensional analysis method.

✔ Solution Using Ratio and Proportion

$$0.2\,\text{mg} : 1\,\text{mL} = 0.1\,\text{mg} : x\,\text{mL} \quad or \quad 200\,\text{mcg} : 1\,\text{mL} = 100\,\text{mcg} : x\,\text{mL}$$

$$\frac{0.2x}{0.2} = \frac{0.1}{0.2} \qquad\qquad \frac{200x}{200} = \frac{100}{200}$$

$$x = \frac{0.1}{0.2} \qquad\qquad x = \frac{100}{200}$$

$$x = 0.5\,\text{mL} \qquad\qquad x = 0.5\,\text{mL}$$

✔ Solution Using the Formula Method

$$\frac{(D)\,0.1\,\text{mg}}{(H)\,0.2\,\text{mg}} \times (Q)\,1\,\text{mL} = x\,\text{mL} \quad or \quad \frac{(D)\,100\,\text{mcg}}{(H)\,200\,\text{mcg}} \times (Q)\,1\,\text{mL} = x\,\text{mL}$$

$$x = \frac{0.1}{0.2} \times 1 \qquad\qquad x = \frac{100}{200} \times 1$$

$$x = 0.5\,\text{mL} \qquad\qquad x = 0.5\,\text{mL}$$

✔ Solution Using Dimensional Analysis

$$x\,\text{mL} = \frac{1\,\text{mL}}{0.2\,\cancel{\text{mg}}} \times \frac{1\,\cancel{\text{mg}}}{1000\,\cancel{\text{mcg}}} \times \frac{100\,\cancel{\text{mcg}}}{1}$$

$$x = \frac{100}{200}$$

$$x = 0.5\,\text{mL}$$

Note that the dosage could be administered in a 3-mL or a 1-mL syringe.

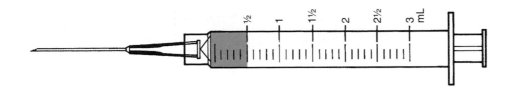

Example: Order: Atropine sulfate 0.6 mg IM stat.

Available: Atropine sulfate in 20-mL vial labelled 0.4 mg per mL

✓ PROBLEM SETUP

1. Note that no conversion is necessary.
2. Think: You will need more than 1 mL to administer the dosage.
3. Calculate the dosage to administer using the ratio and proportion method, the formula method, or the dimensional analysis method.

✔ Solution Using Ratio and Proportion

$$0.4 \text{ mg} : 1 \text{ mL} = 0.6 \text{ mg} : x \text{ mL}$$

$$\frac{0.4x}{0.4} = \frac{0.6}{0.4}$$

$$x = \frac{0.6}{0.4}$$

$$x = 1.5 \text{ mL}$$

Note that some small hypodermics have fraction markings; however, millilitre is metric and should be stated by using a decimal.

✔ Solution Using the Formula Method

$$\frac{(D)\,0.6 \text{ mg}}{(H)\,0.4 \text{ mg}} \times (Q)\,1 \text{ mL} = x \text{ mL}$$

$$x = \frac{0.6}{0.4} \times 1$$

$$x = 1.5 \text{ mL}$$

✔ Solution Using Dimensional Analysis

$$x \text{ mL} = \frac{1 \text{ mL}}{0.4 \text{ mg}} \times \frac{0.6 \text{ mg}}{1}$$

$$x = \frac{0.6}{0.4}$$

$$x = 1.5 \text{ mL}$$

This syringe shows 1.5 mL drawn up:

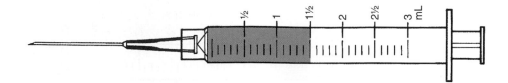

Calculating Dosages for Medications in Units

As previously mentioned, certain medications are measured in units. Some medications measured in units include vitamins, antibiotics, insulin, and heparin. The calculation of insulin will be discussed in Chapter 18. Insulin syringes are used for insulin only. In determining the dosage to administer when medications are measured in units, use the same steps as with other parenteral medications. Dosages of certain medications such as heparin are administered with a tuberculin syringe, as opposed to a hypodermic syringe (3 mL). Because of its effects, **heparin is never rounded off**; exact dosages are given. Heparin will be discussed in more detail in Chapter 21. Let's look at sample problems with units.

Example: Order: Heparin 750 units SUBCUT daily.

Available: Heparin 1 000 units per mL

Calculate the dosage to administer. A 1-mL (tuberculin) syringe will be used.

✔ PROBLEM SETUP

1. Note that no conversion is necessary. No conversion exists for units.
2. Think: The dosage to be given is less than 1 mL. This dosage can be measured accurately in a 1-mL tuberculin syringe. Heparin is administered in exact dosages.
3. Calculate the dosage to administer using the ratio and proportion method, the formula method, or the dimensional analysis method.

 SAFETY ALERT!

Because of the action of heparin, an exact dosage is crucial; the dosage should not be rounded off.

✔ Solution Using Ratio and Proportion

$$1\,000 \text{ units} : 1 \text{ mL} = 750 \text{ units} : x \text{ mL}$$

$$\frac{1\,000x}{1\,000} = \frac{750}{1\,000}$$

$$x = \frac{750}{1\,000}$$

$$x = 0.75 \text{ mL}$$

✔ Solution Using the Formula Method

$$\frac{(D)\,750 \text{ units}}{(H)\,1\,000 \text{ units}} \times (Q)\,1\,\text{mL} = x \text{ mL}$$

$$x = \frac{750}{1\,000} \times 1$$

$$x = 0.75 \text{ mL}$$

✔ Solution Using Dimensional Analysis

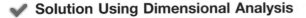

$$x \text{ mL} = \frac{1 \text{ mL}}{100\cancel{0} \cancel{\text{units}}} \times \frac{75\cancel{0} \cancel{\text{units}}}{1}$$

(Note the cancellation of zeros to make numbers smaller.)

$$x = \frac{75}{100}$$

$$x = 0.75 \text{ mL}$$

This syringe shows 0.75 mL drawn up:

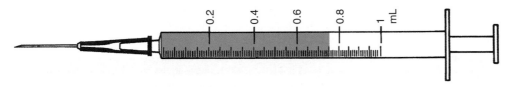

Example: Order: Penicillin G procaine, 500 000 units IM BID.

Available: Penicillin G procaine labelled 300 000 units per mL

☑ PROBLEM SETUP

1. Note that no conversion is necessary.
2. Think: The dosage ordered is more than the available dosage strength. Therefore, more than 1 mL would be required to administer the dosage.
3. Calculate the dosage to administer using the ratio and proportion method, the formula method, or the dimensional analysis method.

✔ Solution Using Ratio and Proportion

$$300\,000 \text{ units} : 1 \text{ mL} = 500\,000 \text{ units} : x \text{ mL}$$

$$300\,000x = 500\,000$$

$$\frac{300\,000x}{300\,000} = \frac{500\,000}{300\,000}$$

$$x = 1.66 = 1.7 \text{ mL}$$

> **NOTE**
> The division here is carried two decimal places. This answer is then rounded off to 1.7 mL. Remember that the 3-mL syringe is marked in tenths of a millilitre.

✔ Solution Using the Formula Method

$$\frac{\text{(D)}\,500\,000 \text{ units}}{\text{(H)}\,300\,000 \text{ units}} \times \text{(Q)}\,1 \text{ mL} = x \text{ mL}$$

$$x = \frac{5\cancel{00}\,\cancel{000}}{3\cancel{00}\,\cancel{000}} \times 1$$

$$x = 1.66 = 1.7 \text{ mL}$$

✔ Solution Using Dimensional Analysis

$$x \text{ mL} = \frac{1 \text{ mL}}{300\,000 \cancel{\text{units}}} \times \frac{500\,000 \cancel{\text{units}}}{1}$$

$$x = \frac{5\cancel{00}\,\cancel{000}}{3\cancel{00}\,\cancel{000}}$$

$$x = 1.66 = 1.7 \text{ mL}$$

This syringe shows 1.7 mL drawn up:

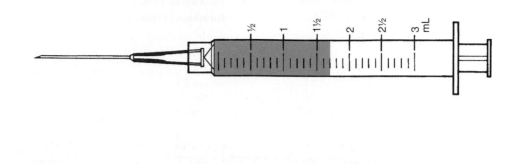

Mixing Medications in the Same Syringe

Two medications may be mixed in one syringe if they are compatible with each other and the total amount does not exceed the amount that can be safely administered in a site. Always consult a drug reference or the pharmacist about the compatibility of medications in a syringe before mixing medications. Some syringe compatibility is time limited; for example, some mixed medication should be given within 15 minutes to ensure stability.

When mixing two medications for administration in one syringe, calculate the dosage to administer in millilitres to the nearest tenth for each of the medications ordered. Then add the results to find the total volume to be combined and administered.

Example: Order: Meperidine 65 mg IM and hydroxyzine 25 mg IM q4h prn for pain.

Available: Meperidine 75 mg per mL and hydroxyzine 50 mg per mL

Solution: Meperidine dose 0.86 = 0.9 mL

hydroxyzine dose 0.5 mL

0.9 mL meperidine + 0.5 mL hydroxyzine = 1.4 mL (total volume)

This syringe shows the doses of the two medications combined:

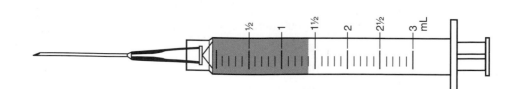

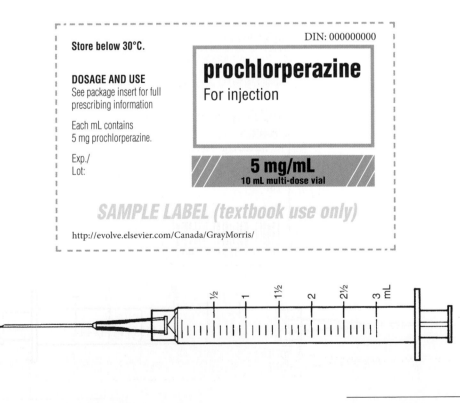

POINTS TO REMEMBER

- Read labels carefully. Do not confuse dosage strength with total volume.
- Know that there is no conversion of units, millimoles, and milliequivalents.
- Do not exceed the dosage administration guidelines for parental administration:
  - IM: maximum volume to administer at one site is 3 mL for average-sized adult (for deltoid muscle, 1 mL), 2 mL for children ages 6–12, and 1 mL for children ages 0–5 years
  - SUBCUT: maximum volume to administer at one site is 1 mL
- Calculate parenteral dosage problems using any of the methods presented (ratio and proportion, the formula method, or dimensional analysis).
- Use the right type of syringe for the medication and dosage ordered.
- Note that two medications can be administered in the same syringe if they are compatible. Calculate the dosage to administer in millilitres to the nearest tenth for each of the medications. Add the result to get the total volume to administer.
- Choose the correct size syringe for the dosage to be administered. Read the calibration carefully.

PRACTICE **PROBLEMS**

Calculate the following dosages using the labels or the information provided. Express your answers in millilitres to the nearest tenth except where indicated. Shade in the dosage on the syringe provided.

28. Order: Prochlorperazine 10 mg IM q4h prn.

    Available:

Store below 30°C.

DIN: 000000000

DOSAGE AND USE
See package insert for full prescribing information

Each mL contains
5 mg prochlorperazine.

Exp./
Lot:

prochlorperazine
For injection

5 mg/mL
10 mL multi-dose vial

SAMPLE LABEL (textbook use only)

http://evolve.elsevier.com/Canada/GrayMorris/

29. Order: Thiamine 75 mg IM daily.

Available:

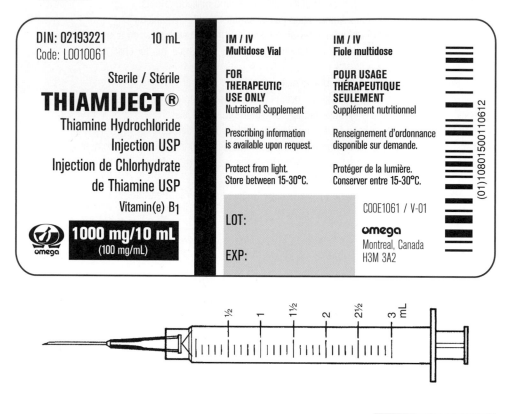

30. Order: Phenobarbital 120 mg IM at bedtime.

Available:

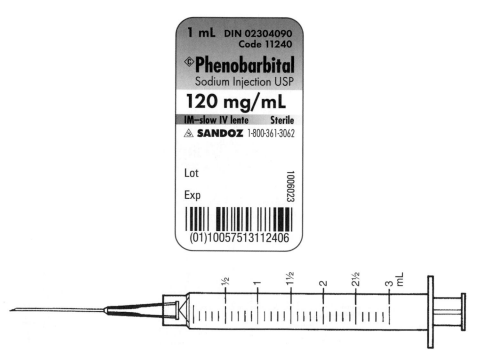

31. Order: Diazepam 8 mg IM q4h prn for agitation.

Available:

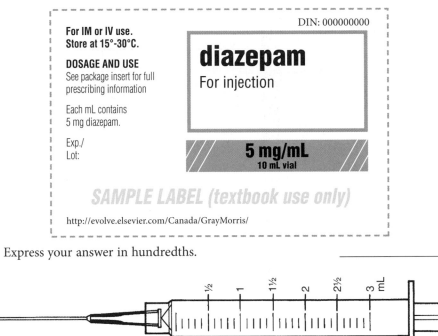

For IM or IV use.
Store at 15°-30°C.

DOSAGE AND USE
See package insert for full
prescribing information

Each mL contains
5 mg diazepam.

Exp./
Lot:

DIN: 000000000

diazepam
For injection

5 mg/mL
10 mL vial

SAMPLE LABEL (textbook use only)

http://evolve.elsevier.com/Canada/GrayMorris/

Express your answer in hundredths.   _____

32. Order: Octreotide acetate 0.25 mg SUBCUT daily.

Available:

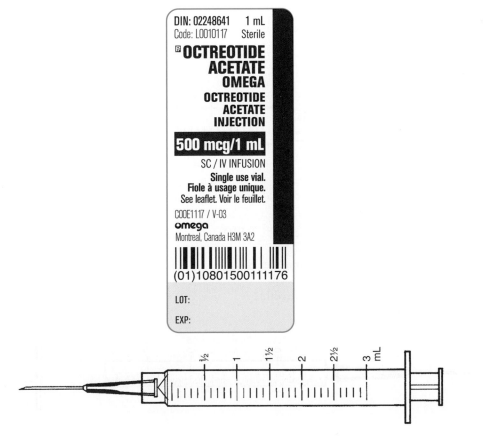

DIN: 02248641   1 mL
Code: L0010117   Sterile

OCTREOTIDE ACETATE
OMEGA
OCTREOTIDE ACETATE INJECTION

500 mcg/1 mL

SC / IV INFUSION

Single use vial.
Fiole à usage unique.
See leaflet. Voir le feuillet.

C00E1117 / V-03
omega
Montreal, Canada H3M 3A2

(01)10801500111176

LOT:

EXP:

33. Order: Meperidine 50 mg IM and hydroxyzine 25 mg IM q4h prn for pain.

    Available: Meperidine labelled 75 mg per mL, hydroxyzine labelled 50 mg per mL

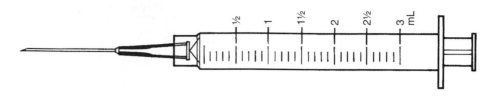

34. Order: Haloperidol decanoate 125 mg IM monthly.

    Available:

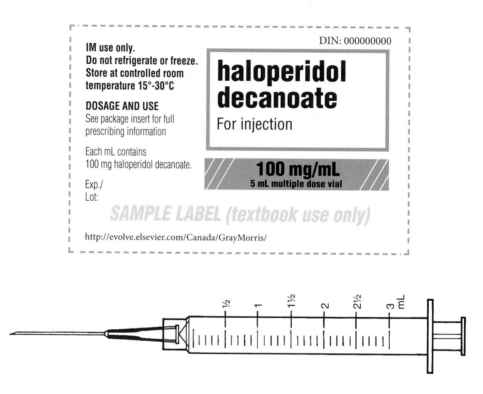

35. Order: Heparin 5 000 units SUBCUT BID.

    Available: Heparin 20 000 units per mL

    Express your answer in hundredths.

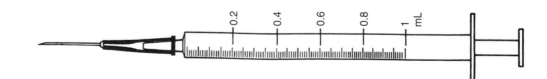

36. Order: Morphine sulfate 15 mg IM q4h prn for pain.

   Available:

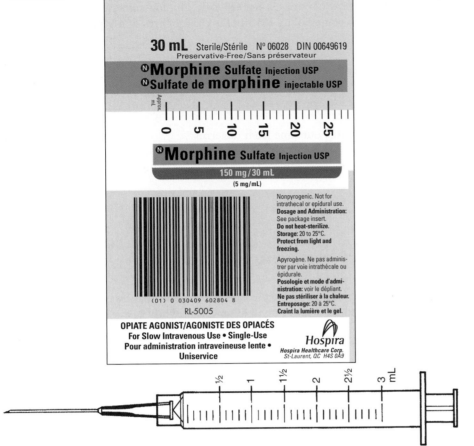

37. Order: Furosemide (Lasix) 20 mg IM stat.

   Available:

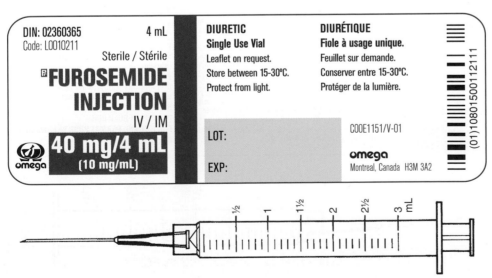

Answers on pages 409–411.

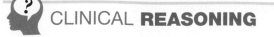 CLINICAL **REASONING**

1. **Scenario:** Order: Hydroxyzine 50 mg IM q4h prn for anxiety. The nurse, in error, administered hydralazine 50 mg IM from a vial labelled 20 mg per mL and gave the patient 2.5 mL.

   a. What patient right was violated? _____

   b. What contributed to the error made? _____

   c. What is the potential outcome from the error? _____

   d. What measures could have been taken to prevent the error? _____

Answers on page 411.

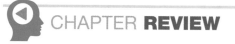 CHAPTER **REVIEW**

Calculate the following dosages using the labels or the information provided. Express your answers in millilitres to the nearest tenth except where indicated. Shade in the dosage on the syringe provided.

1. Order: Clindamycin 0.3 g IM q6h.

   Available:

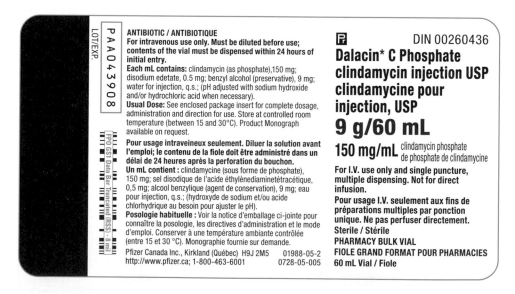

ANTIBIOTIC / ANTIBIOTIQUE
For intravenous use only. Must be diluted before use; contents of the vial must be dispensed within 24 hours of initial entry.
Each mL contains: clindamycin (as phosphate),150 mg; disodium edetate, 0.5 mg; benzyl alcohol (preservative), 9 mg; water for injection, q.s.; (pH adjusted with sodium hydroxide and/or hydrochloric acid when necessary).
Usual Dose: See enclosed package insert for complete dosage, administration and direction for use. Store at controlled room temperature (between 15 and 30°C). Product Monograph available on request.

Pour usage intraveineux seulement. Diluer la solution avant l'emploi; le contenu de la fiole doit être administré dans un délai de 24 heures après la perforation du bouchon.
Un mL contient : clindamycine (sous forme de phosphate), 150 mg; sel disodique de l'acide éthylènediaminetétracétique, 0,5 mg; alcool benzylique (agent de conservation), 9 mg; eau pour injection, q.s.; (hydroxyde de sodium et/ou acide chlorhydrique au besoin pour ajuster le pH).
Posologie habituelle : Voir la notice d'emballage ci-jointe pour connaître la posologie, les directives d'administration et le mode d'emploi. Conserver à une température ambiante contrôlée (entre 15 et 30 °C). Monographie fournie sur demande.

Pfizer Canada Inc., Kirkland (Québec) H9J 2M5   01988-05-2
http://www.pfizer.ca; 1-800-463-6001   0728-05-005

LOT/EXP.
PAA043908
FPO GS1 Data Bar Truncated (RSS) - 8 mil

DIN 00260436
Dalacin* C Phosphate
clindamycin injection USP
clindamycine pour
injection, USP
9 g/60 mL
150 mg/mL clindamycin phosphate de phosphate de clindamycine
For I.V. use only and single puncture, multiple dispensing. Not for direct infusion.
Pour usage I.V. seulement aux fins de préparations multiples par ponction unique. Ne pas perfuser directement.
Sterile / Stérile
PHARMACY BULK VIAL
FIOLE GRAND FORMAT POUR PHARMACIES
60 mL Vial / Fiole

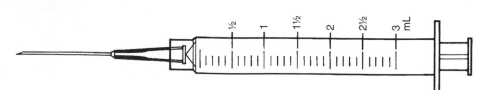

2. Order: Octreotide acetate 175 mcg SUBCUT q12h.

   Available:

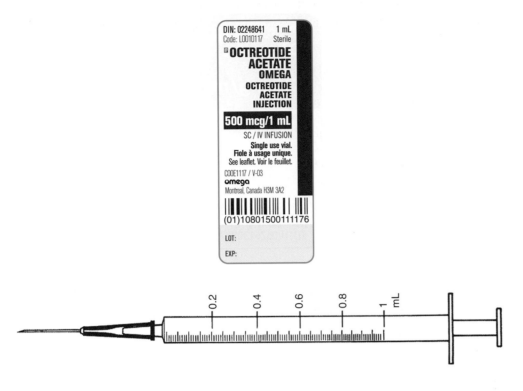

3. Order: Ketorolac 25 mg IM q6h prn for pain.

   Available:

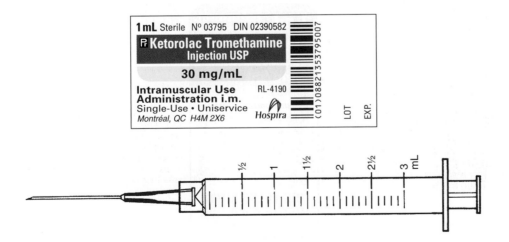

4. Order: Digoxin 100 mcg IM daily.

Available:

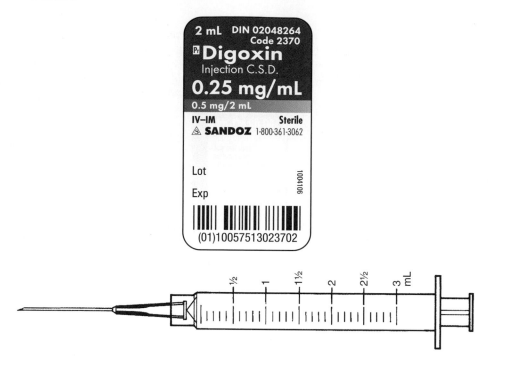

5. Order: Hydromorphone hydrochloride 4 mg SUBCUT q4h prn for pain.

Available:

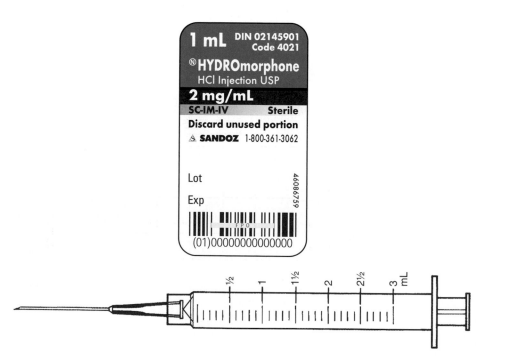

6. Order: Bicillin C-R (900/300) 1 200 000 units IM stat.

    Available:

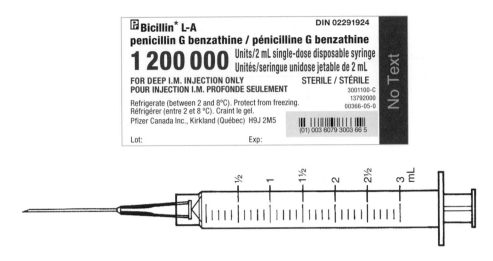

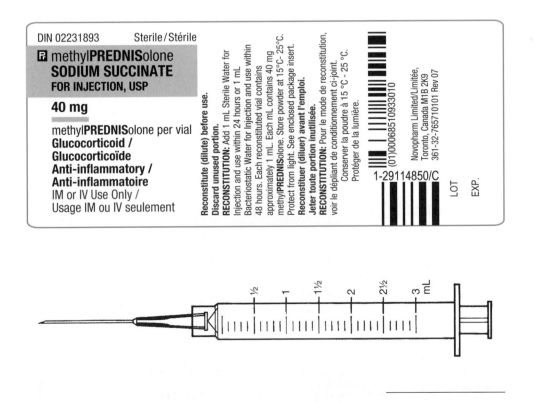

7. Order: Methylprednisolone 100 mg IV q8h for 2 doses.

    Available:

8. Order: Methylergonovine 0.4 mg IM q4h for 3 doses.

   Available: Methylergonovine labelled 0.2 mg per mL

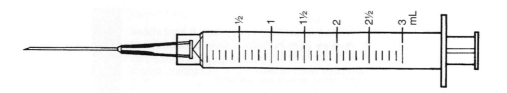

9. Order: Heparin 8 000 units SUBCUT q12h.

   Available:

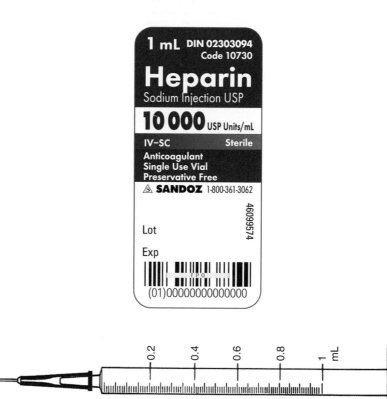

10. Order: Phenytoin sodium 200 mg IV stat.

    Available:

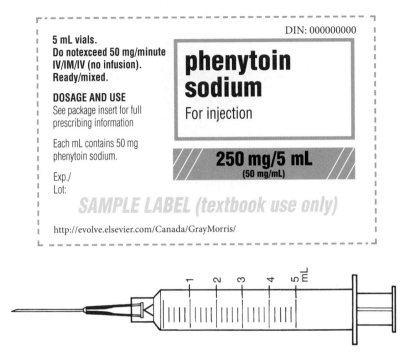

5 mL vials.
**Do notexceed 50 mg/minute
IV/IM/IV (no infusion).
Ready/mixed.**

DOSAGE AND USE
See package insert for full
prescribing information

Each mL contains 50 mg
phenytoin sodium.

Exp./
Lot:

DIN: 000000000

**phenytoin
sodium**
For injection

250 mg/5 mL
(50 mg/mL)

SAMPLE LABEL (textbook use only)

http://evolve.elsevier.com/Canada/GrayMorris/

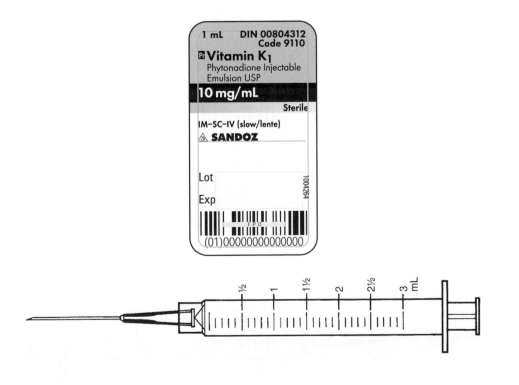

11. Order: Phytonadione 10 mg IM daily for 3 days.

    Available:

1 mL   **DIN 00804312
Code 9110**
℞ **Vitamin K₁**
Phytonadione Injectable
Emulsion USP
10 mg/mL
                        Sterile
IM–SC–IV (slow/lente)
⚠ **SANDOZ**

Lot

Exp

(01)000000000000000

12. Order: Famotidine 40 mg IV at bedtime.

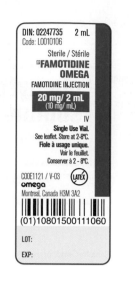

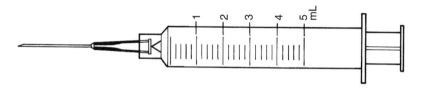

13. Order: Promethazine HCl 25 mg IM q4h prn for nausea.

Available:

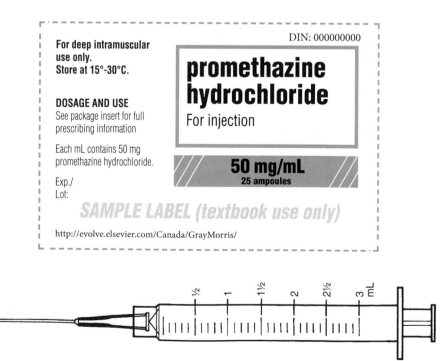

14. Order: Butorphanol 1.5 mg IM q4h prn for pain.

Available: Butorphanol labelled 2 mg per mL

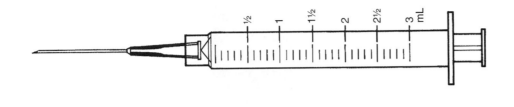

_____

15. Order: Tobramycin 50 mg IM q8h.

Available:

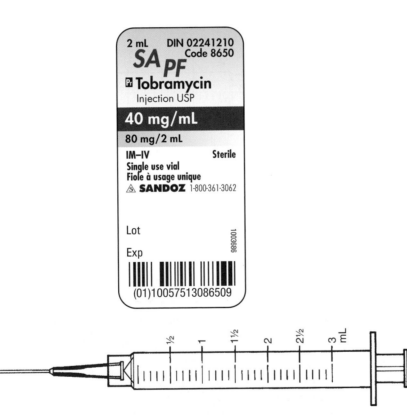

_____

16. Order: Diphenhydramine 25 mg IM q6h prn for itching.

Available:

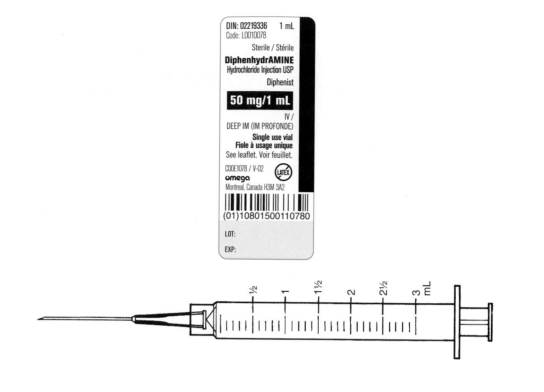

17. Order: Ondansetron 3 mg IV stat.

Available:

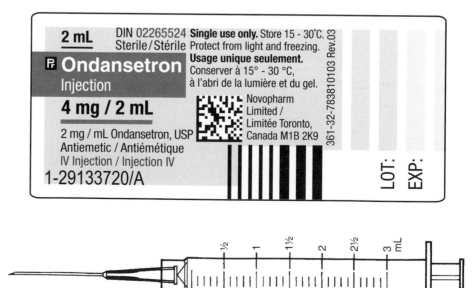

18. Order: Solu-Cortef 400 mg IV daily for a severe inflammation for 5 days.

Available:

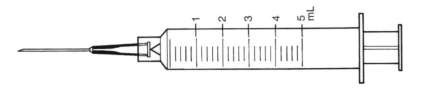

GLUCOCORTICOID / GLUCOCORTICOÏDE
Each Act-O-Vial† contains: / Une fiole Act-O-Vial† contient :
Powder / Poudre
Hydrocortisone (as sodium succinate) .... 250 mg .... hydrocortisone (sous forme de succinate sodique)
Monobasic sodium phosphate anhydrous .... 2 mg .... phosphate monobasique de sodium anhydre
Dibasic sodium phosphate dried .... 21.8 mg .... phosphate dibasique de sodium sec
Diluent / Diluent
Sterile Water for Injection .... q.s. .... eau stérile pour injection

After reconstitution each Act-O-Vial† delivers 2 mL containing 250 mg hydrocortisone (as sodium succinate).
Each mL contains: 125 mg hydrocortisone.
Après la reconstitution de la solution, une fiole Act-O-Vial† fournit 2 mL contenant 250 mg d'hydrocortisone
(sous forme de succinate sodique). Un mL contient : 125 mg d'hydrocortisone.

Usual Adult Dose: See Product Monograph for complete dosage, administration and direction for use.
Posologie habituelle – Adulte : Voir la monographie du produit pour connaître la posologie, les directives
d'administration et le mode d'emploi.

®/M.D. de Pfizer Enterprises S.a.r.l.   † ®/M.D. de Pharmacia & Upjohn Company LLC
Pfizer Canada Inc., Licensee / licencié   Pfizer Canada Inc., Licensee / licencié

Pfizer Canada Inc., Kirkland (Québec) H9J 2M5
http://www.pfizer.ca ; 1-800-463-6001   52241-14-1

Store powder or reconstituted solution
at controlled room temperature
(between 15 and 30°C). Use
reconstituted solution within 3 days.
Single use vial. Discard unused portion.
Protect from light and freezing.
Product Monograph available
on request.

Conserver la poudre ou la solution
reconstituée à une température
ambiante contrôlée (entre 15 et 30 °C).
Utiliser la solution reconstituée dans un
délai de 3 jours. Fiole unidose. Jeter
tout reste de solution.
Craint la lumière et le gel.
Monographie fournie sur demande.

Ⓡ **Solu-CORTEF** ®/MD   DIN 00030619
hydrocortisone sodium succinate for injection USP
succinate sodique d'hydrocortisone pour injection, USP
250 mg /vial / fiole
125 mg/mL (when reconstituted / une fois reconstituée)

For intravenous or intramuscular use
Pour usage intraveineux ou intramusculaire

Sterile Powder / Poudre stérile

SINGLE DOSE ACT-O-VIAL† / FIOLE ACT-O-VIAL† UNIDOSE

10x2 mL vials / fioles

Pfizer Injectables

_____

19. Order: Naloxone 0.2 mg IM stat.

Available:

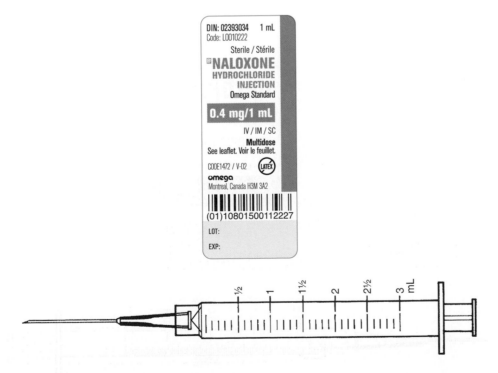

DIN: 02393034   1 mL
Code: L0010222

Sterile / Stérile

Ⓡ **NALOXONE**
HYDROCHLORIDE
INJECTION
Omega Standard

0.4 mg/1 mL

IV / IM / SC

Multidose
See leaflet. Voir le feuillet.

C00E1472 / V-02   LATEX

omega
Montreal, Canada H3M 3A2

(01)10801500112227

LOT:

EXP:

_____

20. Order: Glycopyrrolate 200 mcg IM on call to the OR.

Available:

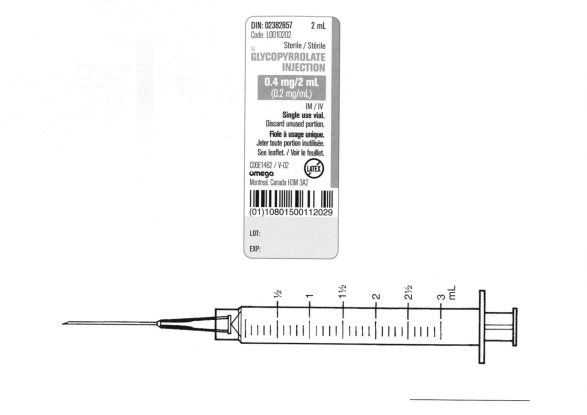

21. Order: Darbepoetin alfa 30 mcg SUBCUT stat.

Available:

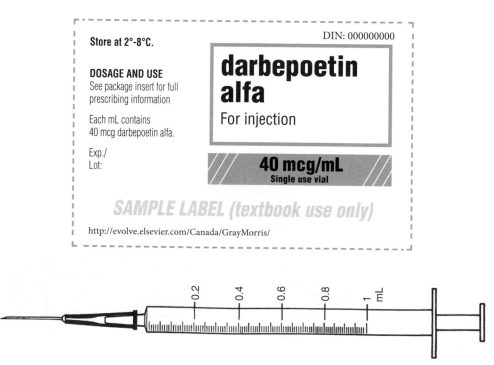

22. Order: Hydroxyzine hydrochloride 35 mg IM stat.

    Available:

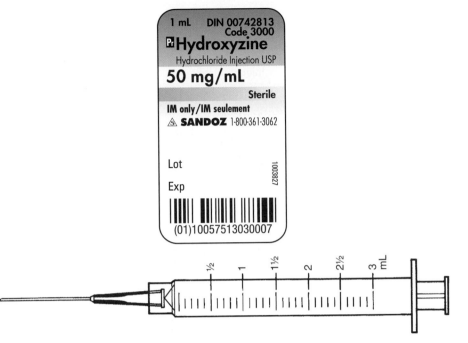

23. Order: Meperidine 60 mg IM q4h prn for pain.

    Available:

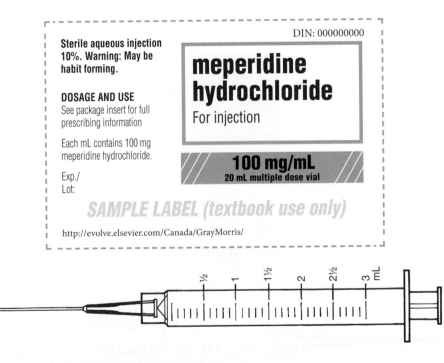

24. Order: Ranitidine 50 mg IV q6h.

Available:

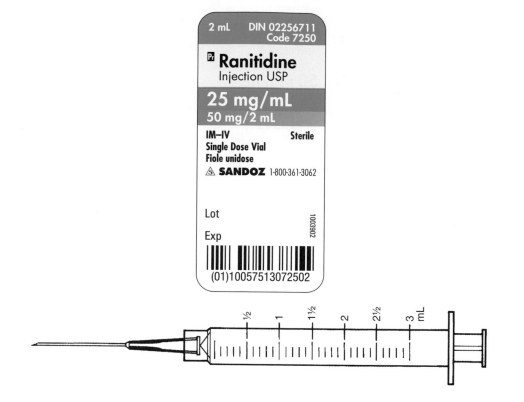

25. Order: Digoxin 0.4 mg IM stat.

Available:

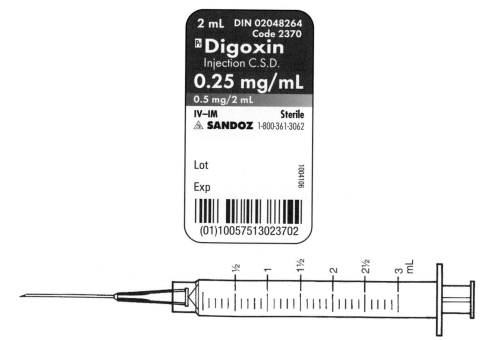

26. Order: Filgrastim 180 mcg SUBCUT daily.

Available:

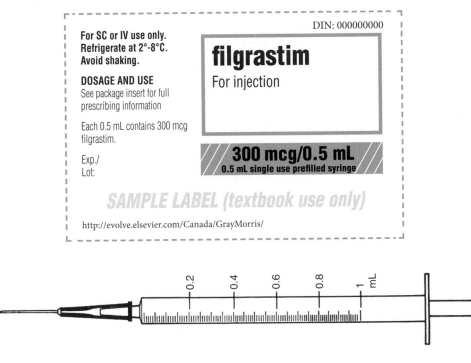

For SC or IV use only.
Refrigerate at 2°-8°C.
Avoid shaking.

DOSAGE AND USE
See package insert for full prescribing information

Each 0.5 mL contains 300 mcg filgrastim.

Exp./
Lot:

DIN: 000000000

filgrastim
For injection

300 mcg/0.5 mL
0.5 mL single use prefilled syringe

SAMPLE LABEL (textbook use only)

http://evolve.elsevier.com/Canada/GrayMorris/

27. Order: Lincocin 500 mg IV q8h.

Available:

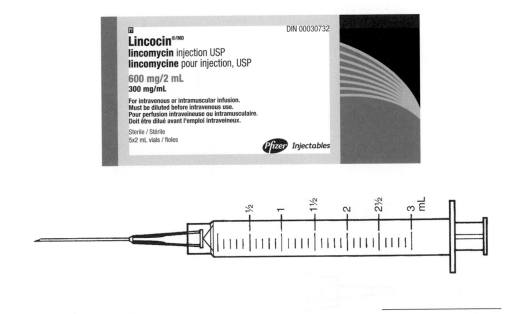

Lincocin®/MD
lincomycin injection USP
lincomycine pour injection, USP

600 mg/2 mL
300 mg/mL

DIN 00030732

For intravenous or intramuscular infusion.
Must be diluted before intravenous use.
Pour perfusion intraveineuse ou intramusculaire.
Doit être dilué avant l'emploi intraveineux.

Sterile / Stérile
5x2 mL vials / fioles

Pfizer Injectables

28. Order: Lorazepam 1.5 mg IM BID prn for agitation.

Available:

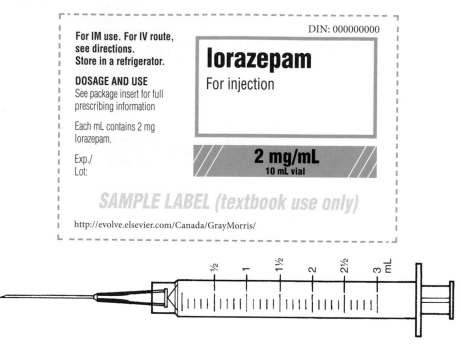

29. Order: Chlorpromazine hydrochloride 65 mg IM q4h prn.

Available:

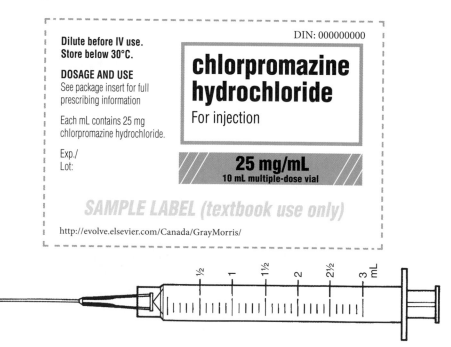

30. Order: Depo-Provera 0.65 g IM once a week (on Thursdays).

    Available:

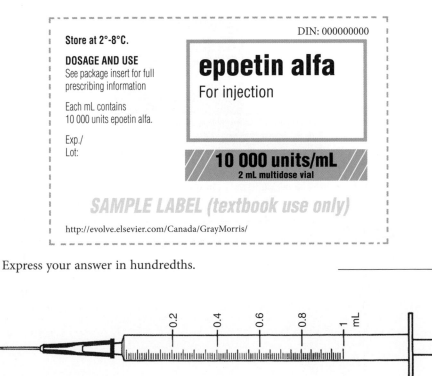

DIN 00585092

DEPO-PROVERA®/MD

MEDROXYPROGESTERONE ACETATE
INJECTABLE SUSPENSION USP
SUSPENSION INJECTABLE D'ACÉTATE DE
MÉDROXYPROGESTÉRONE, USP

150 mg/mL medroxyprogesterone acetate
d'acétate de médroxyprogestérone

Sterile Aqueous Suspension
Suspension aqueuse stérile

Progestogen / Progestatif

For intramuscular use only
Pour usage intramusculaire seulement

1 x 1 mL vial / fiole

Pfizer

31. Order: Epoetin alfa 3 000 units SUBCUT three times per week Monday, Wednesday, and Friday.

    Available:

Store at 2°-8°C.

DOSAGE AND USE
See package insert for full
prescribing information

Each mL contains
10 000 units epoetin alfa.

Exp./
Lot:

DIN: 000000000

epoetin alfa

For injection

10 000 units/mL
2 mL multidose vial

SAMPLE LABEL (textbook use only)

http://evolve.elsevier.com/Canada/GrayMorris/

Express your answer in hundredths. _____

32. Order: Metoclopramide 15 mg IV stat.

Available:

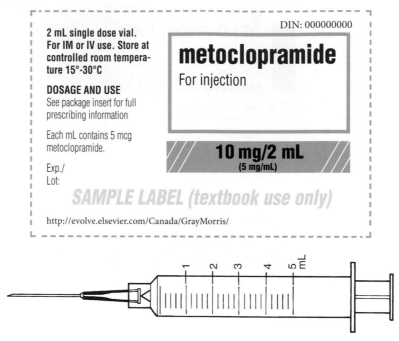

2 mL single dose vial.
For IM or IV use. Store at
controlled room tempera-
ture 15°-30°C

DOSAGE AND USE
See package insert for full
prescribing information

Each mL contains 5 mcg
metoclopramide.

Exp./
Lot:

DIN: 000000000

metoclopramide
For injection

10 mg/2 mL
(5 mg/mL)

SAMPLE LABEL (textbook use only)

http://evolve.elsevier.com/Canada/GrayMorris/

_____

33. Order: Lovenox 30 mg SUBCUT q12h.

Available:

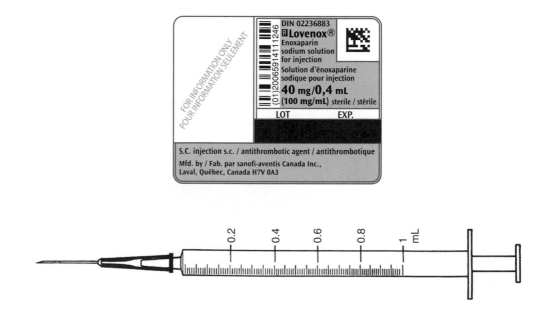

FOR INFORMATION ONLY
POUR INFORMATION SEULEMENT

DIN 02236883
Lovenox®
Enoxaparin
sodium solution
for injection
Solution d'énoxaparine
sodique pour injection
40 mg/0,4 mL
(100 mg/mL) sterile / stérile

| LOT | EXP. |

S.C. injection s.c. / antithrombotic agent / antithrombotique
Mfd. by / Fab. par sanofi-aventis Canada Inc.,
Laval, Québec, Canada H7V 0A3

_____

34. Order: Cimetidine 0.3 g IV TID.

    Available:

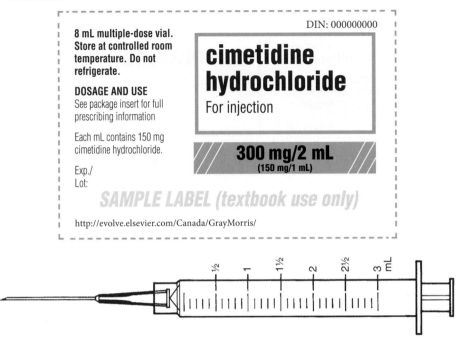

8 mL multiple-dose vial. Store at controlled room temperature. Do not refrigerate.

DOSAGE AND USE
See package insert for full prescribing information

Each mL contains 150 mg cimetidine hydrochloride.

Exp./
Lot:

DIN: 000000000

cimetidine hydrochloride
For injection

300 mg/2 mL
(150 mg/1 mL)

SAMPLE LABEL (textbook use only)

http://evolve.elsevier.com/Canada/GrayMorris/

35. Order: Diazepam 7.5 mg IM stat.

    Available:

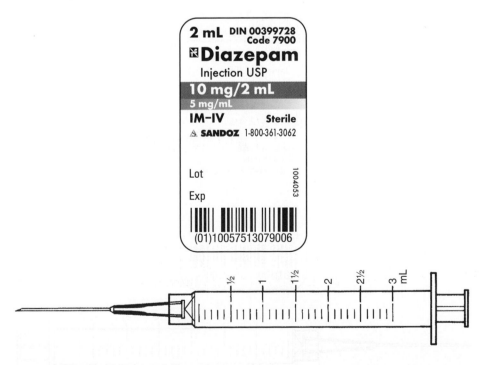

2 mL DIN 00399728
Code 7900
℞ Diazepam
Injection USP
10 mg/2 mL
5 mg/mL
IM–IV Sterile
⚠ **SANDOZ** 1-800-361-3062

Lot 1004053

Exp

(01)10057513079006

36. Order: Bumetanide 1 mg IV daily.

Available:

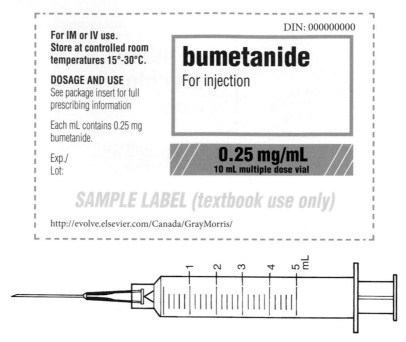

37. Order: Gentamicin 55 mg IV q8h.

Available:

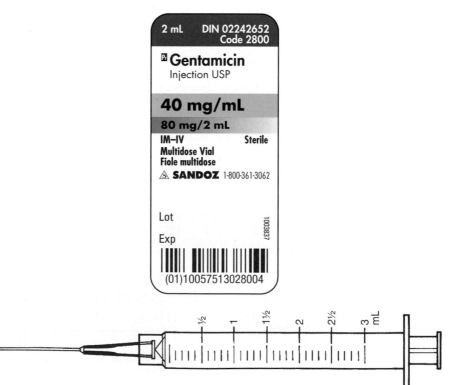

38. Order: Betamethasone 12 mg IM q24h for 2 doses.

    Available:

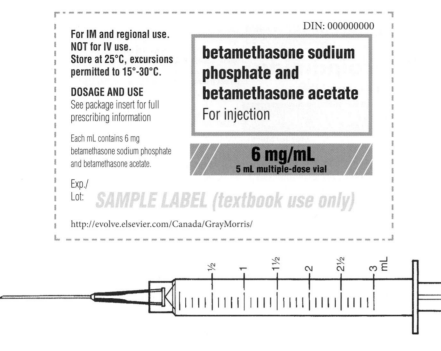

For IM and regional use.
NOT for IV use.
Store at 25°C, excursions
permitted to 15°-30°C.

DOSAGE AND USE
See package insert for full
prescribing information

Each mL contains 6 mg
betamethasone sodium phosphate
and betamethasone acetate.

Exp./
Lot:

DIN: 000000000

betamethasone sodium phosphate and betamethasone acetate
For injection

6 mg/mL
5 mL multiple-dose vial

SAMPLE LABEL (textbook use only)

http://evolve.elsevier.com/Canada/GrayMorris/

39. Order: Aminophylline 0.25 g IV q6h.

    Available:

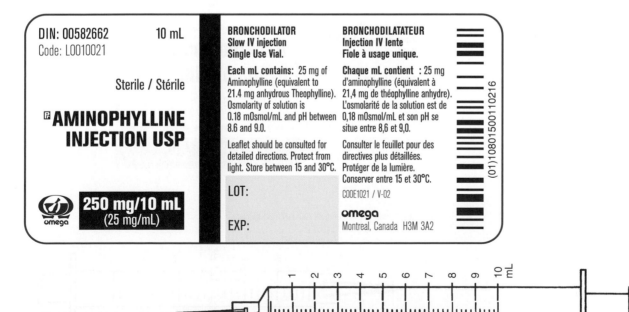

DIN: 00582662   10 mL
Code: L0010021

Sterile / Stérile

℞ **AMINOPHYLLINE INJECTION USP**

250 mg/10 mL
(25 mg/mL)

omega

BRONCHODILATOR
Slow IV injection
Single Use Vial.

Each mL contains: 25 mg of
Aminophylline (equivalent to
21.4 mg anhydrous Theophylline).
Osmolarity of solution is
0.18 mOsmol/mL and pH between
8.6 and 9.0.

Leaflet should be consulted for
detailed directions. Protect from
light. Store between 15 and 30°C.

LOT:

EXP:

BRONCHODILATATEUR
Injection IV lente
Fiole à usage unique.

Chaque mL contient : 25 mg
d'aminophylline (équivalent à
21,4 mg de théophylline anhydre).
L'osmolarité de la solution est de
0,18 mOsmol/mL et son pH se
situe entre 8,6 et 9,0.

Consulter le feuillet pour des
directives plus détaillées.
Protéger de la lumière.
Conserver entre 15 et 30°C.

C00E1021 / V-02

omega
Montreal, Canada H3M 3A2

(01) 1 080 1500 1 10216

40. Order: Procainamide hydrochloride 0.4 g IV stat.

Available:

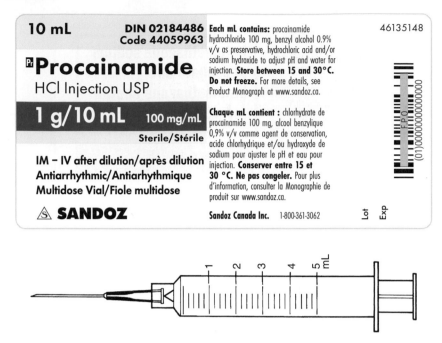

_____

41. Order: Trimethobenzamide hydrochloride 150 mg IM stat.

Available:

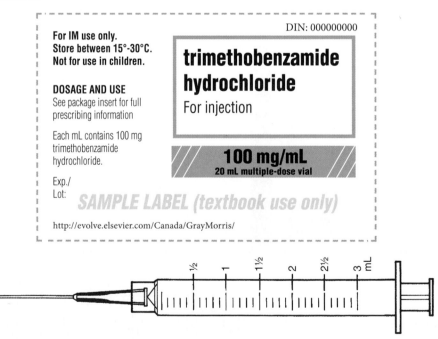

_____

42. Order: Meperidine 65 mg IM and promethazine 25 mg IM q4h prn for pain.

Available:

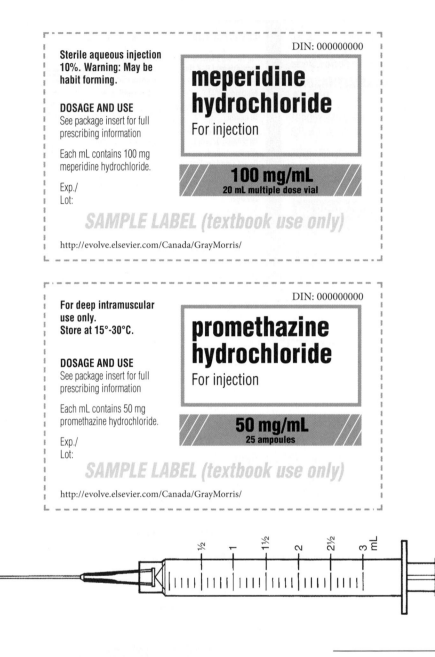

43. Order: Dexamethasone 9 mg IV daily for 4 days.

Available:

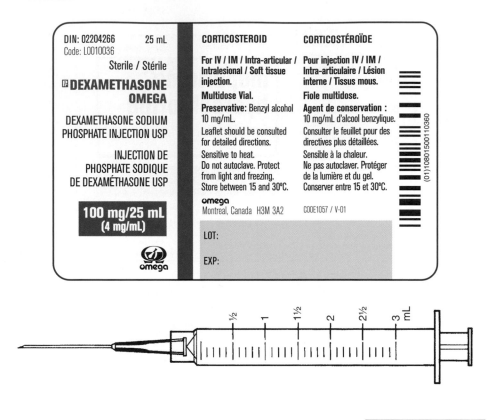

44. Order: Fentanyl 60 mcg IM 30 minutes before surgery.

Available:

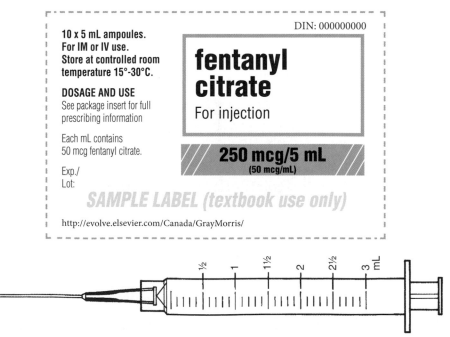

45. Order: Nalbuphine hydrochloride 10 mg IV stat.

Available:

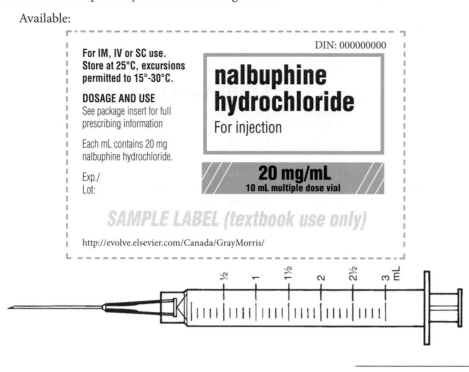

46. Order: Morphine 4 mg IV stat.

Available:

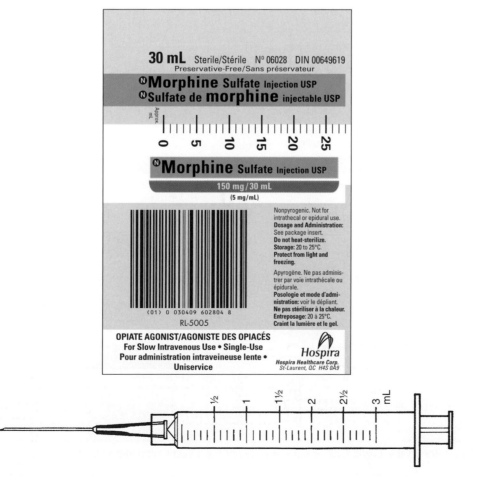

47. Order: Filgrastim 175 mcg SUBCUT daily for 2 weeks.

Available:

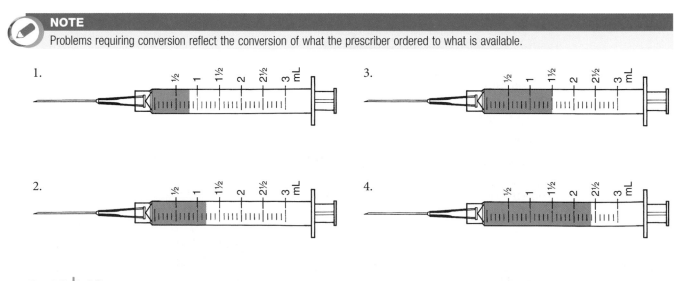

Store at 2°-8°C.

DIN: 000000000

DOSAGE AND USE
See package insert for full
prescribing information

Each mL contains 300 mcg
filgrastim.

Exp./
Lot:

filgrastim
For injection

300 mcg/mL
1.6 mL single use vial

SAMPLE LABEL (textbook use only)

http://evolve.elsevier.com/Canada/GrayMorris/

Answers on pages 411–419.

✳ ANSWERS

Answers to Practice Problems

> **NOTE**
> Problems requiring conversion reflect the conversion of what the prescriber ordered to what is available.

1.

3.

2.

4.

For additional practice problems, refer to the Basic Calculations section of the Drug Calculations Companion,
Version 5 on Evolve.

5. 1.4 mL

6. 1 mL

7. 0.9 mL

8. 0.4 mL

9. 4.4 mL

10. 7 mL

11. 3.2 mL

12. a. 10 mL
    b. 25 mg per mL;
        250 mg per 10 mL
        is also correct.
    c. 10 mL

13. a. 10 mL
    b. 2 mg per mL
    c. IV, IM

14. a. 10 mL
    b. 25 mg per mL
    c. 2 mL

15. a. 20 mL
    b. 100 mg per mL
    c. 0.5 mL

16. a. 2.8 mL
    b. 5 mg per mL
    c. SUBCUT

17. a. 1 mL
    b. 2 mg per mL
    c. N for Narcotic

18. a. SUBCUT
    b. 40 mg per 0.8 mL or
        50 mg per mL

19. a. 2 mL
    b. 20 mg per 2 mL,
        10 mg per 1 mL

20. a. 200 mg per 100 mL,
        2 mg per mL
    b. IV infusion only

21. a. 30 mL
    b. 150 mg per 30 mL,
        5 mg per mL

22. a. 3 mL
    b. 150 mg per 3 mL,
        50 mg per mL
    c. IV use only

23. a. 250 mL
    b. 2 mmol per mL

24. a. 30 mL
    b. 4 mmol per mL

25. a. 2 mL
    b. 10 000 units per mL

26. a. 3 mL
    b. 100 units per mL

27. a. 5 mL
    b. 10 units per mL

28. $5\ \text{mg}:1\ \text{mL} = 10\ \text{mg}:x\ \text{mL}$

or

$$\frac{10\ \text{mg}}{5\ \text{mg}} \times 1\ \text{mL} = x\ \text{mL}$$

Answer: 2 mL. The dosage ordered is more than the available strength; therefore, you will need more than 1 mL to administer the dosage.

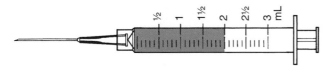

29. $100\ \text{mg}:1\ \text{mL} = 75\ \text{mg}:x\ \text{mL}$

or

$$\frac{75\ \text{mg}}{100\ \text{mg}} \times 1\ \text{mL} = x\ \text{mL}$$

Answer: 0.75 mL = 0.8 mL. The dosage ordered is less than the available strength; therefore, you will need less than 1 mL to administer the dosage. Answer is stated as a decimal (0.8 mL).

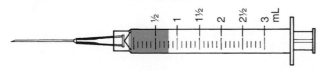

30. $120\ \text{mg}:1\ \text{mL} = 120\ \text{mg}:x\ \text{mL}$

or

$$\frac{120\ \text{mg}}{120\ \text{mg}} \times 1\ \text{mL} = x\ \text{mL}$$

Answer: 1 mL. The dosage ordered is the same as the available strength; therefore, you will need 1 mL to administer the dosage.

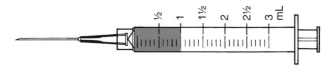

31. $5\ \text{mg}:1\ \text{mL} = 8\ \text{mg}:x\ \text{mL}$

or

$$\frac{8\ \text{mg}}{5\ \text{mg}} \times 1\ \text{mL} = x\ \text{mL}$$

Answer: 1.6 mL. The dosage ordered is more than the available strength; therefore, you will need more than 1 mL to administer the dosage.

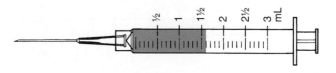

32. Conversion is required. Conversion factor:
    1 000 mcg = 1 mg. Therefore, 0.25 mg = 250 mcg.

    $$500 \text{ mcg} : 1 \text{ mL} = 250 \text{ mcg} : x \text{ mL}$$

    or

    $$\frac{250 \text{ mcg}}{500 \text{ mcg}} \times 1 \text{ mL} = x \text{ mL}$$

    Answer: 0.5 mL. The dosage ordered is less than the available strength; therefore, you will need less than 1 mL to administer the dosage.

    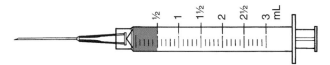

33. Meperidine:

    $$75 \text{ mg} : 1 \text{ mL} = 50 \text{ mg} : x \text{ mL}$$

    or

    $$\frac{50 \text{ mg}}{75 \text{ mg}} \times 1 \text{ mL} = x \text{ mL}$$

    Answer: 0.66 mL = 0.7 mL. The dosage ordered is less than the available strength; therefore, you will need less than 1 mL to administer the dosage.
    Hydroxyzine:

    $$50 \text{ mg} : 1 \text{ mL} = 25 \text{ mg} : x \text{ mL}$$

    or

    $$\frac{25 \text{ mg}}{50 \text{ mg}} \times 1 \text{ mL} = x \text{ mL}$$

    Answer: 0.5 mL. The dosage ordered is less than the available strength; therefore, you will need less than 1 mL to administer the dosage. The total number of millilitres you will prepare to administer is 1.2 mL. This dosage is measurable on a small hypodermic. These two medications are often administered in the same syringe.

    (0.7 mL meperidine + 0.5 mL hydroxyzine = 1.2 mL).

    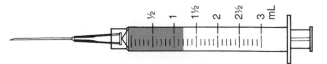

34. $$100 \text{ mg} : 1 \text{ mL} = 125 \text{ mg} : x \text{ mL}$$

    or

    $$\frac{125 \text{ mg}}{100 \text{ mg}} \times 1 \text{ mL} = x \text{ mL}$$

    Answer: 1.25 mL = 1.3 mL. The dosage ordered is more than the available strength; therefore, you will need more than 1 mL to administer the dosage.

    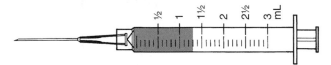

35. $$20\,000 \text{ units} : 1 \text{ mL} = 5\,000 \text{ units} : x \text{ mL}$$

    or

    $$\frac{5\,000 \text{ units}}{20\,000 \text{ units}} \times 1 \text{ mL} = x \text{ mL}$$

    Answer: 0.25 mL. The dosage ordered is less than the available strength; therefore. you will need less than 1 mL to administer the dosage. This dosage can be measured accurately in a 1-mL tuberculin syringe because it is measured in hundredths of a millilitre.

    The dosage to administer is 0.25 mL, which is $\frac{25}{100}$.

    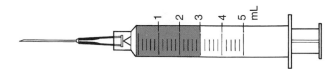

36. $$15 \text{ mg} : 1 \text{ mL} = 5 \text{ mg} : x \text{ mL}$$

    or

    $$\frac{15 \text{ mg}}{5 \text{ mg}} \times 1 \text{ mL} = x \text{ mL}$$

    Answer: 3 mL. The dosage ordered is more than the available strength; therefore, you will need more than 1 mL to administer the dosage.

37. $10 \text{ mg} : 1 \text{ mL} = 20 \text{ mg} : x \text{ mL}$

or

$$\frac{20 \text{ mg}}{10 \text{ mg}} \times 1 \text{ mL} = x \text{ mL}$$

Answer: 2 mL. The dosage ordered is more than the available strength; therefore, you will need more than 1 mL to administer the dosage (if the dosage strength used is 10 mg per mL as indicated on the label).

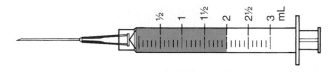

Answers to Clinical Reasoning Questions

1. a. The right medication. Hydroxyzine and hydralazine have similar names but are two different medications.
    b. Not reading the medication label carefully and not comparing it with the order or the medication administration record (MAR).
    c. Hydralazine is an antihypertensive and could cause a fatal drop in the patient's blood pressure.

Answers to Chapter Review

1. Conversion is required. Conversion factor: 1 000 mg = 1 g. Therefore, 0.3 g = 300 mg.

$$9\,000 \text{ mg} : 60 \text{ mL} = 300 \text{ mg} : x \text{ n}$$

or

$$\frac{300 \text{ mg}}{9\,000 \text{ mg}} \times 60 \text{ mL} = x \text{ n}$$

Answer: 2 mL. The dosage ordered is more than the available strength; therefore, you will need less than 60 mL to administer the dosage.

Alternative solution:

$$150 \text{ mg} : 1 \text{ mL} = 300 \text{ mg} : x \text{ mL}$$

or

$$\frac{300 \text{ mg}}{150 \text{ mg}} \times 1 \text{ mL} = x \text{ mL}$$

This setup gives the same answer, 2 mL.

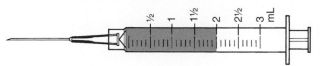

Alternative solution:

$$40 \text{ mg} : 4 \text{ mL} = 20 \text{ mg} : x \text{ mL}$$

or

$$\frac{20 \text{ mg}}{40 \text{ mg}} \times 4 \text{ mL} = x \text{ mL}$$

This setup gives the same answer, 2 mL.

d. Carefully comparing the medication label and dosage with the order or the MAR three times while preparing the medication. Perhaps if the nurse had consulted a reliable drug reference, he or she may have been alerted to the fact that hydralazine is used to treat hypertension and hydroxyzine is used for anxiety, which is what the medication was prescribed for.

2. $500 \text{ mcg} : 1 \text{ mL} = 175 \text{ mcg} : x \text{ mL}$

or

$$\frac{175 \text{ mcg}}{500 \text{ mcg}} \times 1 \text{ mL} = x \text{ mL}$$

Answer: 0.35 mL. The dosage ordered is less than the available strength; therefore, you will need less than 1 mL to administer the dosage.

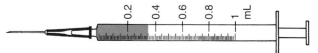

3. $30 \text{ mg} : 1 \text{ mL} = 25 \text{ mg} : x \text{ mL}$

or

$$\frac{25 \text{ mg}}{30 \text{ mg}} \times 1 \text{ mL} = x \text{ mL}$$

Answer: 0.83 mL = 0.8 mL. The dosage ordered is less than the available strength; therefore, you will need less than 1 mL to administer the dosage.

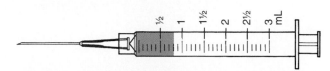

4. Conversion is required. Conversion factor:
   1 000 mcg = 1 mg. Therefore 100 mcg = 0.1 mg.

   $$0.25 \text{ mg} : 1 \text{ mL} = 0.1 \text{ mg} : x \text{ mL}$$

   or

   $$\frac{0.1 \text{ mg}}{0.25 \text{ mg}} \times 1 \text{ mL} = x \text{ mL}$$

   Answer: 0.4 mL. The dosage ordered is less than the available strength.

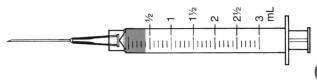

5. $$2 \text{ mg} : 1 \text{ mL} = 4 \text{ mg} : x \text{ mL}$$

   or

   $$\frac{4 \text{ mg}}{2 \text{ mg}} \times 1 \text{ mL} = x \text{ mL}$$

   Answer: 2 mL. The dosage ordered is more than the available strength; therefore, you will need more than 1 mL to administer the dosage.

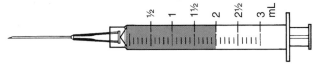

6. $$1\,200\,000 \text{ units} : 2 \text{ mL} = 1\,200\,000 \text{ units} : x \text{ mL}$$

   or

   $$\frac{1\,200\,000 \text{ units}}{1\,200\,000 \text{ units}} \times 2 \text{ mL} = x \text{ mL}$$

   Answer: 2 mL. The dosage ordered is contained in 2 mL; therefore, you will need 2 mL to administer the dosage.

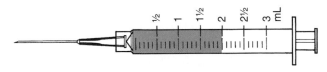

7. $$40 \text{ mg} : 1 \text{ mL} = 100 \text{ mg} : x \text{ mL}$$

   or

   $$\frac{100 \text{ mg}}{40 \text{ mg}} \times 1 \text{ mL} = x \text{ mL}$$

   Answer: 2.5 mL. The amount ordered is more than the available strength; therefore, you will need more than 1 mL to administer the dosage.

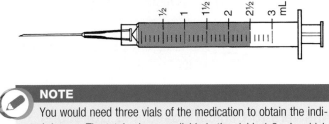

NOTE
You would need three vials of the medication to obtain the indicated dosage. The total volume available in the vial is 1.2 mL, which contains 40 mg.

8. $$0.2 \text{ mg} : 1 \text{ mL} = 0.4 \text{ mg} : x \text{ mL}$$

   or

   $$\frac{0.4 \text{ mg}}{0.2 \text{ mg}} \times 1 \text{ mL} = x \text{ mL}$$

   Answer: 2 mL. The dosage ordered is more than the available strength; therefore, you will need more than 1 mL to administer the dosage.

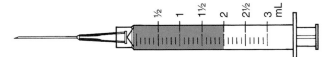

9. $$10\,000 \text{ units} : 1 \text{ mL} = 8\,000 \text{ units} : x \text{ mL}$$

   or

   $$\frac{8\,000 \text{ units}}{10\,000 \text{ units}} \times 1 \text{ mL} = x \text{ mL}$$

   Answer: 0.8 mL. The dosage ordered is less than the available strength; therefore, you will need less than 1 mL to administer the dosage.

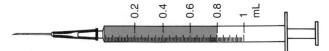

10. $250 \text{ mg} : 5 \text{ mL} = 200 \text{ mg} : x \text{ mL}$

or

$$\frac{200 \text{ mg}}{250 \text{ mg}} \times 5 \text{ mL} = x \text{ mL}$$

Answer: 4 mL. The dosage ordered is less than the available strength; therefore, you will need less than 5 mL to administer the dosage.

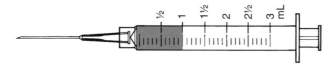

11. $10 \text{ mg} : 1 \text{ mL} = 10 \text{ mg} : x \text{ mL}$

or

$$\frac{10 \text{ mg}}{10 \text{ mg}} \times 1 \text{ mL} = x \text{ mL}$$

Answer: 1 mL. The dosage ordered is the same as the available strength; therefore, you will need 1 mL to administer the dosage.

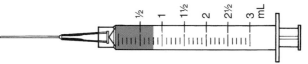

12. $20 \text{ mg} : 2 \text{ mL} = 40 \text{ mg} : x \text{ mL}$

or

$$\frac{40 \text{ mg}}{20 \text{ mg}} \times 2 \text{ mL} = x \text{ mL}$$

Answer: 4 mL. The dosage ordered is more than the available strength; therefore, you will need more than 2 mL to administer the dosage.

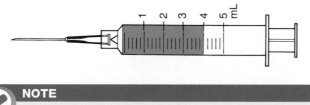

NOTE

You will need two vials of the medication to administer the ordered dosage. The total volume available in the vial is 2 mL, which is equal to 20 mg.

13. $50 \text{ mg} : 1 \text{ mL} = 25 \text{ mg} : x \text{ mL}$

or

$$\frac{25 \text{ mg}}{50 \text{ mg}} \times 1 \text{ mL} = x \text{ mL}$$

Answer: 0.5 mL. The dosage ordered is less than the available strength; therefore, you will need less than 1 mL to administer the dosage.

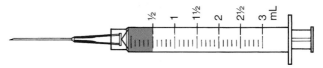

14. $2 \text{ mg} : 1 \text{ mL} = 1.5 \text{ mg} : x \text{ mL}$

or

$$\frac{1.5 \text{ mg}}{2 \text{ mg}} \times 1 \text{ mL} = x \text{ mL}$$

Answer: 0.8 mL. 0.75 mL is rounded to nearest tenth. The dosage ordered is less than the available strength; therefore, you will need less than 1 mL to administer the dosage.

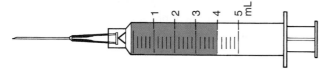

15. $40 \text{ mg} : 1 \text{ mL} = 50 \text{ mg} : x \text{ mL}$

or

$$\frac{50 \text{ mg}}{40 \text{ mg}} \times 1 \text{ mL} = x \text{ mL}$$

Answer: 1.3 mL. 1.25 mL is rounded to nearest tenth. The dosage ordered is more than the available strength per mL if you use 40 mg per mL; therefore, you will need more than 1 mL to administer the dosage.

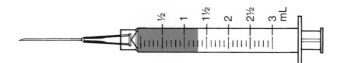

16.   50 mg : 1 mL = 25 mg : x mL

or

$$\frac{25\,mg}{50\,mg} \times 1\,mL = x\,mL$$

Answer: 0.5 mL. The dosage ordered is less than the available strength; therefore, you will need less than 1 mL to administer the dosage.

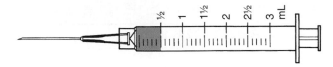

17.   4 mg : 2 mL = 3 mg : x mL

or

$$\frac{3\,mg}{4\,mg} \times 2\,mL = x\,mL$$

Answer: 1.5 mL. The dosage ordered is less than the available strength; therefore, you will need less than 2 mL to administer the dosage.

Alternative solution:

2 mg : 1 mL = 3 mg : x mL

or

$$\frac{3\,mg}{2\,mg} \times 1\,mL = x\,mL$$

This setup gives the same answer, 1.5 mL.

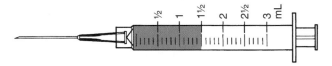

18.   250 mg : 2 mL = 400 mg : x mL

or

$$\frac{400\,mg}{250\,mg} \times 2\,mL = x\,mL$$

Answer: 3.2 mL. The dosage ordered is more than the available strength; therefore, you will need more than 2 mL to administer the dosage.

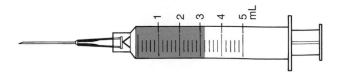

19.   Use the dosage indicated on the label in mg; no conversion required.

0.4 mg : 1 mL = 0.2 mg : x mL

or

$$\frac{0.2\,mg}{0.4\,mg} \times 1\,mL = x\,mL$$

Answer: 0.5 mL. The dosage ordered is less than the available strength; therefore, you will need less than 1 mL to administer the dosage.

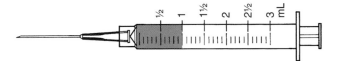

20.   Conversion is required. Conversion factor: 1 000 mcg = 1 mg. Therefore, 200 mcg = 0.2 mg.

0.2 mg : 1 mL = 0.2 mg : x mL

or

$$\frac{0.2\,mg}{0.2\,mg} \times 1\,mL = x\,mL$$

Answer: 1 mL. Because 200 mcg = 0.2 mg, you will need 1 mL to administer the dosage.

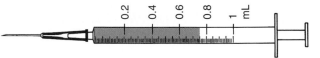

21.   40 mcg : 1 mL = 30 mcg : x mL

or

$$\frac{30\,mcg}{40\,mcg} \times 1\,mL = x\,mL$$

Answer: 0.75 mL. The dosage ordered is less than the available strength; therefore, you will need less than 1 mL to administer the dosage.

22. $50 \text{ mg} : 1 \text{ mL} = 35 \text{ mg} : x \text{ mL}$

or

$$\frac{35 \text{ mg}}{50 \text{ mg}} \times 1 \text{ mL} = x \text{ mL}$$

Answer: 0.7 mL. The dosage ordered is less than the available strength; therefore, you will need less than 1 mL to administer the dosage.

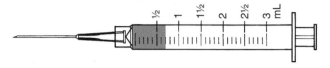

23. $100 \text{ mg} : 1 \text{ mL} = 60 \text{ mg} : x \text{ mL}$

or

$$\frac{60 \text{ mg}}{100 \text{ mg}} \times 1 \text{ mL} = x \text{ mL}$$

Answer: 0.6 mL. The dosage ordered is less than the available strength; therefore, you will need less than 1 mL to administer the dosage.

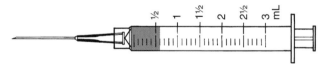

24. $50 \text{ mg} : 2 \text{ mL} = 50 \text{ mg} : x \text{ mL}$

or

$$\frac{50 \text{ mg}}{50 \text{ mg}} \times 2 \text{ mL} = x \text{ mL}$$

Answer: 2 mL. The dosage ordered is contained in 2 mL; therefore, you will need 2 mL to administer the dosage.

Alternative solution:

$25 \text{ mg} : 1 \text{ mL} = 50 \text{ mg} : x \text{ mL}$

or

$$\frac{50 \text{ mg}}{25 \text{ mg}} \times 1 \text{ mL} = x \text{ mL}$$

This setup gives the same answer, 2 mL.

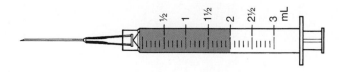

25. $0.5 \text{ mg} : 2 \text{ mL} = 0.4 \text{ mg} : x \text{ mL}$

or

$$\frac{0.4 \text{ mg}}{0.5 \text{ mg}} \times 2 \text{ mL} = x \text{ mL}$$

Answer: 1.6 mL. The dosage ordered is less than the available strength; therefore, you will need less than 2 mL to administer the dosage.

Alternative solution:

$0.25 \text{ mg} : 1 \text{ mL} = 0.4 \text{ mg} : x \text{ mL}$

or

$$\frac{0.4 \text{ mg}}{0.25 \text{ mg}} \times 1 \text{ mL} = x \text{ mL}$$

This setup gives the same answer, 1.6 mL.

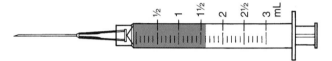

26. $300 \text{ mcg} : 0.5 \text{ mL} = 180 \text{ mcg} : x \text{ mL}$

or

$$\frac{180 \text{ mcg}}{300 \text{ mcg}} \times 0.5 \text{ mL} = x \text{ mL}$$

Answer: 0.3 mL. The dosage ordered is less than the available strength; therefore, you will need less than 0.5 mL to administer the dosage.

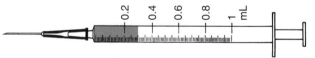

27. $300 \text{ mg} : 1 \text{ mL} = 500 \text{ mg} : x \text{ mL}$

or

$$\frac{500 \text{ mg}}{300 \text{ mg}} \times 1 \text{ mL} = x \text{ mL}$$

Answer: 1.7 mL. 1.66 mL is rounded to the nearest tenth. The dosage ordered is more than the available strength; therefore, you will need more than 1 mL to administer the dosage.

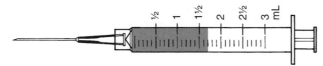

28. $2 \text{ mg} : 1 \text{ mL} = 1.5 \text{ mg} : x \text{ mL}$

or

$$\frac{1.5 \text{ mg}}{2 \text{ mg}} \times 1 \text{ mL} = x \text{ mL}$$

Answer: 0.75 mL = 0.8 mL. The dosage ordered is less than the available strength; therefore, you will need less than 1 mL to administer the dosage.

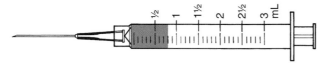

29. $25 \text{ mg} : 1 \text{ mL} = 65 \text{ mg} : x \text{ mL}$

or

$$\frac{65 \text{ mg}}{25 \text{ mg}} \times 1 \text{ mL} = x \text{ mL}$$

Answer: 2.6 mL. The dosage ordered is more than the available strength; therefore, you will need more than 1 mL to administer the dosage.

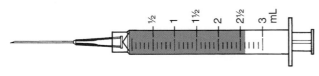

30. Conversion is required. Conversion factor: 1 000 mg = 1 g. Therefore, 0.65 g = 650 mg.

$$150 \text{ mg} : 1 \text{ mL} = 650 \text{ mg} : x \text{ mL}$$

or

$$\frac{650 \text{ mg}}{150 \text{ mg}} \times 1 \text{ mL} = x \text{ mL}$$

Answer: 4.33 mL. 4.3 mL is rounded to the nearest tenth. The dosage ordered is more than the available strength; therefore, you will need more than 1 mL to administer the dosage.

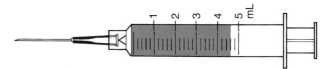

31. $10\,000 \text{ units} : 1 \text{ mL} = 3\,000 \text{ units} : x \text{ mL}$

or

$$\frac{3\,000 \text{ units}}{10\,000 \text{ units}} \times 1 \text{ mL} = x \text{ mL}$$

Answer: 0.3 mL. The dosage ordered is less than the available strength; therefore, you will need less than 1 mL to administer the dosage.

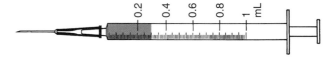

32. $10 \text{ mg} : 2 \text{ mL} = 15 \text{ mg} : x \text{ mL}$

or

$$\frac{15 \text{ mg}}{10 \text{ mg}} \times 2 \text{ mL} = x \text{ mL}$$

Answer: 3 mL. The dosage ordered is more than the available strength; therefore, you will need more than 2 mL to administer the dosage.

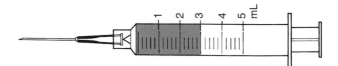

33.   40 mg:0.4 mL = 30 mg:*x* mL

or

$$\frac{30 \text{ mg}}{40 \text{ mg}} \times 0.4 \text{ mL} = x \text{ mL}$$

Answer: 0.3 mL. The dosage ordered is less than the available strength; therefore, you will need less than 0.4 mL to administer the dosage.

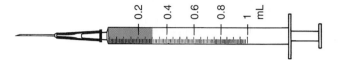

34. Conversion is required. Conversion factor: 1 000 mg = 1 g. Therefore, 0.3 g = 300 mg.

300 mg : 2 mL = 300 mg : *x* mL

or

$$\frac{300 \text{ mg}}{300 \text{ mg}} \times 2 \text{ mL} = x \text{ mL}$$

Answer: 2 mL. The label indicates that the dosage ordered, 300 mg, is contained in a volume of 2 mL.

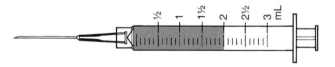

35.   5 mg:1 mL = 7.5 mg:*x* mL

or

$$\frac{7.5 \text{ mg}}{5 \text{ mg}} \times 1 \text{ mL} = x \text{ mL}$$

Answer: 1.5 mL. (State the answer as a decimal; mL is a metric measurement.) The dosage ordered is more than the available strength; therefore, you will need more than 1 mL to administer the dosage.

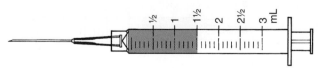

36.   0.25 mg:1 mL = 1 mg:*x* mL

or

$$\frac{1 \text{ mg}}{0.25 \text{ mg}} \times 1 \text{ mL} = x \text{ mL}$$

Answer: 4 mL. The dosage ordered is more than the available strength; therefore, you will need more than 1 mL to administer the dosage.

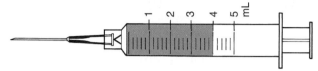

37.   40 mg:1 mL = 55 mg:*x* mL

or

$$\frac{55 \text{ mg}}{40 \text{ mg}} \times 1 \text{ mL} = x \text{ mL}$$

Answer: 1.4 mL; 1.37 rounded to the nearest tenth. The dosage ordered is more than the available strength; therefore, you will need more than 1 mL to administer the dosage.

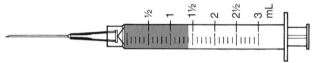

38.   6 mg:1 mL = 12 mg:*x* mL

or

$$\frac{12 \text{ mg}}{6 \text{ mg}} \times 1 \text{ mL} = x \text{ mL}$$

Answer: 2 mL. The dosage ordered is more than the available strength; therefore, you will need more than 1 mL to administer the dosage.

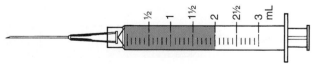

39. Conversion is required. Conversion factor:
1 000 mg = 1 g. Therefore, 0.25 g = 250 mg.

$$25 \text{ mg}:1 \text{ mL} = 250 \text{ mg}:x \text{ mL}$$

or

$$\frac{250 \text{ mg}}{25 \text{ mg}} \times 1 \text{ mL} = x \text{ mL}$$

Answer: 10 mL. The dosage ordered is more than the available strength when using 25 mg per mL; therefore, you will need more than 1 mL to administer the dosage.

Alternative solution:

$$500 \text{ mg}:20 \text{ mL} = 250 \text{ mg}:x \text{ mL}$$

or

$$\frac{250 \text{ mg}}{500 \text{ mg}} \times 20 \text{ mL} = x \text{ mL}$$

This setup gives the same answer, 10 mL.

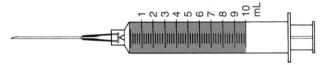

40. Conversion is required. Conversion factor:
1 000 mg = 1 g. Therefore, 0.4 g = 400 mg.

$$100 \text{ mg}:1 \text{ mL} = 400 \text{ mg}:x \text{ mL}$$

or

$$\frac{400 \text{ mg}}{100 \text{ mg}} \times 1 \text{ mL} = x \text{ mL}$$

Answer: 4 mL. The dosage ordered, 400 mg, is more than the available strength when using 100 mg per mL; therefore, you will need more than 1 mL to administer the dosage.

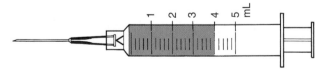

41. $$100 \text{ mg}:1 \text{ mL} = 150 \text{ mg}:x \text{ mL}$$

or

$$\frac{150 \text{ mg}}{100 \text{ mg}} \times 1 \text{ mL} = x \text{ mL}$$

Answer: 1.5 mL. The dosage ordered is more than the available strength; therefore, you will need more than 1 mL to administer the dosage.

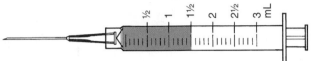

42. Meperidine:

$$100 \text{ mg}:1 \text{ mL} = 65 \text{ mg}:x \text{ mL}$$

or

$$\frac{65 \text{ mg}}{100 \text{ mg}} \times 1 \text{ mL} = x \text{ mL}$$

Answer: 0.7 mL; 0.65 mL rounded to the nearest tenth. The dosage ordered is less than the available strength; therefore, you will need less than 1 mL to administer the dosage.

Promethazine:

$$50 \text{ mg}:1 \text{ mL} = 25 \text{ mg}:x \text{ mL}$$

or

$$\frac{25 \text{ mg}}{50 \text{ mg}} \times 1 \text{ mL} = x \text{ mL}$$

Answer: 0.5 mL. The label indicates that the dosage ordered, 25 mg, is contained in the volume of 1 mL. These two medications are often administered in the same syringe (0.7 mL of meperidine + 0.5 mL of promethazine = 1.2 mL).

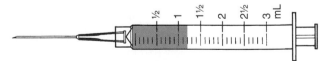

43. $4 \, \text{mg} : 1 \, \text{mL} = 9 \, \text{mg} : x \, \text{mL}$

or

$$\frac{9 \, \text{mg}}{4 \, \text{mg}} \times 1 \, \text{mL} = x \, \text{mL}$$

Answer: 2.3 mL; 2.25 mL rounded to the nearest tenth. The dosage ordered is more than the available strength. You would need more than 1 mL to administer the dosage.

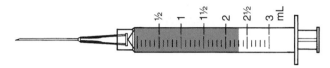

44. $50 \, \text{mcg} : 1 \, \text{mL} = 60 \, \text{mcg} : x \, \text{mL}$

or

$$\frac{60 \, \text{mcg}}{50 \, \text{mcg}} \times 1 \, \text{mL} = x \, \text{mL}$$

Answer: 1.2 mL. The dosage ordered is more than the available strength when using 50 mcg per mL; therefore, you will need more than 1 mL to administer the dosage.

Alternative solution:

$$250 \, \text{mcg} : 5 \, \text{mL} = 60 \, \text{mcg} : x \, \text{mL}$$

or

$$\frac{60 \, \text{mcg}}{250 \, \text{mcg}} \times 5 \, \text{mL} = x \, \text{mL}$$

This setup gives the same answer, 1.2 mL.

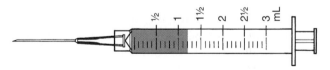

45. $20 \, \text{mg} : 1 \, \text{mL} = 10 \, \text{mg} : x \, \text{mL}$

or

$$\frac{10 \, \text{mg}}{20 \, \text{mg}} \times 1 \, \text{mL} = x \, \text{mL}$$

Answer: 0.5 mL. The dosage ordered is less than the available strength; therefore, you will need less than 1 mL to administer the dosage.

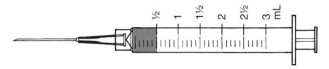

46. $5 \, \text{mg} : 1 \, \text{mL} = 4 \, \text{mg} : x \, \text{mL}$

or

$$\frac{4 \, \text{mg}}{5 \, \text{mg}} \times 1 \, \text{mL} = x \, \text{mL}$$

Answer: 0.8 mL. The dosage ordered is less than the available strength; therefore, you will need less than 1 mL to administer the dosage.

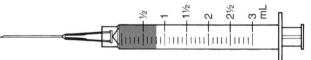

47. $300 \, \text{mcg} : 1 \, \text{mL} = 175 \, \text{mcg} : x \, \text{mL}$

or

$$\frac{175 \, \text{mcg}}{300 \, \text{mcg}} \times 1 \, \text{mL} = x \, \text{mL}$$

Answer: 0.6 mL; 0.58 rounded to the nearest tenth. The dosage ordered is less than the available strength; therefore, you will need less than 1 mL to administer the dosage.

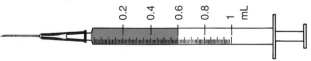

CHAPTER **17**
Reconstitution of Solutions

Objectives

After reviewing this chapter, you should be able to:

1. Prepare a solution from a powdered medication according to directions on the vial or other resources
2. Understand how to label a vial of a medication after it is reconstituted
3. Determine the best concentration of a medication for the dosage ordered when there are several directions for mixing
4. Understand the varying directions for reconstitution of a medication and select the correct directions to prepare the dosage ordered
5. Calculate dosages of reconstituted medications
6. Determine the rate in millilitres per hour for enteral feedings
7. Calculate the amount of solute and solvent needed to prepare a desired strength for enteral feedings

Some medications are unstable when stored in liquid form for long periods of time and, therefore, they are packaged in powdered form. When medications come in powdered form, they must be diluted with a liquid referred to as a *diluent* or *solvent* before they can be administered to a patient. Once a liquid is added to a powdered medication, the solution may be used for only 1 to 14 days, depending on the type of medication. The process of adding a solvent or diluent to a medication in powdered form to dissolve it and form a solution is referred to as *reconstitution*. Reconstitution is necessary for medications that come in powdered form before they can be measured and administered. If you think about it, this process is something you do in everyday situations. For example, when you make iced tea (powdered form), in essence you are reconstituting it. The iced tea, for example, is the powder, and the water you add to it is considered the diluent, or solvent.

In today's health care environment, the pharmacy usually reconstitutes medications unless these are to be given stat or the order was made during the evening or night shift when the pharmacy is not available. Nurses may do more reconstitution in a home care setting, but most prescriptions are prepared by community pharmacies for patient use at home. Nonetheless, nurses must understand the process of reconstitution. There are also times when medications may have to be reconstituted just before administration, so it is the nurse's responsibility to do so safely.

Medications requiring reconstitution can be for oral, parenteral, or enteral use as well as for topical use (such as wound care solutions for cleansing, soaking, and irrigating). Nutritional feedings may be prescribed initially in less than full strength; therefore, the nurse must reconstitute the feeding just before administration to help reduce bacterial growth in the formula over time. Sterile solutions are always used to reconstitute medications for injectable use. Special diluents, when required for reconstitution, are usually packaged with the powdered medication; but oral medications can often be, but are not always, reconstituted with tap water.

Understanding the terminology related to reconstitution is helpful to understanding the process:

- **Solute**—A powdered medication or liquid concentrate to be dissolved or diluted.
- **Solvent (diluent)**—A liquid that is added to the powder or liquid concentrate. The nurse must identify the solvent (diluent) to use. The type of solvent (diluent) varies according to the medication. The package insert or the medication label will indicate the solvent (diluent) to be used and the amount. If the information is not indicated on the label or the package insert is unavailable, consult the pharmacy or a drug reference such as the *Nursing Drug Handbook*. Most institutions now have the *Compendium of Pharmaceuticals and Specialties (CPS): The Canadian Drug Reference for Health Professionals* online for their staff to access.
- **Solution**—The liquid that results when the solvent (diluent) dissolves the solute (powdered medication or liquid concentrate).

Basic Principles of Reconstitution

The first step in reconstitution is to find the reconstitution directions on the vial or the package insert and carefully read them. Medications labelled and packaged with reconstitution directions usually indicate the route of administration: oral, intramuscular (IM), intravenous (IV), or topical. Carefully check the route of administration of the medication and the reconstitution directions. Examples of several directions for reconstitution are shown in this chapter.

> **! SAFETY ALERT!**
>
> Before reconstituting a medication, read and follow the directions on the label or package insert. Also check the expiration date on the medication and diluent. Never make assumptions about the type or amount of diluent to be used. If the information is not available, consult appropriate resources, including the manufacturer's website, before reconstituting the medication.

The basic principles of reconstitution are as follows:

1. The medication manufacturer provides directions for reconstitution, including information regarding the number of millilitres of diluent or solvent that should be added, as well as the type of solution that should be used to reconstitute the medication. The concentration of the medication after it has been reconstituted (the *final concentration*) is also indicated on some medications. The directions for reconstitution must be read and followed carefully.
2. The diluent (solvent, liquid) commonly used for reconstitution is sterile water or sterile 0.9% sodium chloride (normal saline) solution, for injection. Sterile water and normal saline for injection are available in preservative-free diluent used for single-use reconstitution and in bacteriostatic form with preservatives that prevent the growth of microorganisms for multidose vials. Some powdered medications for oral use may be reconstituted with tap water. The manufacturer's directions will tell you which solution to use. If the medication requires a special solution for reconstitution, it is usually supplied by the medication manufacturer and packaged with the medication (e.g., glucagon).

> **! SAFETY ALERT!**
>
> Always use a sterile solution for injection and for mixing to administer a medication by the parenteral route.

3. The reconstitution directions on a label typically provide the following information:
   a. The type of diluent to use for reconstitution.
   b. The amount of diluent to add. This is essential because directions relating to the amount can vary according to the route of administration. There may be different dilution instructions for IV versus IM administration.

c. The length of time the medication is good once it is reconstituted. The length of time a medication can be stored once reconstituted can vary depending on how it is stored. When medications are reconstituted, the solution must be used in a timely fashion. The stability of the medication may be several hours to several days or 2 weeks. Check the medication label, package insert, or appropriate resources for how long a medication may be used after reconstitution.

d. Directions for storing the medication after mixing. Medications must be stored appropriately once reconstituted per manufacturer's instructions to ensure optimal potency and stability of the medication. Medications can become unstable when stored incorrectly and for long periods. Example: A label may state a medication maintains its potency 96 hours at room temperature or 7 days when refrigerated.

e. The strength or concentration of the medication after it has been reconstituted.

   Figure 17-1 shows the ceftriaxone reconstitution procedure for IM. Note that directions on the label say to add 2.1 mL 1% lidocaine hydrochloride injection or sterile water for injection. Sterile water would be the choice of diluent, since you never use medication as a diluent without further orders from the prescriber. The available dosage strength after reconstitution is 350 mg of ceftriaxone per mL of solution.

4. If there are no directions for reconstitution on the label or on the package insert, or if any of the information (listed in number 3) is missing, appropriate resources should be consulted (e.g., a drug reference, the current CPS at the hospital, the pharmacy, or the manufacturer's website).

5. Injectable medications for reconstitution can come in a single-dose vial or a multidose vial. When medications are in single-dose vials, there is enough medication for **one** dose only, and the contents are administered after reconstitution. In the case where the nurse reconstitutes a multidose vial, there is enough medication for **more than one** dose.

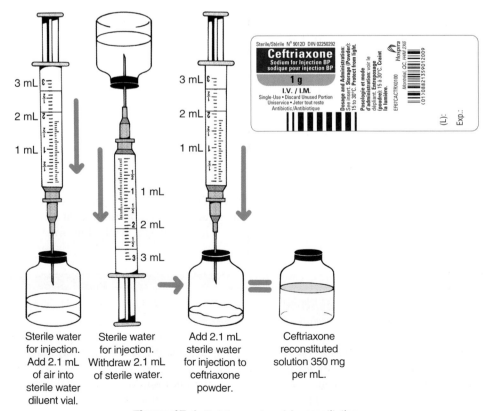

Sterile water for injection. Add 2.1 mL of air into sterile water diluent vial.

Sterile water for injection. Withdraw 2.1 mL of sterile water.

Add 2.1 mL sterile water for injection to ceftriaxone powder.

Ceftriaxone reconstituted solution 350 mg per mL.

Figure 17-1 Ceftriaxone 1-g vial reconstitution.

Therefore, when a multidose vial is reconstituted, it is important to clearly label the vial after reconstitution with the following information:

a. The date and time prepared, dosage strength prepared, and the expiration date and time once reconstituted. *Note:* If all of the solution that is mixed is used, this information is not necessary. Information regarding the date and time of preparation and date and time of expiration is crucial when all of the medication is not used.

b. Storage directions such as "Refrigerate."

c. Your initials.

If the medication label does not have room to clearly write the required information, add a label to the vial and indicate the important information on it. Make certain that the label is applied so that it does not obscure the medication name and dosage.

6. When reconstituting medications that are in multidose vials or have several directions for preparation, **information regarding the dosage strength or final concentration must be on the label; for example, 500 mg per mL. This is important because others who will use the medication after you need this information to determine the dosage.**

TIPS FOR CLINICAL PRACTICE

When reconstituting a multidose medication vial, label it with the required information and store it appropriately. If the vial is not labelled with the date and time the medication was reconstituted, the dosage strength after reconstitution, and the expiration date and time, the medication must be discarded.

7. After the diluent is added to a powder, some medications completely dissolve and there is no additional volume. However, often the powdered medication adds volume to the solution. The powdered medication takes up space as it dissolves and results in an increase in the amount of total (fluid) volume once it has dissolved. This is sometimes referred to as the *displacement factor,* or just *displacement.* The reconstituted material represents the diluent and powder. For example, directions for 1 g of powdered medication may state to add 2.5 mL sterile water for injection to provide an approximate volume of 3 mL (330 mg per mL). When the 2.5 mL of diluent is added, the 1 g of powdered medication displaces an additional 0.5 mL, for a total volume of 3 mL. The available dosage after reconstitution is 330 mg per mL of solution.

SAFETY ALERT!

Always determine both the type and amount of diluent to be used when reconstituting medications. Read and follow the label or package insert directions carefully to ensure that your patient receives the intended dosage. Consult the pharmacist or other appropriate resources if there are any questions. Never assume!

TIPS FOR CLINICAL PRACTICE

If the powder displaces the liquid as it dissolves and increases the volume, the resulting volume and concentration must be considered when the correct dosage of medication is calculated. Whether a medication causes an increase in volume when it is reconstituted will be indicated on the medication label or the package insert.

The two types of reconstituted parenteral solutions are single strength and multiple strength. A single-strength solution has the directions for reconstitution printed on the label, as shown on the 1 g ceftriaxone label in Figure 17-1. A multiple-strength solution usually has several directions for reconstitution and requires that the nurse be even more attentive to the directions to select the best concentration to administer the required dosage. We will discuss reconstitution of multiple-strength solutions later in this chapter.

Let's do some practice problems in relation to single-strength solutions.

+−÷× PRACTICE **PROBLEMS**

Using the label for gemcitabine, answer the following questions.

For IV use only.
Store at controlled room
temperature 20° - 25°C.
Do not refrigerate.

DOSAGE AND USE
See package insert for full
prescribing information

To reconstitute: Add 5 mL of 0.9% Sodium
Chloride Injection (without preservatives)
to make a solution containing 38 mg/
mL. Shake to dissolve. Administer within
24 hours.

Exp./
Lot:

DIN: 000000000

gemcitabine hydrochloride
For injection

200 mg

SAMPLE LABEL (textbook use only)

http://evolve.elsevier.com/Canada/GrayMorris/

1. What is the total dosage strength of
   Gemzar in this vial?   _____

2. How much diluent is added to the vial
   to prepare the medication for IV use?   _____

3. What diluent is recommended for
   reconstitution?   _____

4. What is the final concentration of the
   prepared solution for IV administration?   _____

5. How long will the reconstituted material
   retain its stability?   _____

6. 100 mg IV is ordered for day one of
   treatment. How many mL will
   you give? Shade in the dosage on the
   syringe provided.   _____

Using the label for leucovorin calcium, answer the following questions.

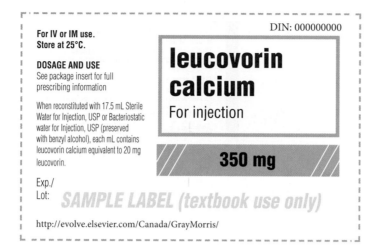

For IV or IM use.
Store at 25°C.

DOSAGE AND USE
See package insert for full
prescribing information

When reconstituted with 17.5 mL Sterile
Water for Injection, USP or Bacteriostatic
water for Injection, USP (preserved
with benzyl alcohol), each mL contains
leucovorin calcium equivalent to 20 mg
leucovorin.

Exp./
Lot:

DIN: 000000000

leucovorin calcium

For injection

350 mg

SAMPLE LABEL (textbook use only)

http://evolve.elsevier.com/Canada/GrayMorris/

7. What is the total dosage strength of
   leucovorin calcium in the vial?
   _____

8. How much diluent is added to the vial to
   reconstitute the medication?
   _____

9. What diluent is recommended for
   reconstitution?
   _____

10. What is the final concentration of the
    reconstituted solution?
    _____

11. For what routes of administration
    is the medication indicated?
    _____

12. Where can you find directions for
    complete prescribing information?
    _____

13. 15 mg IM q6h is ordered. How many
    mL will you give? Shade in the
    dosage on the syringe provided.
    _____

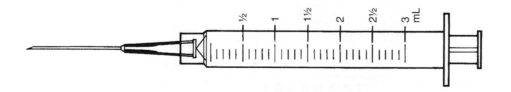

Using the label for methylprednisolone sodium succinate, answer the following questions.

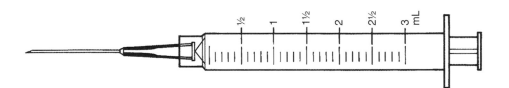

14. What is the total dosage strength of methylprednisolone sodium succinate in the vial?

_____

15. What diluent is recommended to prepare an IV dosage?

_____

16. How many mL of diluent are needed to prepare an IV dosage?

_____

17. What is the final concentration of the solution prepared for IV administration?

_____

18. 35 mg IV daily is ordered. How many mL will you give? Shade in the dosage on the syringe provided.

_____

Using the label for ceftriaxone, answer the following questions.

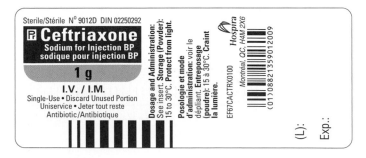

19. What is the total dosage strength of ceftriaxone in this vial?

_____

20. For what routes of administration is the medication indicated?

_____

Using the label for amoxicillin, answer the following questions.

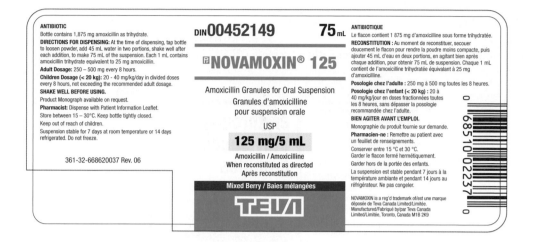

21. How much diluent must be added to prepare the solution?

_____

22. What type of solution is used for the diluent?

_____

23. What is the final concentration of the prepared solution?

_____

24. How should the medication be stored after it is reconstituted?

_____

Using the label for acyclovir and a portion of the package insert, answer the following questions.

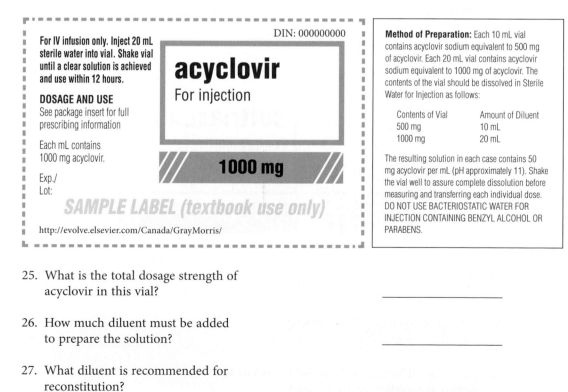

25. What is the total dosage strength of acyclovir in this vial?

_____

26. How much diluent must be added to prepare the solution?

_____

27. What diluent is recommended for reconstitution?

_____

28. What is the final concentration of the prepared solution? _____

29. What is the route of administration? _____

Using the label for erythromycin ethylsuccinate (EES), answer the following questions.

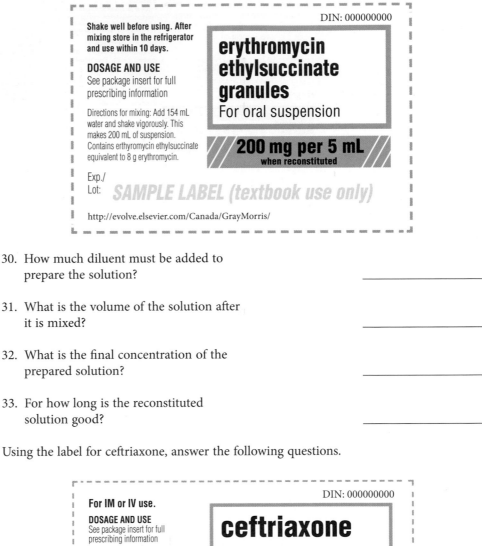

30. How much diluent must be added to prepare the solution? _____

31. What is the volume of the solution after it is mixed? _____

32. What is the final concentration of the prepared solution? _____

33. For how long is the reconstituted solution good? _____

Using the label for ceftriaxone, answer the following questions.

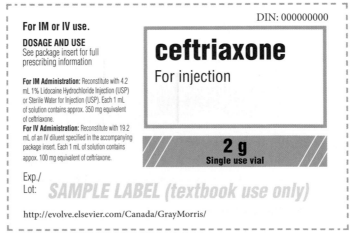

34. What is the total dosage strength of ceftriaxone in this vial? _____

35. How much diluent must be added to the vial to prepare the medication for IM use? _____

36. How much diluent must be added to the vial to prepare the medication for IV use? _____

37. What diluent is recommended for IV reconstitution? _____

38. What is the final concentration of the prepared solution for IV use? _____

Using the label for azithromycin (Zithromax), answer the following questions.

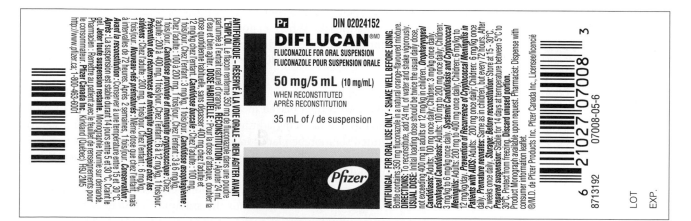

39. What is the total dosage strength of Zithromax in this vial? _____

40. What is the final concentration of the prepared solution? _____

41. What are the directions for use? _____

Using the label for fluconazole, answer the following questions.

42. How much diluent must be added to prepare the solution? _____

43. What diluent is recommended for reconstitution? _____

44. What is the final concentration of the prepared solution? _____

45. How should the medication be stored after it is reconstituted? _____

Answers on page 464.

Calculation of Medications When the Final Concentration (Dosage Strength) Is Not Stated

Sometimes a medication comes with directions for only one way to reconstitute it, and the label does not indicate the final dosage strength after it is mixed, such as "becomes 250 mg per mL." Example: A particular medication is available in 1 g in powder. Directions tell you that adding 2.5 mL of sterile water for injection yields 3 mL of solution. When you add 2.5 mL of sterile water to the powder, the volume expands to 3 mL. The concentration is not changing; you will get 3 mL of solution; however, it will be equal to 1 g. Therefore, the problem is calculated by using 1 g = 3 mL.

Reconstituting Medications with More Than One Direction for Mixing (Multiple Strength)

Remember that the directions for reconstitution can be on the label or a package insert. At times, the vial will contain minimal information. It may only include the dosage strength and state "see package insert for directions for reconstitution or storage."

Some medications, in addition to giving the route of administration, may come with several directions for preparing different solution strengths. In this case, the nurse must choose the dosage strength, or concentration, appropriate for the dosage ordered. A common medication that has a choice of dosage strengths is penicillin. When a medication comes with several directions for preparation or offers a choice of dosage strengths, you must choose the strength most appropriate for the dosage ordered. The guidelines that follow may be used to choose the appropriate concentration of a medication.

Guidelines for Choosing the Appropriate Concentration of a Medication

1. Verify the route of administration. It is essential to know the route of administration before reconstituting:
   a. IM—Intramuscular injections are rarely given today due to the increased use of the IV route of administration for antibiotics, analgesics, and antiemetics. However, if you are administering by IM and have the choice of multiple dosage strengths, ensure that the amount does not exceed the maximum allowed for IM administration. At the same time, you do not want to choose a concentration that will result in irritation when injected into a muscle. When a choice of dosage strengths is offered, do not choose an amount that would exceed the amount allowed for IM administration or one that is very concentrated. Consider the muscle site being used and the age of the patient.
   b. IV—Keep in mind that this medication is usually further diluted because once reconstituted, the medication is then placed in additional fluid of 50 to 100 mL or more, depending on the medication being administered. Example: Erythromycin requires that the reconstituted solution be placed in 250 mL of fluid before administration to a patient. In pediatrics, a medication may be given in a smaller volume of fluid, depending on the child's age, the child's size, and the medication.
2. Choose the concentration or dosage strength that comes closest to what the prescriber has ordered. The dosage strengths are given for the amount of diluent used. Example: If the prescriber orders 300 000 units of a particular medication IM, and the choice of dosage strength is 200 000 units per mL, 250 000 units per mL, and 500 000 units per mL, the strength closest to 300 000 units per mL is 250 000 units per mL. The dosage 250 000 units per mL allows you to administer a dosage within the range allowed for IM administration, and it is not the most concentrated.

⚠ SAFETY ALERT!

When multiple directions are given for reconstituting medications, the smaller the amount of diluent used to reconstitute the medication, the more concentrated the resulting solution will be. Consider the route of administration when reconstituting medications. Always check the route and the directions related to reconstitution.

3. Be aware of the meaning of the word *respectively* on a label. This word appears on some medication labels in the directions on reconstitution. For example, "reconstitute with 23 mL, 18 mL, 8 mL of diluent to provide concentrations of 200 000 units per mL, 250 000 units per mL, 500 000 units per mL, respectively." The word *respectively* means in the order given. In this case, "respectively" indicates that adding 23 mL of diluent will provide 200 000 units per mL, adding 18 mL of diluent will provide 250 000 units per mL, and adding 8 mL of diluent will provide 500 000 units per mL. In other words, the amounts of diluent correspond to the order in which the concentrations are written. **Remember: when you are mixing a medication that is a multiple-strength solution, the dosage strength that you prepare must be written on the vial.**

Keep in mind that some medications for parenteral use come with several directions for mixing to obtain several different solution strengths and require that you select a particular dosage strength. The dosage strength chosen should result in a reasonable amount of solution administered to the patient. Remember that the route of administration is an essential consideration.

Let's look at a sample label that shows a multiple-strength solution. Refer to the label for penicillin G potassium.

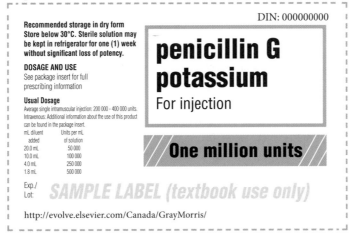

Notice that the label shows "one million units." This means that a total of 1 000 000 units of penicillin G potassium is in the vial. The directions for reconstitution and the dosage strengths that can be obtained are listed on the label. The left column indicates the choices for diluent volume that can be used to reconstitute the medication. The right column indicates the final dosage strengths in units per millilitre that will be made based on the amount of diluent added. If the dosage ordered for the patient was, for example, 250 000 units q6h, the most appropriate strength to mix would be 250 000 units per mL. If you look next to the dosage strength in the directions, you will notice that 4 mL of diluent must be added to obtain a concentration of 250 000 units per mL. Let's assume the order is for 300 000 units IM for an adult. The best concentration in this case would be 250 000 units per mL. Refer to the label and notice that to make this concentration, you will need to add 4 mL of diluent. When calculated, the patient would receive 1.2 mL (3 mL is the maximum for a large adult muscle). Remember that the condition of the intramuscular site and the patient (age and muscle mass) must be considered. Depending on the status of the patient, a different dosage strength may be a better choice. Notice also that when you reconstitute the medication using 4 mL, the total volume will be 4 mL, which means you have enough for approximately two additional doses. Because this medication is a multiple-strength solution, the dosage strength you choose must be indicated on the vial after you reconstitute it. Since the type of diluent is not indicated on the label, other resources, such as hospital (employer, institution) policy or those recommended previously must be consulted.

SAFETY ALERT!

If a multiple-strength solution is prepared and not used in its entirety, the dosage strength (final concentration) you mixed must be indicated on the label to verify the dosage strength of the reconstituted solution. Proper labelling is a crucial detail.

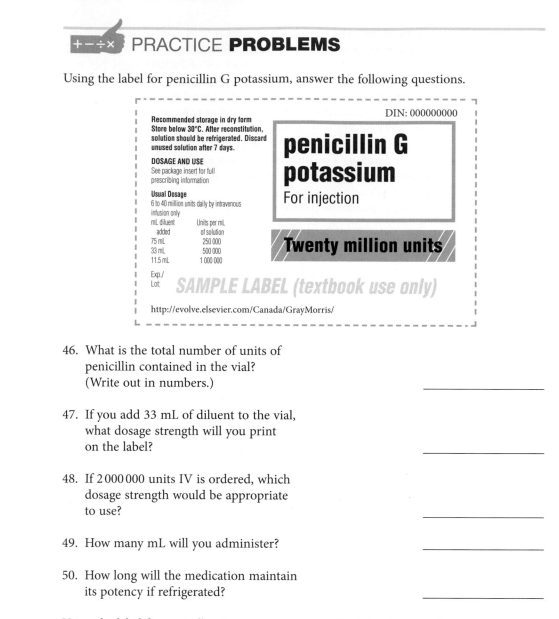

PRACTICE PROBLEMS

Using the label for penicillin G potassium, answer the following questions.

46. What is the total number of units of
penicillin contained in the vial?
(Write out in numbers.)   _____

47. If you add 33 mL of diluent to the vial,
what dosage strength will you print
on the label?   _____

48. If 2 000 000 units IV is ordered, which
dosage strength would be appropriate
to use?   _____

49. How many mL will you administer?   _____

50. How long will the medication maintain
its potency if refrigerated?   _____

Using the label for penicillin G potassium, answer the following questions.

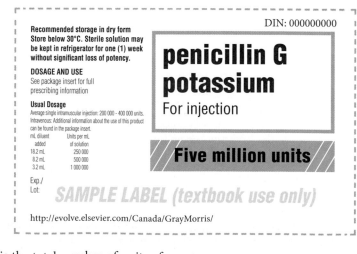

51. What is the total number of units of
penicillin contained in the vial?
(Write out in numbers.)   _____

52. If 700 000 units IM is ordered, which
    dosage strength would be appropriate
    to use?   _____

53. How many mL will you administer?   _____

54. Where will you store any unused
    medication?   _____

55. How long will the medication maintain
    its potency?   _____

56. What concentration strength would be
    obtained if you added 18.2 mL of diluent?
    (Write out in numbers.)   _____

57. Where would the usual dosage for IV
    administration be found?   _____

Answers on pages 464–465.

Reconstituting Medications from Package Insert Directions for Different Routes of Administration

If the label does not contain reconstitution directions, you must obtain directions from the information insert that accompanies the vial. Pay attention to the amount in the vial and the route of administration; there may be different directions based on these factors. Refer to the ceftazidime label (Figure 17-2) and accompanying insert. Note that there are two reconstitution directions for ceftazidime IV infusion: one for a 1-g vial and another for a 2-g vial. Also, note that the ceftazidime label has different directions for IM or IV direct (bolus) injection. Always check the route ordered, and follow the directions corresponding to that route.

> ⚠ **SAFETY ALERT!**
> Carefully check the route of administration ordered before reconstituting a medication and follow the directions corresponding to that route. Do not interchange the dilution instructions for IM or IV because you can harm the patient.

Medication Labels with Instructions to "See Accompanying Literature" (Package Insert) for Reconstitution and Administration

Some medications that require reconstitution may indicate the dosage strength contained in the vial and do not provide the information necessary to reconstitute the medication or information relating to administration on the label. To prepare the powdered medication, you must see the package insert or accompanying literature. Refer to the olanzapine label in Figure 17-3, *A*, and the accompanying package insert information in Figure 17-3, *B*. The label instructs you to "see accompanying literature for dosage, reconstitution instructions, and method of administration."

To reconstitute the medication and calculate a dosage, you need to refer to the package insert. The directions instruct you to add 2.1 mL of sterile water for injection for dosages up to 10 mg, and indicate the number of mL to withdraw to administer specific dosages of the medication IM. For example, notice that if you had to administer 5 mg of olanzapine IM, when the medication has been reconstituted, you would withdraw 1 mL of the medication to administer the ordered dosage of 5 mg.

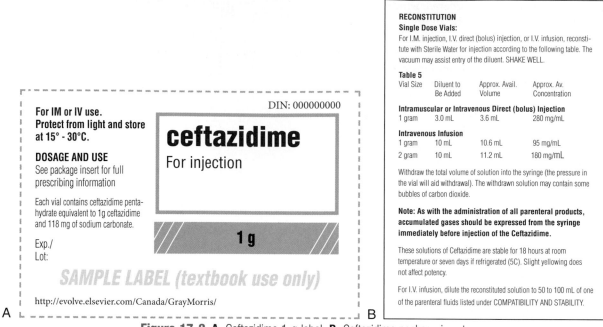

For IM or IV use.
Protect from light and store
at 15° - 30°C.

DOSAGE AND USE
See package insert for full
prescribing information

Each vial contains ceftazidime penta-
hydrate equivalent to 1g ceftazidime
and 118 mg of sodium carbonate.

Exp./
Lot:

DIN: 000000000

ceftazidime
For injection

1 g

SAMPLE LABEL (textbook use only)

http://evolve.elsevier.com/Canada/GrayMorris/

A

RECONSTITUTION
Single Dose Vials:
For I.M. injection, I.V. direct (bolus) injection, or I.V. infusion, reconstitute with Sterile Water for injection according to the following table. The
vacuum may assist entry of the diluent. SHAKE WELL.

Table 5

Vial Size	Diluent to Be Added	Approx. Avail. Volume	Approx. Av. Concentration
Intramuscular or Intravenous Direct (bolus) Injection			
1 gram	3.0 mL	3.6 mL	280 mg/mL
Intravenous Infusion			
1 gram	10 mL	10.6 mL	95 mg/mL
2 gram	10 mL	11.2 mL	180 mg/mL

Withdraw the total volume of solution into the syringe (the pressure in
the vial will aid withdrawal). The withdrawn solution may contain some
bubbles of carbon dioxide.

**Note: As with the administration of all parenteral products,
accumulated gases should be expressed from the syringe
immediately before injection of the Ceftazidime.**

These solutions of Ceftazidime are stable for 18 hours at room
temperature or seven days if refrigerated (5C). Slight yellowing does
not affect potency.

For I.V. infusion, dilute the reconstituted solution to 50 to 100 mL of one
of the parenteral fluids listed under COMPATIBILITY AND STABILITY.

B

Figure 17-2 A, Ceftazidime 1-g label. **B,** Ceftazidime package insert.

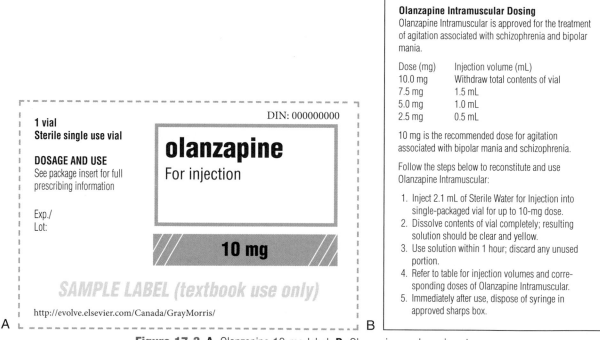

1 vial
Sterile single use vial

DOSAGE AND USE
See package insert for full
prescribing information

Exp./
Lot:

DIN: 000000000

olanzapine
For injection

10 mg

SAMPLE LABEL (textbook use only)

http://evolve.elsevier.com/Canada/GrayMorris/

A

Olanzapine Intramuscular Dosing
Olanzapine Intramuscular is approved for the treatment
of agitation associated with schizophrenia and bipolar
mania.

Dose (mg)	Injection volume (mL)
10.0 mg	Withdraw total contents of vial
7.5 mg	1.5 mL
5.0 mg	1.0 mL
2.5 mg	0.5 mL

10 mg is the recommended dose for agitation
associated with bipolar mania and schizophrenia.

Follow the steps below to reconstitute and use
Olanzapine Intramuscular:

1. Inject 2.1 mL of Sterile Water for Injection into
single-packaged vial for up to 10-mg dose.
2. Dissolve contents of vial completely; resulting
solution should be clear and yellow.
3. Use solution within 1 hour; discard any unused
portion.
4. Refer to table for injection volumes and corresponding doses of Olanzapine Intramuscular.
5. Immediately after use, dispose of syringe in
approved sharps box.

B

Figure 17-3 A, Olanzapine 10-mg label. **B,** Olanzapine package insert.

![+−÷×] PRACTICE **PROBLEMS**

Using the label for olanzapine in Figure 17-3, *A* and *B*, answer the following questions.

58. What is the dosage strength of the total vial?   _____

59. How much diluent must be added to this
    vial to prepare the medication for IM use?   _____

60. What diluent is recommended for
    reconstitution?   _____

61. How long will the reconstituted
    solution be good for?   _____

62. How much would you withdraw
    for a 7.5-mg dose?   _____

63. How much would you withdraw for
    a 2.5-mg dose?   _____

Answers on page 465.

Before we proceed to calculate dosages, let's review the steps to use with medications that have been reconstituted.
1. Use either the ratio and proportion method, the formula method, or the dimensional analysis method to calculate dosages. What is available becomes the dosage strength you obtain after mixing the medication according to the directions.
2. Keep in mind that powdered medications may increase in volume after a liquid is added (diluent + powder). The volume to which the medication expands must be considered when calculations are made.
3. When the final concentration is not stated, use the total weight of the medication in powdered form and the number of millilitres produced after the solvent or liquid has been added.
4. As with all calculation problems, check to make sure that the ordered and the available medications are in the same system and unit of measurement.
5. Do not forget to label your answer.

Calculating Dosages of Reconstituted Medications

To calculate the dosage to administer after reconstituting a medication, the ratio and proportion method, the formula method, or the dimensional analysis method may be used. However, the H (what you have on hand or what is available) is the dosage strength you obtain after you mix the medication according to the directions. If you use ratio and proportion, therefore, the known ratio is also the dosage strength obtained after you mix the medication.

In $\dfrac{D}{H} \times Q = x$, Q is the volume of solution that contains the dosage strength.

In dimensional analysis, the first fraction written is the solution (volume) that contains the dosage strength.

Example: To illustrate, let's calculate the dosage you would administer if you mixed penicillin and made a solution containing 1 000 000 units per mL. Order: 2 000 000 units IM q6h.

✔ PROBLEM SETUP

✔ Solution Using Ratio and Proportion

$$1\,000\,000 \text{ units} : 1\text{ mL} = 2\,000\,000 \text{ units} : x\text{ mL}$$

$$\text{(known)} \qquad\qquad \text{(unknown)}$$

$$\frac{1\,\cancel{000}\,\cancel{000}\,x}{1\,\cancel{000}\,\cancel{000}} = \frac{2\,\cancel{000}\,\cancel{000}}{1\,\cancel{000}\,\cancel{000}} \quad \begin{array}{l}\text{(Note cancellation}\\ \text{of zeros to make}\\ \text{numbers smaller.)}\end{array}$$

$$x = \frac{2}{1}$$

$$x = 2\text{ mL}$$

✔ Solution Using the Formula Method

$$\frac{D}{H} \times Q = x$$

$$\frac{2\,000\,000 \text{ units}}{1\,000\,000 \text{ units}} \times 1\text{ mL} = x\text{ mL}$$

$$x = \frac{2\,\cancel{000}\,\cancel{000}}{1\,\cancel{000}\,\cancel{000}}$$

$$x = 2\text{ mL}$$

✔ Solution Using Dimensional Analysis

$$x\text{ mL} = \frac{1\text{ mL}}{1\,000\,000 \,\cancel{\text{units}}} \times \frac{2\,000\,000\,\cancel{\text{units}}}{1}$$

$$x = \frac{2\,\cancel{000}\,\cancel{000}}{1\,\cancel{000}\,\cancel{000}}$$

$$x = \frac{2}{1}$$

$$x = 2\text{ mL}$$

Example: Order: 0.2 g of a medication IV q6h.

Available: 500 mg of the medication in powdered form that states add 8 mL of diluent to yield a solution 500 mg per 8 mL.

✔ PROBLEM SETUP

1. Note that a conversion is necessary. Conversion factor: 1 000 mg = 1 g. Convert what is ordered into the available units. This will eliminate a decimal point. Therefore, 0.2 g = 200 mg.
2. Think: What would a logical answer be? You will need more than 1 mL but less than 8 mL.

✔ Solution Using Ratio and Proportion

$$500 \text{ mg} : 8 \text{ mL} = 200 \text{ mg} : x \text{ mL}$$

(known)   (unknown)

$$\frac{\cancel{500}\,x}{\cancel{500}} = \frac{200 \times 8}{500}$$

$$x = \frac{1\,600}{500}$$

$$x = 3.2 \text{ mL}$$

✔ Solution Using the Formula Method

$$\frac{D}{H} \times Q = x$$

$$\frac{200 \text{ mg}}{500 \text{ mg}} \times 8 \text{ mL} = x \text{ mL}$$

$$x = \frac{200 \times 8}{500}$$

$$x = \frac{1\,600}{500}$$

$$x = 3.2 \text{ mL}$$

✔ Solution Using Dimensional Analysis

$$x \text{ mL} = \frac{8 \text{ mL}}{500 \text{ } \cancel{mg}} \times \frac{1\,000 \text{ } \cancel{mg}}{1 \text{ } \cancel{g}} \times \frac{2 \text{ } \cancel{g}}{1}$$

$$x = \frac{8\,000 \times 0.2}{500}$$

$$x = \frac{1\,600}{500}$$

$$x = 3.2 \text{ mL}$$

POINTS TO REMEMBER

- If the medication is not used in its entirety after it is mixed, clearly label the vial after reconstitution with the following information:
  a. Date and time of preparation, dosage strength prepared, and date and time of expiration
  b. Storage directions
  c. Initials of the preparer
- Read all directions carefully; if there are no reconstitution instructions on the vial, then the package insert, the pharmacy, or other reliable resources may be used to find the information needed for reconstitution.
- When directions on the label are for IM and IV reconstitution, read the label carefully for the solution you are preparing.
- Follow the type and amount of diluent to be used for reconstitution exactly.
- Read the directions relating to storage (room temperature, refrigeration) and the time period for maintaining potency.
- When the dilution of powdered medication results in an increase in volume, take into consideration this increased volume when calculating the dosage.

- Read instructions carefully. There may be different directions for mixing according to the amount in the vial and the route. Always check the route ordered and follow the directions corresponding to the route. Interchanging the dilution instructions for IV and IM administration can have serious outcomes for the patient.
- Do **not** use lidocaine to mix a medication (even if it is an option for reconstitution on a label), without checking with the prescriber.

Reconstituting Noninjectable Solutions

Nurses or other health care providers may be required to dilute a concentrated liquid or powder (solute) with a solution such as water or saline (solvent) so as to make a less concentrated solution. For example, they may need to prepare nutritional liquids, topical cleansing solutions, or irrigants and soaks. Aseptic preparation as well as the storage and use of reconstituted topical solutions are vital to patient safety. To promote patient safety, the pharmacy is primarily responsible for preparing irrigating and soaking solutions, while nurses are generally responsible for preparing nutritional feedings that are not full strength, with some involvement from dietary department. Therefore, for this section, the reconstitution of nutritional feeding is the focus.

The principles of reconstitution can be applied to noninjectable solutions. Enteral feeding solutions are formulated to be administered in full strength; however, when prescribed, the nurse may need to dilute the enteral solution before administering it. Before beginning calculations, let's discuss enteral feedings.

Enteral Feeding

Enteral feeding involves the provision of nutrients to the gastrointestinal tract. It is provided to patients who are unable to ingest food safely or are having difficulty eating. Enteral nutrition may be provided with a nasogastric, jejunal, or gastric tube. It may consist of blended foods or tube feeding formulas. Tube feedings can be administered in several ways, depending on the patient's needs. They may be given as a bolus amount by means of gravity several times per day by using a large-volume syringe, as a continuous gravity drip over a period of a $\frac{1}{2}$ hour to 1 hour several times per day by using a pouch to hang the feeding, or as a continuous drip per infusion pump. When patients receive a continuous feeding, the feeding is placed in a special pouch or container and attached to a feeding pump. A common feeding pump is the Kangaroo pump (Figure 17-4). When the feeding pump is used, the feeding is delivered at a rate expressed in millilitres per hour (mL/h). For the purpose of this chapter, we will focus on administering a feeding by the continuous drip method with an enteral infusion pump.

When an order is written for feedings by continuous infusion, the nurse attaches the feeding to a special pump and administers it at the prescribed rate in millilitres per hour. A sample order is Jevity at 65 mL per hour by PEG (percutaneous endoscopic gastrostomy) or NG (nasogastric) tube. The feeding order also includes a certain volume of water with feeding (100–250 mL). Some orders may be written as follows: Pulmo Care 400 mL q8h followed by 100 mL of water after each feed. When the prescriber does not indicate millilitres per hour, the nurse uses the same formula as with IV calculation to determine the rate. In pediatrics, the order often specifies the formula and the rate. Example: Similac 24 at 20 mL per hour continuously by NG tube.

Example: Order: Pulmocare 400 mL q8h followed by 100 mL of water after each feed. Determine the rate in millilitres per hour.

Solution: $$\frac{400\,\text{mL}}{8\,\text{h}} = 50\,\text{mL/h}$$

The pump would be set to deliver 50 mL per hour.

Figure 17-4 Kangaroo pump. (From Potter, P. A., Perry, A. G., Stockert, P., et al. (2013). *Fundamentals of nursing* (8th ed.). St. Louis: Mosby.)

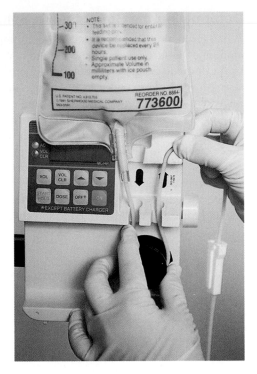

Example: Order: Isosource 1 200 mL over 16 hours. Determine the rate in millilitres per hour.

Solution:
$$\frac{1\,200\,\text{mL}}{16\,\text{h}} = 75\,\text{mL/h}$$

NOTE
The amount of water given with a tube feeding and how it is administered vary from one institution to the next. Check the institution's policy relating to administering enteral feedings.

The pump would be set to deliver 75 mL per hour.

In addition to nutrients, medications may be given through a tube. Liquid medications are preferred; however, some tablets may be crushed, dissolved in water, and administered.

Never assume. Not all medications are designed for administration through a tube, so check with the pharmacist or other appropriate resources. A medication's effectiveness could depend on the location of the tube (e.g., stomach, jejunum).

! SAFETY ALERT!

Always verify that the medications to be administered are not sublingual, enteric-coated, or timed-release medications because such medications are absorbed differently and the effects of the medication may be altered. Consult the pharmacist or drug reference before tablets are crushed and before capsules are opened and dissolved for tube feeding administration.

+−÷× PRACTICE PROBLEMS

Determine the rate in millilitres per hour for the following continuous feedings.

64. Ensure 480 mL by NG tube over 8 h.
    Follow with 100 mL of water after each feeding.   _____

65. Peptamen 1 600 mL over 24 h by gastrostomy
    tube (GT). Follow with 250 mL of water.   _____

Answers on page 465.

Determining the Strength of a Solution

When reconstituting solutions that are noninjectable, it is essential to understand that the amount of liquid (solvent) that is used to make a substance less concentrated is determined by the desired strength of the solution. Therefore, if you add more solvent, the final solution strength will be less concentrated; the less solvent that is added, the more concentrated the final solution strength will be. An example to illustrate this concept is the directions for making 1 litre of iced tea from a powder. Directions call for 4 cups (960 mL) of water to 1 packet of powdered iced tea. If you prefer a stronger tea taste, you might add 480 mL of water (solvent) to the powder (solute) to make it more concentrated. However, if you add 960 mL of water (solvent) to the powder (solute), the final solution will be more diluted and less concentrated because you added more water (solvent).

The strength of a solution can be expressed using ratios, fractions, or percentages. The fraction format is usually preferred to explain the ratio of solute to the total solution. For example, a $\frac{1}{3}$-strength solution indicates 1 part solute for 3 parts of the total solution. This strength solution could also be expressed as $1:3$ solution or $33\frac{1}{3}$ solution.

Calculation of Solutions

Because of special circumstances in both adults and children, nutritional liquids may require dilution before they are used. These nutritional liquids may be administered orally or through feeding tubes. Nutritional solutions can be supplied in ready-to-use form, powder for reconstitution, or liquid concentrate. Nutritional formulas may be diluted with sterile or tap water, however, tap water is used most often for adult patients. **Always consult a drug reference or institutional policy regarding what should be used to reconstitute a nutritional formula.**

Before preparing a solution of a specific strength from a solute (see the steps in Box 17-1), review the definitions of *solute, solvent,* and *solution* on page 417.

BOX 17-1	**Steps in Preparing a Solution of a Specific Strength**

1. Determine the amount of solute needed using this formula:

$$\text{Desired solution strength} \times \text{Amount of desired solution} = \text{Solute (solution to be dissolved)}$$

Note: The strength of the desired solution is written as a fraction; the amount of desired solution is expressed in millilitres or ounces, depending on the problem. This will give you the amount of solute you will need to add to the solvent to prepare the desired solution.

2. Determine the amount of solvent needed using this formula:

$$\text{Amount of desired solution} - \text{Solute} = \text{Amount of liquid needed to dissolve substance (solvent)}$$

Example: Order: $\frac{1}{3}$-strength Ensure 900 mL by NG tube over 8 h.

Solution:

$$\underset{\substack{\text{(desired} \\ \text{strength)}}}{\frac{1}{3}} \times \underset{\substack{\text{(amount of} \\ \text{solution)}}}{900\,\text{mL}} = \underset{\text{(solute)}}{x}$$

Step 1:

$$x = \frac{900}{3}$$

$$x = 300\,\text{mL}$$

You need 300 mL of the formula (solute).

Step 2:

$$\underset{\substack{\text{(amount of} \\ \text{solution)}}}{900\,\text{mL}} - \underset{\text{(solute)}}{300\,\text{mL}} = \underset{\substack{\text{(amount needed to} \\ \text{dissolve solvent)}}}{600\,\text{mL}}$$

Therefore, you would add 600 mL water to 300 mL of Ensure to make 900 mL of $\frac{1}{3}$-strength Ensure.

Example: $\frac{3}{4}$-strength Isomil 4 oz PO q4h for 24 h

Note: 4 oz q4h = 6 feedings; 4 oz × 6 = 24 oz

Solution: 1 oz = 30 mL; therefore, 24 oz = 720 mL

$$\frac{3}{4} \times 720 \text{ mL} = x \text{ mL}$$

$$x = \frac{2160}{4}$$

$$x = 540 \text{ mL of the formula (solute)}$$

$$720 \text{ mL} - 540 \text{ mL} = 180 \text{ mL}$$
(amount of   (solute)   (amount needed
solution)   to dissolve) solvent

Therefore, you would add 180 mL water to 540 mL of Isomil to make 720 mL of $\frac{3}{4}$-strength Isomil for a 24-hour period.

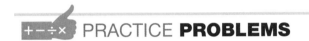 PRACTICE **PROBLEMS**

Prepare the following strength solutions. For questions in ounces, provide answers in ounces and millilitres.

66. $\frac{2}{3}$-strength Sustacal 300 mL PO QID.   _____

67. $\frac{3}{4}$-strength Ensure 16 oz by NG tube over 8 h.   _____

68. $\frac{1}{2}$-strength Ensure 20 oz by GT over 5 h.   _____

Answers on page 465.

POINTS TO REMEMBER
- Place enteral feedings (continuous) in an infusion pump and administer them at a rate expressed in millilitres per hour. The prescriber usually orders the feeding rate in millilitres per hour. If not, the nurse must calculate the rate at which to deliver the feeding.
- To prepare a solution of a specific strength, write the desired solution strength as a fraction and multiply it by the amount of desired solution. This will give you the amount of solute needed.
- Calculate the solvent with this formula: The amount of desired solution − solute = amount of liquid needed to dissolve the substance (solvent).
- Think and calculate with accuracy to avoid making errors in determining the dilution for a required solution strength.

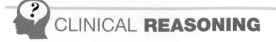

CLINICAL **REASONING**

1. **Scenario:** Order: Ceftazidime 250 mg IM q8h. The nurse had the package insert that follows and a 1-g vial.

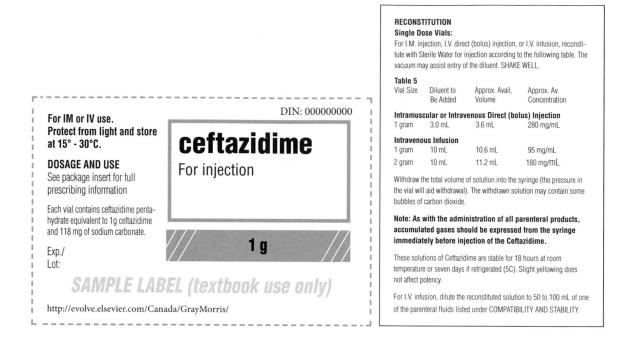

For IM or IV use.
Protect from light and store at 15° - 30°C.

DOSAGE AND USE
See package insert for full prescribing information

Each vial contains ceftazidime penta-hydrate equivalent to 1g ceftazidime and 118 mg of sodium carbonate.

Exp./
Lot:

DIN: 000000000

ceftazidime
For injection

1 g

SAMPLE LABEL (textbook use only)

http://evolve.elsevier.com/Canada/GrayMorris/

RECONSTITUTION
Single Dose Vials:
For I.M. injection, I.V. direct (bolus) injection, or I.V. infusion, reconstitute with Sterile Water for injection according to the following table. The vacuum may assist entry of the diluent. SHAKE WELL.

Table 5

Vial Size	Diluent to Be Added	Approx. Avail. Volume	Approx. Av. Concentration
Intramuscular or Intravenous Direct (bolus) Injection			
1 gram	3.0 mL	3.6 mL	280 mg/mL
Intravenous Infusion			
1 gram	10 mL	10.6 mL	95 mg/mL
2 gram	10 mL	11.2 mL	180 mg/mL

Withdraw the total volume of solution into the syringe (the pressure in the vial will aid withdrawal). The withdrawn solution may contain some bubbles of carbon dioxide.

Note: As with the administration of all parenteral products, accumulated gases should be expressed from the syringe immediately before injection of the Ceftazidime.

These solutions of Ceftazidime are stable for 18 hours at room temperature or seven days if refrigerated (5C). Slight yellowing does not affect potency.

For I.V. infusion, dilute the reconstituted solution to 50 to 100 mL of one of the parenteral fluids listed under COMPATIBILITY AND STABILITY.

The nurse reconstituted the medication ceftazidime with 10.6 mL of diluent and administered 2.6 mL to the patient.

a. What error occurred here? _____

b. What concentration should have been made? _____

c. What concentration did the nurse make and for which route? _____

d. What is the potential outcome of the error? _____

e. What measures could have been taken to prevent the error? _____

Answers on page 465.

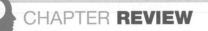

CHAPTER **REVIEW**

Use the labels provided to answer the questions. Round your answers to the nearest tenth where indicated. Shade in the dosage on the syringe provided.

1. Order: Cefazolin 250 mg IM q4h.

   Available:

   Sterile/Stérile   DIN 02108127

   ℞ **CEFAZOLIN**
   FOR INJECTION, USP

   1 g

   Cefazolin per vial
   Antibiotic / Antibiotique

   IM or IV use only
   Usage IM ou IV seulement

   Single use. Discard unused portion. Reconstitute (dilute) before use. **RECONSTITUTION: Adult Dosage:** 500 mg to 1 g every 6 to 8 hours. **IM:** Add 2.5 mL Sterile Water for Injection for a 334 mg/mL solution. **Direct IV (Bolus):** Further dilute reconstituted solution to a minimum of 10 mL using Sterile Water for Injection. **Shake well.** Reconstituted solution stable 24 hours at room temperature or 72 hours refrigerated. Consult package insert for dosage and prescribing information. Store powder between 15 – 30°C. Protect from light.

   Emploi unique. Jeter toute portion inutilisée. Reconstituer (diluer) avant l'emploi. Pour la posologie, le mode de reconstitution et les renseignements thérapeutiques, consulter le dépliant de conditionnement. Conserver la poudre entre 15 °C et 30 °C, à l'abri de la lumière.

   Teva Canada Limited/Limitée, Toronto, Canada M1B 2K9
   361-32-693970110 Rev 06   E33CACEFAZ101

   (01)00006851086310 2   Lot   EXP.

   a. How much diluent must be added to
      the vial for IM administration?   _____

   b. What is the final concentration of the
      solution prepared for IM administration?   _____

   c. How many mL will you administer to
      provide the dosage ordered?   _____

   d. Shade in the dosage calculated on the syringe provided.

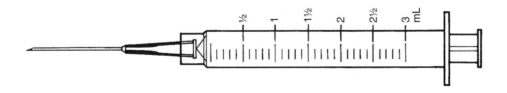

2. Order: Methylprednisolone sodium succinate 165 mg IV daily.

    Available:

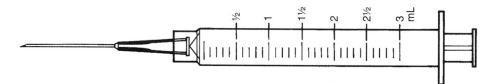

GLUCOCORTICOID
Each vial contains:
Methylprednisolone (as sodium succinate) . . . . 500 mg
Monobasic sodium phosphate anhydrous . . . . 6.4 mg
Dibasic sodium phosphate dried . . . . 69.6 mg
(pH adjusted with sodium hydroxide when needed)
Reconstitute each vial with 8 mL of Bacteriostatic Water for Injection
USP (benzyl alcohol as preservative). After reconstitution each vial
delivers 8 mL.
1 mL contains: 62.5 mg methylprednisolone.
Usual Adult Dose: See Product Monograph for complete dosage,
administration and direction for use.
Store powder or reconstituted solution at room temperature
(between 15 and 30°C). Use reconstituted solution within 48 hours.
Single dose vial. Discard unused portion.
Protect from light and freezing.
Product Monograph available on request.
Pharmacist: Dispense with Consumer Information leaflet
(www.pfizer.ca).

08826-14-3

GLUCOCORTICOÏDE
Une fiole contient :
Méthylprednisolone (sous forme de succinate sodique) . . . 500 mg
Phosphate monosodique anhydre . . . . 6,4 mg
Phosphate disodique séché . . . . 69,6 mg
(ajout d'hydroxyde de sodium au besoin pour ajuster le pH)
Reconstituer le contenu de chaque fiole avec 8 mL d'eau bactériostatique
pour injection, USP (alcool benzylique comme agent de conservation).
Après la reconstitution, chaque fiole fournit 8 mL.
Un mL contient : 62,5 mg de méthylprednisolone.
Posologie habituelle – Adulte : Voir la monographie du produit pour
connaître la posologie, les directives d'administration et le mode d'emploi.
Conserver la poudre ou la solution reconstituée à la température ambiante
(entre 15 et 30 °C). Utiliser la solution reconstituée dans un délai de
48 heures. Fiole unidose. Jeter tout reste de solution.
Craint la lumière et le gel.
Monographie fournie sur demande.
Pharmacien : Remettre avec le feuillet de renseignements pour le
consommateur (www.pfizer.ca).

IB/M.D. de
Pfizer Enterprises S.a.r.l.
Pfizer Canada Inc.,
licensee / licencié
Pfizer Canada Inc.
Kirkland (Québec) H9J 2M5
http://www.pfizer.ca
1-800-463-6001

DIN 00030678

℞ Solu-**MEDROL** ®/MD
methylprednisolone sodium succinate
succinate sodique de méthylprednisolone
for injection USP / pour injection, USP
500 mg / vial / fiole
62.5 mg/mL after / après reconstitution
For intravenous or intramuscular use / Pour usage intraveineux ou intramusculaire
Sterile Powder / Poudre stérile
5 Single Dose Vials / Fioles unidoses
Pfizer Injectables

    a. How many mL will you administer? _____

    b. Shade in the dosage calculated on the syringe provided.

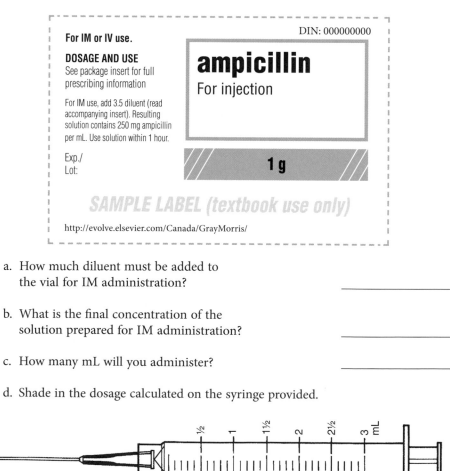

3. Order: Ampicillin 375 mg IM q6h.

    Available:

```
For IM or IV use.                                    DIN: 000000000

DOSAGE AND USE                    ┌─────────────────────────┐
See package insert for full       │                         │
prescribing information           │   ampicillin            │
                                  │   For injection         │
For IM use, add 3.5 diluent (read │                         │
accompanying insert). Resulting   └─────────────────────────┘
solution contains 250 mg ampicillin
per mL. Use solution within 1 hour.  ///////    1 g    ///////

Exp./
Lot:

          SAMPLE LABEL (textbook use only)

       http://evolve.elsevier.com/Canada/GrayMorris/
```

    a. How much diluent must be added to
        the vial for IM administration?   _____

    b. What is the final concentration of the
        solution prepared for IM administration?   _____

    c. How many mL will you administer?   _____

    d. Shade in the dosage calculated on the syringe provided.

4. Order: Doxycycline 100 mg IVPB q12h.

Available:

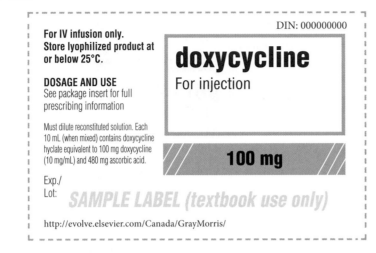

For IV infusion only.
Store lyophilized product at
or below 25°C.

DOSAGE AND USE
See package insert for full
prescribing information

Must dilute reconstituted solution. Each
10 mL (when mixed) contains doxycycline
hyclate equivalent to 100 mg doxycycline
(10 mg/mL) and 480 mg ascorbic acid.

Exp./
Lot:

DIN: 000000000

doxycycline
For injection

100 mg

SAMPLE LABEL (textbook use only)

http://evolve.elsevier.com/Canada/GrayMorris/

How many mL will you administer? _____

5. Order: Amoxicillin 0.4 g PO q8h.

Available:

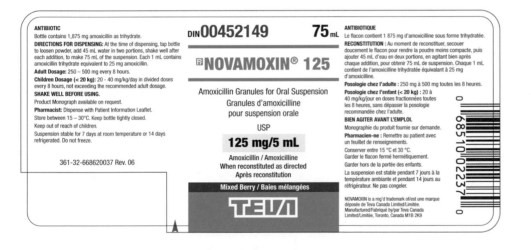

ANTIBIOTIC
Bottle contains 1,875 mg amoxicillin as trihydrate.
DIRECTIONS FOR DISPENSING: At the time of dispensing, tap bottle
to loosen powder, add 45 mL water in two portions, shake well after
each addition, to make 75 mL of the suspension. Each 1 mL contains
amoxicillin trihydrate equivalent to 25 mg amoxicillin.
Adult Dosage: 250 – 500 mg every 8 hours.
Children Dosage (< 20 kg): 20 – 40 mg/kg/day in divided doses
every 8 hours, not exceeding the recommended adult dosage.
SHAKE WELL BEFORE USING.
Product Monograph available on request.
Pharmacist: Dispense with Patient Information Leaflet.
Store between 15 – 30°C. Keep bottle tightly closed.
Keep out of reach of children.
Suspension stable for 7 days at room temperature or 14 days
refrigerated. Do not freeze.

361-32-668620037 Rev. 06

DIN **00452149**   **75** mL

℞**NOVAMOXIN® 125**

Amoxicillin Granules for Oral Suspension
Granules d'amoxicilline
pour suspension orale
USP

125 mg/5 mL

Amoxicillin / Amoxicilline
When reconstituted as directed
Après reconstitution

Mixed Berry / Baies mélangées

TEVA

ANTIBIOTIQUE
Le flacon contient 1 875 mg d'amoxicilline sous forme trihydratée.
RECONSTITUTION : Au moment de reconstituer, secouer
doucement le flacon pour rendre la poudre moins compacte, puis
ajouter 45 mL d'eau en deux portions, en agitant bien après
chaque addition, pour obtenir 75 mL de suspension. Chaque 1 mL
contient de l'amoxicilline trihydratée équivalent à 25 mg
d'amoxicilline.
Posologie chez l'adulte : 250 mg à 500 mg toutes les 8 heures.
Posologie chez l'enfant (< 20 kg) : 20 à
40 mg/kg/jour en doses fractionnées toutes
les 8 heures, sans dépasser la posologie
recommandée chez l'adulte.
BIEN AGITER AVANT L'EMPLOI.
Monographie du produit fournie sur demande.
Pharmacien-ne : Remettre au patient avec
un feuillet de renseignements.
Conserver entre 15 °C et 30 °C.
Garder le flacon fermé hermétiquement.
Garder hors de la portée des enfants.
La suspension est stable pendant 7 jours à la
température ambiante et pendant 14 jours au
réfrigérateur. Ne pas congeler.

NOVAMOXIN is a reg'd trademark of/est une marque
déposée de Teva Canada Limited/Limitée.
Manufactured/Fabriqué by/par Teva Canada
Limited/Limitée, Toronto, Canada M1B 2K9

a. How much diluent must be added to prepare the solution? _____

b. What diluent is recommended for reconstitution? _____

c. What is the dosage strength of the reconstituted solution? _____

d. How many mL will you administer? _____

e. How long will the medication maintain its potency? _____

6. Order: Penicillin G potassium 275 000 units IM q6h.

Available:

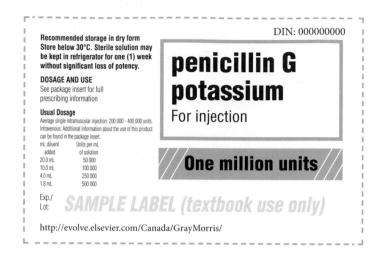

a. Which dosage strength would be best to administer? _____

b. How many mL of diluent would be needed to make the dosage strength? _____

c. How many mL will you administer? _____

d. Shade in the dosage calculated on the syringe provided.

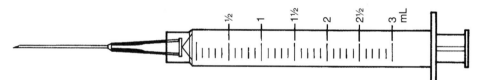

7. Order: Cytarabine 200 mg IV daily for 1 week.

Available:

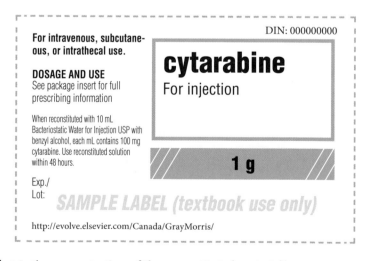

a. What is the concentration of the reconstituted material? _____

b. How many mL will you add to the IV? _____

c. Shade in the dosage calculated on the syringe provided.

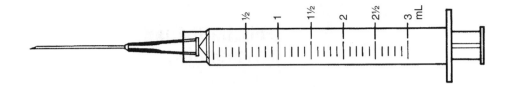

8. Order: Methylprednisolone sodium succinate 175 mg IV q6h.

Available:

DIN 02231893   Sterile/Stérile

℗ methylPREDNISolone
SODIUM SUCCINATE
FOR INJECTION, USP

40 mg

methylPREDNISolone per vial
Glucocorticoid /
Glucocorticoïde
Anti-inflammatory /
Anti-inflammatoire
IM or IV Use Only /
Usage IM ou IV seulement

Reconstitute (dilute) before use.
Discard unused portion.
RECONSTITUTION: Add 1 mL Sterile Water for Injection and use within 24 hours or 1 mL Bacteriostatic Water for Injection and use within 48 hours. Each reconstituted vial contains approximately 1 mL. Each mL contains 40 mg methylPREDNISolone. Store powder at 15°C- 25°C. Protect from light. See enclosed package insert.
Reconstituer (diluer) avant l'emploi.
Jeter toute portion inutilisée.
RECONSTITUTION: Pour le mode de reconstitution, voir le dépliant de conditionnement ci-joint.
Conserver la poudre à 15 °C - 25 °C.
Protéger de la lumière.

(01)00068510933010

Novopharm Limited/Limitée,
Toronto, Canada M1B 2K9
361-32-765710101 Rev 07

1-29114850/C

LOT

EXP.

a. What is the total dosage strength of methylprednisolone sodium succinate in this vial? _____

b. What diluent is recommended for reconstitution? _____

c. How many mL will you add to the IV? _____

d. Shade in the dosage calculated on the syringe provided.

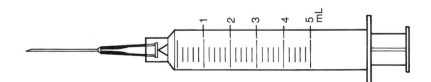

9. Order: Amoxicillin/clavulanate 0.5 g PO q12h (calculation based on amoxicillin).

Available:

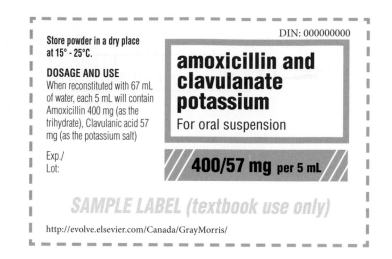

a. How many mL of diluent must be added? _____

b. What is the dosage strength after reconstitution? _____

c. How many mL are needed to administer
the required dosage? _____

10. Order: Cefotan 1.2 g IM q12h.

Available: Read the medication label and the portion of the package insert.

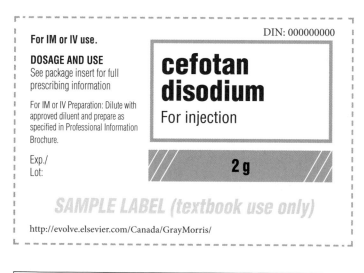

Vial Size	Volume of Diluent Added (mL)	Approximate Withdrawal Vol (mL)	Approximate Average Concentration (mg/mL)
1 gram	2	2.5	400
2 gram	3	4	500

a. How many mL will you administer?   _____

b. Shade in the dosage calculated on the syringe provided.

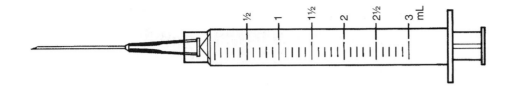

11. Order: Nafcillin 0.5 g IM q6h.

Available:

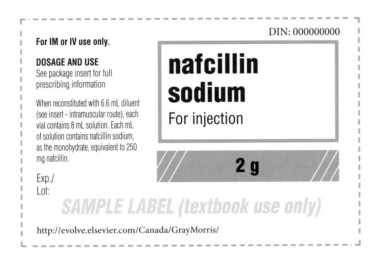

For IM or IV use only.

DOSAGE AND USE
See package insert for full
prescribing information

When reconstituted with 6.6 mL diluent
(see insert - intramuscular route), each
vial contains 8 mL solution. Each mL
of solution contains nafcillin sodium,
as the monohydrate, equivalent to 250
mg nafcillin.

Exp./
Lot:

DIN: 000000000

nafcillin sodium
For injection

2 g

SAMPLE LABEL (textbook use only)

http://evolve.elsevier.com/Canada/GrayMorris/

a. What is the dosage strength of the reconstituted nafcillin?   _____

b. How many mL will you administer?   _____

c. Shade in the dosage calculated on the syringe provided.

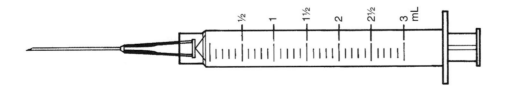

12. Order: Clavulin 350 mg PO q12h for 10 days.

    Available:

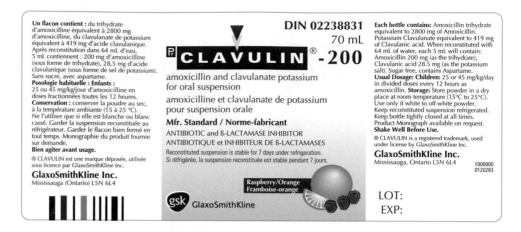

    a. How many mL of diluent must be added?   _____

    b. What is the dosage strength after reconstitution?   _____

    c. How many mL will you administer?   _____

13. Order: Claforan 1 g IV q8h.

    Available:

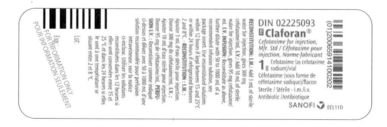

Guide for reconstitution of Claforan®			
	Diluent to be added (mL)	Approximate withdrawable volume (mL)	Approximate average conc. (mg cefotaxime/mL)
Intramuscular			
1 g vial	3	3.4	300
Intravenous			
1 g vial	10	10.4	95

Intramuscular: Reconstitute with sterile water for injection or bacteriostatic water for injection.
Intravenous: Reconstitute with sterile water for injection.
I.V. Infusion: Reconstitute as above, further dilute with 50 to 1000 mL of a recommended infusion solution, see package insert.
Use reconstituted solutions within 12 hours if kept between 15 and 25°C or within 24 hours if stored between 2 and 8°C.
Please refer to the enclosed information leaflet for directions and precautions.
Product Monograph available to health professionals upon request or at www.sanofi.ca.
Store powder between 15 and 25°C.
Protect from light and heat.

a. How much diluent must be added
   to the vial for IV administration? _____

b. What is the dosage strength of the solution
   prepared for IV administration? _____

c. How many mL will you add to the IV? _____

14. Order: Penicillin G potassium 400 000 units IM q4h.

   Available:

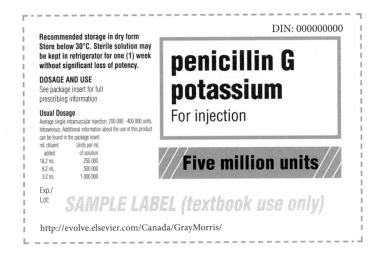

a. How many mL will you administer? _____

b. Shade in the dosage calculated on the syringe provided.

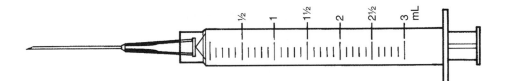

15. Order: Ceftazidime 250 mg IM q12h.

Available:

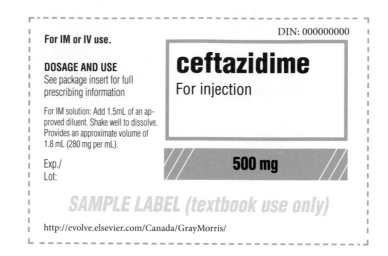

For IM or IV use.

DOSAGE AND USE
See package insert for full prescribing information

For IM solution: Add 1.5mL of an approved diluent. Shake well to dissolve. Provides an approximate volume of 1.8 mL (280 mg per mL).

Exp./
Lot:

DIN: 000000000

ceftazidime
For injection

500 mg

SAMPLE LABEL (textbook use only)

http://evolve.elsevier.com/Canada/GrayMorris/

a. How many mL will you administer? _____

b. Shade in the dosage calculated on the syringe provided.

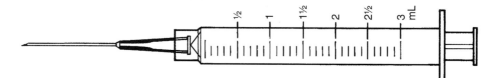

16. Order: Ticarcillin disodium 0.5 g IM q6h.

Available:

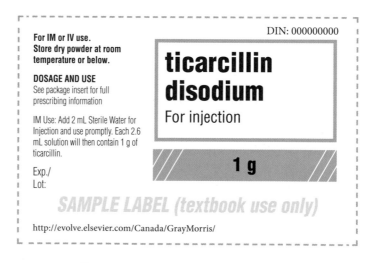

For IM or IV use.
Store dry powder at room temperature or below.

DOSAGE AND USE
See package insert for full prescribing information

IM Use: Add 2 mL Sterile Water for Injection and use promptly. Each 2.6 mL solution will then contain 1 g of ticarcillin.

Exp./
Lot:

DIN: 000000000

ticarcillin disodium
For injection

1 g

SAMPLE LABEL (textbook use only)

http://evolve.elsevier.com/Canada/GrayMorris/

a. How many mL will you administer? _____

b. Shade in the dosage calculated on the syringe provided.

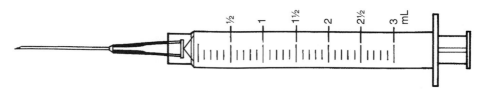

17. Order: Cytarabine 150 mg IV daily for 7 days.

Available:

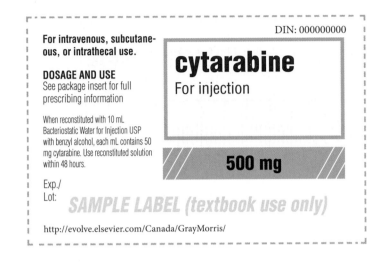

a. How many mL will you administer? _____

b. Shade in the dosage calculated on the syringe provided.

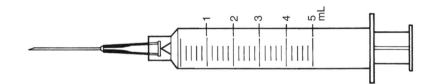

18. Order: Vancomycin 0.45 g IV q8h.

Available:

Vial Size / Flacon de	Volume to add / Volume à ajouter	Approx. Vol. / Vol. approx.	Vancomycin Conc. / Conc. de vancomycine
500 mg	10 mL	10.3 mL	50 mg/mL

a. How many mL of diluent must be added to the vial? _____

b. What is the final concentration of the prepared solution? _____

c. How many mL will you add to the IV? _____

d. Shade in the dosage calculated on the syringe provided.

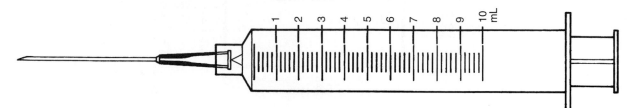

19. Order: Levothyroxine sodium 0.05 mg IV daily.

Available:

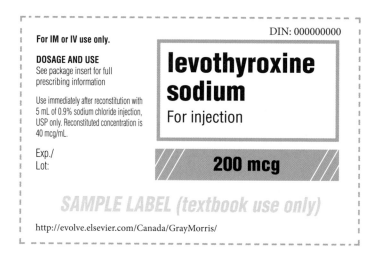

For IM or IV use only.

DOSAGE AND USE
See package insert for full
prescribing information

Use immediately after reconstitution with
5 mL of 0.9% sodium chloride injection,
USP only. Reconstituted concentration is
40 mcg/mL.

Exp./
Lot:

DIN: 000000000

levothyroxine sodium

For injection

200 mcg

SAMPLE LABEL (textbook use only)

http://evolve.elsevier.com/Canada/GrayMorris/

a. How many mL will you add to the IV? _____

b. Shade in the dosage calculated on the syringe provided.

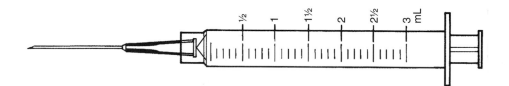

20. Order: Acyclovir 0.25 g IV q8h for 5 days.

    Use the directions from the package insert.

    Available:

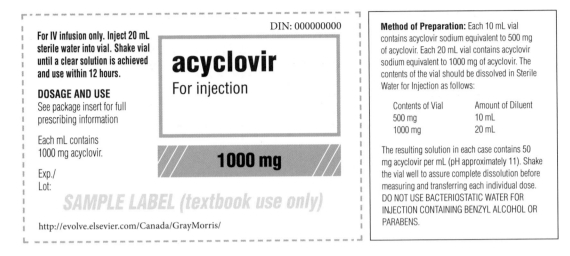

DIN: 000000000

For IV infusion only. Inject 20 mL sterile water into vial. Shake vial until a clear solution is achieved and use within 12 hours.

DOSAGE AND USE
See package insert for full prescribing information

Each mL contains 1000 mg acyclovir.

Exp./
Lot:

SAMPLE LABEL (textbook use only)

http://evolve.elsevier.com/Canada/GrayMorris/

acyclovir
For injection

1000 mg

Method of Preparation: Each 10 mL vial contains acyclovir sodium equivalent to 500 mg of acyclovir. Each 20 mL vial contains acyclovir sodium equivalent to 1000 mg of acyclovir. The contents of the vial should be dissolved in Sterile Water for Injection as follows:

Contents of Vial	Amount of Diluent
500 mg	10 mL
1000 mg	20 mL

The resulting solution in each case contains 50 mg acyclovir per mL (pH approximately 11). Shake the vial well to assure complete dissolution before measuring and transferring each individual dose. DO NOT USE BACTERIOSTATIC WATER FOR INJECTION CONTAINING BENZYL ALCOHOL OR PARABENS.

    a.　How many mL will you add to the IV?　　_____

    b.　Shade in the dosage calculated on the syringe provided.

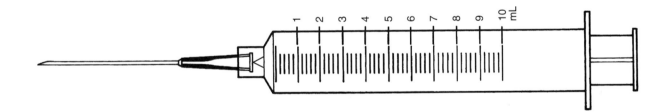

21. Order: Cefpodoxime proxetil 200 mg PO q12h.

    Available:

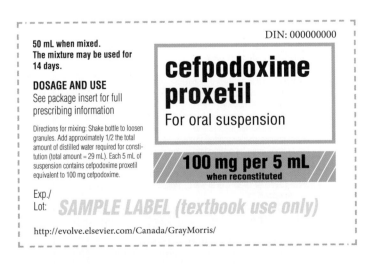

DIN: 000000000

50 mL when mixed. The mixture may be used for 14 days.

DOSAGE AND USE
See package insert for full prescribing information

Directions for mixing: Shake bottle to loosen granules. Add approximately 1/2 the total amount of distilled water required for constitution (total amount = 29 mL). Each 5 mL of suspension contains cefpodoxime proxetil equivalent to 100 mg cefpodoxime.

Exp./
Lot:

cefpodoxime proxetil
For oral suspension

100 mg per 5 mL
when reconstituted

SAMPLE LABEL (textbook use only)

http://evolve.elsevier.com/Canada/GrayMorris/

    How many mL will you administer using an oral syringe?　　_____

22. Order: Cefazolin 0.5 g IM q8h.

Available:

Sterile/Stérile   DIN 02108127

℗ **CEFAZOLIN**
FOR INJECTION, USP

1 g

Cefazolin per vial
Antibiotic / Antibiotique

IM or IV use only
Usage IM ou IV seulement

Single use. Discard unused portion. **Reconstitute (dilute) before use. RECONSTITUTION: Adult Dosage:** 500 mg to 1 g every 6 to 8 hours. **IM:** Add 2.5 mL Sterile Water for Injection for a 334 mg/mL solution. **Direct IV (Bolus):** Further dilute reconstituted solution to a minimum of 10 mL using Sterile Water for Injection. **Shake well.** Reconstituted solution stable 24 hours at room temperature or 72 hours refrigerated. Consult package insert for dosage and prescribing information. Store powder between 15 – 30ºC. Protect from light.

Emploi unique. Jeter toute portion inutilisée. Reconstituer (diluer) avant l'emploi. Pour la posologie, le mode de reconstitution et les renseignements thérapeutiques, consulter le dépliant de conditionnement. Conserver la poudre entre 15 °C et 30 °C, à l'abri de la lumière.

Teva Canada Limited/Limitée, Toronto, Canada M1B 2K9
361-32-693970110 Rev 06   E33CACEFAZ101

(01)00068510863102

Lot   EXP.

a. How many mL will you administer?   _____

b. Shade in the dosage on the syringe provided.

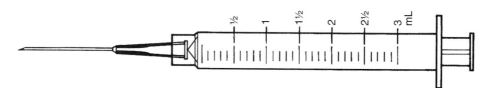

23. Order: Cefepime hydrochloride 1.5 g IV q12h.

Available:

℗ Sterile/Stérile   DIN 02319039

Cefepime
for/pour injection
House Standard / Norme - maison

2.0 g

2.0 g per vial / par fiole
Single Use Vial / Fiole unidose
ANTIBIOTIC / ANTIBIOTIQUE
For IV use / Pour usage IV

Dose should be individualized.
Dosage and Administration: See outer carton and package insert. **RECONSTITUTION: I.V. / I.V. INFUSION:** See outer carton and package insert. **Store powder at 15-30°C or at 2-8°C. Protect from light.** Discard unused portion. Each single use vial contains 2 g cefepime (as cefepime HCl) and 1450 mg L-arginine.
La dose doit être adaptée à chaque patient.
Posologie et mode d'administration: Lire l'emballage et la notice ci-incluse. **RECONSTITUTION: I.V. / PERFUSION I.V.:** Lire l'emballage et la notice ci-incluse. **Conserver la poudre à 15 à 30°C ou à 2 à 8°C. Protéger de la lumière.** Jeter toute portion inutilisée. Une fiole unidose contient 2 g de céfépime (comme chlorhydrate de céfépime) et 1450 mg L-arginine.
Dist. by / dist. par: Apotex Inc.,Toronto, Canada

948006079

TN/DRUGS/763   M.L. No. 763

(01)0(07)71313191104

FOR INTRAVENOUS USE ONLY
Dose should be individualized.
Adult Dose: 0.5 to 2 g every 8-12 hours.
Pediatric Dose: ages 2 months to 12 years, ≤ 40 kg:
50 mg/kg every 8-12 hours.
RECONSTITUTION: Intravenous: Add 10 mL of recommended diluent.
Intravenous infusion: Reconstitute as above and further dilute with a recommended infusion solution to obtain 10 or 20 mg/mL.
See package insert for detailed information and reconstitution instructions.
Product Monograph available to health professionals upon request.
Store powder at 15-30°C or at 2-8°C. Protect from light. Discard unused portion.
Each single use vial contains 2 g cefepime (as cefepime HCl) and 1450 mg L-arginine.

Dist. by / dist. par: Hospira Healthcare Corporation
Apotex Inc.   Corporation de soins de la santé Hospira
Toronto, Canada   Montréal, QC H4M 2X6

Note: Package insert indicates final dosage strength as 160 mg per mL.

a. How many mL will you add to the IV?   _____

b. Shade in the dosage on the syringe provided.

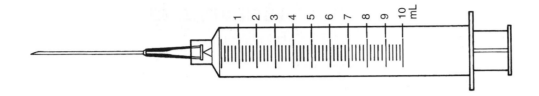

24. Order: Penicillin G sodium 425 000 units IV daily.

    Available:

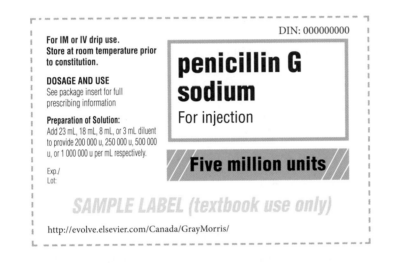

For IM or IV drip use.
Store at room temperature prior
to constitution.

DOSAGE AND USE
See package insert for full
prescribing information

Preparation of Solution:
Add 23 mL, 18 mL, 8 mL, or 3 mL diluent
to provide 200 000 u, 250 000 u, 500 000
u, or 1 000 000 u per mL respectively.

Exp./
Lot:

DIN: 000000000

penicillin G sodium

For injection

Five million units

SAMPLE LABEL (textbook use only)

http://evolve.elsevier.com/Canada/GrayMorris/

a. Which dosage strength would be best to choose?   _____

b. How many mL of diluent would be
   needed to make the dosage strength?   _____

c. How many mL will you add to the IV?   _____

d. Shade in the dosage calculated on the syringe provided.

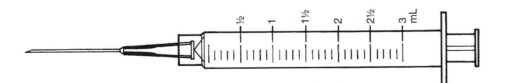

25. Order: Voriconazole 200 mg IV q12h.

    Available:

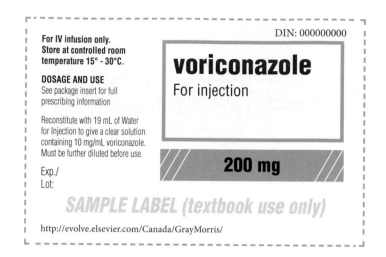

    a. How many mL of diluent must be added to the vial? _____

    b. How many mL will you add to the IV? _____

26. Order: Cefprozil 500 mg PO q12h for 10 days.

    Available:

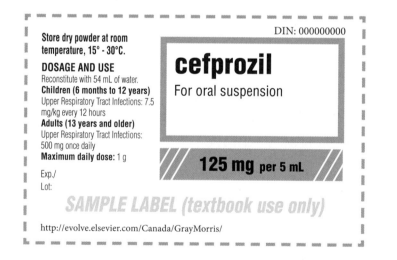

    a. How many mL of diluent are
       recommended for reconstitution? _____

    b. How many mL will you administer? _____

27. Order: Piperacillin sodium and tazobactam sodium 2.25 g q8h IV.

    Available:

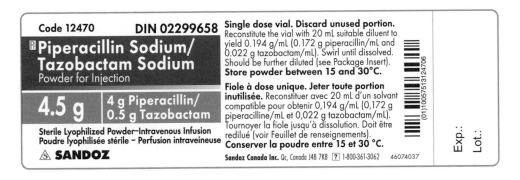

    a. How many mL of diluent are recommended
    for reconstitution?   _____

    b. What is the dosage strength of the vial?   _____

    c. How many mL will you add to the IV?   _____

28. Order: Zithromax 500 mg PO stat for 1 dose.

    Available:

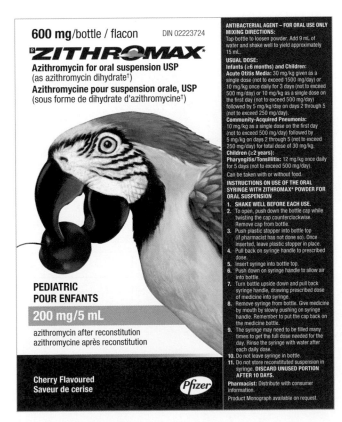

    How many mL will you administer?   _____

29. Order: Cefobid 1 g IM q12h for 5 days.

    Available: Cefoperazone (Cefobid) 1 g with directions to add 1.4 mL of sterile water for injection. Each 2 mL yields 1 g.

    a. How many mL will you administer? _____

    b. Shade in the dosage on the syringe provided.

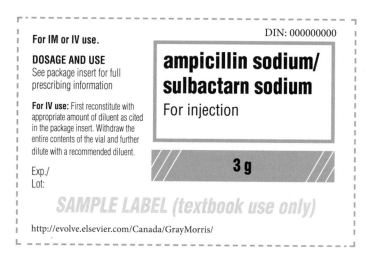

30. Order: Ampicillin sodium/sulbactarn sodium 1.5 g IV q6h.

    Available:

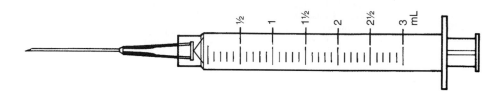

Refer to the portion of the package insert.

Vial Size	Volume of Diluent to Be Added	Withdrawal Volume
1.5 g	3.2 mL	4 mL
3 g	6.4 mL	8 mL

How many mL will you add to the IV? _____

31. Order: Famotidine 20 mg PO BID.

    Available:

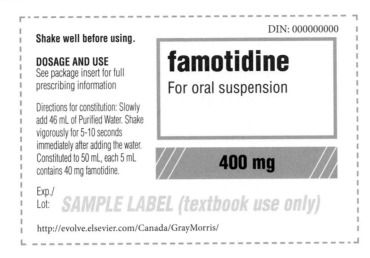

Shake well before using.

DOSAGE AND USE
See package insert for full prescribing information

Directions for constitution: Slowly add 46 mL of Purified Water. Shake vigorously for 5-10 seconds immediately after adding the water. Constituted to 50 mL, each 5 mL contains 40 mg famotidine.

Exp./
Lot:

DIN: 000000000

famotidine
For oral suspension

400 mg

SAMPLE LABEL (textbook use only)

http://evolve.elsevier.com/Canada/GrayMorris/

   How many mL will you administer using an oral syringe? _____

32. Order: Ceftriaxone 125 mg IM stat.

    Available:

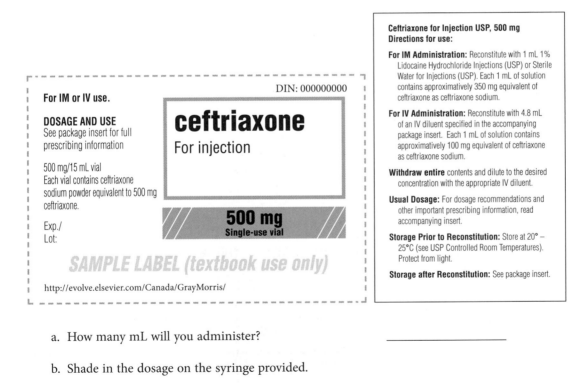

For IM or IV use.

DOSAGE AND USE
See package insert for full prescribing information

500 mg/15 mL vial
Each vial contains ceftriaxone sodium powder equivalent to 500 mg ceftriaxone.

Exp./
Lot:

DIN: 000000000

ceftriaxone
For injection

500 mg
Single-use vial

SAMPLE LABEL (textbook use only)

http://evolve.elsevier.com/Canada/GrayMorris/

Ceftriaxone for Injection USP, 500 mg
Directions for use:

For IM Administration: Reconstitute with 1 mL 1% Lidocaine Hydrochloride Injections (USP) or Sterile Water for Injections (USP). Each 1 mL of solution contains approximatively 350 mg equivalent of ceftriaxone as ceftriaxone sodium.

For IV Administration: Reconstitute with 4.8 mL of an IV diluent specified in the accompanying package insert. Each 1 mL of solution contains approximatively 100 mg equivalent of ceftriaxone as ceftriaxone sodium.

Withdraw entire contents and dilute to the desired concentration with the appropriate IV diluent.

Usual Dosage: For dosage recommendations and other important prescribing information, read accompanying insert.

Storage Prior to Reconstitution: Store at 20° – 25°C (see USP Controlled Room Temperatures). Protect from light.

Storage after Reconstitution: See package insert.

   a. How many mL will you administer? _____

   b. Shade in the dosage on the syringe provided.

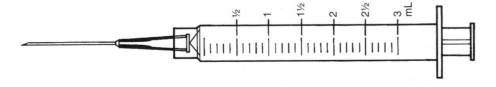

33. Order: Amphotericin B 45.5 mg IV daily.

   Available:

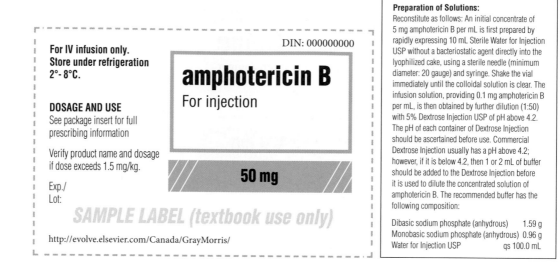

For IV infusion only.
Store under refrigeration
2°- 8°C.

DOSAGE AND USE
See package insert for full
prescribing information

Verify product name and dosage
if dose exceeds 1.5 mg/kg.

Exp./
Lot:

DIN: 000000000

amphotericin B
For injection

50 mg

SAMPLE LABEL (textbook use only)

http://evolve.elsevier.com/Canada/GrayMorris/

Preparation of Solutions:
Reconstitute as follows: An initial concentrate of
5 mg amphotericin B per mL is first prepared by
rapidly expressing 10 mL Sterile Water for Injection
USP without a bacteriostatic agent directly into the
lyophilized cake, using a sterile needle (minimum
diameter: 20 gauge) and syringe. Shake the vial
immediately until the colloidal solution is clear. The
infusion solution, providing 0.1 mg amphotericin B
per mL, is then obtained by further dilution (1:50)
with 5% Dextrose Injection USP of pH above 4.2.
The pH of each container of Dextrose Injection
should be ascertained before use. Commercial
Dextrose Injection usually has a pH above 4.2;
however, if it is below 4.2, then 1 or 2 mL of buffer
should be added to the Dextrose Injection before
it is used to dilute the concentrated solution of
amphotericin B. The recommended buffer has the
following composition:

Dibasic sodium phosphate (anhydrous)   1.59 g
Monobasic sodium phosphate (anhydrous) 0.96 g
Water for Injection USP   qs 100.0 mL

Use the information from the portion of the package insert to answer the questions and calculate the number of mL you will administer.

a. How many mL of diluent must be
   added for the initial concentration?   _____

b. What is the recommended diluent?   _____

c. What is the final concentration of
   the prepared solution per mL?   _____

d. How many mL will you administer?   _____

34. Order: Cephalexin 300 mg PO q12h for 5 days.

   Available:

ANTIBIOTIC
Each bottle contains 5000 mg cephalexin
(as the monohydrate).
DIRECTIONS FOR DISPENSING:
At the time of dispensing, add two portions of 30 mL
water to a total of 60 mL of water to the dry mixture in
the bottle to make 100 mL of the suspension. Shake well
after each addition. Each 1 mL contains cephalexin
monohydrate equivalent to 50 mg cephalexin.
Adult Dosage: 250 mg every 6 hours.
Children Dosage: 25 – 50 mg/kg of body weight per day,
in equally divided doses at 6 hour intervals. For more
severe infections, dose may be doubled.
Product Monograph available on request.
Store between 15 - 30°C.

TEVA is a reg'd trademark of / est une marque déposée
de TEVA Pharmaceutical Industries Ltd. used under
license by / utilisée sous licence par TEVA Canada
Limited/Limitée, Toronto, Canada M1B 2K9

SHAKE WELL BEFORE USING.
When reconstituted, suspension is stable for
14 days under refrigeration 2 - 8°C. Do not freeze.

DIN **00342092**   **100 mL**

℞ **TEVA-CEPHALEXIN 250**

**250 mg/
5 mL**

Cephalexin for Oral Suspension
Suspension orale de céphalexine
USP

Cephalexin/Céphalexine
When reconstituted as directed
Après reconstitution

TEVA

ANTIBIOTIQUE
Le flacon renferme 5000 mg de céphalexine
(sous forme monohydratée).
MODE DE RECONSTITUTION :
Pour reconstituer, ajouter deux portions de
30 mL d'eau, soit un total de 60 mL d'eau, à
la préparation en poudre que contient le flacon
afin d'obtenir 100 mL de suspension. Bien
agiter après chaque addition. Chaque mL de
suspension contient de la céphalexine
monohydratée équivalent à 50 mg de
céphalexine.
Posologie chez l'adulte : 250 mg toutes les
6 heures.
Posologie chez l'enfant : 25 à 50 mg/kg de
poids corporel par jour, fractionnés en doses
égales à des intervalles de 6 heures. Dans les
cas d'infection grave, on peut doubler la
posologie.
Monographie de produit fournie sur demande.
Conserver entre 15 °C et 30 °C.

361-32-756630040 Rev 09   333-32-100886

BIEN AGITER AVANT L'EMPLOI.
La suspension reconstituée est stable pendant 14 jours
au réfrigérateur (2 °C à 8 °C). Mettre à l'abri du gel.

0 68510 32440 5

a. How many mL of diluent must be
   added to the bottle for
   reconstitution?   _____

b. What is the final concentration of the
prepared solution?   _____

c. How many mL will you administer?   _____

35. Order: Zithromax 250 mg PO daily.

Available:

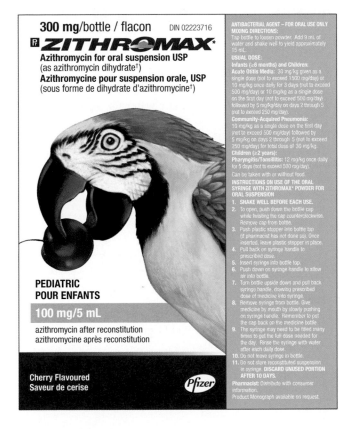

a. How many mL of diluent
must be added to the bottle?   _____

b. What is the final concentration
of the prepared solution?   _____

c. How many mL will you administer?   _____

Prepare the following solutions from the nutritional formulas. For questions in ounces,
provide answers in ounces and millilitres.

36. Order: $\frac{1}{4}$-strength Ensure 12 oz by nasogastric tube over 6 h. _____

37. Order: $\frac{2}{3}$-strength Isomil 6 oz PO q4h for 24 h. _____

38. A patient has an order for Jevity 1 200 mL by continuous feeding through a gastrostomy tube over 16 hours, followed by 250 mL of free water. The feeding is placed on
an infusion pump. Calculate the mL per hour to set the pump at. _____

39. Order: $\frac{1}{8}$-strength Ensure 4 oz by nasogastric tube q4h for 24 h. _____

Answers on pages 466–472.

evolve _____

For additional practice
problems, refer to the
Basic Calculations section
of the Drug Calculations
Companion, Version 5
on Evolve.

✳ ANSWERS

Answers to Practice Problems

1. 200 mg per vial

2. 5 mL

3. 0.9% sodium chloride injection without preservatives

4. 38 mg per mL

5. 24 h

6. 2.6 mL

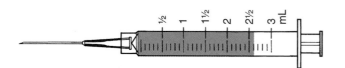

7. 350 mg per vial

8. 17.5 mL

9. Sterile water for injection or bacteriostatic water for injection preserved with benzyl alcohol

10. 20 mg per mL

11. IV or IM use

12. See package insert

13. 0.8 mL

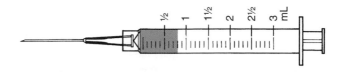

14. 500 mg per vial

15. Bacteriostatic water for injection with benzyl alcohol

16. 8 mL

17. 62.5 mg per mL

18. 0.6 mL

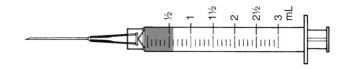

19. 1 g per vial (1 gram per vial)

20. IM or IV use

21. 45 mL

22. Water

23. 125 mg per 5 mL

24. Store at room temperature or refrigerate and keep tightly closed.

25. 1 000 mg (1 g) per vial

26. 20 mL

27. Sterile water for injection

28. 50 mg per mL

29. IV infusion only

30. 154 mL

31. 200 mL

32. 200 mg per 5 mL

33. 10 days (refrigerated)

34. 2 g per vial

35. 4.2 mL

36. 19.2 mL

37. IV diluents specified in the accompanying package insert

38. 100 mg per mL

39. 500 mg per vial

40. 100 mg per mL

41. IV infusion only

42. 24 mL

43. Water

44. 50 mg per 5 mL; 10 mg per mL

45. Store reconstituted suspension between 5°C and 30°C. Protect from freezing.

46. 20 000 000 units

47. 500 000 units per mL

48. 1 000 000 units per mL; this dosage strength is closest to what is ordered.

49. 2 mL

50. 7 days (1 week)

51. 5 000 000 units

52. 500 000 units per mL

53. 1.4 mL

54. Refrigerator

55. 7 days (1 week)

56. 250 000 units per mL

57. Package insert

58. 10 mg per vial

59. 2.1 mL

60. Sterile water for injection

61. 1 hour

62. 1.5 mL

63. 0.5 mL

64. $\dfrac{480\,\text{mL}}{8\,\text{h}} = 60\,\text{mL/h}$

65. $\dfrac{1\,600\,\text{mL}}{24\,\text{h}} = 66.6 = 67\,\text{mL/h}$

66. 300 mL PO QID = 300 mL × 4 = 1 200 mL

$$\frac{2}{3} \times 1\,200\,\text{mL} = x\,\text{mL}$$

$$x = \frac{2\,400}{3}$$

x = 800 mL of formula needed.

1 200 mL − 800 mL = 400 mL (water)

Therefore, you will add 400 mL of water to 800 mL of Sustacal to make 1 200 mL of $\frac{2}{3}$-strength Sustacal.

67. 1 oz = 30 mL   20 oz = 600 mL

$$\frac{1}{2} \times 600\,\text{mL} = x\,\text{mL} \qquad or \qquad \frac{1}{2} \times 20\,\text{oz} = x\,\text{oz}$$

$$x = \frac{600}{2} \qquad\qquad\qquad x = \frac{20}{2}$$

$$x = 300\,\text{mL} \qquad\qquad\quad x = 10\,\text{oz}$$

x = 300 mL; you need 10 oz of Ensure.

600 mL (20 oz) − 300 mL (10 oz) Ensure = 300 mL (10 oz of water)

10 oz Ensure + 10 oz water = 20 oz $\frac{1}{2}$-strength Ensure.

68. 1 oz = 30 mL; therefore, 16 oz = 480 mL

$$\frac{3}{4} \times 480\,\text{mL} = x\,\text{mL} \qquad or \qquad \frac{3}{4} \times 16\,\text{oz} = x\,\text{oz}$$

$$x = \frac{1\,440}{4} \qquad\qquad\qquad x = \frac{48}{4}$$

$$x = 360\,\text{mL} \qquad\qquad\quad x = 12\,\text{oz}$$

x = 12 oz (360 mL) of formula needed.

16 oz (480 mL) − 12 oz (360 mL) = 4 oz water (120 mL). You would need 360 mL of formula and 120 mL of water.

Answers to Clinical Reasoning Questions

1. a. The wrong dosage was administered because the nurse chose the incorrect dilution instructions. The dilution instructions used were for IV instead of IM.
   b. The concentration for IM should have been made (add 3 mL of diluents to give a concentration of 280 mg per mL).
   c. The nurse added 10.6 mL of a diluent and made the concentration for IV administration 95 mg per mL.
   d. The patient received three times the dose of medication IM (2.6 mL instead of 0.9 mL).

   Interchanging dilution instructions for IV and IM administration can have serious outcomes ranging from irritation of muscles to formation of a sterile abscess.
   e. This type of error could have been prevented by the nurse by reading the label carefully for the correct amount of diluents for the route ordered. Nurses must always check the route ordered and follow the directions that correspond to that route. The dilution instructions for IV and IM should never be interchanged.

✎ **NOTE**

For problems in which conversion is indicated, answers are shown with the order converted to what is available. Calculations could also be performed using the dimensional analysis method.

Answers to Chapter Review

1. a. 2.5 mL
   b. 334 mg per mL
   c.   334 mg : 1 mL = 250 mg : x mL

   $$\frac{334x}{334} = \frac{250}{334}$$

   $$x = 0.74 = 0.7 \text{ mL}$$

   or

   $$\frac{250 \text{ mg}}{334 \text{ mg}} \times 1 \text{ mL} = x \text{ mL}$$

   Answer: 0.7 mL. The dosage ordered is less than the available strength; therefore, you will need less than 1 mL to administer the dosage.

   d.

   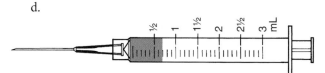

2. a.   500 mg : 8 mL = 165 mg : x mL

   $$\frac{500x}{500} = \frac{1\,320}{500}$$

   $$x = 2.64 = 2.6 \text{ mL}$$

   or

   $$\frac{165 \text{ mg}}{500 \text{ mg}} \times 8 \text{ mL} = x \text{ mL}$$

   Answer: 2.6 mL. The dosage ordered is less than the available strength; therefore, you will need less than 8 mL to administer the dosage.

   b.

   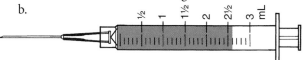

3. a. 3.5 mL
   b. 250 mg per mL
   c.   250 mg : 1 mL = 375 mg : x mL

   $$\frac{250x}{250} = \frac{375}{250}$$

   $$x = 1.5 \text{ mL}$$

   or

   $$\frac{375 \text{ mg}}{250 \text{ mg}} \times 1 \text{ mL} = x \text{ mL}$$

Answer: 1.5 mL. The dosage ordered is more than the available strength; you will need more than 1 mL to administer the dosage.

d.

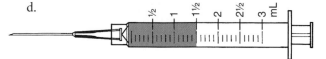

4.   10 mg : 1 mL = 100 mg : x mL

   $$\frac{10x}{10} = \frac{100}{10}$$

   $$x = 10 \text{ mL}$$

   or

   $$\frac{100 \text{ mg}}{10 \text{ mg}} \times 1 \text{ mL} = x \text{ mL}$$

Answer: 10 mL. The dosage ordered is more than the available strength; therefore, you will need more than 1 mL to administer the dosage. 10 mL IV can be administered.

5. a. Conversion is required. Conversion factor: 1 g = 1 000 mg. Therefore, 0.4 g = 400 mg. Answer: 45 mL
   b. Water
   c. 125 mg per 5 mL
   d.   125 mg : 5 mL = 400 mg : x mL

   $$\frac{125x}{125} = \frac{2\,000}{125}$$

   $$x = 16 \text{ mL}$$

   or

   $$\frac{400 \text{ mg}}{125 \text{ mg}} \times 5 \text{ mL} = x \text{ mL}$$

   Answer: 16 mL. The dosage ordered is more than the available strength; therefore, you will need more than 5 mL to administer the dosage. 16 mL PO can be administered; sometimes large volumes are administered PO.
   e. 14 days if refrigerated (7 days at room temperature)

6. a. 250 000 units per mL
   b. 1.1 mL
   c. 250 000 units : 1 mL = 275 000 units : x mL

$$\frac{250\,000x}{250\,000} = \frac{275\,\cancel{000}}{275\,\cancel{000}}$$

$$x = \frac{275}{250}$$

$$x = 1.1\,\text{mL}$$

or

$$\frac{275\,000\,\text{units}}{250\,000\,\text{units}} \times 1\,\text{mL} = x\,\text{mL}$$

Answer: 1.1 mL. The dosage ordered is more than what is available; therefore, you will need more than 1 mL to administer the dosage.
   d.

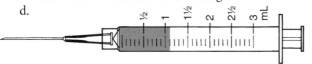

7. a. 100 mg per mL
   b. 100 mg : 1 mL = 200 mg : x mL

$$\frac{100x}{100} = \frac{200}{100}$$

$$x = 2\,\text{mL}$$

or

$$\frac{200\,\text{mg}}{100\,\text{mg}} \times 1\,\text{mL} = x\,\text{mL}$$

Answer: 2 mL. The dosage ordered is more than what is available; therefore, you will need more than 1 mL to administer the dosage.
   c.

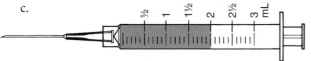

8. a. 40 mg per vial
   b. Bacteriostatic water for injection
   c. 40 mg : 1 mL = 175 mg : x mL

$$\frac{40x}{40} = \frac{175}{40}$$

$$x = 4.37 = 4.4\,\text{mL}$$

or

$$\frac{175\,\text{mg}}{40\,\text{mg}} \times 1\,\text{mL} = x\,\text{mL}$$

Answer: 4.4 mL. When mixed according to directions, the dosage is 40 mg per mL; therefore, you will need more than 1 mL to administer the dosage ordered.

d.

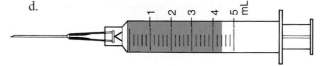

9. a. Conversion is required. Conversion factor: 1 000 mg = 1 g. Therefore, 0.5 g = 500 mg.
      Answer: 67 mL
   b. 400 mg per 5 mL
   c. 400 mg : 5 mL = 500 mg : x mL

$$\frac{400x}{400} = \frac{2\,500}{400}$$

$$x = 6.25 = 6.3\,\text{mL}$$

or

$$\frac{500\,\text{mg}}{400\,\text{mg}} \times 5\,\text{mL} = x\,\text{mL}$$

Answer: 6.3 mL. The dosage ordered is more than the available strength; therefore, you will need more than 5 mL to administer the dosage.

10. a. Conversion is required. Conversion factor: 1 000 mg = 1 g. Therefore, 1.2 g = 1 200 mg.

$$500\,\text{mg} : 1\,\text{mL} = 1\,200\,\text{mg} : x\,\text{mL}$$

$$\frac{500x}{500} = \frac{1\,200}{500}$$

$$x = 2.4\,\text{mL}$$

or

$$\frac{1\,200\,\text{mg}}{500\,\text{mg}} \times 1\,\text{mL} = x\,\text{mL}$$

Answer: 2.4 mL. The dosage ordered is more than the available strength; therefore, you will need more than 1 mL to administer the dosage.
    b.

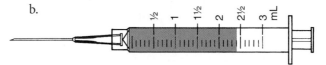

11. a. 250 mg per mL
    b. Conversion is required. Conversion factor: 1 000 mg = 1 g. Therefore, 0.5 g = 500 mg.

$$250\,\text{mg} : 1\,\text{mL} = 500\,\text{mg} : x\,\text{mL}$$

$$\frac{250x}{250} = \frac{500}{250}$$

$$x = 2\,\text{mL}$$

or

$$\frac{500\,\text{mg}}{250\,\text{mg}} \times 1\,\text{mL} = x\,\text{mL}$$

d.

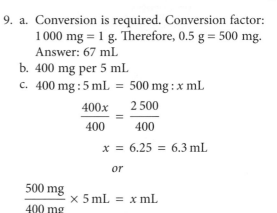

Answer: 2 mL. The dosage ordered is more than the available strength; therefore, you will need more than 1 mL to administer the dosage.

c.

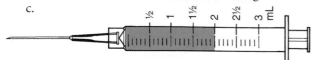

12. a. 64 mL
    b. 200 mg per 5 mL
    c. 200 mg : 5 mL = 350 mg : x mL

$$\frac{200x}{200} = \frac{1750}{200}$$

$$x = 8.75 = 8.8 \text{ mL}$$

or

$$\frac{350 \text{ mg}}{200 \text{ mg}} \times 5 \text{ mL} = x \text{ mL}$$

Answer: 8.8 mL; 8.75 rounded to the nearest tenth. The dosage ordered is more than the available strength; therefore, you will need more than 5 mL to administer the dosage.

13. a. 10 mL
    b. 95 mg per mL
    c. Conversion is required. Conversion factor: 1 000 mg = 1g.

$$95 \text{ mg} : 1 \text{ mL} = 1\,000 \text{ mg} : x \text{ mL}$$

or

$$\frac{1\,000 \text{ mg}}{95 \text{ mg}} \times 1 \text{ mL} = x \text{ mL}$$

Answer: 10.5 mL. The dosage ordered is more than the available strength; therefore, you will need more than 10 mL to administer the dosage and two vials.

14. a.   500 000 units : 1 mL = 400 000 units : x mL

or

$$\frac{400\,000 \text{ units}}{500\,000 \text{ units}} \times 1 \text{ mL} = x \text{ mL}$$

Answer: 0.8 mL. The dosage ordered is less than the available strength; therefore, you will need less than 1 mL to administer the dosage. *Note:* 500 000 units per mL was used because it is closest to the dosage ordered.

b.

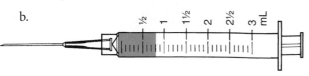

15. a.   280 mg : 1 mL = 250 mg : x mL

or

$$\frac{250 \text{ mg}}{280 \text{ mg}} \times 1 \text{ mL} = x \text{ mL}$$

Answer: 0.9 mL; 0.89 mL rounded to the nearest tenth. The dosage ordered is less than the available strength; therefore, you will need less than 1 mL to administer the dosage.

b.

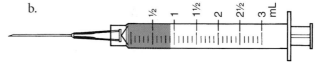

16. a.   1 g : 2.6 mL = 0.5 g : x mL

or

$$\frac{0.5 \text{ g}}{1 \text{ g}} \times 2.6 \text{ mL} = x \text{ mL}$$

Answer: 1.3 mL. The dosage ordered is one half of the available strength; therefore, you will need less than 2.6 mL to administer the dosage.

b.

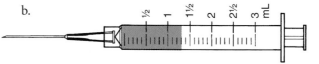

17. a.   50 mg : 1 mL = 150 mg : x mL

or

$$\frac{150 \text{ mg}}{50 \text{ mg}} \times 1 \text{ mL} = x \text{ mL}$$

Answer: 3 mL. The dosage ordered is more than the available strength; you will need more than 1 mL to administer the dosage.

b.

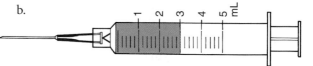

18. a. Conversion is required. Conversion factor:
    1 000 mg = 1 g. Therefore, 0.45 g = 450 mg.
    Answer: 10 mL.
    b. 50 mg per mL
    c.   50 mg : 1 mL = 450 mg : x mL

    $$x = 9 \text{ mL}$$

    or

    $$\frac{450 \text{ mg}}{50 \text{ mg}} \times 1 \text{ mL} = x \text{ mL}$$

    Answer: 9 mL. The dosage ordered is more than
    the available strength; therefore, you will need
    more than 1 mL to administer the dosage.

    d.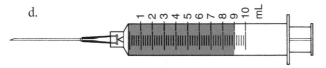

19. a. Conversion is required. Conversion factor:
    1 000 mcg = 1 mg. Therefore, 0.05 mg = 50 mcg.

    40 mcg : 1 mL = 50 mcg : x mL

    $$\frac{40x}{40} = \frac{50}{40}$$

    $$x = 1.3 \text{ mL}$$

    or

    $$\frac{50 \text{ mcg}}{40 \text{ mcg}} \times 5 \text{ mL} = x \text{ mL}$$

    Answer: 1.3 mL; 1.25 mL rounded to the nearest
    tenth. The dosage ordered is less than the available
    strength; therefore, you will need less than 5 mL to
    administer the dosage.

    b.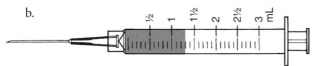

20. a. Conversion is required. Conversion factor:
    1 000 mg = 1 g. Therefore, 0.25 g = 250 mg.

    50 mg : 1 mL = 250 mg : x mL

    $$\frac{50x}{50} = \frac{250}{50}$$

    $$x = 5 \text{ mL}$$

    or

    $$\frac{250 \text{ mg}}{50 \text{ mg}} \times 1 \text{ mL} = x \text{ mL}$$

Answer: 5 mL. The dosage ordered is more than
the available strength; therefore, you will need
more than 1 mL to administer the dosage.

b.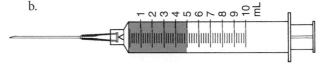

21.   100 mg : 5 mL = 200 mg : x mL

    or

    $$\frac{200 \text{ mg}}{100 \text{ mg}} \times 5 \text{ mL} = x \text{ mL}$$

Answer: 10 mL. The dosage ordered is more than the
available strength; therefore, you will need more than
5 mL to administer the dosage.

22. a. Conversion is required. Conversion factor:
    1 000 mg = 1 g. Therefore, 0.5 g = 500 mg.

    330 mg : 1 mL = 500 mg : x mL

    or

    $$\frac{500 \text{ mg}}{330 \text{ mg}} \times 1 \text{ mL} = x \text{ mL}$$

    Answer: 1.5 mL. The dosage ordered is more than
    what is available; therefore, you will need more
    than 1 mL to administer the dosage.

    b.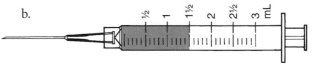

23. a. Conversion is required. Conversion factor:
    1 000 mg = 1 g. Therefore, 1.5 g = 1 500 mg.

    160 mg : 1 mL = 1 500 mg : x mL

    or

    $$\frac{1 500 \text{ mg}}{160 \text{ mg}} \times 1 \text{ mL} = x \text{ mL}$$

    Answer: 9.4 mL; 9.37 mL rounded to the nearest
    tenth. The dosage ordered is more than the
    available strength; therefore, you will need more
    than 1 mL to administer the dosage.

    b.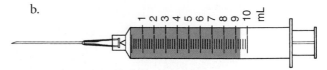

24. a. 500 000 units per mL
    b. 8 mL
    c.   500 000 units : 1 mL = 425 000 units : x mL

or

$$\frac{425\,000 \text{ units}}{500\,000 \text{ units}} \times 1\,\text{mL} = x\,\text{mL}$$

Answer: 0.9 mL; 0.85 mL rounded to the nearest tenth. The dosage ordered is less than the available dosage strength; therefore, you will need less than 1 mL to administer the dosage. 500 000 units per mL is closer to what prescriber ordered.

d.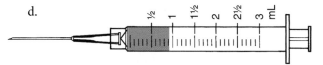

25. a. 19 mL
    b. 10 mL : 1 mL = 200 mg : x mL

$$\frac{10x}{10} = \frac{200}{10}$$

$$x = 20\,\text{mL}$$

or

$$\frac{200 \text{ mg}}{10 \text{ mg}} \times 1\,\text{mL} = x\,\text{mL}$$

Answer: 20 mL. The dosage ordered is more than the available strength; therefore, you will need more than 1 mL to administer the dosage.

26. a. 54 mL
    b.   125 mg : 5 mL = 500 mg : x mL

$$\frac{125x}{125} = \frac{2\,500}{125}$$

$$x = 20\,\text{mL}$$

or

$$\frac{500 \text{ mg}}{125 \text{ mg}} \times 5\,\text{mL} = x\,\text{mL}$$

Answer: 20 mL. The dosage ordered is more than the available strength; therefore, you will need more than 5 mL to administer the dosage.

27. a. 20 mL
    b. 4.5 g per vial
    c. Conversion is required. Conversion factor: 1 000 mg = 1 g. Therefore, 2.25 g = 2 250 mg.

$$194 \text{ mg} : 1\,\text{mL} = 2\,250 \text{ mg} : x\,\text{mL}$$

$$\frac{194x}{194} = \frac{2\,250}{194}$$

$$x = 11.3\,\text{mL}$$

or

$$\frac{2\,250 \text{ mg}}{194 \text{ mg}} \times 61\,\text{mL} = x\,\text{mL}$$

Answer: 11.6 mL; 11.59 mL rounded to the nearest tenth. The dosage ordered is more than the available strength; therefore, you will need more than 1 mL to administer the dosage.

28.   200 mg : 5 mL = 500 mg : x mL

$$\frac{200x}{200} = \frac{2\,500}{200}$$

$$x = 12.5\,\text{mL}$$

or

$$\frac{500 \text{ mg}}{200 \text{ mg}} \times 5\,\text{mL} = x\,\text{mL}$$

Answer: 12.5 mL. The dosage ordered is more than what is available; therefore, you will need more than 5 mL to administer the dosage.

29. a.   1 g : 2 mL = 1 g : x mL

$$x = 2\,\text{mL}$$

or

$$\frac{1\,\text{g}}{1\,\text{g}} \times 2\,\text{mL} = x\,\text{mL}$$

Answer: 2 mL. When mixed according to directions, the solution gives 1 g in 2 mL; therefore, you will need 2 mL to administer the dosage ordered.

b.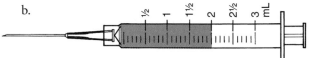

30.   3 g:8 mL = 1.5 g:x mL

or

$$\frac{1.5\,g}{3\,g} \times 8\,mL = x\,mL$$

Answer: 4 mL. The dosage ordered is less than the available strength; therefore, you will need less than 8 mL to administer the dosage. (The dosage ordered is half of the available strength.)

31.   40 mg:5 mL = 20 mg:x mL

$$\frac{40x}{40} = \frac{100}{40}$$

$$x = 2.5\,mL$$

or

$$\frac{20\,mg}{40\,mg} \times 5\,mL = x\,mL$$

Answer: 2.5 mL. The dosage ordered is less than the available strength; you will need less than 5 mL to administer the dosage.

32. a.   350 mg:1 mL = 125 mg:x mL

$$\frac{350x}{350} = \frac{125}{350}$$

$$x = 0.4\,mL$$

or

$$\frac{125\,mg}{350\,mg} \times 1\,mL = x\,mL$$

Answer: 0.4 mL; 0.35 mL rounded to the nearest tenth. The dosage ordered is less than what is available; therefore, you will need less than 1 mL to administer the dosage.

b.

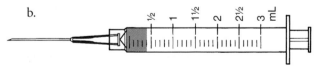

33. a. 10 mL
    b. Sterile water for injection without a bacteriostatic agent
    c. 5 mg per mL
    d.   5 mg:1 mL = 45.5 mg:x mL

or

$$\frac{45.5\,mg}{5\,mg} \times 1\,mL = x\,mL$$

Alternative solution:

50 mg:10 mL = 45.5 mg:x mL

or

$$\frac{45.5\,mg}{50\,mg} \times 10\,mL = x\,mL$$

This setup would net the same answer of 9.1 mL. Answer: 9.1 mL. The dosage ordered is more than the available strength; therefore, you will need more than 1 mL to administer the dosage.

34. a. 60 mL
    b. 250 mg per 5 mL
    c.   250 mg:1 mL = 300 mg:x mL

or

$$\frac{300\,mg}{250\,mg} \times 5\,mL = x\,mL$$

Answer: 6 mL. The dosage ordered is more than the available strength; therefore, you will need more than 5 mL to administer the dosage.

35. a. 9 mL
    b. 100 mg per 5 mL
    c.   100 mg:5 mL = 250 mg:x mL

or

$$\frac{250\,mg}{100\,mg} \times 5\,mL = x\,mL$$

Answer: 12.5 mL. The dosage ordered is more than what is available; therefore, you will need more than 5 mL to administer the dosage.

36. 1 oz = 30 mL; 12 oz = 360 mL

$$\frac{1}{4} \times 360\,mL = x\,mL$$

$$\frac{360}{4} = x$$

$$x = 90\,mL$$

or

$$\frac{1}{4} \times 12\,oz = x\,oz$$

$$\frac{12}{4} = x$$

$$x = 3\,oz$$

$x = 90$ mL; you need 3 oz of Ensure.

360 mL (12 oz) − 90 mL (3 oz) Ensure = 270 mL (9 oz of water)

Answer: 3 oz (90 mL) of Ensure + 9 oz (270 mL) water = 12 oz (360 mL) of $\frac{1}{4}$-strength Ensure.

37. *Note:* 6 oz q4h = 6 feedings; 6 oz × 6 = 36 oz

1 oz = 30 mL; therefore, 36 oz = 1 080 mL

$\frac{2}{3} \times 1080\,\text{mL} = x\,\text{mL}$

$\frac{2160}{3} = x$

x = 720 mL of the formula (Isomil) needed

1 080 mL − 720 mL = 360 mL (water)

Answer: 24 oz (720 mL) of Isomil + 12 oz (360 mL) of water = 36 oz (1 080 mL) $\frac{2}{3}$-strength Isomil.

38. Answer: $\frac{1\,200\,\text{mL}}{16\,\text{h}} = 75\,\text{mL/h}$

39. 4 oz q4h would be 24 oz

$\frac{1}{8} \times 24\,\text{oz} = 3\,\text{oz}$ (90 mL) Ensure

24 oz − 3 oz = 21 oz

1 oz = 30 mL; therefore, 21 oz × 30 = 630 mL

Answer: 3 oz (90 mL) of Ensure + 21 oz (630 mL) of water = 24 oz (720 mL) of $\frac{1}{8}$-strength Ensure.

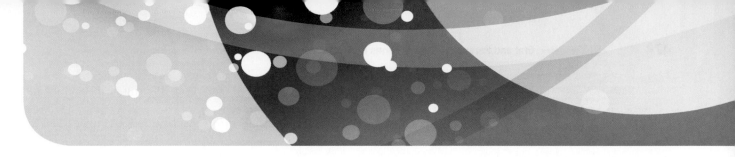

CHAPTER 18

Insulin

Objectives

After reviewing this chapter, you should be able to:

1. Identify important information on insulin labels
2. Identify various methods for insulin administration
3. Read calibrations on 30-, 50-, and 100-unit syringes
4. Measure insulin in single doses
5. Measure combined insulin dosages

Insulin, which is used in the treatment of diabetes mellitus (DM), is a hormone secreted by the islets of Langerhans in the pancreas. It is a necessary hormone for glucose use by the body. Individuals who do not produce adequate insulin experience an increase in their blood sugar (glucose) level. These individuals may require the administration of insulin. Accuracy in insulin administration is extremely important because inaccurate dosages can lead to serious or life-threatening emergencies. Insulin is one of the top five "high-alert" medications, according to Institute for Safe Medication Practices Canada (ISMP Canada, 2012). High-alert medications have a high risk of causing injury or death to a patient. They are also medications with which health care providers often make errors. The consequences of errors associated with these medications are usually more devastating than those that occur with other medications. Medications classified as high-alert require safeguards to protect patient safety. Always follow the policy of your health care facility for administering any high-alert medication to decrease the chance of error.

ISMP Canada (2003) and Cohen (2010) have identified some common causes of insulin errors:

- Miscommunication of insulin orders
- Abbreviations "U," "IU," or "u" written for "units" and misinterpreted as a zero (0) or another number
- Look-alike medication names (e.g., Humulin and Humalog) in similar packaging
- Use of a tuberculin syringe to prepare a dose, which has resulted in tenfold overdoses
- Use of an insulin syringe to prepare a nonstandard concentration (insulin syringes are accurate only for the most common concentration, 100 units per millilitre [mL])
- Incorrect preparation of insulin suspensions (e.g., Insulin NPH) for dose withdrawal and administration; suspensions must be re-suspended according to protocol prior to use
- Incorrect rates programmed into infusion pumps, sometimes due to a patient receiving multiple pump infusions
- Insulin being mistakenly administered to patients who do not have diabetes, leading to profound hypoglycemia

- Misreading of a blood glucose (BG) meter (see Figure 18-4, *B*) result or the faulty functioning of meters

This list is just a sample of the causes of insulin errors that have serious implications for nurses.

> **! SAFETY ALERT!**
>
> Accuracy in insulin preparation and administration is crucial. Inaccurate dosages can lead to serious adverse or life-threatening effects. Nurses must correctly interpret insulin orders and use the correct syringe to measure insulin for administration.

Insulin dosages are measured in units and administered with syringes that correspond to U-100 insulin as written on the package and the syringe itself; U-100 insulin means 100 units per mL. The most common types of insulin are supplied in 10-mL vials and labelled U-100. In the spring of 2015, Health Canada approved a new basal insulin analogue (insulin glargine [rDNA origin]) injection, U-300 (Sanofi Canada, 2015). The trade name for insulin glargine U-300 is Toujeo, and it is manufactured by Sanofi Canada. Insulin glargine U-300 is 300 units per mL in a disposable prefilled pen.

Insulin is also available in the United States as U-500 (500 units per mL). U-500 is a more concentrated strength and is sometimes used for people who are highly insulin resistant. The use of this U-500 concentration of insulin remains controversial mainly because of reported medication errors that have resulted in patient injury (ISMP, 2013). The 2013 Canadian Diabetes Association Clinical Practice Guidelines (CDA CPG) for the prevention and management of diabetes in Canada do not endorse the use of this higher concentration of insulin (Canadian Diabetes Association [CDA] Clinical Practice Guidelines Expert Committee, 2013). **Discussion of insulin in this chapter refers to the standard concentration of 100 units per mL.**

> **! SAFETY ALERT!**
>
> U-100 = 100 units per mL
> U-300 = 300 units per mL
> U-300 insulin is three times as concentrated as U-100. It is **crucial** that the nurse use extreme **caution** when administering U-300 insulin **to prevent an unintentional overdose, which can result in irreversible insulin shock and death for a patient.**

Labels

Reading insulin labels is basically the same as reading any other medication label. It is essential that the nurse know the significant information on an insulin label and where to locate it. That information includes the origin and type of insulin, the brand and generic names, the dosage strength or concentration, and storage information. Figure 18-1 shows information that can be found on an insulin label. Notice the following:

- The letter *N* that follows the trade name Novolin identifies the type of insulin by action and time. N = NPH (intermediate acting). These letters are important identifiers for insulin.
- An upper case *N* is used for NPH. You will also see *R* for regular insulin.
- Concentration (dosage strength) of the insulin is also indicated; notice U-100 (100 units per mL)
- The expiration date is also indicated on insulin labels and is important to check.

> **! SAFETY ALERT!**
>
> Carefully read insulin labels to avoid a medication error that could be life threatening. Always read the label and compare it with the medication order three times. Insulin dosages must be checked by two nurses. Reading the label carefully ensures selection of the correct action time and type of insulin.

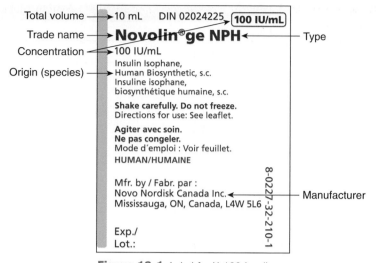

Figure 18-1 Label for U-100 insulin.

Types of Insulin and Their Action

"Insulin preparations are primarily produced by recumbent DNA technology and are formulated either as structurally identical to human insulin or as a modification of human insulin (insulin analogues) to alter pharmacokinetics" (CDA Clinical Practice Guidelines Expert Committee, 2013, p. S56). Most adults with type 1 diabetes use the preferred human insulin and insulin analogues. Although rarely used, preparations of animal-sourced insulin are still accessible in Canada (p. S56).

The various types of insulin (with trade names) used to treat patients with diabetes appear in Table 18-1. Notice the onset, peak, and duration of action for each type. These action times are estimates only: the patient, the site of injection, and the type of insulin used influence insulin action.

Rapid-acting insulin analogues (insulin aspart, insulin glulisine, and insulin lispro) are to be administered at the main mealtimes as bolus (prandial) insulin in the basal-bolus regimen of multiple daily injections (MDI). Rapid-acting insulin analogues are preferred over short-acting regular insulin, especially in continuous subcutaneous insulin infusion (CSII), as they have been shown to lower the risk of hypoglycemia and have better patient outcomes overall.

Short-acting regular insulins are also used as prandial/bolus insulin for mealtimes. Regular insulin is the only type of insulin that is currently administered intravenously in Canada, and it must be administered in a hospital.

Intermediate-acting insulins are known as insulin NPH, of which there are two kinds. Refer to Table 18-1 for the trade names of these two types of insulin. Insulin NPH is used as basal insulin in the basal-bolus regimen and is now recommended to be given at bedtime (at around 10:00 PM) to help prevent nocturnal hypoglycemia. Sometimes, NPH may be given twice per day, in the morning before breakfast and at bedtime.

Long-acting basal insulin analogues (insulin detemir and insulin glargine) are usually given at bedtime for the basal insulin as well to help reduce nocturnal hypoglycemia. They should not be mixed with any other insulin. You will note in Table 18-1 that long-acting basal insulin analogues have no peak time and have a duration of action of up to 30 hours.

Premixed insulins are available in fixed preparations, as shown in Table 18-1 and Figure 18-3. Premixed regular insulins combine regular and insulin NPH in percentages. For

TABLE 18-1 Types of Insulin Available in Canada			
Types of Insulin			
Insulin Type (Trade Name)	**Onset**	**Peak**	**Duration**
Bolus (Prandial) Insulins			
Rapid-acting insulin analogues (clear):			
• Insulin aspart (NovoRapid®)	10–15 min	1–1.5 h	3–5 h
• Insulin glulisine (Apidra™)	10–15 min	1–1.5 h	3–5 h
• Insulin lispro (Humalog®)	10–15 min	1–2 h	3.5–4.75 h
Short-acting insulins (clear):			
• Insulin regular (Humulin®-R)	30 min	2–3 h	6.5 h
• Insulin regular (Novolin®geToronto)			
Basal Insulins			
Intermediate-acting insulins (cloudy):			
• Insulin NPH (Humulin®-N)	1–3 h	5–8 h	Up to 18 h
• Insulin NPH (Novolin®ge NPH)			
Long-acting basal insulin analogues (clear):			
• Insulin detemir (Levemir®)	90 min	Not applicable	Up to 24 h (detemir 16–24 h)
• Insulin glargine (Lantus®)	90 min		Up to 24 h (glargine 24 h)
• Insulin glargine U-300 (Toujeo®)	Up to 6 h		Up to 30 h
Premixed Insulins			
Premixed regular insulin—NPH (cloudy):		A single vial or cartridge contains a fixed ratio of insulin	
• 30% insulin regular/70% insulin NPH (Humulin® 30/70)		(% of rapid-acting or short-acting insulin to % of	
• 30% insulin regular/70% insulin NPH (Novolin®ge 30/70)		intermediate-acting insulin)	
• 40% insulin regular/60% insulin NPH (Novolin®ge 40/60)			
• 50% insulin regular/50% insulin NPH (Novolin®ge 50/50)			
Premixed insulin analogues (cloudy):			
• 30% Insulin aspart/70% insulin aspart protamine crystals (NovoMix® 30)			
• 50% Insulin aspart/50% insulin aspart protamine crystals (NovoMix® 50)			
• 25% insulin lispro/75% insulin lispro protamine (Humalog® Mix25®)			
• 50% insulin lispro/50% insulin lispro protamine (Humalog® Mix50®)			

Reprinted from Canadian Journal of Diabetes, 37/S1, Angela McGibbon, Cindy Richardson, Cheri Hernandez, John Dornan, "Pharmacotherapy in Type 1 Diabetes," S56–S60, Copyright 2013, with permission from Elsevier.

h, hour; *min,* minute.

> **NOTE**
>
> The premixed insulin analogue 50% insulin aspart/50% insulin aspart protamine crystals (NovoMix 50) and the basal insulin glargine U-300 (Toujeo) were approved for use in Canada **after** the CDA CPG were published in 2013.

example, Humulin 30/70 has 30% regular **short-acting** insulin and 70% **intermediate-acting** insulin NPH. Premixed insulin analogues, on the other hand, combine **rapid-acting** insulin analogues with **intermediate-acting** insulin NPH. The onset of action of premixed insulin analogues is 5 to 15 minutes, while the onset of premixed regular insulins is around 30 to 45 minutes. Premixed regular insulins or insulin analogues should **not** be prescribed to patients who have type 1 diabetes. For best patient outcomes, an MDI regimen (four times per day) of **basal-bolus** insulin is recommended. Premixed insulins are available in vials and pens. Figure 18-2 shows samples of labels grouped by action times.

Regular and insulin NPH may be mixed together for one injection as was the norm for many years. However, with the influx of premixed insulins/analogues, the need to mix insulin has drastically decreased. Moreover, while rapid-acting insulin is the preferred/first choice for bolus insulin, it may also be mixed with NPH if a patient who has type 2 diabetes requires amounts that are not available as premixed analogue combinations. It is important for the nurse to know that rapid-acting insulin analogues (e.g., lispro) bind quickly with insulin NPH and must be injected immediately (within 5 minutes) after mixing.

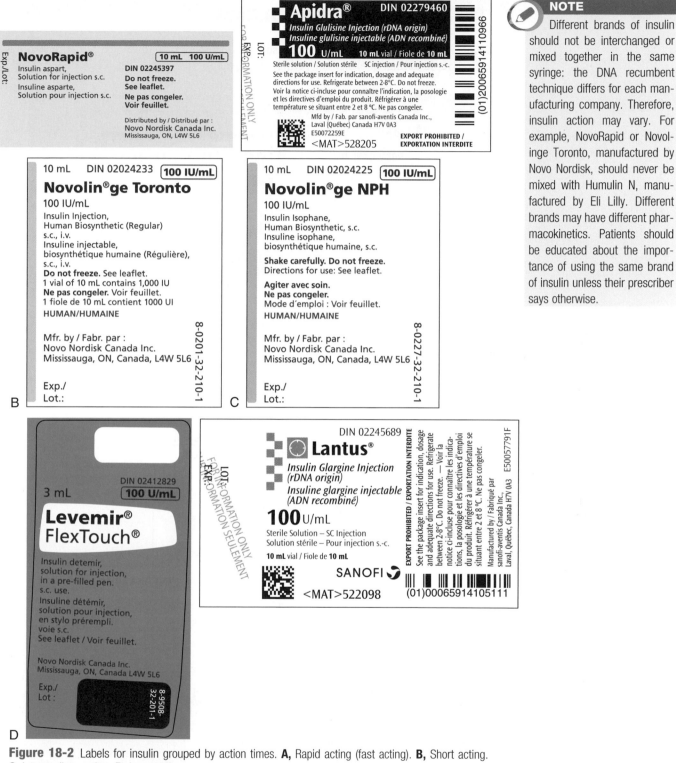

Figure 18-2 Labels for insulin grouped by action times. **A,** Rapid acting (fast acting). **B,** Short acting. **C,** Intermediate acting. **D,** Long acting.

> **NOTE**
>
> Different brands of insulin should not be interchanged or mixed together in the same syringe: the DNA recumbent technique differs for each manufacturing company. Therefore, insulin action may vary. For example, NovoRapid or Novolinge Toronto, manufactured by Novo Nordisk, should never be mixed with Humulin N, manufactured by Eli Lilly. Different brands may have different pharmacokinetics. Patients should be educated about the importance of using the same brand of insulin unless their prescriber says otherwise.

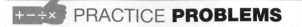 PRACTICE **PROBLEMS**

Using the labels provided, identify the insulin trade or generic name and action time (short acting, rapid acting, intermediate acting, or long acting).

DIN: 000000000

10 mL.

DOSAGE AND USE
See package insert for full prescribing information

Each mL contains 100 units insulin lispro.

Exp./
Lot:

insulin lispro (rDNA)
For injection

100 units/mL

SAMPLE LABEL (textbook use only)

http://evolve.elsevier.com/Canada/GrayMorris/

1. Generic name: _____   Action time: _____

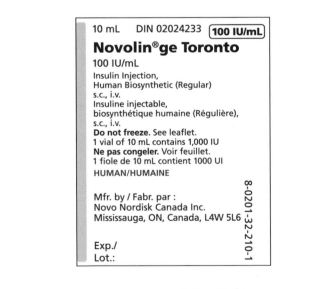

10 mL   DIN 02024233   100 IU/mL

Novolin®ge Toronto

100 IU/mL

Insulin Injection,
Human Biosynthetic (Regular)
s.c., i.v.
Insuline injectable,
biosynthétique humaine (Régulière),
s.c., i.v.
Do not freeze. See leaflet.
1 vial of 10 mL contains 1,000 IU
Ne pas congeler. Voir feuillet.
1 fiole de 10 mL contient 1000 UI
HUMAN/HUMAINE

Mfr. by / Fabr. par :
Novo Nordisk Canada Inc.
Mississauga, ON, Canada, L4W 5L6

Exp./
Lot.:

8-0201-32-210-1

2. Trade name: _____   Action time: _____

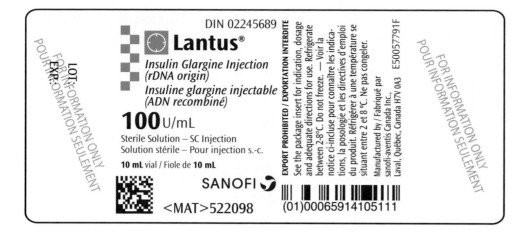

DIN 02245689

Lantus®

*Insulin Glargine Injection
(rDNA origin)*

*Insuline glargine injectable
(ADN recombiné)*

100 U/mL

Sterile Solution – SC Injection
Solution stérile – Pour injection s.-c.

10 mL vial / Fiole de **10 mL**

SANOFI

<MAT>522098

(01)00065914105111

See the package insert for indication, dosage and adequate directions for use. Refrigerate between 2-8°C. Do not freeze. — Voir la notice ci-incluse pour connaître les indications, la posologie et les directives d'emploi du produit. Réfrigérer à une température se situant entre 2 et 8 °C. Ne pas congeler.

Manufactured by / Fabriqué par sanofi-aventis Canada Inc., Laval, Québec, Canada H7V 0A3   E50057791F

3. Trade name: _____   Action time: _____

---

10 mL   DIN 02024225   **100 IU/mL**

Novolin®ge NPH

100 IU/mL

Insulin Isophane,
Human Biosynthetic, s.c.
Insuline isophane,
biosynthétique humaine, s.c.

Shake carefully. Do not freeze.
Directions for use: See leaflet.

Agiter avec soin.
Ne pas congeler.
Mode d´emploi : Voir feuillet.

HUMAN/HUMAINE

Mfr. by / Fabr. par :
Novo Nordisk Canada Inc.
Mississauga, ON, Canada, L4W 5L6

Exp./
Lot.:

8-0227-32-210-1

4. Trade name: _____   Action time: _____

Answers on page 505.

Appearance of Insulin

All rapid-acting, short-acting, and long-acting insulins are clear. All intermediate-acting (NPH) insulins and premixed insulin/insulin analogues are cloudy (see Table 18-1). Figure 18-3 presents some premixed combination insulin labels.

> **⚠ SAFETY ALERT!**
>
> Remember: insulin has been identified as a high-alert medication. Avoid an error that could be life threatening to the patient. Carefully read all labels to ensure that you select the correct type of insulin. The action time of insulin varies.

Insulin Administration Methods

Insulin is administered by syringe, pen, or pump. The major route of insulin administration is by subcutaneous (SUBCUT) injection; insulin is never administered intramuscularly. Regular insulin is also administered intravenously when blood glucose levels are extremely elevated. Figure 18-4 shows the various delivery systems used to administer insulin. The

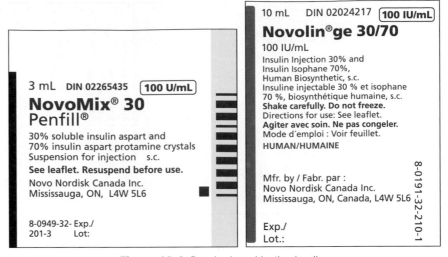

Figure 18-3 Premixed combination insulins.

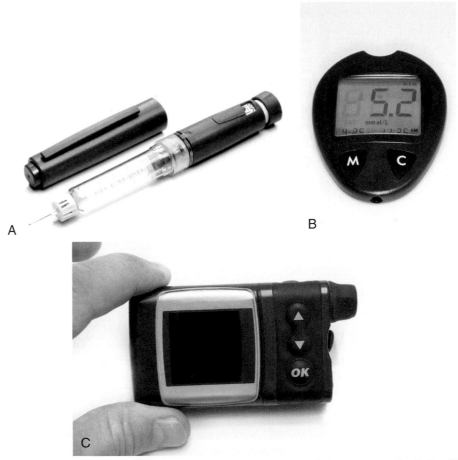

Figure 18-4 A, Insulin pen with cap off. **B,** Blood glucose meter. **C,** Insulin pump. (**A,** © Can Stock Photo Inc./piedmont photo. **B,** © Can Stock Photo Inc./Bob Betenia. **C,** © Can Stock Photo Inc./HdcPhoto.)

2013 CDA CPG recommend that insulin regimens be tailored to the patient's "treatment goals, lifestyle, diet, age, general health, motivation, hypoglycemia awareness status and ability for self-management" (CDA Clinical Practice Guidelines Expert Committee, 2013, p. S56).

Insulin Pump

Insulin can also be administered by a pump. A CSII pump provides a low dose of continuous insulin over 24 hours a day through a catheter placed under the skin. This process mimics the physiological basal insulin secretion along with additional bolus doses for meals and blood glucose elevations. Pumps have become more popular today and are used by children and adults alike. CSII uses rapid-acting insulin analogues or short-acting insulin, but rapid-acting insulin analogues are the insulin of choice for use in pump therapy (CDA Clinical Practice Guidelines Expert Committee, 2013). In addition to eliminating the need for multiple daily injections, CSII therapy may be superior to MDI in reducing the rates of severe hypoglycemia. Despite its high cost, the CSII pump has been gaining popularity because it not only allows flexibility in timing of meals and activity but also offers an improved quality of life to the patient. Figure 18-4, *C* shows an example of an insulin pump. The pump is implantable and external (portable).

Insulin Pen

Insulin can also be delivered by an insulin pen. When capped, the insulin pen looks very much like an ink pen. Some pens are disposed of after one use, whereas others have replaceable insulin cartridges. All insulin pens minimize the discomfort from an injection because the needles in insulin pens are extremely short and thin. Figure 18-4, *A* shows the parts of an insulin pen. The insulin pen has a dose selector knob used to "dial" the desired dose of insulin. Once the pen has been cleared of any air in the cartridge (primed) and the dose set, the insulin is injected by pressing on the injection button. When injection is completed, the needle is removed and the cap replaced. Insulin pens are available in many styles (and colours): a prefilled, disposable model; a smaller low-dose model; and a refillable model, in which a new cartridge can be inserted when needed. Patient education on the use of the insulin pen (the correct method to hold the pen and read the dosing dial) is a must. It will help in the prevention of dosage errors.

Measuring Insulin in a U-100 Syringe

Syringes are still the preferred means of insulin administration for many patients with diabetes. Insulin is less expensive in vials than in cartridges used in pens. As mentioned in Chapter 16, syringes are available in three volumes and graduations. Most health care providers who work with adult patients will only see the standard U-100 (1-mL) insulin syringe in the health care setting.

1. **Lo-Dose syringes:** The 50-unit Lo-Dose insulin syringe has a capacity of 50 units (0.5 mL). It is calibrated in 1-unit increments. The 30-unit Lo-Dose insulin syringe has a capacity of 30 units (0.3 mL). It is also calibrated in 1-unit increments and is mostly used to measure very small amounts of insulin for children.
2. **Standard U-100 insulin syringes:** The 100-unit syringe comes with even and odd numbers. Two types of 1-mL syringes are in current use:
   a. The single-scale 1-mL syringe is calibrated in 2-unit increments. Any dosage measured in an odd number of units is measured between the even calibrations. This syringe would not be recommended for patients receiving odd number (e.g., 25, 33) units of insulin, because the insulin dose cannot be accurately measured.
   b. The dual-scale 1-mL syringe has a scale with even-numbered 2-unit increments (2, 4, etc.) on one side and a scale with odd-numbered 2-unit increments (1, 3, etc.) on the other. To avoid confusion, odd-numbered doses (e.g., 13 units) should be measured on the scale with the odd-numbered calibration, and even-numbered doses (e.g., 26 units) should be measured on the scale with the even-numbered calibration. When even numbers of units are measured, each calibration is then measured as 2 units.

To review what the different types of insulin syringes look like, see Figure 18-5.

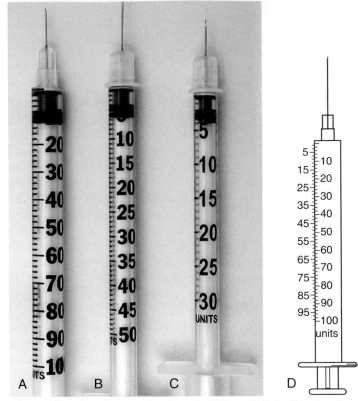

Figure 18-5 Types of insulin syringes. **A,** Single-scale (100 units). **B,** Lo-Dose insulin syringe (50 units). **C,** Lo-Dose insulin syringe (30 units). **D,** Dual-scale syringe (100 units).

> ## SAFETY ALERT!
> Administer insulin in an insulin syringe used only for the administration of U-100 insulin. Do not use an insulin syringe to measure other medications that are measured in units. Syringes of 30 and 50 units measure a smaller volume of insulin but are intended for the measurement of U-100 insulin only. Use the smallest capacity insulin syringe available to ensure the accuracy of dosage preparation.

Lo-Dose Syringe

Let's look at some insulin dosages measured in the syringes to help you visualize the amounts in a syringe. Syringe *A* shows 30 units and syringe *B* shows 37 units in a Lo-Dose syringe.

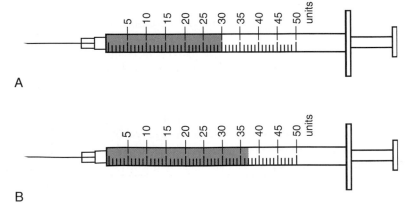

PRACTICE **PROBLEMS**

Indicate the dosage shown by the arrow on each syringe.

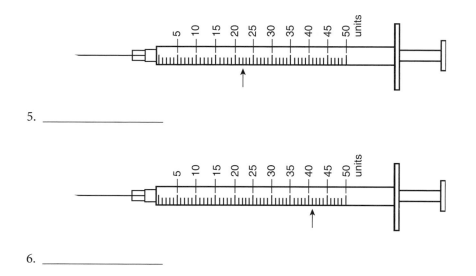

5. _____

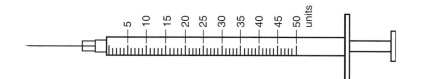

6. _____

Shade in the specified dosage on each syringe.

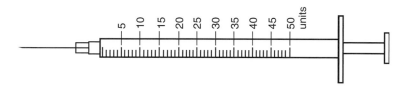

7. 17 units

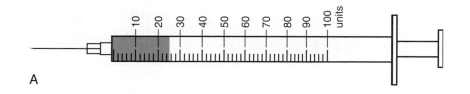

8. 47 units

Answers on page 505.

Single-Scale 1-Millilitre Syringe

Now let's look at what dosages would look like on a single-scale 1-mL syringe. Syringe *A* shows 25 units and Syringe *B* shows 55 units. Notice that the dosages are drawn up between the even calibrations.

A

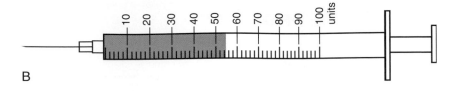

B

Dual-Scale 1-Millilitre Syringe

Now let's look at what dosages would look like on a dual-scale 1-mL syringe. Syringe *C* shows 37 units; notice that the scale on the left is used. Syringe *D* shows 54 units; notice that the scale on the right is used.

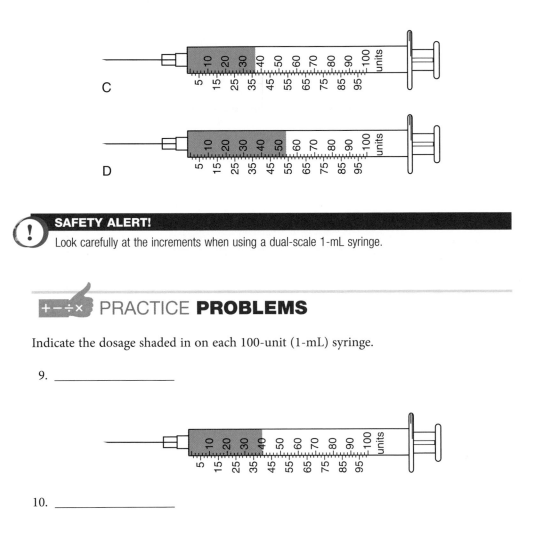

C

D

> **(!) SAFETY ALERT!**
> Look carefully at the increments when using a dual-scale 1-mL syringe.

PRACTICE **PROBLEMS**

Indicate the dosage shaded in on each 100-unit (1-mL) syringe.

9. _____

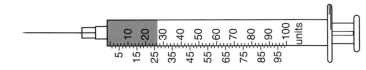

10. _____

11. _____

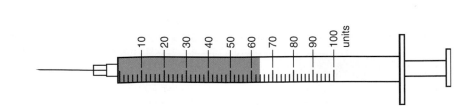

12. _____

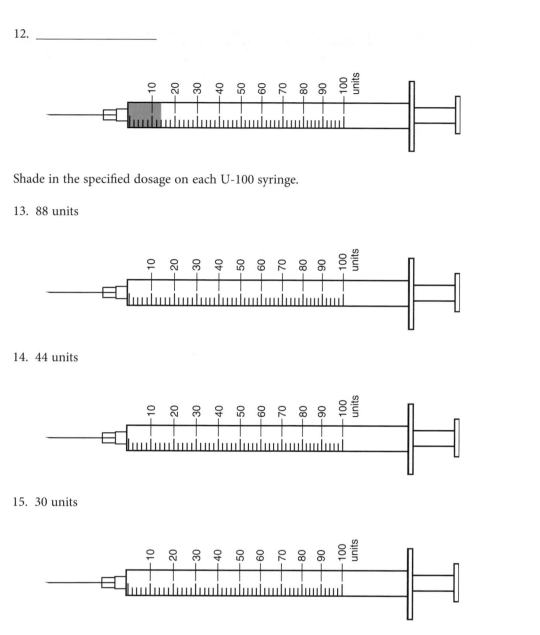

Shade in the specified dosage on each U-100 syringe.

13. 88 units

14. 44 units

15. 30 units

Answers on page 505.

Insulin Orders

Like any written medication order, an insulin order must be written clearly and contain certain information to prevent errors in administration. Box 18-1 presents insulin-specific guidelines for clinical order sets.

These guidelines only apply to subcutaneous insulin injections and not to orders for intravenous (IV) or CSII therapy. Although these guidelines have been published for some time, not all institutions and prescribers follow them completely. However, many institutions have incorporated most of the components in their various insulin order sets. For example, Figure 18-6 shows a sample of an order set for subcutaneous insulin. Based on hospital policy, the prescriber (a physician or endocrinologist in most hospitals) would select from the prewritten types of insulin and write the amount of units as warranted by the individual patient's condition. An example of an order for insulin for a patient in hospital is indicated on the patient care order set in Figure 18-6. Insulin orders are as follows:

Basal insulin NPH (Novolin ge NPH) 30 units at bedtime and bolus with insulin aspart (NovoRapid) 8 units before breakfast, 7 units before lunch, and 10 units before dinner.

BOX 18-1	ISMP Canada Guidelines for Subcutaneous Insulin Order Sets

- Where possible, include both the brand and generic names for insulin
- If both the brand and generic names can be included, list the brand name first, followed by the generic name in brackets
- Present choices of insulin products organized in the following categories:

Scheduled Insulin
- Basal:
  - Intermediate acting
  - Long acting
- Bolus (mealtime or prandial):
  - Rapid acting
  - Short acting
- Premixed:
  - Rapid- + intermediate-acting analogues
  - Short- + intermediate-acting human insulin

Correction Dose Insulin
- Rapid- or short-acting insulin used to correct hyperglycemia
- Scheduled basal insulin orders:
  - List orders for basal insulin before orders for bolus insulin
  - Require prescribers to indicate whether basal insulin is deliberately omitted
    - Include a reminder to reassess "no standing basal insulin order required" after 24–48 hours
- Schedule bolus insulin orders with any directions to be followed
- Provide parameters and guidance on frequency and timing of insulin doses
- Correction dose insulin:
  - Use only rapid- or short-acting insulin
  - Provide different correction dose insulin algorithms (refer to the sample **Diabetes Management Record** for subcutaneous insulin in Appendix B)
  - Provide an option to order an individualized algorithm
- Consider providing guidelines for when to consult other members on the interprofessional team

Adapted from ISMP Canada (2013). ISMP Canada Guidelines for Subcutaneous Insulin Order Sets (pp. 2–4). Retrieved from http://www.ismp-canada.org/download/insulin/ISMP_Guidelines_SC_InsulinOrderSets.pdf. Reprinted with permission from ISMP Canada.

*Administer insulin aspart subcutaneously **in addition** to scheduled insulin dose to correct hyperglycemia premeal.*

According to the patient blood glucose, extra rapid acting insulin may be administered according to the **correction dose insulin algorithm** section of Figure 18-6. For example, if this patient's blood glucose before breakfast is 8.4 millimoles per litre (mmol/L), then the nurse should administer an extra unit of insulin aspart along with the prescribed 8 units. In this case, the patient should receive a total of 9 units of insulin aspart before breakfast. Correction insulin is discussed later is this chapter. Remember that orders may be individualized based on patient medical presentation and history. For the majority of noncritically ill patients in hospital who are treated with insulin, the premeal glucose target should be less than 7.8 millimoles (mmol) per litre (L), and the random glucose target should be less than 10.0 mmol per L (CDA Clinical Practice Guidelines Expert Committee, 2013). The aim of treatment is to meet individual targets without recurrent hypoglycemia.

> **SAFETY ALERT!**
>
> If correction dose insulin is required at bedtime, the current practice is to give half (50%) of the premeal correction dose to lower the risk of nocturnal hypoglycemia.

Correction Insulin

When the recommended blood glucose targets are not met by basal-bolus subcutaneous insulin at home or in hospital, patients may receive a correctional dose to lower blood glucose. This concept and practice has now replaced the previous treatment option called *sliding scale insulin*.

Adult Subcutaneous Insulin Order Set				
Monitor Blood Glucose (BG) before breakfast, before lunch, before dinner, at bedtime (2200) & prn				
	Before Breakfast	**Before Lunch**	**Before Dinner**	**Bedtime (2200)**
Bolus Insulin: ☑ insulin aspart ☐ insulin lispro ☐ insulin Regular	Administer ____8____units SUBCUT	Administer ____7____units SUBCUT	Administer ____10____units SUBCUT	
Basal Insulin: ☑ insulin NPH ☐ insulin detemir ☐ insulin glargine	Administer _____units SUBCUT		Administer _____units SUBCUT	Administer ____30____units SUBCUT
Supplemental (Correction) Dose Insulin Algorithm	Administer according to Supplemental (correction) dose algorithm: ☑ Insulin aspart **OR** insulin lispro SUBCUT TID before meals Do **NOT** use Supplemental insulin scale for blood glucose taken at bedtime Notify physician if bedtime BG is greater than 19 mmol/L **OR** ☐ Insulin aspart **OR** insulin lispro SUBCUT _____(frequency)			

Capillary Blood Glucose (mmol/L)	Supplemental Insulin Dose (Give along with routine bolus pre-meal insulin above)
Less than 4	Follow protocol for treatment of hyoglycemia
____4__to__6__	____0___units SUBCUT
__6.1__to__8__	__0.5___units SUBCUT
__8.1__to__10__	____1___units SUBCUT
__10.1__to__12__	____2___units SUBCUT
__12.1__to__14__	____3___units SUBCUT
__14.1__to__16__	____5___units SUBCUT
__16.1__to__19__	____8___units SUBCUT
Greater than 19	Notify Physician

Printed Name of Prescriber	Signature, Designation	License #	Date YYYY/MM/DD	Time
Samuel Richardson	Samuel Richardson, MD	83-67890	2015/04/11	1800

Figure 18-6 Sample Adult Subcutaneous Insulin Order Set.

The 2013 CDA CPG discourage the use of sliding scale insulin, which is the administration of rapid- or short-acting insulin alone without basal insulin and only if blood glucose is above a certain level. Research has revealed that this reactive practice has been linked with not only worse glycemic results but also poor clinical outcomes for people with diabetes. By contrast, a supplemental (correction) insulin dose, in addition to scheduled basal +/− bolus insulin is recommended (Miller et al., 2014, p. 4).

The basal insulin component uses longer-acting insulin analogues to control the fasting blood glucose (FBG) level, and the nutritional component uses rapid- or short-acting insulin to cover nutritional intake and correct hyperglycemia. The basal plus rapid- or short-acting insulin is referred to as *basal-bolus insulin therapy,* which closely approximates normal physiological insulin production and controls hyperglycemia. The correction dose is determined by the patient's insulin sensitivity and current blood glucose level.

Box 18-2 provides another example of a correction dose insulin algorithm and a graph from the 2013 CDA CPG. The y axis of the graph reflects a patient's blood glucose (BG) and the x axis reflects mealtimes.

For this patient example, blood glucose before breakfast and lunch is 6 mmol per L, and therefore no supplemental insulin is required according to the correction dose algorithm. However, at dinner, along with routine bolus of 6 units, 2 extra units of bolus insulin are required because blood glucose increased to 12 mmol per L, which falls within the 10.1 to 13 mmol per L range shown. At bedtime, the patient receives only basal insulin of 18 units as prescribed.

It is important that nurses understand that patients with type 2 diabetes whose blood glucose remains in target range on their oral antihyperglycemic medication(s) may be

BOX 18-2 Sample Basal + Bolus + Correction

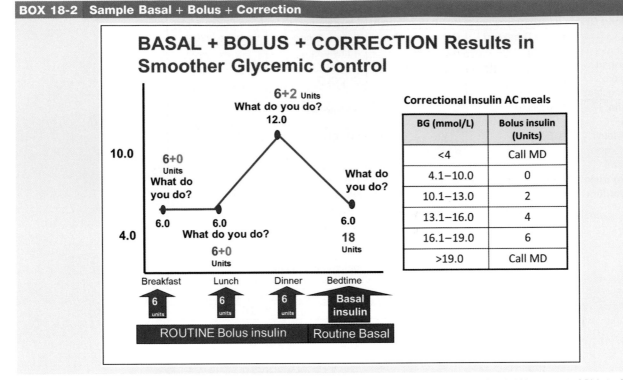

Reprinted from *Canadian Journal of Diabetes*, 37/S1, Robyn Houlden, Sara Capes, Maureen Clement, David Miller, "In-hospital Management of Diabetes," S77–S81, Copyright 2013, with permission from Elsevier.
BG, blood glucose; *L*, litre; *MD*, medical doctor; *mmol*, millimole.

prescribed correction insulin algorithm alone. As long as their oral medication remains effective in keeping their blood glucose within target, basal-bolus insulin may not be required. For most people with diabetes who require insulin, the basal-bolus insulin therapy is a regimen that has proven to be optimal for achieving glycemic control in patients with diabetes.

> ### *i* TIPS FOR **CLINICAL PRACTICE**
>
> Nurses must understand and practise according to hospital protocol. When a patient's condition changes, insulin requirements may also change and the physician as well as others on the interprofessional team should be informed accordingly.

Preparing a Single Dose of Insulin in an Insulin Syringe

Measuring insulin in an insulin syringe is different from measuring most other injectable medications. There is no calculation or conversion required because the syringe measures units of insulin, rather than volume of solution. An order that includes the components of a medication order must be written as described in Chapter 9.

Frequent errors have occurred with insulin doses. As a result, special attention should be used when preparing doses of insulin. Insulin dosage errors can be avoided by following two important rules to ensure safe administration of insulin.

> ### → RULE
>
> **Avoiding Insulin Dosage Errors**
> 1. Insulin doses **MUST** be checked by two nurses. To be considered an independent verification, the check by the second nurse must occur independently away from the first nurse, with no prior knowledge of the calculations used to verify the dosage.
> 2. In the preparation of combination dosages (two insulins), two nurses must verify each step of the process.

The examples that follow and the Practice Problems and Chapter Review problems are intended to help you practise preparing a dose of insulin in an insulin syringe. The orders are for practice purposes only and do not reflect the current guidelines discussed in this chapter. Review Appendix C for current guidelines regarding possible orders. The examples and problems are based on U-100 (100 units per mL) insulin. All preparations of insulin will use a U-100 syringe, which may be Lo-Dose or the standard syringe. The standard syringe is used in most institutions.

Example: Order: Insulin Humulin R 40 units SUBCUT in AM $\frac{1}{2}$ hour before breakfast.

Available: Humulin R

To measure 40 units, withdraw insulin to the 40 mark on the syringe. A Lo-Dose syringe can also be used to draw up this dose, as the following syringe shows.

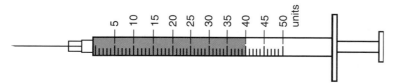

Example: Order: Insulin Humulin N 70 units SUBCUT daily at 7:30 AM.

Available: Humulin N

Draw up the ordered amount in a standard insulin syringe.

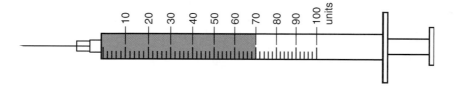

Example: Order: Insulin Humulin R 5 units SUBCUT stat.

Available: Humulin R

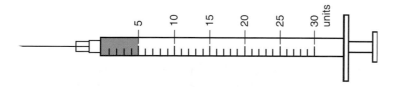

Measuring Two Types of Insulin in the Same Syringe

Sometimes individuals may require two different types of insulin for control of their blood glucose levels, for example, NPH and regular insulin. To reduce the number of injections, it is common to mix two insulins in a single syringe. The need to mix insulin has decreased due to the availability of a variety of premixed combinations. However, not all patients can achieved glycemic control with premixes. To mix insulin in one syringe, remember the rule that follows.

Drawing up rapid- or short-acting insulin first prevents contamination of the clear insulin with the intermediate (cloudy) insulin. This sequence is extremely important.

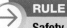

> **RULE**
>
> **Safety When Combining Two Insulins in Same Syringe**
>
> Draw up clear insulin first, and then draw up cloudy insulin. Rapid- and short-acting insulins are clear (regular, aspart, lispro). Intermediate-acting insulins (NPH) are cloudy.
>
> THINK: First rapid-acting or short-acting insulin, then intermediate-acting insulin.
>
> THINK: The insulin that acts **first** is drawn up **first.**

To prepare insulin in one syringe (mixing insulin), complete the following steps (Figures 18-7 and 18-8):

1. Cleanse the tops of both vials with an alcohol wipe.
2. Inject air equal to the amount being withdrawn into the vial of cloudy insulin first. When the air is injected, the tip of the needle should not touch the solution.
3. Remove the needle from the vial of cloudy insulin.
4. Using the same syringe, inject an amount of air into the regular insulin (clear) equal to the amount to be withdrawn, invert or turn the bottle up in the air, and draw up the desired amount.
5. Remove the syringe from the regular insulin, and check for air bubbles. If air bubbles are present, gently tap the syringe to remove them.
6. Next withdraw the desired dosage from the vial of cloudy insulin.
7. The total number of units in the syringe will be the sum of the two insulin orders.

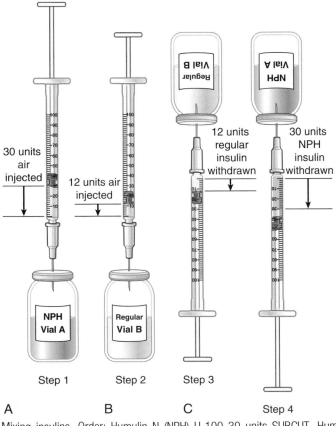

Figure 18-7 Mixing insulins. Order: Humulin N (NPH) U-100 30 units SUBCUT, Humulin R (Regular) U-100, 12 units SUBCUT. **A,** Inject 30 units of air into Humulin N (NPH) first; do not allow needle to touch insulin. **B,** Inject 12 units of air into Humulin R (Regular). **C,** Withdraw 12 units of Humulin R; withdraw needle. Insert needle into vial of Humulin N and withdraw 30 units. Total 30 units Humulin N (NPH) + 12 units Humulin R (Regular) = 42 units. (Modified from Harkreader, H., & Hogan, M. A. (2007). *Fundamentals of nursing: Caring and clinical judgment* (3rd ed.). St. Louis: Saunders.)

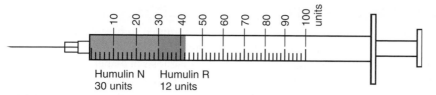

Humulin N
30 units

Humulin R
12 units

Figure 18-8 Total of two insulins combined. Total = 42 units (30 units Humulin NPH + 12 units Humulin R).

⚠ SAFETY ALERT!

DO NOT combine long-acting basal insulin analogues or dilute them with any other insulin preparation. The effects can be life threatening.

ⓘ TIPS FOR CLINICAL PRACTICE

- Cloudy insulin should be rolled gently between the palms of the hands to mix it before it is drawn up. **Do not** shake insulin. Shaking creates bubbles in addition to breaking down the particles and causing clumping.
- Insulins mix instantly; they do not remain separated. Therefore, insulin that has been overdrawn cannot be returned to the vial. You must discard the entire medication and start over.

Example: Order: 18 units of regular insulin and 22 units of NPH SUBCUT.

The total amount of insulin is 40 units (18 units [regular] + 22 units [NPH] = 40 units).

To administer this dose, a Lo-Dose syringe or a U-100 (1-mL) syringe can be used. However, because the dose is 40 units, the Lo-Dose would be more desirable. (See the syringes that follow, illustrating this dosage.) Note that most institutions do not carry Lo-Dose syringes on adult units. Use the syringe that is available to you as long as it is safe to do so.

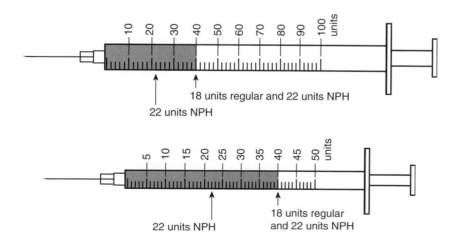

18 units regular and 22 units NPH

22 units NPH

22 units NPH

18 units regular and 22 units NPH

ⓘ TIPS FOR CLINICAL PRACTICE

When mixing insulins, follow the steps outlined. Committing one of the following phrases to memory may help you remember the steps: (1) last injected is **first** drawn up; (2) run fast first (regular), then slow down (NPH); (3) clear to cloudy; or (4) clear, cloudy (in alphabetical order). Also remember, when mixing insulins, only the same type should be mixed together, for example, Humulin R and Humulin NPH.

Intravenous Insulin

Most patients with diabetes of any type who are admitted to hospital can be treated successfully with subcutaneous insulin. However, some patients will require IV insulin therapy. These include patients who are critically ill with a diagnosis of diabetic ketoacidosis (DKA), hyperosmolar hyperglycemic state (HHS), myocardial infarction (MI), or acute coronary syndrome (ACS). Patients with diabetes who are undergoing a surgical procedure and others who are unable to eat may also require IV insulin to control hyperglycemia (Miller et al., 2014, p. 2). Some critically ill patients who require IV insulin may not have had pre-existing diabetes but presented with hyperglycemia with their current illness.

The 2013 CDA CPG recommend that hospitals develop IV insulin clinical order sets that are specific to different categories of illness. For example, patients with DKA in intensive care would have a different insulin clinical order set than adult patients in an acute medical unit. Blood glucose targets for patients with different categories of illness are not the same. For example, the blood glucose target for a noncritically ill patient is about 5 to 10 mmol per L. By contrast, the target for a critically ill patient on insulin infusion is between 7.8 and 10 mmol per L. A starting insulin infusion rate is calculated based on current blood glucose, patient weight, or a patient's previous subcutaneous insulin requirements (if applicable).

Table 18-2 presents a maintenance insulin IV infusion clinical order set for an adult inpatient in acute care. The IV insulin requirement is calculated based on the patient's weight. The physician completes the clinical order set, which includes the frequency of bedside blood glucose monitoring (BBGM), the starting insulin dose, and the maintenance infusion based on responding blood glucose levels.

Calculating an Intravenous Insulin Infusion

Calculating an IV insulin infusion is similar to calculating a heparin infusion in units per hour and millilitres per hour. All methods used previously for calculating oral and parenteral medications may be used for IV insulin rates: the ratio and proportion method, the formula method, and the dimensional analysis method.

Let's use this patient profile and Table 18-2 to calculate IV insulin drip adjustments in the example that follows:

A 23-year-old patient with type 1 diabetes was admitted to hospital due to bronchial pneumonia. The IV insulin requirement is calculated based on the patient's weight of 55 kg.

TABLE 18-2 Sample Maintenance Insulin Intravenous Infusion Clinical Order Set for Adult Inpatient Care

Adjustment based on current and previous glucose values as follows:

Current Value Bedside Blood Glucose (mmol/L)	Increase in Glucose Current Value Higher Than Previous	Small Decrease in Glucose Current Value Lower Than Previous by Less Than 3 mmol/L	Moderate to Large Decrease in Glucose Current Value Lower Than Previous by 3 mmol/L or Greater
<4	Stop infusion, treat per hospital hypoglycemia protocol. Repeat blood glucose monitoring in 20 minutes, Resume infusion at 50% of previous rate once blood glucose greater than 5 mmol/L		
4–5.9	Reduce rate by 1 unit/h	Reduce rate by 1 unit/h	Reduce rate by 50%
6–10 (target)	No change in rate	No change	Reduce rate by 50%
10.1–12	Increase rate by 0.5 unit/h	Increase rate by 0.5 unit/h	Reduce rate by 1unit/h
12.1–15	Increase rate by 1 unit/h	Increase rate by 1 unit/h	No change in rate
15.1–18	Increase rate by 2 unit/h	Increase rate by 2 unit/h	No change in rate
>18	Increase rate by 3 unit/h Notify physician ordering insulin	Increase rate by 3 unit/h	No change in rate

Signature, Designation:	College Licence#	Date:	Time:

Millar et al. (2013). Blood glucose lowering working group, CPG Dissemination & Implementation Committee. In-hospital Management of Diabetes: Clinical Order Sets. Retrieved from http://guidelines.diabetes.ca/CDACPG_resources/Summary_In-hospital_mgmt_of_diabetes_FINAL_July_8-2014.pdf. Reproduced with permission by the Canadian Diabetes Association. April 2016.

h, hour; *L*, litre; *mmol*, millimole.

Example: Order: Mix 50 units regular human insulin (Humulin R) in 250 mL 0.9% sodium chloride for 0.2 units/mL. Initiate the IV insulin infusion at 0.1 units/kg/h.

1. What is the initial insulin IV infusion rate in units per hour? The frequency of BBGM is between q20min and q4h, depending on the results. The patient profile indicates that weight is 55 kg. Blood glucose is currently 14 .5 mmol per L.

Answer: 0.1 unit per kg per hour = 0.1 unit × 55 kg = 5.5 units per hour = initial infusion rate.

2. The patient's blood glucose was 13.3 mmol per L 2 hours post infusion. What should the nurse do according to the protocol in Table 18-2?

Answer: The patient's blood glucose is 13.3 mmol per L now. It was 14.5 mmol per L before. According to the protocol in Table 18-2, it is a small decrease (less than 3 mmol per L) and falls between the range of 12.1 to 15 mmol per L. Therefore, the nurse should increase the infusion rate by 1 unit per hour.

3. What is the new infusion rate in units per hour?

Answer: The new infusion rate is 5.5 unit per hour + 1 unit per hour = 6.5 unit per hour.

4. What rate in millilitres per hour will the nurse program the infusion pump to deliver the new rate of 6.5 units per hour?

✔ PROBLEM SETUP

✔ Solution Using Ratio and Proportion

We know that the insulin concentration is 50 units in 250 mL of normal saline (NS). Set up the equation with what is known on the left:

$$50 \, \text{units} : 250 \, \text{mL} = 6.5 \, \text{units} : x$$

$$50x = 1625$$

$$x = \frac{1625}{50} = 32.5 \, \text{mL}$$

✔ Solution Using the Formula Method

$$\frac{6.5 \, \text{units}}{50 \, \text{units}} \times 250 \, \text{mL} = 32.5 \, \text{mL}$$

Because insulin is a high-alert medication, it should be set up on a pump that has decimal calibration to the tenth of a millilitre, so answers may be rounded to the nearest tenth. Delivering an incorrect dosage of insulin in even small increments of 0.5 mL can have a significant impact on a patient's blood glucose. Again, it is important for the nurse to know the policy of the hospital regarding insulin infusion. Be sure to follow protocol.

Hypoglycemia

Insulin administration cannot be discussed without addressing hypoglycemia. In fact, the most common adverse effect of insulin therapy is hypoglycemia, otherwise known as low blood glucose. According to the 2013 CDA CPG, hypoglycemia is "the development of autonomic or neuroglycopenic symptoms, a low plasma glucose level" of less than 4 mmol per L and "symptoms responding to the administration of carbohydrate" (CDA Clinical Practice Guidelines Expert Committee, 2013, p. S69). Hypoglycemia caused by insulin and other insulin secretagogues (e.g., sulfonylureas) is a major challenge for people with diabetes.

The aim of diabetes management is to achieve positive patient outcomes without increasing the risk of hypoglycemia. The risk of hypoglycemia for all patients who take antihyperglycemic medications must be anticipated and monitored, and any resulting hypoglycemia must be treated immediately. All clinical order sets for insulin (SUBCUT and IV) must include a protocol for the management of hypoglycemia. Recurrent hypoglycemia, even mild episodes, can negatively impact the quality of life of people who have diabetes.

POINTS TO REMEMBER

- Note that when insulins are mixed, regular insulin (clear) is always drawn up first, then cloudy.
- Do not shake insulin. Roll the insulin gently between the palms of the hands to mix.
- Read insulin labels to ensure that you have the correct type of insulin to avoid medication errors. Only mix the same types of insulin (e.g., Humulin R and Humulin N).
- Write insulin orders with "units" spelled out. Do not use the abbreviations "U," "IU," or "u."
- Do not mix long-acting basal insulin analogues with any other insulin or dilute with any other insulin preparation.
- Avoid insulin dosage errors; always obtain an independent verification by a second nurse.
- Note that current evidence supports basal-prandial insulin therapy, which improves patient outcomes and is an optimal strategy for achieving glycemic control in patients who have diabetes.
- When administering insulin IV, use only regular insulin (as recommended by the 2013 CDA CPG).
- Follow institution clinical order sets for SUBCUT and IV insulin administration.
- Know the hypoglycemia management protocol and treat patients accordingly.
- Include in all insulin orders an algorithm for some form of basal-bolus regimen as well as a correction insulin dose.
- Avoid using sliding scale insulin alone to treat hyperglycemia.

PRACTICE **PROBLEMS**

16. A patient who has type 1 diabetes was admitted to the emergency department with abdominal pain. She weighs 76 kg. The emergency physician used her total daily SUBCUT insulin dose from home as well as her weight and BG, which is 17.6 mmol per L to decide on the initial insulin infusion concentration.

    Order: Mix 100 units insulin regular (Novolin ge Toronto) in 100 mL NS (1 unit per mL). Start the insulin infusion at a rate of 0.1 unit/kg/h. Check BG q1h–q4h according to protocol and make insulin adjustment according to schedule.

    For this Practice Problem use Table 18-2 for direction on insulin adjustment based on the blood glucose values provided.
    a. What is the initial insulin infusion dose according to the patient's weight? Round answers to the nearest tenth for increased accuracy.
    b. Four hours after the infusion started, the patient's BG is 14.2 mmol per L. What should the nurse do?
    c. What is the mL per hour for the rate on 7.6 units per hour?

17. A patient has type 1 diabetes and is on a SUBCUT basal-bolus insulin regimen of rapid-acting insulin analogue before meals and long-acting basal insulin analogue at bedtime. Doses of rapid-acting insulin analogue are 8 units, 6 units, and 12 units before breakfast, lunch, and dinner, respectively. Long-acting basal insulin analogue is 29

units at bedtime. In addition, a correction scale is implemented for supplemental rapid-acting insulin analogue as follows:

BG (mmol/L)	Bolus Insulin (units)
less than 4	Call MD
4.1–10	0
10.1–13	2
13.1–16	4
16.1–19	6
greater than 19	Call MD

If the patient's BG is 10.5 mmol per L before lunch, what is the total amount of rapid-acting insulin analogue that should be administered at that time?

 CLINICAL **REASONING**

1. **Scenario:** The prescriber wrote the following insulin order:
   Humulin U-100 10 0 SUBCUT ac breakfast.
   The nurse assumed that the order was for regular insulin 100 units and administered the insulin to the patient. Later, it was discovered the insulin dose desired was insulin NPH 10 units.

   a. What error occurred here? _____

   b. What patient medication rights were violated? _____

   c. What is the potential outcome of the error? _____

   d. What measures could have been taken to prevent the error that

   occurred? _____

2. **Scenario:** A patient is to receive Humulin R 10 units SUBCUT and Humulin N 14 units SUBCUT before breakfast. In drawing up the insulins in the same syringe, the nurse used the following technique:
   - Injected 10 units of air into the regular vial.
   - Injected 14 units of air into the NPH vial.
   - Withdrew 14 units of Insulin NPH, then the 10 units of regular insulin.
     a. What is the error in the technique of drawing up the two insulins?

     _____

     b. What is the potential outcome from the technique used? _____

Answers on pages 505–506.

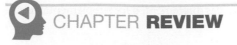

CHAPTER **REVIEW**

Using the labels or the information provided, indicate the dosage you would prepare and shade it in on the syringe provided.

1. Order: Novolin ge Toronto 35 units SUBCUT daily at 0730.

   Available:

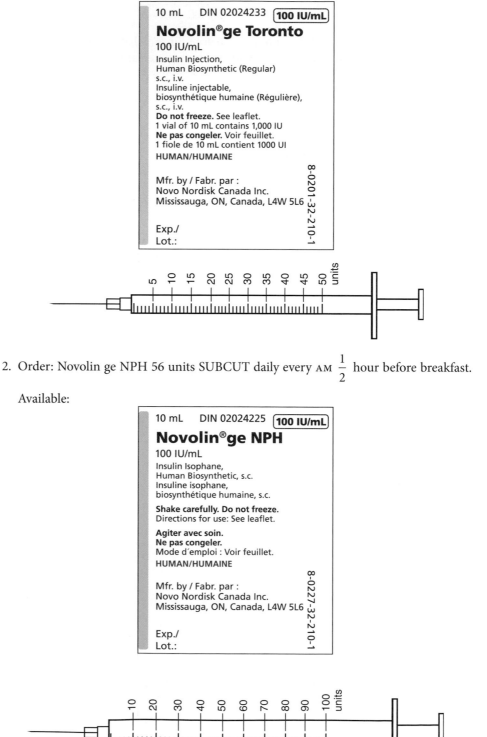

10 mL   DIN 02024233   **100 IU/mL**

Novolin®ge Toronto

100 IU/mL

Insulin Injection,
Human Biosynthetic (Regular)
s.c., i.v.
Insuline injectable,
biosynthétique humaine (Régulière),
s.c., i.v.
Do not freeze. See leaflet.
1 vial of 10 mL contains 1,000 IU
Ne pas congeler. Voir feuillet.
1 fiole de 10 mL contient 1000 UI
HUMAN/HUMAINE

Mfr. by / Fabr. par :
Novo Nordisk Canada Inc.
Mississauga, ON, Canada, L4W 5L6

8-0201-32-210-1

Exp./
Lot.:

2. Order: Novolin ge NPH 56 units SUBCUT daily every AM $\frac{1}{2}$ hour before breakfast.

   Available:

10 mL   DIN 02024225   **100 IU/mL**

Novolin®ge NPH

100 IU/mL

Insulin Isophane,
Human Biosynthetic, s.c.
Insuline isophane,
biosynthétique humaine, s.c.

Shake carefully. Do not freeze.
Directions for use: See leaflet.

Agiter avec soin.
Ne pas congeler.
Mode d´emploi : Voir feuillet.
HUMAN/HUMAINE

Mfr. by / Fabr. par :
Novo Nordisk Canada Inc.
Mississauga, ON, Canada, L4W 5L6

8-0227-32-210-1

Exp./
Lot.:

3. Order: Novolin ge Toronto 18 units SUBCUT and Novolin ge NPH 40 units SUBCUT daily at 0730.

   Available:

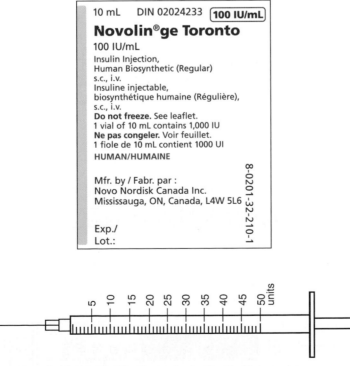

10 mL DIN 02024233 [100 IU/mL]	10 mL DIN 02024225 [100 IU/mL]
Novolin®ge Toronto 100 IU/mL Insulin Injection, Human Biosynthetic (Regular) s.c., i.v. Insuline injectable, biosynthétique humaine (Régulière), s.c., i.v. **Do not freeze.** See leaflet. 1 vial of 10 mL contains 1,000 IU **Ne pas congeler.** Voir feuillet. 1 fiole de 10 mL contient 1000 UI HUMAN/HUMAINE Mfr. by / Fabr. par : Novo Nordisk Canada Inc. Mississauga, ON, Canada, L4W 5L6 Exp./ Lot.:	**Novolin®ge NPH** 100 IU/mL Insulin Isophane, Human Biosynthetic, s.c. Insuline isophane, biosynthétique humaine, s.c. **Shake carefully. Do not freeze.** Directions for use: See leaflet. **Agiter avec soin.** **Ne pas congeler.** Mode d'emploi : Voir feuillet. HUMAN/HUMAINE Mfr. by / Fabr. par : Novo Nordisk Canada Inc. Mississauga, ON, Canada, L4W 5L6 Exp./ Lot.:

4. Order: Novolin ge Toronto 9 units SUBCUT daily.

   Available:

10 mL   DIN 02024233 [100 IU/mL]
Novolin®ge Toronto 100 IU/mL Insulin Injection, Human Biosynthetic (Regular) s.c., i.v. Insuline injectable, biosynthétique humaine (Régulière), s.c., i.v. **Do not freeze.** See leaflet. 1 vial of 10 mL contains 1,000 IU **Ne pas congeler.** Voir feuillet. 1 fiole de 10 mL contient 1000 UI HUMAN/HUMAINE Mfr. by / Fabr. par : Novo Nordisk Canada Inc. Mississauga, ON, Canada, L4W 5L6 Exp./ Lot.:

Indicate the number of units measured in the following syringes.

5. Units measured: _____

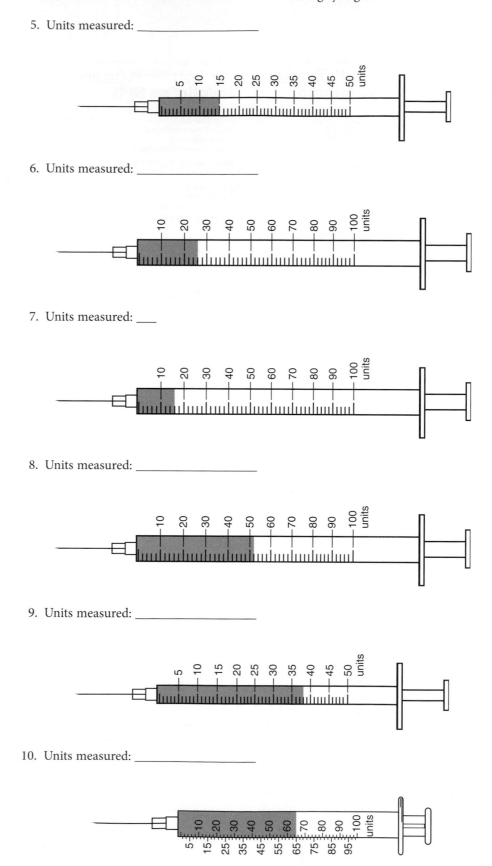

6. Units measured: _____

7. Units measured: ____

8. Units measured: _____

9. Units measured: _____

10. Units measured: _____

11. Units measured: _____

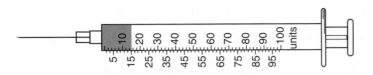

Calculate the dosage of insulin where necessary, and shade in the dosage on the syringe provided. Labels have been included with some problems.

12. Order: Humulin R 10 units SUBCUT at 0730.

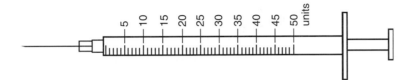

13. Order: Humulin R 16 units SUBCUT and Humulin N 24 units SUBCUT ac breakfast.

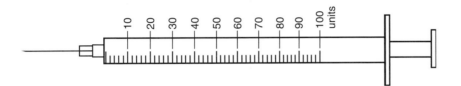

14. Order: Humulin R 10 units SUBCUT and Humulin N 15 units SUBCUT ac breakfast.

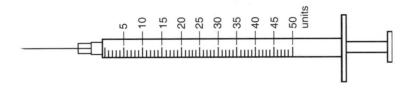

15. Order: Humulin R 5 units SUBCUT and Humulin N 25 units SUBCUT ac breakfast.

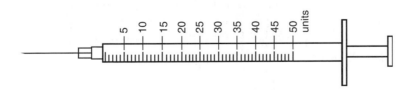

16. Order: Novolin ge Toronto 40 units SUBCUT and Novolin ge NPH 10 units SUBCUT at 0730.

10 mL DIN 02024233	100 IU/mL
Novolin®ge Toronto	
100 IU/mL	
Insulin Injection,	
Human Biosynthetic (Regular)	
s.c., i.v.	
Insuline injectable,	
biosynthétique humaine (Régulière),	
s.c., i.v.	
Do not freeze. See leaflet.	
1 vial of 10 mL contains 1,000 IU	
Ne pas congeler. Voir feuillet.	
1 fiole de 10 mL contient 1000 UI	
HUMAN/HUMAINE	
Mfr. by / Fabr. par :	
Novo Nordisk Canada Inc.	
Mississauga, ON, Canada, L4W 5L6	
Exp./	
Lot.:	

8-0201-32-210-1

10 mL DIN 02024225	100 IU/mL
Novolin®ge NPH	
100 IU/mL	
Insulin Isophane,	
Human Biosynthetic, s.c.	
Insuline isophane,	
biosynthétique humaine, s.c.	
Shake carefully. Do not freeze.	
Directions for use: See leaflet.	
Agiter avec soin.	
Ne pas congeler.	
Mode d'emploi : Voir feuillet.	
HUMAN/HUMAINE	
Mfr. by / Fabr. par :	
Novo Nordisk Canada Inc.	
Mississauga, ON, Canada, L4W 5L6	
Exp./	
Lot.:	

8-0227-32-210-1

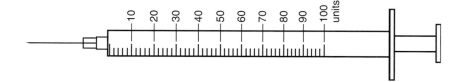

17. Order: Humulin N 48 units SUBCUT and Humulin R 30 units SUBCUT 30 minutes ac breakfast.

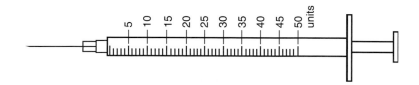

18. Order: Novolin R 16 units SUBCUT and Novolin N 12 units SUBCUT 0730.

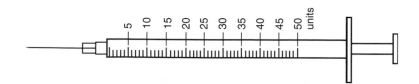

19. Order: Novolin R 17 units SUBCUT 1700.

20. Order: Insulin lispro 15 units SUBCUT daily at 0730.

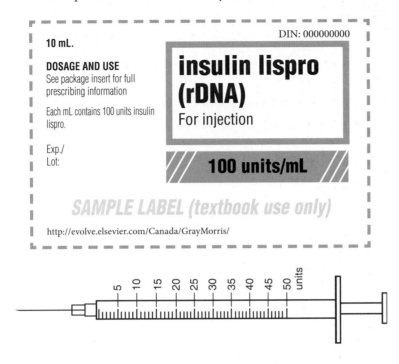

10 mL.

DOSAGE AND USE
See package insert for full
prescribing information

Each mL contains 100 units insulin
lispro.

Exp./
Lot:

DIN: 000000000

**insulin lispro
(rDNA)**
For injection

100 units/mL

SAMPLE LABEL (textbook use only)

http://evolve.elsevier.com/Canada/GrayMorris/

21. Order: Humulin R 26 units SUBCUT and Humulin N 48 units SUBCUT daily.

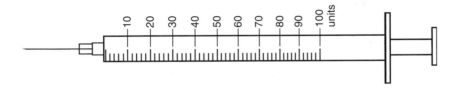

22. Order: Novolin ge 30/70 27 units SUBCUT at 1700.

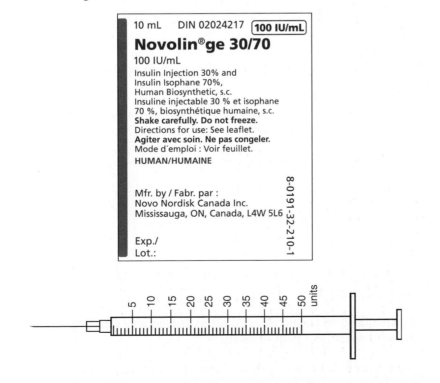

10 mL   DIN 02024217   **100 IU/mL**
Novolin®ge 30/70
100 IU/mL
Insulin Injection 30% and
Insulin Isophane 70%,
Human Biosynthetic, s.c.
Insuline injectable 30 % et isophane
70 %, biosynthétique humaine, s.c.
Shake carefully. Do not freeze.
Directions for use: See leaflet.
Agiter avec soin. Ne pas congeler.
Mode d'emploi : Voir feuillet.
HUMAN/HUMAINE

Mfr. by / Fabr. par :
Novo Nordisk Canada Inc.
Mississauga, ON, Canada, L4W 5L6

8-0191-32-210-1

Exp./
Lot.:

23. Order: Novolin ge Toronto 21 units SUBCUT and Novolin ge NPH 35 units SUBCUT daily at 0730.

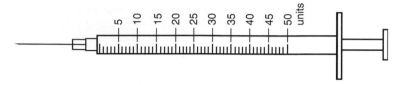

24. Order: Novolin ge Toronto 5 units SUBCUT and Novolin ge NPH 35 units SUBCUT 0730.

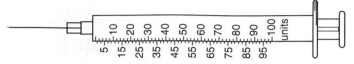

25. Order: NovoRapid 36 units SUBCUT 0730 before breakfast.

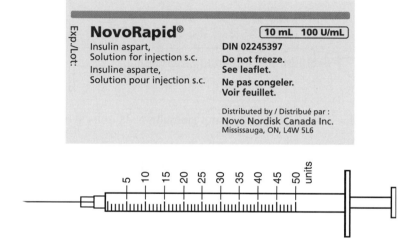

26. A patient is taking a basal-bolus regimen of insulin NPH (Humulin N) 25 units at bedtime and insulin lispro (Humalog) 6 units before breakfast, 5 units before lunch, and 7 units before dinner. The patient also has a correction insulin with insulin lispro scheduled if needed to reach target BG levels. Use the following correction scale to answer the questions. The patient is taking the standard algorithm of 40 to 80 units per day.

If BG <4 mmol/L, Use Hypoglycemia Protocol	Insulin Sensitive <40 Units/Day		Standard 40–80 Units/Day		Insulin Resistant >80 Units/Day	
BBGM (mmol/L)	Meal	Bedtime	Meal	Bedtime	Meal	Bedtime
8–10	0	0	1	0	2	0
10.1–12	1	0	2	0	4	2
12.1–14	2	0	3	2	6	3
14.1–16	2	0	4	2	8	4
greater than 16	3	2	5	3	10	5
greater than 18	Contact physician for orders if BG is greater than 18 mmol/L					

a. How many units of correction insulin are needed if the patient's BG is 13.9 mmol per L before dinner?

b. What is the total amount of rapid-acting insulin analogue needed if the patient's BG is 10 mmol per L before breakfast?

c. What is the total amount of rapid-acting insulin analogue plus intermediate-acting insulin required at bedtime if the patient's BG is 9.7 mmol per L?

27. Order: Humulin N 66 units SUBCUT 2200.

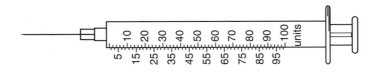

28. Order: Humulin R 32 units SUBCUT every morning at 0730.

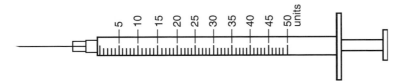

29. Order: Humulin N 35 units SUBCUT daily at 0730.

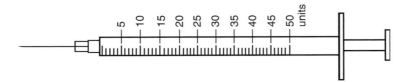

30. Order: Humulin R 9 units SUBCUT 1700.

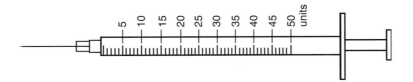

31. Order: Humulin N 24 units SUBCUT 2200.

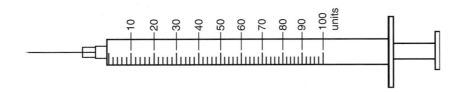

32. Order: Humulin R 8 units SUBCUT, and Humulin N 18 units SUBCUT at 0730.

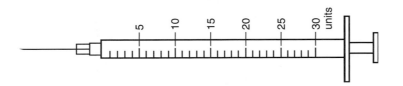

33. Order: Humulin N 11 units SUBCUT at bedtime.

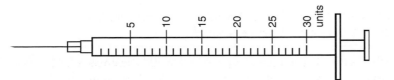

34. Order: Humulin 30/70 20 units SUBCUT $\frac{1}{2}$ hour before breakfast.

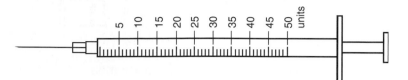

35. Order: Humulin R 10 units SUBCUT and Humulin N 42 units SUBCUT at 1630.

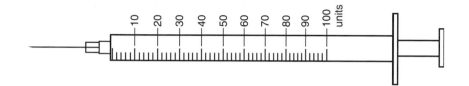

36. Order: Novolin R 8 units SUBCUT and Novolin N 15 units SUBCUT at 0730.

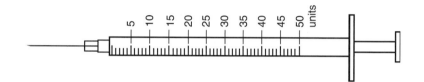

37. Order: Humalog insulin 35 units SUBCUT at 0730.

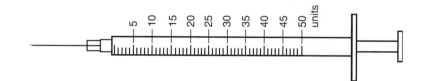

38. Order: Humulin R 30 units SUBCUT and Humulin N 40 units SUBCUT daily at 0800.

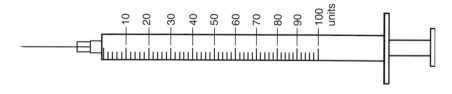

Answers on pages 506–507.

✳ ANSWERS

Answers to Practice Problems

1. Generic name: insulin lispro
   Action time: Rapid acting

2. Trade name: Novolin ge Toronto
   Action time: Short acting

3. Trade name: Lantus
   Action time: Long acting

4. Trade name: Noveolin ge NPH
   Action time: Intermediate acting

5. 22 units

6. 41 units

7.

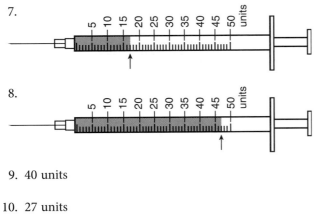

8.

9. 40 units

10. 27 units

11. 64 units

12. 14 units

13.

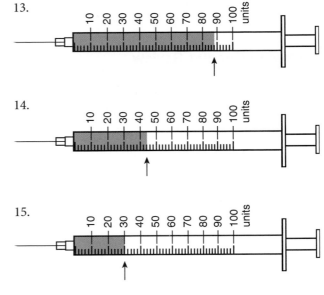

14.

15.

16. a. The insulin infusion rate in units per hour is 0.1 unit per kg per hour × 76 kg = 7.6 units per hour.
    b. The BG has dropped from 17.6 mmol per L to 14.2 mmol per L, a decrease of 3.4 mmol per L. According to Table 18-2, no change is necessary. The infusion rate remains at 7.6 units per hour.
    c. $\dfrac{7.6 \text{ units}}{100 \text{ units}} \times 100 \text{ mL} = 7.6 \text{ mL/h}$

17. The patient receives routine rapid-acting insulin analogue of 6 units before lunch. A correction dose of 2 units is added for a BG reading of 10.5, according to the supplemental schedule.
    6 units + 2 correction units = 8 units in total.

Answers to Clinical Reasoning Questions

1. a. Failure to clarify an insulin order when the type of insulin was not specified and the dosage was not clear because "U" was used for units. The almost closed "U" caused it to be mistaken for "0."
   b. The right medication, the right dose.
   c. The patient received 10 times the dose of an insulin (regular) that was not ordered. Regular insulin is short acting, and NPH is intermediate acting and was desired. Administering the insulin would likely cause a dangerously low glucose level (hypoglycemia). Results could be tremors, confusion, sweating, and death. This incident constitutes malpractice.
   d. The error could have been prevented by remembering that all the essential components of an insulin order should have been in the order (name of insulin, number of units to be administered, route, frequency, and strength). When one element is missing, never assume. The order should have been clarified with the prescriber. Further, the dosage should have been double-checked with another nurse. In addition, units should have been written out in the order to avoid misinterpretation of "U" as a zero. Many insulin errors occur when the nurse fails to clarify an incomplete order or misinterprets the dosage when *units* is abbreviated.

2. a. The nurse should have injected the 14 units of air into the NPH vial and then injected 10 units of air into the regular vial and drawn up the 10 units of regular insulin first. First regular, then NPH. Another nurse should have been present during the mixing and to verify the dosage drawn.

b. Contamination of insulins. Regular (short-acting) insulin is drawn up first to prevent it from becoming contaminated with intermediate-acting insulin. Reversing the order in which the doses of the two insulins are drawn up can also result in incorrect insulin doses.

Answers to Chapter Review

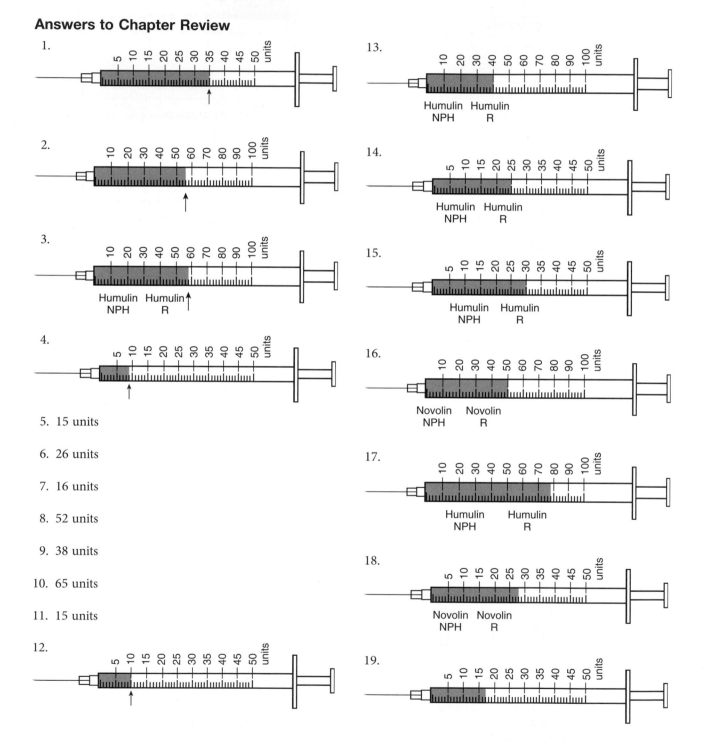

1.

2.

3.

4.

5. 15 units

6. 26 units

7. 16 units

8. 52 units

9. 38 units

10. 65 units

11. 15 units

12.

13.

14.

15.

16.

17.

18.

19.

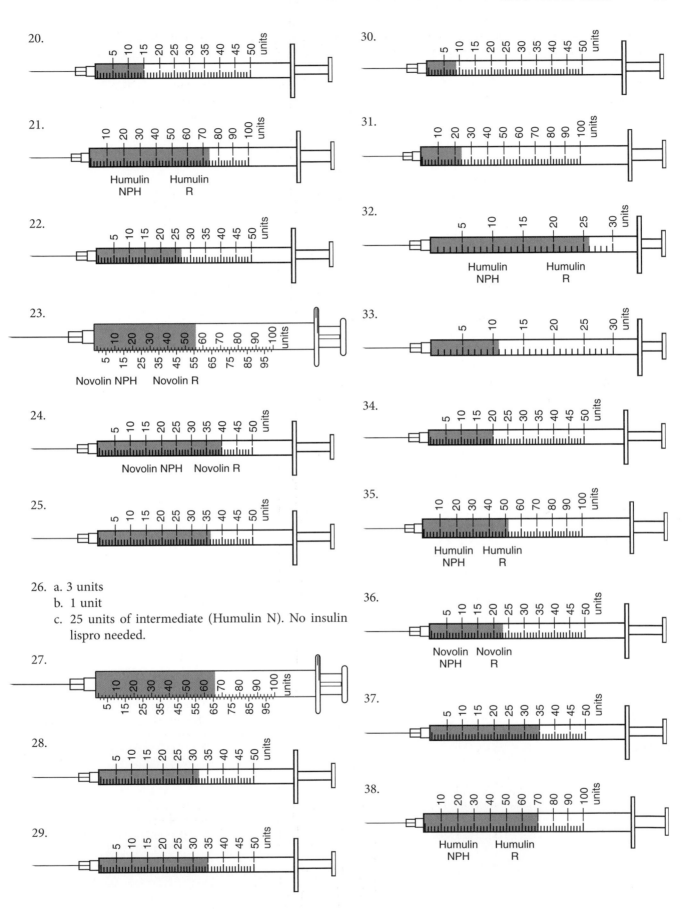

20.

21. Humulin   Humulin
    NPH   R

22.

23. Novolin NPH   Novolin R

24. Novolin NPH   Novolin R

25.

26. a. 3 units
    b. 1 unit
    c. 25 units of intermediate (Humulin N). No insulin
    lispro needed.

27.

28.

29.

30.

31.

32. Humulin   Humulin
    NPH   R

33.

34.

35. Humulin   Humulin
    NPH   R

36. Novolin   Novolin
    NPH   R

37.

38. Humulin   Humulin
    NPH   R

Intravenous and Heparin Calculations, Pediatric Dosage Calculations, and Critical Care Calculations

The ability to accurately calculate intravenous flow rates is essential to the safe administration of intravenous medications to patients.

CHAPTER **19**
Intravenous Solutions and Equipment

Objectives

After reviewing this chapter, you should be able to:

1. Identify common intravenous (IV) solutions and their abbreviations
2. Define the following terms associated with IV therapy: *peripheral line, central line, primary line, secondary line, IV piggyback, saline and heparin locks, IV push,* and *IV bolus*
3. Identify best practices to prevent IV administration errors and ensure patient safety
4. Differentiate among various devices used to administer IV solutions (e.g., volumetric pumps, syringe pumps, patient-controlled analgesia pumps)
5. Describe how technology related to IV therapy can enhance patient safety

A general discussion of intravenous therapy will make it easier to understand the calculations associated with intravenous (IV) therapy that will be discussed in Chapter 20. *Intravenous* refers to the administration of fluids, nutrients, or medications through a vein. Medications, electrolyte solutions, blood, and blood products are frequently ordered and administered directly into the vein. The reasons for the administration of IV fluids are varied. Fluids administered directly into the bloodstream have a rapid effect that is necessary during emergencies or other critical care situations when medications are needed. The advantage of administering medications by this route is the immediate availability of the medication to the body and the rapidity of action. However, IV administration of medications can be rapidly fatal to the patient if the incorrect medication or dosage is administered. Numerous medications are available for IV use. Each medication has guidelines relating to its use. Health care providers are responsible for knowing about the medications they administer.

The reasons for ordering IV fluids include the following:

- To restore or maintain fluid and electrolyte balance
- To replace lost fluids
- To act as a medium for administering medications directly into the bloodstream

Maintenance fluids help to sustain normal levels of fluids and electrolytes. They may also be ordered for patients at risk for depletion, such as the patient who is NPO (nothing by mouth). *Replacement* fluids are ordered for a patient who has lost fluids as a result of vomiting, diarrhea, or hemorrhage.

Intravenous Delivery Methods

IV fluids and medications can be administered by continuous and intermittent infusion.

- *Continuous IV infusions* replace or maintain fluids and electrolytes. As the name implies, a continuous infusion is an IV solution that flows continuously until it is changed.

- *Intermittent IV infusions* (e.g., IV piggyback, IV push) are used to administer medications and supplemental fluids. Intermittent peripheral infusion devices, known as saline or heparin locks, are used to maintain venous access without the need for continuous infusion.

> **!** **SAFETY ALERT!**
>
> Nursing responsibility includes administering IV fluids to the right patient at the right rate and monitoring the patient during therapy. Follow the rights of medication administration when administering IV therapy to patients (see Chapter 8).

In IV therapy, nurses calculate infusion rates in drops per minute (gtt/min) or millilitres per hour (mL/h). The calculations necessary for the safe administration of IV fluids will be presented in Chapter 20.

> **!** **SAFETY ALERT!**
>
> If a patient receives an IV infusion too rapidly and is not monitored closely, reactions can vary from mild to severe.

Intravenous Solutions

There are several types of IV solutions. The type of solution used is individualized according to the patient and the reason for its use. IV solutions come prepared in plastic bags or glass bottles, and they range in volume from 50 mL (bags only) to 1 000 mL. IV plastic bags are most commonly used. IV solutions are clearly labelled with the exact components and amount of solution. When IV solutions are written in orders and charts, abbreviations are used. You may encounter various abbreviations: "D" is for dextrose, "W" is for water, "S" is for saline, and "NS" is for normal saline. Ringer's lactate solution (or lactated Ringer's solution), a commonly used electrolyte solution, is abbreviated as "RL" or "LR." Refer to Box 19-1, and learn the common abbreviations for IV solutions. Figures 19-1 to 19-6 show various IV solutions. Abbreviations are often used when health care providers discuss IV solutions. Nurses must know the common IV solution components and the solution concentration strengths represented by such abbreviations.

BOX 19-1 **Abbreviations for Common Intravenous Solutions**	
NS	Normal saline (sodium chloride 0.9%)*
$\frac{1}{2}$ NS	Sodium chloride 0.45%
D5W or 5% D/W	Dextrose 5% in water
$\frac{2}{3} - \frac{1}{3}$ NS	3.3% dextrose and 0.3% sodium chloride ($\frac{2}{3}$ dextrose- $\frac{1}{3}$ NaCl)
D5RL	Dextrose 5% and lactated Ringer (Ringer's lactate)
RL or RLS	Lactated Ringer's solution (electrolytes)
D5NS	Dextrose 5% in sodium chloride
D5 and $\frac{1}{2}$ NS (0.45%)	Dextrose 5% in $\frac{1}{2}$ 0.45% sodium chloride

From Brown, M., & Mulholland, J. (2008). *Drug calculations: Process and problems for clinical practice* (8th ed.). St. Louis: Mosby.
*IV bags are labelled as "sodium chloride" but frequently referred to as "normal saline" or "NS."

Intravenous Solution Components

Intravenous solutions generally contain glucose (dextrose), sodium chloride (NaCl), water, and/or electrolytes. The components of IV solutions are indicated on the label of the IV solution.

Solution Strength

The abbreviation letters indicate the components in the IV solution, and the numbers indicate the solution strength or concentration of the components in the IV solution. The numbers may be written as subscripts: for example, D_5W (dextrose 5% in water).

Normal saline solutions are written with 0.9 and the percent sign (e.g., D_5 0.9% NS). Saline is available in different percentages. *Normal saline* is the common term used for 0.9% sodium chloride. Another common saline IV concentration is 0.45% NaCl, often written as $\frac{1}{2}$ NS (0.45% is half of 0.9%). Other saline solution strengths include 0.33% NaCl, also abbreviated as $\frac{1}{3}$ NS, and 0.225% NaCl, also abbreviated as $\frac{1}{4}$ NS. Some IV orders, therefore, may be written as $\frac{1}{2}$ NS, $\frac{1}{4}$ NS, or $\frac{1}{3}$ NS. IV solutions can contain saline only (see Figure 19-6) or saline mixed with dextrose, which would be indicated with the percentage of dextrose (e.g., D_5 0.9% sodium chloride) (see Figures 19-3 and 19-4).

> **! SAFETY ALERT!**
>
> Pay close attention to the abbreviations used for IV solutions. The letters indicate the solution components, whereas the numbers indicate the solution strength.

Let's examine some IV labels. Recall from Chapter 4 that solutions are ordered in percentage strengths and that the percentage indicates the number of grams (g) per 100 millilitres (mL) of diluent.

- D5W: This abbreviation means dextrose 5% in water, which indicates that each 100 mL of solution contains 5 g of dextrose (Figure 19-1).
- D5RL: This abbreviation means 5% dextrose in Ringer's lactate solution. Ringer's lactate solution contains electrolytes, including potassium chloride (KCl) and calcium chloride (Figure 19-2).
- 5% dextrose and 0.9% sodium chloride: This solution contains 5 g of dextrose and 0.9 g (or 900 mg) of normal saline or NaCl per 100 mL solution (Figure 19-3).
- 5% dextrose and 0.45% sodium chloride: This solution contains 5 g of dextrose and 0.45 g (or 450 mg) of normal saline or NaCl per 100 mL solution (Figure 19-4).
- 20 mEq potassium chloride in 5% dextrose and 0.45% sodium chloride (Figure 19-5): Notice that the solution in this figure contains 5% dextrose and 0.45% sodium chloride like the IV label shown in Figure 19-4, but it also contains 20 milliequivalents (mEq) of potassium chloride (KCl). Potassium chloride is a high-alert medication. Notice that "20 mEq potassium" is written in red on the label. **Do not confuse these two solutions. Always read labels carefully.**
- 0.9% sodium chloride: This solution contains 0.9 g (or 900 mg) of sodium chloride per 100 mL solution (Figure 19-6).

Intravenous Orders

The prescriber is responsible for writing the order. However, administering and monitoring an IV is a nursing responsibility. An IV order (Figure 19-7) **must** specify the following:
- Name of the IV solution
- Name of the medication to be added, if any
- Amount (volume) to be administered
- Time period during which the IV is to infuse

Intravenous Solution Additives

Potassium chloride is a common additive to IV fluids. Potassium chloride is measured in millimoles or milliequivalents. The order is usually written to indicate the amount of millimoles or milliequivalents per litre (1 000 mL) to be added to the IV fluid. In many institutions, IV solutions are available premixed with potassium.

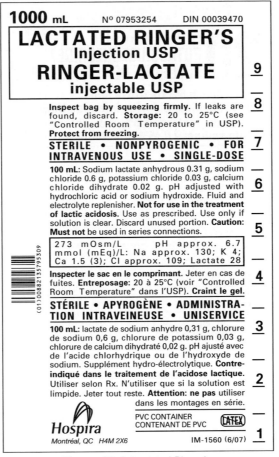

Figure 19-1 5% dextrose (D5W).

LOT   EXP   DIN 000000000   1

5% Dextrose Injection USP   2

1000 mL   3

EACH 100 mL CONTAINS   5 g DEXTROUS HYDROUS   3
USP pH 4.0 (3.2 TO 6.5)   OSMOLARITY 252 mOs-
mol/L (CALC) STERILE NONPYROGENIC   SINGLE
DOSE CONTAINER   ADDITIVES MAY BE INCOMPAT-   4
IBLE   CONSULT WITH PHARMACIST IF AVAILABLE
WHEN INTRODUCING ADDITIVES USE ASEPTIC
TECHNIQUE   MIX THOROUGHLY   DO NOT STORE
DOSAGE   INTRAVENOUSLY AS DIRECTED BY A PHY-   5
SICIAN   SEE DIRECTIONS   CAUTIONS   SQUEEZE AND
INSPECT INNER BAG WHICH MAINTAINS PRODUCT
STERILITY   DISCARD IF LEAKS ARE FOUND   MUST   6
NOT BE USED IN SERIES CONNECTIONS   DO NOT
ADMINISTER SIMULTANEOUSLY WITH BLOOD   DO
NOT USE UNLESS SOLUTION IS CLEAR   FEDERAL
LAW PROHIBITS DISPENSING WITHOUT PRESCRIP-   7
TION   STORE UNIT IN MOISTURE BARRIER OVER-
WRAP AT ROOM TEMPERATURE (25C) UNTIL READY
TO USE   AVOID EXCESSIVE HEAT   SEE INSERT   8

SAMPLE LABEL (textbook use only)

http://evolve.elsevier.com/Canada/GrayMorris/   9

Figure 19-1 5% dextrose (D5W).

LOT   EXP   DIN 000000000   1

5% Dextrose and 0.9% Sodium
Chloride Injection USP   2

1000 mL   3

EACH 100 mL CONTAINS DEXTROUS HYDROUS 5 g;
SODIUM CHLORIDE 900 mg IN WATER FOR INECTION.   4
ELECTROLYTES PER 1000 mL; SODIUM 154 mEq;
CHLORIDE 154 mEq.
560 mOsmol/LITRE (CALC),   5
pH 4.3 (3.5 to 6.5)
ADDITIVES MAY BE INCOMPATIBLE   CONSULT WITH
PHARMACIST, IF AVAILABLE, WHEN INTRODUCING   6
ADDITIVES. USE ASEPTIC TECHNIQUE,   MIX THOR-
OUGHLY   AND DO NOT STORE.   SINGLE DOSE CON-
TAINER. FOR IV USE.   USUAL DOSAGE: SEE INSERT.   7
STERILE, NONPYROGENIC   USE ONLY IF SOLUTION
IS CLEAR AND CONTAINER IS UNDAMAGED. MUST
NOT BE USED IN SERIES CONNECTIONS.   8

SAMPLE LABEL (textbook use only)

http://evolve.elsevier.com/Canada/GrayMorris/   9

Figure 19-3 5% dextrose and 0.9% sodium
chloride (D5NS).

1000 mL   Nº 07953254   DIN 00039470

LACTATED RINGER'S
Injection USP
RINGER-LACTATE
injectable USP   9

Inspect bag by squeezing firmly. If leaks are
found, discard. **Storage:** 20 to 25°C (see
"Controlled Room Temperature" in USP).
Protect from freezing.   8

STERILE • NONPYROGENIC • FOR
INTRAVENOUS USE • SINGLE-DOSE   7

100 mL: Sodium lactate anhydrous 0.31 g, sodium
chloride 0.6 g, potassium chloride 0.03 g, calcium
chloride dihydrate 0.02 g. pH adjusted with   6
hydrochloric acid or sodium hydroxide. Fluid and
electrolyte replenisher. **Not for use in the treatment**
of lactic acidosis. Use as prescribed. Use only if
solution is clear. Discard unused portion. **Caution:**   5
Must not be used in series connections.

273 mOsm/L   pH approx. 6.7
mmol (mEq)/L: Na approx. 130; K 4;
Ca 1.5 (3); Cl approx. 109; Lactate 28

Inspecter le sac en le comprimant. Jeter en cas de
fuites. **Entreposage:** 20 à 25°C (voir "Controlled   4
Room Temperature" dans l'USP). **Craint le gel.**

STÉRILE • APYROGÈNE • ADMINISTRA-
TION INTRAVEINEUSE • UNISERVICE   3

100 mL: lactate de sodium anhydre 0,31 g, chlorure
de sodium 0,6 g, chlorure de potassium 0,03 g,
chlorure de calcium dihydraté 0,02 g. pH ajusté avec
de l'acide chlorhydrique ou de l'hydroxyde de
sodium. Supplément hydro-électrolytique. **Contre-**   2
indiqué dans le traitement de l'acidose lactique.
Utiliser selon Rx. N'utiliser que si la solution est
limpide. Jeter tout reste. **Attention: ne pas** utiliser
dans les montages en série.

Hospira
Montréal, QC   H4M 2X6

PVC CONTAINER
CONTENANT DE PVC   LATEX   1

IM-1560 (6/07)

Figure 19-2 Lactated Ringer's.

LOT   EXP   DIN 000000000   1

5% Dextrose and 0.45% Sodium
Chloride Injection USP   2

1000 mL   3

EACH 100 mL CONTAINS DEXTROUS HYDROUS 5 g;
SODIUM CHLORIDE 450 mg IN WATER FOR INECTION.
ELECTROLYTES PER 1000 mL; SODIUM 77 mEq;   4
CHLORIDE 77 mEq.
406 mOsmol/LITRE (CALC),
pH 4.3 (3.5 to 6.5)
ADDITIVES MAY BE INCOMPATIBLE.   CONSULT WITH   5
PHARMACIST, IF AVAILABLE, WHEN INTRODUCING
ADDITIVES. USE ASEPTIC TECHNIQUE,   MIX
THOROUGHLY   AND DO NOT STORE.   SINGLE DOSE   6
CONTAINER. FOR INTRAVENOUS USE.   USUAL
DOSAGE: SEE INSERT. STERILE, NONPYROGENIC
FEDERAL LAW PROHIBITS DISPENSING WITHOUT   7
PRESCRIPTION. USE ONLY IF SOLUTION IS CLEAR
AND CONTAINER IS UNDAMAGED. MUST NOT BE
USED IN SERIES CONNECTIONS.   8

SAMPLE LABEL (textbook use only)

http://evolve.elsevier.com/Canada/GrayMorris/   9

Figure 19-4 5% dextrose and 0.45%
sodium chloride (D5 and $\frac{1}{2}$ NS).

1000 mL N° 07902254 DIN 00466670

20 (mEq) mmol/L **POTASSIUM CHLORIDE/ CHLORURE DE POTASSIUM**

in 5% Dextrose and 0.45% Sodium Chloride Injection USP/ dans du dextrose à 5% et du chlorure de sodium à 0,45% injectable USP

Inspect bag by squeezing firmly. If leaks are found, discard. **Storage:** 15 to 30°C. **Protect from freezing.**

STERILE • NONPYROGENIC • HYPERTONIC • FOR INTRAVENOUS USE • SINGLE-USE

100 mL: Potassium chloride 0.15 g, dextrose monohydrate 5 g, sodium chloride 0.45 g. Fluid, nutrient and electrolyte replenisher. Use as prescribed. Use only if solution is clear. Discard unused portion. **Caution: Must not** be used in series connections.

447 mOsm/L   pH approx. 5
mmol (mEq)/L: K 20; Na 76; Cl approx. 96

Inspecter le sac en le comprimant. Jeter en cas de fuites. **Entreposage:** 15 à 30°C. **Craint le gel.**

STÉRILE • APYROGÈNE • HYPERTONIQUE • ADMINISTRATION INTRAVEINEUSE • UNISERVICE

100 mL: chlorure de potassium 0,15 g, dextrose monohydraté 5 g, chlorure de sodium 0,45 g. Supplément nutritif et hydro-électrolytique. Respecter la prescription. N'utiliser que si la solution est limpide. Jeter tout reste. **Attention: ne pas** utiliser dans les montages en série.

Hospira

PVC CONTAINER
CONTENANT DE PVC **LATEX**

Hospira Healthcare Corporation
Montréal, QC H4S 0A9   IM-3627

Figure 19-5 20 mmol potassium chloride in 5% dextrose and 0.45% sodium chloride.

LOT   EXP   DIN 000000000

0.9% Sodium Chloride Injection USP

1000 mL

EACH 100 mL CONTAINS SODIUM CHLORIDE 900 mg IN WATER FOR INECTION.
ELECTROLYTES PER 1000 mL; SODIUM 154 mEq; CHLORIDE 154 mEq.
308 mOsmol/LITRE (CALC),
pH 5.6 (4.5 to 7)
ADDITIVES MAY BE INCOMPATIBLE   CONSULT WITH PHARMACIST, IF AVAILABLE, WHEN INTRODUCING ADDITIVES. USE ASEPTIC TECHNIQUE,   MIX THOROUGHLY AND DO NOT STORE. SINGLE DOSE CONTAINER. FOR INTRAVENOUS USE. USUAL DOSAGE: SEE INSERT. STERILE, NONPYROGENIC
USE ONLY IF SOLUTION IS CLEAR AND CONTAINER IS UNDAMAGED. MUST NOT BE USED IN SERIES CONNECTIONS.

SAMPLE LABEL (textbook use only)

http://evolve.elsevier.com/Canada/GrayMorris/

Figure 19-6 0.9% sodium chloride (NS).

Order	Interpretation
D₅W 1 000 mL IV q8h	Infuse 1 000 mL 5% dextrose in water intravenously every 8 hours.
0.9% NS 1 000 mL IV with 20 mEq KCl per L q8h.	Infuse 1 000 mL 0.9% normal saline IV solution with 20 milliequivalents of potassium chloride added per litre every 8 hours.

Figure 19-7 Sample IV orders. D_5W, dextrose 5% in water; *IV*, intravenous; *KCl*, potassium chloride; *mEq*, milliequivalent; *mL*, millilitres; *NS*, normal saline; *q8h*, every 8 hours.

(!) SAFETY ALERT!

Remember the following when adding potassium chloride to an IV:

- Ensure that it is compatible with the solution and well-diluted.
- Monitor the patient during infusion; rapid infusion of potassium can cause death due to cardiac depression, arrhythmias, and arrest.
- Check the IV site frequently; this medication is extremely irritating.
- Administer IV using an infusion control device.
- Never administer potassium concentrate in an IV push.
- **DO NOT** add potassium to an IV bag that is already infusing. Injecting potassium into an upright infusing IV solution causes the medication to concentrate in the lower portion of the IV bag resulting in the patient receiving a concentrated medication solution, which can be harmful.

Charting Intravenous Solutions

IV solutions are charted on the intake and output (I&O) flow sheet; in some institutions, they are also charted on the medication administration record (MAR). Figure 19-8 is a sample I&O charting record. In institutions where there is computer charting, this information is entered into the electronic record.

Parenteral Nutrition

Parenteral nutrition is a form of nutritional support in which nutrients are provided by the IV route. Parenteral nutrition solutions consist of glucose, amino acids, minerals, vitamins, and/or fat emulsions. The nutrients are infused by a peripheral or central line. Solutions less than 10% dextrose may be given through a peripheral vein; parenteral nutrition with greater than 10% dextrose requires administration by a central venous catheter. A central venous catheter is placed into a high-flow central vein, such as the superior vena cava, by the health care provider. Lipid emulsions are sometimes given when the patient is receiving parenteral nutrition. When lipids are being infused, there is a noticeable difference in the colour of the fluid: it has an opaque white colour. Lipids provide supplemental kilocalories and prevent fatty acid deficiencies. These emulsions can be administered through a separate peripheral line, through a central line by Y-connector tubing, or as mixtures with the parenteral nutrition solution.

Patients who are unable to digest or absorb enteral nutrition are candidates for parenteral nutrition. Parenteral nutrition is also referred to as *total parenteral nutrition* and *hyperalimentation*. The same principles relating to IV therapy are applicable to parenteral nutrition, but more emphasis is placed on care for the site to prevent infection. Further discussion of parenteral nutrition can be found in nursing reference books. The calculation of IV flow rates and infusion times, which will be discussed in this chapter, are also applicable to parenteral nutrition solutions.

IV medication protocols are valuable references, often posted in the medication room of an institution. They provide nurses with specifics about usual medication dosage, dilution for IV administration, compatibility, and the specific patient observations that need to be made during medication administration. **Always adhere to the protocol for administering IV medications.**

Juice glass – 180 mL   Small water cup – 120 mL
Water glass – 210 mL   Jello cup – 150 mL
Coffee cup – 240 mL   Ice cream – 120 mL
Soup bowl – 180 mL   Creamer – 30 mL

Client information

Date: 8/17/16

INTAKE					OUTPUT				
Time	Type	Amt	Time	IV/ Blood type	Amount absorbed	Time	Urine	Stool	Other
			7A	1 000 mL D5W	800 mL	9A	400 mL		
			12P	IVPB	100 mL	1P	500 mL		
8 h total					900 mL		900 mL		

Figure 19-8 Sample of charting IV fluids on an I&O record. *D₅W,* dextrose 5% in water; *IVPB,* intravenous piggyback; *mL,* millilitres.

> **(!) SAFETY ALERT!**
>
> Before placing any additives in an IV solution (vitamins, medications, electrolytes), be sure the additives are compatible with the solution. Some incompatible additives may cause the solution to become cloudy or crystallize. Always verify the compatibility of the additive and the solution.

Administration of Blood and Blood Products

Blood and blood products are also administered intravenously. When blood is administered, specific protocols must be followed. They can be found in parenteral policies/guidelines in the patient care environment. Most patient care policies and procedures within an institution can be accessed electronically. IV flow rates and infusion times are also calculated for blood and blood products. When blood is administered, a standard blood set or Y-type blood set is commonly used. The *Y* refers to two spikes above the drip chamber of the IV tubing. One spike is attached to the blood container, and the other is attached to a container of normal saline solution. Normal saline is used to flush the IV tubing at the start and at the end of the transfusion. Blood may be administered by gravity (Figure 19-9) or electronic pump. Tubing for blood administration has an in-line filter.

Administration of Intravenous Solutions

IV solution is administered by an IV infusion set, which includes a sealed bag containing the solution. A drip chamber is connected to the IV bag or bottle. The flow rate is adjusted to drops per minute (gtt/min) by use of a roller clamp. Some IV tubings have a

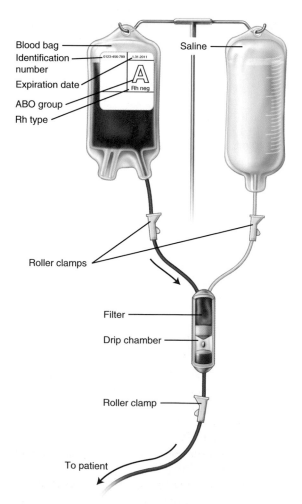

Figure 19-9 Setup for blood administration. (From Harkreader, H., & Hogan, M. A. (2007). *Fundamentals of nursing: Caring and clinical judgment* (3rd ed.). St. Louis: Saunders.)

Blood bag
Identification number
Expiration date
ABO group
Rh type
0123-456-789   1.31.2011
A
Rh neg
Saline
Roller clamps
Filter
Drip chamber
Roller clamp
To patient

sliding clamp attached, which can be used to temporarily stop the IV infusion. Injection ports are located on the IV tubing and on most IV solution bags. Injection ports allow for medications to be injected directly into the bag of solution or line. The injection ports also allow for the attachment of secondary IV lines that contain fluids or medications to the primary line. Figure 19-10 shows a primary line infusion set. IV fluids infuse by gravity flow. This means that for the IV solution to infuse, it must be hung above the level of the patient's heart, which will allow for adequate pressure to be exerted for the IV to infuse. The height of the IV bag, therefore, has a relationship to the flow rate. The higher the IV bag is hung, the greater the pressure; therefore, the IV will infuse at a faster rate. Of course, the roller clamp ultimately controls the flow rate of an IV infused by gravity.

Intravenous Sites

IV lines are referred to as either *peripheral* or *central lines.* The infusion site of a **peripheral line** is a vein in the arm, hand, or scalp (in an infant); or, if other sites are not accessible and on rare occasions, a vein in the leg. For a **central line,** a special catheter is used to access a large vein such as the subclavian or jugular vein. The special catheter is threaded through a large vein into the superior vena cava. Examples of central catheters include triple-lumen, Hickman, Broviac, and Groshong catheters. When a peripheral vein is used to access a central vein, you may see the term *peripherally inserted central catheter,* or *PICC,* line. A PICC line is usually inserted into the antecubital vein in the arm and is advanced into the superior vena cava.

Primary and Secondary Lines

The primary IV is the patient's main source for IV fluids and electrolytes such as potassium chloride, which is added in specific amounts *per litre* of solution. Since potassium chloride is a high-alert medication, different strengths are added by the manufacturer. IV solutions with and without potassium chloride are usually stocked by each unit and selected as needed, according to IV orders. Units usually have packages of primary IV sets and secondary IV sets. **Secondary lines** are usually used to administer intermittent medications and are attached to the primary line at an injection port. They can also be used to infuse other IV solutions, as long as they are compatible with the solution on the primary line. A secondary line is referred to as an IV piggyback (IVPB). Notice that the IVPB is hanging higher than the primary line in Figure 19-11.

The IVPB is hung higher than the primary line so that it gives it greater pressure than the primary line, thereby allowing it to infuse first. Most secondary IV sets come with an extender that allows the nurse to lower the primary bag. Notice that the secondary bags are smaller than the primary bags; the secondary bags are most often seen in 50 to 100 mL. The amount of solution used for the IVPB is determined by the medication being added. Some medications may have to be mixed in 250 mL of fluid for administration. IVPB medications can come premixed by the manufacturer or pharmacist, depending on the institution, or the nurse may have to prepare them. The flow rate for an IVPB to infuse should be checked. The manufacturer's insert provides recommended times for infusion. This information may also be obtained from a drug reference or parenteral manual (electronic or otherwise) on the unit.

Systems for Administering Medications by Intravenous Piggyback

Several systems are available for piggybacking medication. You may have the opportunity to see or use such a system in your institution or unit. It is important to note, however, that not all patient care areas use these systems: medication can be administered safely by IVPB on both a gravity IV system and an electronic pump system without any special piggyback system.

One type of IVPB system used in some institutions is the **ADD-Vantage system.** This system requires a special type of IV bag that has a port for inserting medication (usually in powdered form and mixed with the IV solution as a diluent). In this system, the contents of the vial are mixed into the total solution and then infused (Figure 19-12).

Baxter's MINI-BAG Plus Container System is also used to administer medication by IVPB. The MINI-BAG Plus Container System, which is dispensed by the pharmacy, has a

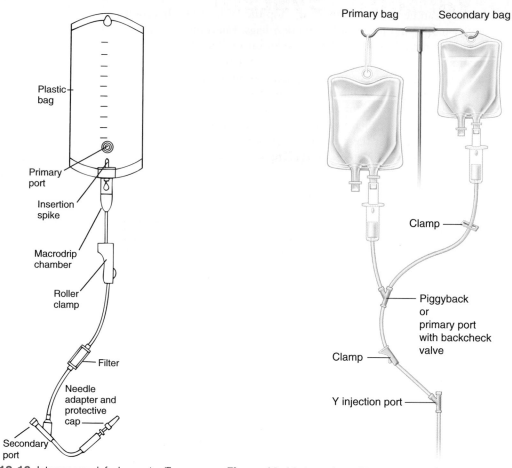

Figure 19-10 Intravenous infusion set. (From Clayton, B. D., & Willihnganz, M. (2013). *Basic pharmacology for nurses* (16th ed.). St. Louis: Mosby.)

Figure 19-11 Intermittent IV medication administration can be accomplished with the use of IV piggyback. (From Harkreader, H., & Hogan, M. A. (2007). *Fundamentals of nursing: Caring and clinical judgment* (3rd ed.). St. Louis: Saunders.)

vial of unreconstituted medication attached to a special port. The internal seal is broken and the medication and diluent are mixed just before administration. The medication vial remains attached to the MINI-BAG Container System (Figure 19-13).

Volume-control devices are used for accurate measurement of small-volume medications and fluids. Most volume-control devices have a capacity of 100 to 150 mL and can be used with secondary or primary lines. They are also used intermittently for medication purposes. They have a port that allows medication to be injected and a certain amount of IV fluid to be added as a diluent (Figure 19-14). Volume-control devices are referred to by their trade names (Soluset or Buretrol), depending on the institution. They are used mostly in pediatrics and critical care settings. These devices allow for precise control of the infusion and the medication.

Saline and Heparin Intravenous Locks

Intermittent venous access devices (Figure 19-15) are used for the purpose of administering IV medication intermittently or for access to a vein in an emergency situation. Intermittent venous access devices are referred to as *saline locks* or *heparin locks*. The line is usually kept free from blockage or clotting by flushing it with sterile saline solution or heparin (anticoagulant). It is important to note that heparin locks are no longer used routinely for keeping patency. Normal saline locks have replaced heparin locks, except for central-line locks.

Various institutions have purchased a needleless system (Figure 19-16) for administration of medications through the primary line and for access devices such as saline locks. The needleless system does not require attachment of a needle by the nurse. The system allows for administration by IV push, IV bolus, or by IVPB.

ADD-Vantage™ System

Instructions for use

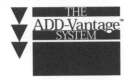

1. Assemble - Use Aseptic Technique

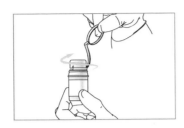

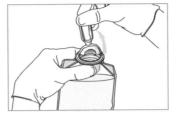

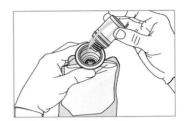

Swing the pull ring over the top of the vial and pull down far enough to start the opening. Then pull straight up to remove the cap. Avoid touching the rubber stopper and vial threads.

Hold diluent container and gently grasp the tab on the pull ring. Pull up to break the tie membrane. Pull back to remove the cover. Avoid touching the inside of the vial port.

Screw the vial into the vial port until it will go no further. Recheck the vial to assure that it is tight. Label appropriately.

2. Activate - Pull Plug/Stopper to Mix Drug with Diluent

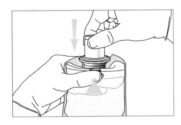

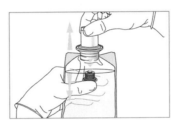

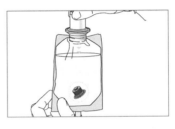

Hold the vial as shown. Push the drug vial down into container and grasp the inner cap of the vial through the walls of the container.

Pull the inner plug from the drug vial: allow drug to fall into diluent container for fast mixing. Do not force stopper by pushing on one side of inner cap at a time.

Verify that the plug and rubber stopper have been removed from the vial. The floating stopper is an indication that the system has been activated.

If the rubber stopper is not removed from the vial and medication is not released on the first attempt, the inner cap may be manipulated back into the rubber stopper without removing the drug vial from the diluent container. After repositioning the inner cap, repeat the "Activate" step.

3. Mix and Administer - Within Specified Time

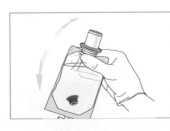

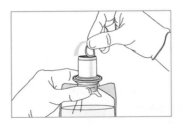

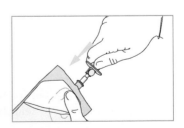

Mix container contents thoroughly to assure complete dissolution. Look through bottom of vial to verify complete mixing. Check for leaks by squeezing container firmly. If leaks are found, discard unit.

Pull up hanger on the vial.

Remove the white administration port cover and spike (pierce) the container with the piercing pin. Administer within the specified time.

For more information, contact your Hospira representative at 1-877-9Hospira (946-7747) or visit www.hospira.com

Hospira, Inc., 275 North Field Drive, Lake Forest, IL 60045   P12-3781/R1-Apr. 13

World's leading provider of injectable drugs and infusion technologies

Figure 19-12 Assembling and administering medication with the ADD-Vantage system. (From Hospira, Inc., Lake Forest, IL.)

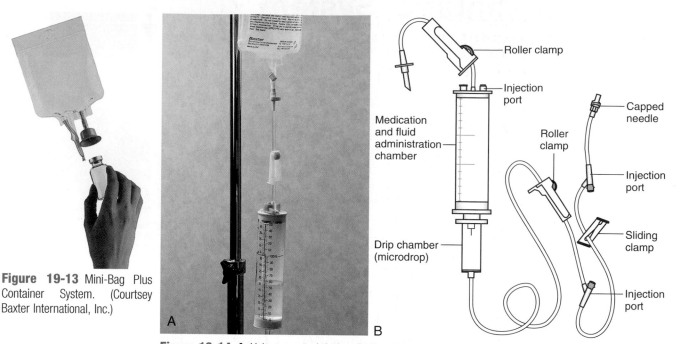

Figure 19-13 Mini-Bag Plus Container System. (Courtsey Baxter International, Inc.)

Figure 19-14 A, Volume-control device. **B,** Parts of a volume-control set. (**A,** From Potter, P. A., Perry, A. G., Stockert, P., et al. (2013). *Fundamentals of nursing* (8th ed.). St. Louis: Mosby.)

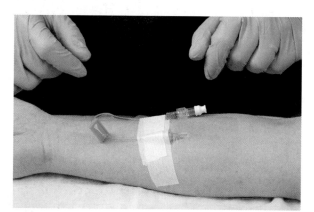

Figure 19-15 Intermittent lock covered with a rubber diaphragm. (From Potter, P. A., Perry, A. G., Stockert, P., et al. (2013). *Fundamentals of nursing* (8th ed.). St. Louis: Mosby.)

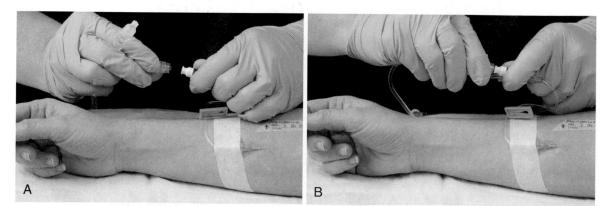

Figure 19-16 A, Needleless infusion system. **B,** Connection into an injection port. (From Potter, P. A., Perry, A. G., Stockert, P., et al. (2013). *Fundamentals of nursing* (8th ed.). St. Louis: Mosby.)

When medications are administered through a venous access device (VAD) that is accessed intermittently, the nurse should consider the proper flushing and maintenance of the device. The volume of normal saline used or the choice of heparin depends on the type of VAD. Check your institution's policy!

> **! SAFETY ALERT!**
>
> Remember that heparin is a high-alert medication that comes in many dosage strengths (concentrations). The concentration for a heparin lock flush is 10 units per mL or 100 units per mL. The average heparin lock flush dosage is 10 units and **never** exceeds 100 units. If heparin is used in your institution, always check the concentration carefully. To increase patient safety and prevent adverse effects from heparin lock flushes, saline lock flushes are used to maintain peripheral IV catheter patency on general care units. Heparin lock flushes are still used to maintain central venous access devices in general and specialty care areas. Always refer to the policy at your health care facility regarding the frequency, volume, and concentration of saline or heparin to be used to maintain the IV lock.

Medications can be administered through an IV port used for direct injection of medication by syringe. This type of administration is referred to as **IV push** or **IV bolus.** *IV push* indicates that a syringe is attached to the port and the medication is pushed in. *IV bolus* indicates that a volume of IV fluid is infused over a specific period of time through an IV administration set. There are guidelines, however, relating to who may administer IV push medications and in which patient care area. The nurse should check the institution's policy regarding IV push or IV bolus.

Electronic Infusion Devices

Several electronic infusion devices are available today (Figure 19-17 shows two types). These devices are also referred to as electronic controllers or pumps and are designed to deliver measured amounts of IV solution or IV medication through IV injection over time. Special tubing is supplied by the manufacturers of these electronic devices. Each device can be set for a specific flow rate, and typically the device activates an alarm if the rate is interrupted. The use of electronic infusion devices is based on the need to strictly regulate the IV. Electronic infusion devices are essential in pediatrics and the critical care setting, where they provide for infusion of small amounts of fluids or medications with precision.

Most of the electronic infusion devices in current use are powered by direct current (from a wall unit) and have an internal rechargeable battery. When the device is unplugged, for example, to allow patient ambulation, the battery becomes the power source. Infusion pumps present significant threats to patient safety, with various performance problems that have resulted in both over- and under-infusion. Although electronic infusion devices are a great improvement in patient health outcomes, medications errors still arise with them.

In 2003, a national infusion pump survey was undertaken by the Institute for Safe Medication Practices Canada (ISMP Canada) in collaboration with the Canadian Healthcare Association (now HealthCareCAN), Health Canada, Healthcare Insurance Reciprocal of Canada (HIROC), and University of Toronto researchers (ISMP Canada, 2004). Based on the survey results, ISMP Canada made a number of recommendations for actions hospitals can take to improve infusion pump safety:

- Conduct a failure mode and effects analysis (FMEA) when acquiring new pumps and when assessing pumps in current use.
- Label each infusion line when using multiple-channel pumps.
- Conduct frequent rounds to double-check IV solutions and to detect device programming errors.
- Perform independent double-checks of infusions of high-alert medications before administration.
- Prominently display IV fluid and medication labels on the infusion pump and the tubing at the port of entry.
- Double-check all programming of infusion devices. Because of the errors that have occurred with infusion devices due to incorrect programming, this safeguard is mandatory.
- Educate all health care providers on how to use infusion devices.

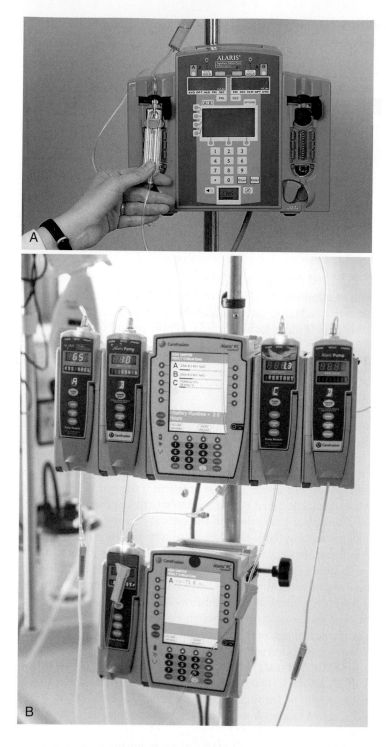

Figure 19-17 A, Dual-channel infusion pump. **B,** Multiple channel infusion pump. (**A,** From Potter, P. A., Perry, A. G., Stockert, P., et al. (2013). *Fundamentals of nursing* (8th ed.). St. Louis: Mosby. **B,** © Marshall Ikonography/Alamy Stock Photo.)

- Ensure free-flow protection on all infusion devices and patient-controlled analgesia pumps. *Free-flow protection* means that the tubing has a built-in mechanism similar to a clamp that is mobilized when the tubing is removed from the pump, therefore preventing the flow of fluid into the patient when the pump is stopped or the tubing is taken out of the infusion pump.

A specific aim of ISMP Canada (2004) and the collaborating organizations in undertaking the national survey on infusion pump use was to develop strategies for safer infusion pump use—related to both equipment and practice.

Available on the market today are programmable infusion pumps called *smart pumps* that have safety features designed to help prevent medication errors. Smart pumps have customized software that has a reference library of medications indicating the minimum and maximum rates at which medications should safely infuse. It is expected that over time, smart pumps will replace infusion devices in all institutions.

> **⚠ SAFETY ALERT!**
>
> An institution may use a variety of infusion pumps. Nurses must know how to use them correctly to prevent patient harm and a fatal outcome.

Electronic Volumetric Pumps. Electronic volumetric pumps infuse fluids into the vein under pressure and against resistance and do not depend on gravity. The pumps are programmed to deliver a set amount of fluid per hour (see Figure 19-17). There is a wide range of electronic pumps. Because these pumps deliver millilitres per hour (mL/h), any millilitre calculation that results in a decimal fraction is rounded to a whole millilitre, unless the pump has decimal capability and the IV medication is a high-alert medication, such as insulin and heparin. These pumps are common in critical care settings, pediatrics, and oncology.

Syringe Pumps. Syringe pumps are electronic devices that deliver medications or fluids by use of a syringe. The medication is measured in a syringe and attached to the special pump, and the medication is infused at the flow rate set (Figure 19-18). These pumps are useful in pediatrics and critical care settings, as well as in labour and delivery areas.

Patient-Controlled Analgesia Devices. Patient-controlled analgesia (PCA) is a form of pain management that allows the patient to self-administer IV analgesics. In PCA, a computerized infuser pump that contains a syringe of pain medication is connected to the IV line of a patient (Figure 19-19, *B*). The PCA pump is programmed to allow dosages of narcotics only within specific limits to be delivered to prevent overdosage. The dosage and frequency of administration are ordered by the prescriber and set on the pump. The patient self-medicates by use of a control button. The pump also keeps a record of the number of times the patient uses the device. The display on the pump lets patients know when they are able to medicate themselves and when it is impossible to give themselves another dose. The pump therefore has what is called "a lockout interval." In this interval, no pain medication is delivered. A medication commonly administered by PCA is morphine (30 mg morphine per 30 mL). Portable PCA pumps are also available and are battery operated (see Figure 19-19, *A*).

Nurses must be familiar with the infusion devices used at their institution; in-service education is essential in the use of all infusion devices.

Figure 19-18 A, Syringe inserted into syringe pump. **B,** Freedom 60 syringe infusion pump system. (**A,** From Perry, A. G., Potter, P. A., & Elkin, M. K. (2012). *Nursing interventions and clinical skills* (5th ed.). St. Louis: Mosby. **B,** Courtesy Repro-Med Systems, Inc., Chester, NY.)

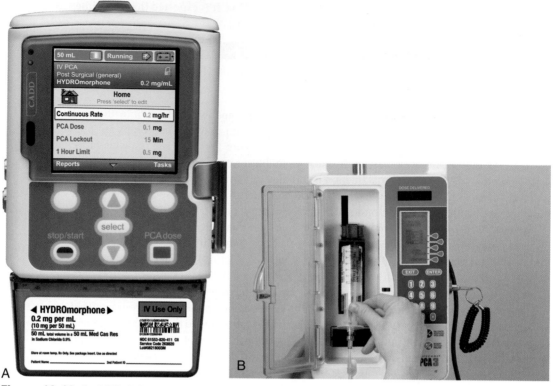

Figure 19-19 A, CADD-Solis pain management pump. **B,** Patient-controlled analgesia ambulatory infusion pump. (**A,** From Smiths Medical ASD, Inc., St. Paul, MN. **B,** From Perry, A. G., Potter, P. A., & Elkin, M. K. (2012). *Nursing interventions and clinical skills* (5th ed.). St. Louis: Mosby.)

> ⚠️ **SAFETY ALERT!**
>
> Many infusion pumps look similar, but their functions are different. Because of the wide variation in infusion pumps and their functions, caution is mandatory when they are used. It has been estimated that a significant number of IV medication errors result from errors in pump programming. It is mandatory to double-check the programming of all infusion devices and monitor patients receiving an infusion.

> ⚙️ **POINTS TO REMEMBER**
>
> - IV orders are written by the physician or other prescriber certified to do so (e.g., nurse practitioner, physician's assistant).
> - IV orders must specify the name of the IV solution, medications (if any are to be added), the amount to be administered, and the infusion time.
> - Several electronic devices are on the market for infusing IV solutions. Always familiarize yourself with the equipment before use.
> - The institution's protocol for IV administration must be followed.
> - The nurse is primarily responsible for monitoring the patient during IV therapy.
> - The nurse is responsible for any errors that occur in the administration of IV fluids (e.g., inadequate dilution, too rapid infusion).
> - In IV abbreviations, the letters indicate the solution components, and the numbers indicate the solution strength.
> - Solution strength expressed as a percentage (%) indicates grams of solute per 100 mL of fluid.
> - Principles relating to IV flow rates and infusion times are also applicable to parenteral nutrition solutions and blood and blood products.

+−÷× PRACTICE **PROBLEMS**

Answer the following questions as briefly as possible.

1. What does PCA stand for? _____

2. An IV initiated in a patient's lower arm is called what type of line?

   _____

3. IVPB means _____.

4. A patient has an IV of 1000 mL 0.9% NS. The abbreviation identifies what type of solution?

   _____

5. A secondary line is hung _____ than the primary line.

6. Volumetric pumps infuse fluids into the vein by _____.

Identify the components and percentage strength of the following IV solutions.

7. D20W _____

8. D5W 10 mmol KCl _____

Answers on page 527.

? CLINICAL **REASONING**

Scenario: A patient returned to the unit after surgery connected to a PCA pump. An order was written to attach a solution of 100 mL 0.9% NS with morphine 100 mg to the pump and infuse at a rate of 1 mg per 6 min. The solution ordered was inserted into the device and the flow rate set. The patient had been instructed on the use of the PCA pump. The patient continued to complain of severe pain on each shift, despite the pump indicating that medication was being received at the set flow rate. The patient received intermittent boluses of morphine to relieve pain.

Twenty-four hours later, a nurse opened the PCA pump, found the full amount of IV solution in place, and noticed that the tubing had not been primed.

What should have been done in this situation?

_____

_____

_____

Answer on page 527.

◀ CHAPTER **REVIEW**

Using IV solution labels *A* to *D* below and on page 527, specify the letter of the label that corresponds with the fluid abbreviation.

1. D5$\frac{1}{2}$NS _____

2. D5W_____

3. RL _____

4. D5NS _____

Answer the following questions.

5. A patient has a PCA pump in use following surgery. What is this device used to control?

_____

6. When an IV medication is injected directly into the vein through a port, it is called an

_____ or _____ .

7. The two major intravenous access sites are _____ and _____ .

8. A patient is to receive an antibiotic IVPB. In order for the antibiotic to infuse first, how

must it be hung in relation to the existing IV solution bag? _____

1000 mL   Nº 07953254   DIN 00039470

LACTATED RINGER'S
Injection USP
RINGER-LACTATE
injectable USP

9

Inspect bag by squeezing firmly. If leaks are found, discard. **Storage:** 20 to 25°C (see "Controlled Room Temperature" in USP). **Protect from freezing.**

8

STERILE • NONPYROGENIC • FOR INTRAVENOUS USE • SINGLE-DOSE

7

100 mL: Sodium lactate anhydrous 0.31 g, sodium chloride 0.6 g, potassium chloride 0.03 g, calcium chloride dihydrate 0.02 g. pH adjusted with hydrochloric acid or sodium hydroxide. Fluid and electrolyte replenisher. **Not for use in the treatment of lactic acidosis.** Use as prescribed. Use only if solution is clear. Discard unused portion. **Caution: Must not** be used in series connections.

6

5

273 mOsm/L   pH approx. 6.7
mmol (mEq)/L: Na approx. 130; K 4;
Ca 1.5 (3); Cl approx. 109; Lactate 28

Inspecter le sac en le comprimant. Jeter en cas de fuites. **Entreposage:** 20 à 25°C (voir "Controlled Room Temperature" dans l'USP). **Craint le gel.**

4

STÉRILE • APYROGÈNE • ADMINISTRA-TION INTRAVEINEUSE • UNISERVICE

100 mL: lactate de sodium anhydre 0,31 g, chlorure de sodium 0,6 g, chlorure de potassium 0,03 g, chlorure de calcium dihydraté 0,02 g. pH ajusté avec de l'acide chlorhydrique ou de l'hydroxyde de sodium. Supplément hydro-électrolytique. **Contre-indiqué dans le traitement de l'acidose lactique.** Utiliser selon Rx. N'utiliser que si la solution est limpide. Jeter tout reste. **Attention: ne pas** utiliser dans les montages en série.

3

2

Hospira
Montréal, QC H4M 2X6

PVC CONTAINER
CONTENANT DE PVC   LATEX

IM-1560 (6/07)

1

A

(01)00882135795509

LOT   EXP   DIN 000000000   1

5% Dextrose and 0.45% Sodium Chloride Injection USP   2

1000 mL

3

EACH 100 mL CONTAINS DEXTROUS HYDROUS 5 g; SODIUM CHLORIDE 450 mg IN WATER FOR INECTION. ELECTROLYTES PER 1000 mL; SODIUM 77 mEq; CHLORIDE 77 mEq. 406 mOsmol/LITRE (CALC), pH 4.3 (3.5 to 6.5)   4

ADDITIVES MAY BE INCOMPATIBLE. CONSULT WITH PHARMACIST, IF AVAILABLE, WHEN INTRODUCING ADDITIVES. USE ASEPTIC TECHNIQUE, MIX THOROUGHLY AND DO NOT STORE. SINGLE DOSE CONTAINER. FOR INTRAVENOUS USE. USUAL DOSAGE: SEE INSERT. STERILE, NONPYROGENIC FEDERAL LAW PROHIBITS DISPENSING WITHOUT PRESCRIPTION. USE ONLY IF SOLUTION IS CLEAR AND CONTAINER IS UNDAMAGED. MUST NOT BE USED IN SERIES CONNECTIONS.   5 6 7

8

SAMPLE LABEL (textbook use only)

http://evolve.elsevier.com/Canada/GrayMorris/   9

B

```
 ___ LOT        EXP         DIN 000000000   1
                                            ─

 5% Dextrose Injection USP                  2
 ─  1000 mL                                 ─

    EACH 100 mL CONTAINS   5 g DEXTROUS HYDROUS   3
 ─  USP pH 4.0 (3.2 TO 6.5)  OSMOLARITY 252 mOs-  ─
    mol/L (CALC) STERILE NONPYROGENIC    SINGLE
    DOSE CONTAINER   ADDITIVES MAY BE INCOMPAT-   4
 ─  IBLE   CONSULT WITH PHARMACIST IF AVAILABLE   ─
    WHEN INTRODUCING ADDITIVES USE ASEPTIC
    TECHNIQUE  MIX THOROUGHLY  DO NOT STORE
    DOSAGE  INTRAVENOUSLY AS DIRECTED BY A PHY-   5
 ─  SICIAN   SEE DIRECTIONS  CAUTIONS  SQUEEZE AND ─
    INSPECT INNER BAG WHICH MAINTAINS PRODUCT
    STERILITY   DISCARD IF LEAKS ARE FOUND    MUST 6
 ─  NOT BE USED IN SERIES CONNECTIONS   DO NOT     ─
    ADMINISTER SIMULTANEOUSLY WITH BLOOD   DO
    NOT USE UNLESS SOLUTION IS CLEAR  FEDERAL
    LAW PROHIBITS DISPENSING WITHOUT PRESCRIP-     7
 ─  TION   STORE UNIT IN MOISTURE BARRIER OVER-    ─
    WRAP AT ROOM TEMPERATURE (25C) UNTIL READY
    TO USE  AVOID EXCESSIVE HEAT  SEE INSERT       8
                                                   ─

    SAMPLE LABEL (textbook use only)
 ─  http://evolve.elsevier.com/Canada/GrayMorris/  9
 C                                                 ─
```

```
 ___ LOT        EXP         DIN 000000000   1
                                            ─

 5% Dextrose and 0.9% Sodium                2
 ─ Chloride Injection USP                   ─

    1000 mL                                 3
 ─                                          ─

    EACH 100 mL CONTAINS DEXTROUS HYDROUS 5 g;
    SODIUM CHLORIDE 900 mg IN WATER FOR INJECTION.  4
 ─  ELECTROLYTES PER 1000 mL; SODIUM 154 mEq;       ─
    CHLORIDE 154 mEq.
    560 mOsmol/LITRE (CALC),                        5
 ─  pH 4.3 (3.5 to 6.5)                             ─
    ADDITIVES MAY BE INCOMPATIBLE   CONSULT WITH
    PHARMACIST, IF AVAILABLE, WHEN INTRODUCING      6
 ─  ADDITIVES. USE ASEPTIC TECHNIQUE,  MIX THOR-    ─
    OUGHLY  AND DO NOT STORE.  SINGLE DOSE CON-
    TAINER. FOR IV USE.   USUAL DOSAGE: SEE INSERT. 7
 ─  STERILE, NONPYROGENIC   USE ONLY IF SOLUTION    ─
    IS CLEAR AND CONTAINER IS UNDAMAGED. MUST
    NOT BE USED IN SERIES CONNECTIONS.              8
                                                    ─

    SAMPLE LABEL (textbook use only)
 ─  http://evolve.elsevier.com/Canada/GrayMorris/   9
 D                                                  ─
```

Answers below.

✳ ANSWERS

Answers to Practice Problems

1. patient-controlled analgesia

2. peripheral

3. intravenous piggyback

4. 0.9% normal saline or 0.9% sodium chloride

5. higher

6. pressure

7. 20% dextrose in water

8. 5% dextrose in water with 10 mmol potassium chloride (KCl)

Answer to Clinical Reasoning Question

Troubleshooting should have been done by the nurses caring for the patient. If the patient's pain was not being relieved, the device should have been checked for possible malfunctioning and to determine whether the machine had been set up properly. It is mandatory that all programming be double-checked by nurses and the pump be monitored frequently to ensure that it is functioning. The patient's continual complaint of severe pain with no relief should have been a key concern to the nurses caring for the patient.

Answers to Chapter Review

1. B

2. C

3. A

4. D

5. Pain

6. IV push; IV bolus

7. Peripheral; central

8. Higher

*e*volve

For additional practice problems, refer to the Advanced Calculations section of the Drug Calculations Companion, Version 5 on Evolve.

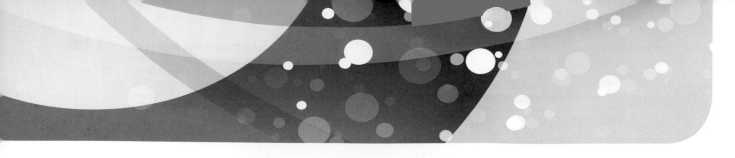

CHAPTER **20**
Intravenous Calculations

Objectives

After reviewing this chapter, you should be able to:

1. Calculate the intravenous (IV) flow rate in millilitres per hour
2. Identify the two types of tubing used to administer IV fluids
3. Identify the drop factor in drops per millilitres from IV tubing packages
4. Calculate the IV flow rate in millilitres per hour and in drops per minute using different formulas
5. Calculate the IV flow rate in drops per minute using the shortcut method (mL/h and constant drop factor)
6. Calculate the flow rate for medications ordered intravenously over a specified time period
7. Calculate infusion times and completion times
8. Recalculate IV flow rates and determine the percentage of increase or decrease

This chapter presents the calculations performed in intravenous (IV) therapy. Nurses are responsible for ensuring that patients receive the correct IV flow rate. Several methods to calculate IV flow rates are presented in this chapter: the ratio and proportion method, the formula method, the dimensional analysis method, and the shortcut method.

Intravenous Flow Rate Calculation

Today, IV fluids are usually ordered to be administered at flow rates expressed in millilitres per hour (mL/h). Consider this example: IV NS with 20 mmol KCl/L 125 mL/h. The nurse would program an electronic infusion device to administer the IV ordered at 125 mL per hour. If the IV is to be manually regulated by gravity (without a pump), then the nurse would convert the 125 mL per hour into drops per minute (gtt/min). Although electronic infusion devices are used routinely, IV flow rates (primary and secondary) are still regulated manually: pumps are not always available for every patient at a given time. A simple IV order like the one in the example can be administered by gravity flow instead of a pump. However, complex IV orders as well as certain high-alert IV medications (e.g., heparin infusion) must be administered via pump to increase patient safety.

IV fluids may also be ordered in large volumes to infuse over several hours: for example, 1 000 mL over 8 hours. Alternatively, a large volume can be ordered by total volume to infuse at a rate of infusion in millilitres per hour: for example, 1 000 mL D5W at a flow rate of 125 mL/h.

Calculating Flow Rates for Infusion Pumps in Millilitres per Hour

The nurse is responsible for programming the infusion pump to deliver the volume ordered.

With technological advances, some infusion pumps are capable of delivering IV fluids in tenths of a millilitre. Always be familiar with the IV equipment being used at your institution before rounding millilitres per hour to the nearest *whole* millilitre per hour.

Most electronic infusion devices that regulate the flow of IV solutions are programmed in millilitres per hour (mL/h). For the purpose of this text, the equipment being used is programmable in whole millilitres per hour; therefore, millilitres per hour should be rounded to a whole number unless indicated that the infusion pump has decimal capability. Let's begin with the calculation of IV flow rates in millilitres per hour.

To calculate an IV flow rate in millilitres per hour, the nurse needs to know the following:
- The volume (amount) of solution in millilitres to infuse
- The infusion time, expressed in hours
- The formula used to calculate the flow rate in millilitres per hour:

$$x \, \text{mL/h} = \frac{\text{Amount of solution (mL)}}{\text{Time (h)}}$$

Round the resulting flow rate to the nearest whole number or tenth, depending on the equipment.

Example 1: Order: IV D5W 3 000 mL over 24 hours. Determine the flow rate in millilitres per hour.

✔ Solution Using the Formula Method

1. Think: The pump infuses in millilitres per hour (mL/h).
2. Set up the problem and solve.

$$x \, \text{mL/h} = \frac{3\,000 \, \text{mL}}{24 \, \text{h}}$$

$$x = 125 \, \text{mL/h}$$

The pump would be set to deliver 125 mL per hour.

✔ Solution Using Ratio and Proportion

$$3\,000 \, \text{mL} : 24 \, \text{h} = x \, \text{mL} : 1 \, \text{h}$$

$$\frac{24x}{24} = \frac{3\,000}{24}$$

$$x = 125 \, \text{mL/h}$$

Remember, as stated in Chapter 12, ratio and proportion can be set up in several formats. This problem could have been set up with the desired time for the infusion (usually 1 hour) over the total time ordered in hours on one side of the equation, and the hourly amount in millilitres labelled "*x*" over the total volume to be infused in millilitres on the other side:

NOTE
When using ratio and proportion, units of measurement must be stated in the same sequence.

$$\frac{1 \, \text{h}}{24 \, \text{h}} = \frac{x \, \text{mL}}{3\,000 \, \text{mL}} \quad or \quad 1 \, \text{h} : 24 \, \text{h} = x \, \text{mL} : 3\,000 \, \text{mL}$$

When a medication is added to an IV, such as in an IV piggyback (IVPB), it may be ordered to infuse in less than an hour (which is often the case when an antibiotic is administered). When the time period for infusion by an electronic infusion device is less than an hour, the flow rate must still be determined in millilitres per hour. Use the ratio proportion method to determine millilitres per hour or use this formula:

$$x \text{ mL/h} = \frac{\text{Total mL to infuse}}{\text{Number of min to infuse}} \times 60 \text{ min/h}$$

Let's look at an example illustrating this formula.

Example 2: Order: Cefazolin 500 mg in 50 mL NS over 30 min.

1. Think: The pump infuses in millilitres per hour (mL/h).
2. Use the ratio and proportion method to determine mL per hour. Remember: 1 h = 60 min.

✔ Solution Using Ratio and Proportion

$$50 \text{ mL} : 30 \text{ min} = x \text{ mL} : 60 \text{ min}$$

$$30x = 50 \times 60$$

$$\frac{30x}{30} = \frac{3\,000}{30}$$

$$x = 100 \text{ mL/h}$$

The pump would be set to deliver 100 mL per hour for 50 mL to infuse within 30 minutes.

An alternative formula that can be used to determine the flow rate in millilitres per hour for an infusion time period that is less than an hour is as follows:

$$x \text{ mL/h} = \frac{\text{Total mL to infuse}}{\text{Number of min to infuse}} \times 60 \text{ min/h}$$

Let's look at Example 2 using this formula.

$$x \text{ mL/h} = \frac{50 \text{ mL}}{\overset{}{\underset{1}{30 \text{ min}}}} \times \frac{\overset{2}{60 \text{ min}} / h}{1}$$

Notice that minutes can be cancelled here.

$$x = \frac{100}{1}$$

$$x = 100 \text{ mL/h}$$

Calculating Millilitres per Hour Using the Dimensional Analysis Method

Calculating millilitres per hour using the dimensional analysis method is similar to using the formula method.

Steps:
1. Identify what you are looking for and write it on the left side of the equation in a fraction format.
2. Write the starting fraction using the information from the problem.

Example 1: A patient with an infusion pump has an order for 3 000 mL of D5W over 24 hours.

Label factor: $\dfrac{x \text{ mL}}{h} =$

Starting fraction: $\dfrac{3\,000 \text{ mL}}{24 \text{ h}}$

$$\dfrac{x \text{ mL}}{h} = \dfrac{3\,000 \text{ mL}}{24 \text{ h}}$$ *Note*: No cancellation of
units is required here.

$$x = 125 \text{ mL/h}$$

Medications such as antibiotics or other supplemental fluids can also be infused **inter-mittently** by adding a **secondary line** to the primary IV. Let's say a physician wants to prescribe an antibiotic for a patient postoperatively. The prescription may read like the order in Example 2.

Example 2: Order: Cefazolin 1 g IV q8h x 3 doses.

In most institutions, the medication administration record (MAR) may indicate a solution, an amount, and the rate at which to infuse a medication. The volume of the IVPB solution is usually 50 to 250 mL and should infuse over 20, 30, or 60 minutes or more, depending on the type and amount of medication added. A drug reference indicates that after recon-stitution, the IV cefazolin should be further diluted with 50 to 100 mL of normal saline (NS) or dextrose 5% in water (D5W) and run over 10 minutes to 1 hour. The nurse uses critical thinking and decides to use 50 mL NS and infuse the medication over 30 minutes. Notice that the infusion time is less than 1 hour. The pump delivers millilitres per hour. Therefore, the fraction for 1 h = 60 min is added to the equation.

> **NOTE**
>
> At some institutions, when **10 mL** or more of medication is added to the dilution fluid, it must be added to the volume of solution when calculating the flow rate. Be aware of your institution's policy.

$$\dfrac{x \text{ mL}}{h} = \dfrac{50 \text{ mL}}{\overset{}{\underset{1}{30 \text{ min}}}} \times \dfrac{\overset{2}{60 \text{ min}}}{1}$$ *Note*: Minutes are cancelled here so that you are left with mL per hour.

$$x = 100 \text{ mL/h}$$

> **SAFETY ALERT!**
>
> The usual flow rate in millilitres per hour ranges from 50 to 200 mL per hour. If the flow rate you have calculated exceeds this amount, double-check the order and your calculation. Remember to use the correct information from the order for the dosage calculation method you are using. Choose the dosage calculation method that is easiest for you.

> **POINTS TO REMEMBER**
>
> - Calculate the flow rate for an electronic infusion device in millilitres per hour.
> - To determine the flow rate for an electronic infusion device (e.g., pumps and controllers) in millilitres per hour, use the following formula:
>
> $$x \text{ mL/h} = \dfrac{\text{Amount of solution (mL)}}{\text{Time (h)}}$$
>
> - If the infusion time is less than 1 hour, use the ratio and proportion method or the dimensional analysis method to determine the flow rate in millilitres per hour.
> - Remember: 60 min = 1 h.
> - Note that an alternative formula can be used to determine the flow rate in millilitres per hour for an infusion time period that is less than 1 hour:
>
> $$x \text{ mL/h} = \dfrac{\text{Total mL to infuse}}{\text{Number of min to infuse}} \times 60 \text{ min/h}$$
>
> - Round millilitres per hour to a whole number or the nearest tenth, depending on the equipment used.
> - Always know the equipment being used by the institution before rounding to a whole number.

PRACTICE **PROBLEMS**

Calculate the flow rate in millilitres per hour using an electronic pump. For convenience, the solution and infusion time are provided. Understand that in the real world, you may be the one to decide the solution and infusion time, based on various factors, including patient condition, the institution's policy, or other influences.

1. 1 800 mL $\frac{2}{3} - \frac{1}{3}$ NS in 24 h by infusion pump _____

2. 2 000 mL D5W in 24 h by infusion pump _____

3. 500 mL RL in 12 h by infusion pump _____

4. 100 mL 0.45% NS in 45 min by infusion pump _____

5. 1 500 mL D5RL in 24 h by infusion pump _____

6. 750 mL D5W in 16 h by infusion pump _____

7. Ampicillin 750 mg IV in 30 mL NS over 20 min by infusion pump _____

8. Ceftizoxime 500 mg IV in 50 mL NS over 15 min by infusion pump _____

9. Ceftriaxone 1500 mg IV in 100 mL over 1 h by infusion pump _____

10. Ondansetron 4 mg IV in 50 mL D5W over 15 min by infusion pump _____

Answers on page 554.

Calculating Flow Rates in Drops per Minute

When an electronic infusion device is not used, the nurse manually regulates the IV flow rate. For a manually regulated IV, the nurse must calculate the flow rate as the number of drops per minute (gtt/min).

IV flow rates in drops per minute are determined by the type of IV administration tubing. The drop size is regulated by the size of the tubing (the larger the tubing, the larger the drops). The first step in calculating the IV flow rate in drops per minute is to identify the type of tubing and its calibration. The calibration of the tubing is printed on each IV administration package (Figure 20-1). It is essential to know the size of tubing when an IV is manually regulated.

The same tubing used to manually regulate an IV is usually compatible with the electronic infusion devices used by an institution. Once the tubing is set up on an electronic infusion device, the infusion rate is expressed in millilitres per hour.

Intravenous Tubing

IV tubing has a drop chamber. The nurse determines the flow rate by adjusting the clamp and observing the drop chamber to count the drops per minute (Figure 20-2). The size of the drop depends on the type of IV tubing used. The calibration of IV tubing in **drops per millilitre (gtt/mL)** is known as the *drop factor* and is indicated on the box in which the IV tubing is packaged. The drop factor, which is necessary to calculate flow rates, is also shown on the packaging of IV administration sets (see Figure 20-1).

The two common types of tubing used to administer IV fluids are discussed next.

Macrodrop Tubing

Macrodrop (macrogtt) is the standard type of tubing used for general IV administration. This type of tubing delivers a certain number of drops per millilitre, as specified by the manufacturer. Macrodrop tubing delivers 10, 15, or 20 drops equal to 1 mL. Macrodrops

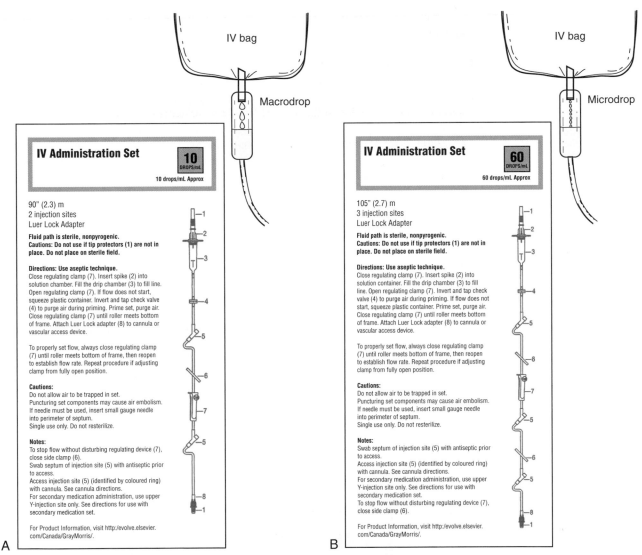

IV bag

Macrodrop

IV Administration Set **10** DROPS/mL

10 drops/mL Approx

90" (2.3) m
2 injection sites
Luer Lock Adapter

Fluid path is sterile, nonpyrogenic.
Cautions: Do not use if tip protectors (1) are not in
place. Do not place on sterile field.

Directions: Use aseptic technique.
Close regulating clamp (7). Insert spike (2) into
solution chamber. Fill the drip chamber (3) to fill line.
Open regulating clamp (7). If flow does not start,
squeeze plastic container. Invert and tap check valve
(4) to purge air during priming. Prime set, purge air.
Close regulating clamp (7) until roller meets bottom
of frame. Attach Luer Lock adapter (8) to cannula or
vascular access device.

To properly set flow, always close regulating clamp
(7) until roller meets bottom of frame, then reopen
to establish flow rate. Repeat procedure if adjusting
clamp from fully open position.

Cautions:
Do not allow air to be trapped in set.
Puncturing set components may cause air embolism.
If needle must be used, insert small gauge needle
into perimeter of septum.
Single use only. Do not resterilize.

Notes:
To stop flow without disturbing regulating device (7),
close side clamp (6).
Swab septum of injection site (5) with antiseptic prior
to access.
Access injection site (5) (identified by coloured ring)
with cannula. See cannula directions.
For secondary medication administration, use upper
Y-injection site only. See directions for use with
secondary medication set.

For Product Information, visit http://evolve.elsevier.
com/Canada/GrayMorris/.

A

IV bag

Microdrop

IV Administration Set **60** DROPS/mL

60 drops/mL Approx

105" (2.7) m
3 injection sites
Luer Lock Adapter

Fluid path is sterile, nonpyrogenic.
Cautions: Do not use if tip protectors (1) are not in
place. Do not place on sterile field.

Directions: Use aseptic technique.
Close regulating clamp (7). Insert spike (2) into
solution container. Fill the drip chamber (3) to fill
line. Open regulating clamp (7). Invert and tap check
valve (4) to purge air during priming. If flow does not
start, squeeze plastic container. Prime set, purge air.
Close regulating clamp (7) until roller meets bottom
of frame. Attach Luer Lock adapter (8) to cannula or
vascular access device.

To properly set flow, always close regulating clamp
(7) until roller meets bottom of frame, then reopen
to establish flow rate. Repeat procedure if adjusting
clamp from fully open position.

Cautions:
Do not allow air to be trapped in set.
Puncturing set components may cause air embolism.
If needle must be used, insert small gauge needle
into perimeter of septum.
Single use only. Do not resterilize.

Notes:
Swab septum of injection site (5) with antiseptic prior
to access.
Access injection site (5) (identified by coloured ring)
with cannula. See cannula directions.
For secondary medication administration, use upper
Y-injection site only. See directions for use with
secondary medication set.
To stop flow without disturbing regulating device (7),
close side clamp (6).

For Product Information, visit http://evolve.elsevier.
com/Canada/GrayMorris/.

B

Figure 20-1 IV administration sets. **A,** Set with drop factor of 10 (10 gtt = 1 mL). **B,** Set with drop factor of 60 (60 gtt = 1 mL).

Figure 20-2 Observing the drop chamber to count drops per minute. (From Potter, P. A., Perry, A. G., Stockert, P., et al. (2013). *Fundamentals of nursing* (8th ed.). St. Louis: Mosby.)

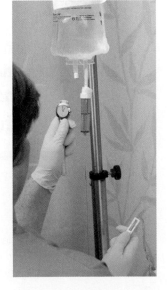

are large drops; therefore, large amounts of fluid are administered in macrodrops (see Figure 20-1, *A*). Most institutions stock one type of macrodrop tubing for routine IV adult administration (e.g., 10 gtt per mL). Always read the IV tubing package and identify the drop factor of the tubing.

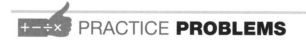

SAFETY ALERT!

The nurse must be aware of the drop factor to accurately administer IV fluids at the correct flow rate to a patient. Never assume the drop factor for macrodrop tubing; it can be 10, 15, or 20 gtt per mL. Knowing the drop factor of the IV tubing used can avoid an error in IV flow rate determination and prevent the patient from receiving IV fluid at the incorrect flow rate.

Microdrop Tubing

Microdrop (microgtt) tubing delivers tiny drops, which can be inferred from the prefix *micro*. It is used when small amounts and more exact measurements are needed, such as in pediatrics, for older adults, and in critical care settings. Microdrop tubing delivers 60 gtt equal to 1 mL. Because there are 60 minutes in an hour, the number of microdrops per minute is equal to the number of millilitres per hour. For example, if a patient is receiving 100 mL per hour, he or she is receiving 100 microgtt per min (see Figure 20-1, *B*).

Notice the size of the drops in Figure 20-1, *A* (macrodrop) and 20-1, *B* (microdrop).

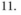 PRACTICE **PROBLEMS**

Identify the drop factor for the IV tubing label provided.

**Vented Basic Set
10 drops/mL** **10**

11. _____

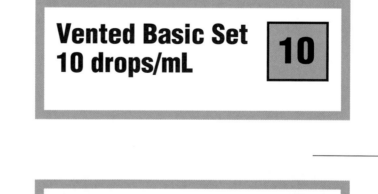

**Microdrip
Primary I.V. Set,
Vented, 178 cm** **60 DROPS/mL**

12. _____

**Non-Vented Burette Set
with Microbore Tubing
and Luer-Lock**

Macrodrop Set: Approx. 20 drops/mL

13. _____

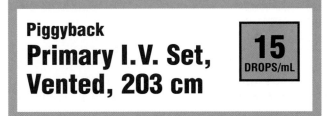

**Piggyback
Primary I.V. Set,
Vented, 203 cm**

**15
DROPS/mL**

14. _____

Answers on page 554.

POINTS TO REMEMBER

- Knowing the drop factor is the *FIRST* step in the accurate administration of IV fluids in drops per minute.
- The drop factor always appears on the package of IV tubing.
- Macrodrops are large and deliver 10, 15, or 20 gtt per mL.
- Microdrops are small and deliver 60 gtt per mL.
- Drop factor = drops per millilitre.

Calculating Flow Rates in Drops per Minute Using a Formula

The calculation of flow rates in drops per minute can be done by using a formula method or the dimensional analysis method. Although several formulas can be used, this chapter will focus on the most popular formula. The most common calculation necessary when an IV is manually regulated, or an electronic infusion device is not used, involves solving to determine the flow rate in drops per minute.

To calculate the flow rate at which an IV is to infuse, regardless of the method used (formula method or dimensional analysis), the nurse needs to know the following:

- The volume (amount) of solution in millilitres to infuse
- The drop factor (gtt/mL) of the IV tubing
- The time (minutes or hours) for the infusion

The Formula Method

This formula is used most often to calculate the flow rate in drops per minute, and the flow rate can be expressed as 60 minutes or less:

$$x \, \text{gtt/min} = \frac{\text{Amount of solution (mL)} \times \text{Drop factor (gtt/mL)}}{\text{Time (min)}}$$

Before calculating, let's review some basic principles:

1. Drops per minute are always expressed in whole numbers. Think: You cannot regulate an IV to half a drop, **you can only count whole drops;** therefore, drops are expressed in whole numbers.

2. The principles of rounding are applied if a calculation for drops per minute does not result in a whole number. Carry the calculation one decimal place and round the drops per minute to the nearest whole number. For example, 19.5 gtt per min is rounded to 20 gtt per min.

3. Answers must be labelled. The label is usually drops per minute unless otherwise specified. Examples: 100 gtt per min, 17 gtt per min.

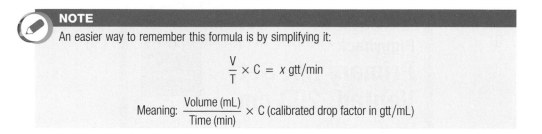

> **NOTE**
>
> An easier way to remember this formula is by simplifying it:
>
> $$\frac{V}{T} \times C = x \text{ gtt/min}$$
>
> Meaning: $\dfrac{\text{Volume (mL)}}{\text{Time (min)}} \times C \text{ (calibrated drop factor in gtt/mL)}$

Let's look at some sample problems step by step.

Example 1: Order: D5W to infuse at 100 mL/h. Drop factor: 10 gtt/mL. At what flow rate in drops per minute should the IV be regulated?

1. Set up the problem, placing the information given in the correct position in the formula.

$$x \text{ gtt/min} = \frac{100 \text{ mL} \times 10 \text{ gtt/mL}}{60 \text{ min}}$$

2. Reduce where possible to make numbers smaller and easier to manage. Note that the labels are dropped when performing mathematical steps.

$$x = \frac{100 \times \overset{1}{\cancel{10}}}{\underset{6}{\cancel{60}}} = \frac{100 \times 1}{6} = \frac{100}{6}$$

3. Divide $\dfrac{100}{6}$ to obtain the flow rate in drops per minute. Carry division one decimal place and round off to the nearest whole number.

$$x = \frac{100}{6} = 16.6$$

$$x = 17 \text{ gtt/min}$$

To deliver 100 mL per hour with a drop factor of 10 gtt per mL, the flow rate should be adjusted to 17 gtt per min.

Example 2: Order: IV medication in 50 mL NS in 20 min. Drop factor: microdrop (60 gtt/mL). At what flow rate in drops per minute should the IV be regulated?

$$x \text{ gtt/min} = \frac{50 \text{ mL} \times \overset{3}{\cancel{60}} \text{ gtt/mL}}{\underset{1}{\cancel{20}} \text{ min}}$$

$$x = \frac{50 \times 3}{1} = \frac{150}{1}$$

$$x = 150 \, \text{gtt}/\text{min}$$

To deliver 50 mL in 20 minutes with a drop factor of 60 gtt per mL, the IV should be adjusted to 150 gtt per min. This may sound like a lot; however, remember the type of IV tubing used is a microdrop, which always delivers 60 gtt per mL. It is a good idea to memorize this fact.

The Dimensional Analysis Method

Let's look at calculating the flow rate in drops per minute using the dimensional analysis method. Remember that IV fluids are ordered in small volumes of fluid that usually contain medication or in large volumes to infuse over several hours. Let's solve Examples 1 and 2 in the preceding section using the dimensional analysis method.

Example 1: Order: D5W to infuse at 100 mL/h. Drop factor: 10 gtt/mL. At what flow rate in drops per minute should the IV be regulated?

1. Set up the problem. You are calculating drops per minute, so write gtt/min to the left of the equation, followed by the equal sign (=), and label gtt/min with x since that is what you are looking for:

$$\frac{x \, \text{gtt}}{\text{min}} =$$

2. Extract the information that contains gtt from the problem; the drop factor is 10 gtt/1 mL. Write this factor into the equation, placing gtt in the numerator.

$$\frac{x \, \text{gtt}}{\text{min}} = \frac{10 \, \text{gtt}}{1 \, \text{mL}}$$

3. The next fraction is written so that the denominator matches the previous fraction (what you are looking for). Go back to the problem, and you will see that the order is to infuse 100 mL in 1 hour. Enter the 1 hour as 60 min in the denominator because you are calculating drops per minute (100 mL/60 min).

$$\frac{x \, \text{gtt}}{\text{min}} = \frac{10 \, \text{gtt}}{1 \, \text{mL}} \times \frac{100 \, \text{mL}}{60 \, \text{min}}$$

4. Now that you have the equation completed, cancel the units and notice that you are left with the desired drops per minute.

$$\frac{x \, \text{gtt}}{\text{min}} = \frac{10 \, \text{gtt}}{1 \, \cancel{\text{mL}}} \times \frac{100 \, \cancel{\text{mL}}}{60 \, \text{min}}$$

$$x = \frac{100 \times \cancel{10}^{1}}{\cancel{60}_{6}} = \frac{100}{6}$$

$$x = 16.6 = 17 \, \text{gtt}/\text{min}$$

Note: This example could have been solved without changing the hourly flow rate to 60 min, but it would have required the addition of a 1 h = 60 min conversion factor to the equation.

$$\frac{x \, \text{gtt}}{\text{min}} = \frac{10 \, \text{gtt}}{1 \, \text{mL}} \times \frac{100 \, \text{mL}}{1 \, \text{h}} \times \frac{1 \, \text{h}}{60 \, \text{min}}$$

The next step would have been to cancel the denominator/numerator mL and h, leaving the desired drops per minute.

$$\frac{x \text{ gtt}}{\text{min}} = \frac{10 \text{ gtt}}{1 \text{ mL}} \times \frac{100 \text{ mL}}{1 \text{ h}} \times \frac{1 \text{ h}}{60 \text{ min}}$$

$$x = \frac{100 \times \overset{1}{\cancel{10}}}{\underset{6}{\cancel{60}}} = \frac{100}{6}$$

$$x = 16.6 = 17 \text{ gtt/min}$$

Remember that reducing can make numbers smaller.

Example 2: Order: IV medication in 50 mL NS in 20 min. Drop factor: microdrop (60 gtt/mL). At what flow rate in drops per minute should the IV be regulated?

1. Set up the problem. You are calculating drops per minute, so write gtt/min to the left of the equation, followed by the equal sign (=), and label gtt/min with x, since that is what you are looking for:

$$\frac{x \text{ gtt}}{\text{min}} =$$

2. Extract the information that contains gtt from the problem; the drop factor is 60 gtt/1 mL. Write this factor in the equation, placing gtt in the numerator.

$$\frac{x \text{ gtt}}{\text{min}} = \frac{60 \text{ gtt}}{1 \text{ mL}}$$

3. The next fraction is written so that the denominator matches the previous fraction (what you are looking for). Go back to the problem, and you will see that the order is to infuse 50 mL in 20 min. Enter the third fraction so that 50 mL is in the numerator and 20 min is in the denominator.

$$\frac{x \text{ gtt}}{\text{min}} = \frac{60 \text{ gtt}}{1 \text{ mL}} \times \frac{50 \text{ mL}}{20 \text{ min}}$$

4. Now that you have the equation completed, cancel the units and notice that you are left with the desired drops per minute.

$$\frac{x \text{ gtt}}{\text{min}} = \frac{60 \text{ gtt}}{1 \text{ mL}} \times \frac{50 \text{ mL}}{20 \text{ min}}$$

$$x = \frac{60 \times \overset{5}{\cancel{50}}}{\underset{2}{\cancel{20}}} = \frac{300}{2}$$

$$x = 150 \text{ gtt/min}$$

In the rest of this chapter, the formula method is used in examples. Use the method of calculation you are comfortable with to calculate dosages.

PRACTICE **PROBLEMS**

Calculate the flow rate in drops per minute using any method of calculation.

15. Administer D5W at 75 mL/h.
    The drop factor is 10 gtt/mL.   _____

16. Administer D5 $\frac{1}{2}$ NS at 30 mL/h.

    The drop factor is a microdrop.   _____

17. Administer RL at 125 mL/h.
    The drop factor is 15 gtt/mL.   _____

18. Administer 1 000 mL D5 0.33% NS
    in 6 h. The drop factor is 15 gtt/mL.   _____

19. An IV medication in 60 mL of
    0.9% NS is to be administered in 45 min.
    The drop factor is a microdrop.   _____

20. 1 000 mL of Ringer's lactate solution
    (RL) is to infuse in 16 h. The drop
    factor is 15 gtt/mL.   _____

21. Infuse 150 mL of $\frac{2}{3} - \frac{1}{3}$ NS in 2 h.

    The drop factor is 20 gtt/mL.   _____

22. Administer 3 000 mL D5 and $\frac{1}{2}$ NS in 24 h.
    The drop factor is 10 gtt/mL.   _____

23. Infuse 2 000 mL D5W in 12 h.
    The drop factor is 15 gtt/mL.   _____

24. An IV medication in 60 mL D5W is to be administered
    in 30 min. The drop factor is a microdrop.   _____

Answers on pages 554–555.

Calculating Flow Rates in Drops per Minute Using the Shortcut Method

A shortcut method can be used to calculate drops per minute only in settings where the IV sets have the same drop factor. Example: an institution where all the macrodrop sets deliver 10 gtt per mL. This method can also be used with microdrop sets (60 gtt/mL). It is important to note that this method can be used only if the rate of the IV infusion ordered is expressed in millilitres per hour (or mL/60 min). It is imperative that nurses become familiar with the administration equipment at the institution where they work.

To use the shortcut method, you must know the drop factor constant for the administration set you are using. The drop factor constant is sometimes referred to as the *division factor*. To obtain the drop factor constant (division factor) for the IV administration set being used, divide 60 by the drop factor calibration. Box 20-1 shows the drop factor constant calculated based on the drop factor of tubing.

BOX 20-1 Drop Factor Constants	
Drop Factor of Tubing	**Drop Factor Constant**
10 gtt/mL	$\dfrac{60}{10} = 6$
15 gtt/mL	$\dfrac{60}{15} = 4$
20 gtt/mL	$\dfrac{60}{20} = 3$
60 gtt/mL	$\dfrac{60}{60} = 1$

Example: The drop factor for an IV administration set is 15 gtt/mL. Obtain the drop factor constant.

Solution: $\dfrac{60}{15} = 4$

The drop factor constant is 4.

RULE

After the drop factor constant is determined, the drops per minute can be calculated in one step:

$$x \text{ gtt/min} = \frac{\text{mL/h}}{\text{gtt factor constant}}$$

PRACTICE **PROBLEMS**

Calculate the drop factor constant for the following IV sets.

25. 20 gtt/mL _____

26. 10 gtt/mL _____

27. 60 gtt/mL _____

Answers on page 556.

Now that you know how to determine the drop factor constant, let's look at examples that use the shortcut method to calculate drops per minute.

Example: Administer 0.9% NS at 100 mL/h. The drop factor is 20 gtt/mL. The drop factor constant is 3.

✔ Solution Using the Shortcut Method

This problem can be solved by using the shortcut method once you know the drop factor constant (division factor).

$$x \text{ gtt}/\text{min} = \frac{100 \text{ mL/h}}{3} = 33.3 = 33 \text{ gtt}/\text{min}$$

$$x = 33 \text{ gtt}/\text{min}$$

Notice that the 100 mL per hour rate divided by the drop factor constant gives the same answer.

Example: Administer 0.9% NS at 75 mL/h. The drop factor is 60 gtt/mL. The drop factor constant is 1.

✔ Solution Using the Shortcut Method

Calculate the drops per minute.

$$x \, \text{gtt}/\text{min} = \frac{75 \, \text{mL}/\text{h}}{1} = 75 \, \text{gtt}/\text{min}$$

$$x = 75 \, \text{gtt}/\text{min}$$

 PRACTICE **PROBLEMS**

Calculate the flow rate in drops per minute using the shortcut method.

28. Order: D5W 200 mL/h.
    Drop factor: 10 gtt/mL. _____

29. Order: $\dfrac{2}{3} - \dfrac{1}{3}$ NS 50 mL/h.
    Drop factor: 15 gtt/mL. _____

30. Order: 0.45% NS 80 mL/h.
    Drop factor: 60 gtt/mL. _____

31. Order: 0.9% NS 140 mL/h.
    Drop factor: 20 gtt/mL. _____

Answers on page 556.

Remember that the shortcut method (using the drop factor constant) can be used to calculate the drops per minute for any volume of fluid that can be stated in millilitres per hour (or mL/60 min).

> **RULE**
>
> The shortcut method can be used if the volume is large, as is the case in the example that follows. However, an additional step of converting the order to millilitres per hour must be done first. Then, you can proceed to calculate the drops per minutes using the shortcut method.

Example: Order: RL 1 500 mL in 12 h. Drop factor: 15 gtt/mL. Drop factor constant: 4.

$$1\,500 \, \text{mL} \div 12 = 125 \, \text{mL}/\text{h}$$

✔ Solution Using the Shortcut Method

Now that you have the millilitres per hour, you can proceed with the shortcut method, using the drop factor constant.

$$x \, \text{gtt}/\text{min} = \frac{125 \, \text{mL}}{4} = 31.2 = 31 \, \text{gtt}/\text{min}$$

$$x = 31 \, \text{gtt}/\text{min}$$

Example: Order: 20 mL D5W in 30 min. Drop factor: 15 gtt/mL. Drop factor constant: 4.

NOTE

It is important to realize that with a microdrop, which delivers 60 gtt per mL, the drops per minute will be the same as the millilitres per hour. This is because the set calibration is 60, and the drop factor constant is based on 60 minutes (1 h); therefore, the drop factor constant is 1.

✔ Solution Using the Shortcut Method

If the volume of fluid to be infused is small, the volume and the time must each be multiplied to get millilitres per hour. To express this order in millilitres per hour, you multiply by 2.

$$2 \, \text{mL}/30 \, \text{min} = (20 \times 2)/(2 \times 30 \, \text{min}) = 40 \, \text{mL/h}$$

$$x \, \text{gtt/min} = \frac{40 \, \text{mL}}{4} = 10 \, \text{gtt/min}$$

$$x = 10 \, \text{gtt/min}$$

✚−÷✕ PRACTICE **PROBLEMS**

Calculate the flow rate in drops per minute using the shortcut method.

32. Order: 1 000 mL D5W in 10 h.
    Drop factor: 10 gtt/mL.   _____

33. Order: 1 500 mL RL in 12 h.
    Drop factor: 15 gtt/mL.   _____

34. Order: 40 mL D5W in 20 min.
    Drop factor: 10 gtt/mL.   _____

35. Order: $\frac{2}{3}$ dextrose − $\frac{1}{3}$ NaCl with 20 units
    Pitocin for 2 L at 125 mL/h.
    Drop factor: 15 gtt/mL.   _____

36. Order: 1 000 mL D5 0.9% NS
    for 3 L at 100 mL/h.
    Drop factor: microdrop.   _____

Answers on pages 556–557.

NOTE

In hospitals, IV solutions and medications are regulated by electronic pumps more often than they are regulated manually by gravity. Electronic infusion devices are set to deliver a specific flow rate per hour. Special IV tubing is usually required for the device, and calculations are based on that tubing. Institutions usually use the same primary and secondary IV tubing for electronic infusion devices as they do for manually regulated IVs.

⚙ POINTS TO REMEMBER

- To calculate the IV flow rate in drops per minute, begin by identifying the volume of solution, the time factor for the IV to infuse, and the drop factor of the IV tubing.
- Note that the drop factor is expressed as drops per millilitre (gtt/mL) and indicated on the package of the IV tubing.
- Calculate drops per minute by using the formula method or the dimensional analysis method.
- Use this formula to calculate drops per minute:

$$x \, \text{gtt/min} = \frac{\text{Amount of solution (mL)} \times \text{Drop factor (gtt/mL)}}{\text{Time (min)}}$$

- The formula is used for any time period that can be expressed as 60 minutes or less.
- For a time period greater than 60 minutes, find the millilitres per hour first, and then use the formula to determine drops per minute.
- Round drops per minute to the nearest whole number (division carried one decimal place).
- Note that the shortcut method can be used to calculate flow rates in millilitres per hour. It cannot be used if the infusion time period is less than 1 hour and is calculated in minutes.
- To determine the drop constant factor for an IV set, divide 60 by the calibration of the set.

✛－÷✕ PRACTICE **PROBLEMS**

Practice Problems and Chapter Review problems state the main volume for the medication ordered. Keep in mind that this is not usually the case when medication is ordered.

Calculate the flow rate in millilitres per hour or drops per minute as indicated for the following medications being administered IV. Use the labels where provided. (Add the volume of medication being added to the IV solution if it is 10 mL or greater.)

37. Order: Doxycycline 50 mg IV in
    D5W 100 mL over 1 h via infusion
    pump. What is the flow rate of the
    infusion in mL per hour?   _____

38. Order: Erythromycin 200 mg in
    250 mL D5W to infuse over 1 h.
    Drop factor: 10 gtt/mL. What is the
    flow rate of the infusion in gtt per min?   _____

39. Order: Ampicillin 1 g is added to 50 mL D5W to infuse over 45 minutes. Drop factor: 10 gtt/mL. For the IV, reconstitute with 10 mL of diluent to get 1 g per 10 mL. (Consider the medication added in the volume of fluid.)

    a. If the medication is to be infused
       via pump, at what flow rate in mL
       per hour should the nurse program
       the pump?   _____

    b. At what flow rate in gtt per min
       should the nurse infuse the IV
       if it is manually regulated?   _____

40. Order: Clindamycin 900 mg in 75 mL D5W over 30 min. Drop factor: 10 gtt/mL.

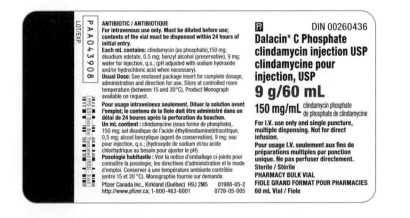

    a. How many mL of medication
       must be added to the solution?   _____

    b. Calculate the flow rate in mL
       per hour at which the IV
       should infuse.   _____

41. Order: Cimetidine 300 mg IVPB q8h. The medication has been added to 50 mL D5W to infuse over 30 min. Drop factor: 10 gtt/mL.

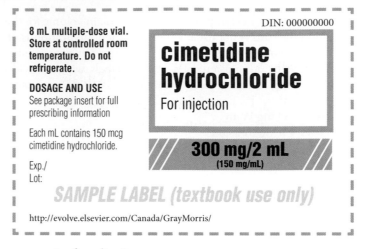

8 mL multiple-dose vial. Store at controlled room temperature. Do not refrigerate.

DOSAGE AND USE
See package insert for full prescribing information

Each mL contains 150 mcg cimetidine hydrochloride.

Exp./
Lot:

DIN: 000000000

cimetidine hydrochloride

For injection

300 mg/2 mL
(150 mg/mL)

SAMPLE LABEL (textbook use only)

http://evolve.elsevier.com/Canada/GrayMorris/

a. How many mL of medication must be added to the solution? _____

b. Calculate the flow rate in mL per hour at which the IV should infuse. _____

42. Order: Vancomycin 500 mg IVPB q24h. The reconstituted vancomycin provides 50 mg/mL. The medication is placed in 100 mL of D5W to infuse over 60 minutes. Drop factor: 15 gtt/mL.

a. At what flow rate in mL per hour should the nurse set the infusion pump to administer the medication? _____

b. At what flow rate in gtt per min should the nurse infuse the IV medication? _____

43. Order: Amphotericin B 20 mg IV Soluset (IVSS) in 300 mL D5W over 6 h. The reconstituted material contains 50 mg/10 mL. Drop factor: 60 gtt/mL.

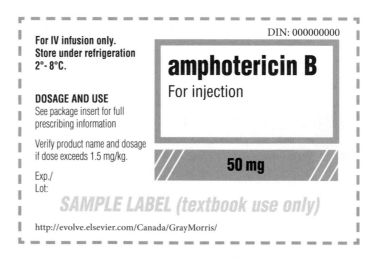

For IV infusion only. Store under refrigeration 2°- 8°C.

DOSAGE AND USE
See package insert for full prescribing information

Verify product name and dosage if dose exceeds 1.5 mg/kg.

Exp./
Lot:

DIN: 000000000

amphotericin B

For injection

50 mg

SAMPLE LABEL (textbook use only)

http://evolve.elsevier.com/Canada/GrayMorris/

a. What should be the flow rate of the medication infusion in mL per hour? _____

b. At what flow rate in gtt per min should the IV be infused? _____

44. Order: Sulfamethoxazole and trimethoprim 300 mg in 300 mL D5W over 1 h q6h. Drop factor: 10 gtt/mL. Calculate the dose using trimethoprim.

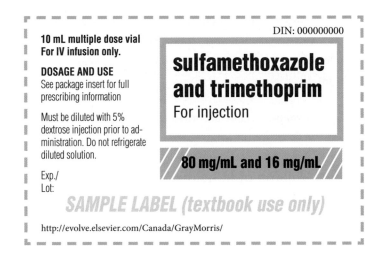

   a. How many mL of medication will be added to the IV? (Round answer to nearest tenth.)   _____

   b. Consider the medication added to the volume of IV fluid. Calculate the flow rate in gtt per min at which the IV should infuse.   _____

45. Order: Zidovudine (Retrovir) 100 mg IV q4h over 1 h. Available medication states each mL contains 10 mg of zidovudine. The medication is placed in 100 mL of D5W. Drop factor: 10 gtt/mL. What is the flow rate in mL per hour if infused via pump?

Answers on pages 557–558.

Determining Infusion Time and Volume

You may need to calculate the following:
- **Infusion time in hours**—How long it will take a certain amount of fluid to infuse or how long it may last.
- **Volume of infusion**—The total number of millilitres a patient will receive in a certain time period.

   These unknown elements can be determined by the use of the formula method or the dimensional analysis method.

Calculating Total Infusion Time in Hours
Formula

$$\text{Total infusion time in hours:} \quad \frac{\text{Total volume (mL)}}{\text{mL/h}} = \text{Total time (h)}$$

Example: Order: IV NS 500 mL infusing at 125 mL/h. How many hours will it take for the 500 mL to infuse?

Solution: $\dfrac{500 \ \cancel{mL}}{125 \ \cancel{mL}/h} = 4\,h$

> **NOTE**
> When you are calculating time intervals and the answer is in hours and minutes, express the entire time in hours. For example, 1 hour and 30 minutes = 1.5 h or $1\frac{1}{2}$ h; $1\frac{1}{2}$ h is the preferred term.

The infusion will take 4 hours to complete.

Example: Order: IV $\frac{2}{3} - \frac{1}{3}$ NS 1 000 mL at 80 mL/h starting at the beginning of shift at 0800. At what time should the total volume be absorbed?

Solution: $\frac{1\,000\ \text{mL}}{80\ \text{mL/h}} = 12.5\,\text{h} = 12\frac{1}{2}\,\text{h}$

The total volume will be absorbed at $0800 + 12\frac{1}{2} = 2030$.

Calculating Total Volume of Infusion
Formula

Total volume of infusion: Total time (h) × mL/h = Total volume (mL)

Example: A patient's IV D5W is infusing via electronic pump at 150 mL/h. How many mL should infuse in the next 12-h shift?

Solution: 12 h × 150 mL/h = 1 800 mL

The total volume of the infusion is 1 800 mL.

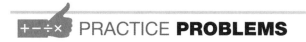 PRACTICE **PROBLEMS**

Calculate the infusion time or infusion volume as indicated.

46. You find that there is 150 mL of D5W left in an IV. The IV is infusing at 60 mL/h. How many hours will the fluid last?   _____

47. 0.9% NS is infusing at 140 mL/h. How many mL of fluid will the patient receive in 5 hours?   _____

48. 180 mL of $\frac{2}{3} - \frac{1}{3}$ NS is left in an IV that is infusing at 180 mL/h. How many hours will the fluid last?   _____

49. D5 $\frac{1}{2}$ NS is infusing at 180 mL/h. How many mL will the patient receive in 8 hours?   _____

50. There is 90 mL of D5 0.33% NS left in an IV that is infusing at 60 mL/h. How many hours will the fluid last?   _____

Answers on page 558.

Recalculating an Intravenous Flow Rate

Flow rates on IVs change when a patient stands, sits, or is repositioned in bed if IVs are infusing by gravity. Therefore, nurses must frequently check flow rates. IVs are generally labelled with a start and finish time as well as markings with specific time periods. Sometimes IVs infuse ahead of schedule, or they may be behind schedule if they are not monitored closely. When this happens, the IV flow rate must be recalculated. To recalculate the flow rate, the nurse uses the volume remaining and the time remaining. Recalculation may be done with uncomplicated infusions. IVs that require exact infusion rates should be monitored by an electronic infusion device.

> **⚠ SAFETY ALERT!**
>
> Never arbitrarily increase or decrease an IV to get it back on schedule without assessing a patient and checking with the prescriber. Increasing or decreasing the flow rate without thought can result in serious harm to a patient. Check the institution's policy. Avoid off-schedule IV flow rates by regularly monitoring the IV at least every 30 to 60 minutes.

When an IV is significantly ahead of or behind schedule, you may need to notify the prescriber, depending on the patient's condition and the use of appropriate nursing judgment. **Always assess the patient** before making any change to an IV flow rate. Changes depend on the patient's condition. Check the institution's policy regarding the percentage of adjustment that can be made. Each situation must be individually evaluated, and appropriate action must be taken.

A safe rule is that the recalculated flow rate should not vary from the original flow rate by more than 25%. If the recalculated flow rate varies by more than 25% from the original flow rate, the prescriber should be notified. The order may require revision. If a patient is stable, recalculate the IV flow rate, using the remaining volume and time, and then proceed to calculate millilitres per hour using the formula method or the dimensional analysis method.

Let's go over the steps to recalculate an IV flow rate, if allowed by the institution's policy and the patient is stable.

To recalculate an IV flow rate:

1. Use the remaining volume and remaining hours, and calculate the flow rate in millilitres per hour.

$$x\,\text{mL/h} = \frac{\text{Remaining volume (mL)}}{\text{Remaining time (h)}}$$

2. Determine whether the new flow rate calculation is greater or less than 25%. Use the amount of increase or decrease divided by the original flow rate.

$$\frac{\text{Amount of} \uparrow \text{or} \downarrow}{\text{Original rate}} = \%\ \text{of variation of original rate (round to nearest whole percent)}$$

Let's look at some examples. *Note:* all examples assume that the institution allows a 25% IV flow rate variation and the patient is stable.

Example: **IV Behind Schedule.** 1 000 mL of D5RL was to infuse in 8 hours at 125 mL per hour. After 4 hours, you notice 700 mL of fluid left in the IV. Recalculate the flow rate for the remaining solution. *Note:* The infusion is behind schedule. After 4 hours, half of the volume (or 500 mL) should have infused.

Solution: Time remaining: 8 h − 4 h = 4 h

$$\text{Volume remaining: } 1\,000\text{ mL} - 300\text{ mL} = 700\text{ mL}$$

$$700\text{ mL} \div 4 = 175\text{ mL/h}$$

$$x\text{ mL/h} = \frac{700\text{ mL}}{4\text{ h}} = 175\text{ mL/h}$$

Determine the percentage of change:

$$\frac{175\text{ mL} - 125\text{ mL}}{125\text{ mL}} = \frac{50}{125} = 0.4 = 40\%$$

In this situation, the flow rate must be increased from 125 to 175 mL per hour, which is more than 25% of the original flow rate. Always assess the patient first to determine the patient's ability to tolerate an increase in fluid. In addition to assessing the patient's status, you should notify the prescriber. A new order is needed since the recalculated flow rate is 40%, which exceeds the 25% benchmark.

Course of Action: Assess the patient; notify the prescriber. This increase could result in serious consequences for the patient. Do not increase the flow rate. The increase is greater than 25%.

Example: **IV Ahead of Schedule.** An IV of 1 000 mL D5W is to infuse from 0800 to 1600 (8 h). The flow rate is set at 125 mL per hour. In 5 hours, you notice that 700 mL has infused. Recalculate the flow rate for the remaining solution.

Solution: Time remaining: 8 h − 5 h = 3 h

$$\text{Volume remaining: } 1\,000\text{ mL} - 700\text{ mL} = 300\text{ mL}$$

$$300\text{ mL} \div 3 = 100\text{ mL/h}$$

Determine the percentage of change:

$$\frac{100\text{ mL} - 125\text{ mL}}{125\text{ mL}} = \frac{-25}{125} = -0.2 = -20\%$$

In this situation, the flow rate must be decreased from 125 to 100 mL per hour, but this is not a change greater than 25% of the original; −20% is within the acceptable 25% range of change. However, the patient's condition must still be assessed to determine the ability to tolerate the change, and the prescriber may still require notification.

Course of Action: This is an acceptable decrease; it is less than 25%. Assess the patient, adjust the flow rate, and assess the patient during the remainder of the infusion.

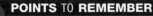

POINTS TO REMEMBER

- Monitor IV therapy every 30 to 60 minutes to maintain the IV flow rate ordered.
- Do not arbitrarily speed up or slow down an IV that is behind or ahead of schedule.
- Know your institution's policy regarding the recalculation of IV flow rates. An IV should not vary more than 25% from its original flow rate.
- To recalculate an IV flow rate:
- Determine millilitres per hour:

$$x \, mL/h = \frac{Remaining \; volume \, (mL)}{Remaining \; time \, (h)}$$

- Determine the % of change:

$$\frac{Amount \; of \uparrow or \downarrow}{Original \; rate} = \% \; of \; variation \; of \; original \; rate \, (round \; to \; nearest \; whole \; percent)$$

- Contact the prescriber for a new IV order if the recalculated flow rate exceeds 25% of the original flow rate.

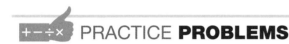

PRACTICE **PROBLEMS**

For each of the problems, recalculate the IV flow rates in millilitres per hour. Determine the percentage of change, and state your course of action. *Note:* The institution allows 25% IV flow rate variation and patients are stable.

51. 500 mL of 0.9% NS was to infuse in 8 h at 63 mL/h.

    After 5 hours, you find 250 mL of fluid left.

    a. _____ mL per hour

    b. _____ %

    c. _____ Course of action

52. 250 mL of D5W was to infuse in 3 h at 83 mL/h. With $1\frac{1}{2}$ hours remaining, you find 200 mL left.

    a. _____ mL per hour

    b. _____ %

    c. _____ Course of action

53. 1 500 mL $\frac{2}{3} - \frac{1}{3}$ NS was to infuse in 12 h at 125 mL/h. After 6 hours, 650 mL has infused.

    a. _____ mL per hour

    b. _____ %

    c. _____ Course of action

54. 1 000 mL D5 0.33% NS was to infuse in 12 h at 83 mL/h. After 4 hours, 250 mL has infused.

    a. _____ mL per hour

    b. _____ %

    c. _____ Course of action

55. 500 mL D5 0.9% NS was to infuse in 5 h at 100 mL/h. After 2 hours, 250 mL has infused.

    a. _____ mL per hour

    b. _____ %

    c. _____ Course of action

Answers on pages 558–559.

Charting Intravenous Therapy

At some institutions, continuous IV therapy may be charted on a special IV record or IV flow sheet. Medications that are administered intermittently by IVPB are charted on the MAR. The forms used to chart IV therapy (whether a patient is receiving an IV solution that contains medications or a solution without medications) vary from institution to institution.

Labelling Solution Bags

The markings on IV solution bags are not as precise as, for example, those on a syringe. Most IV bags are marked in increments of 50 to 100 mL. After calculating the amount of solution to infuse in 1 hour, the nurse may mark the bag to indicate where the level of fluid should be at each hour. Marking the IV bag allows the nurse to check that the fluid is infusing on time, especially if the IV is regulated manually. Many institutions have commercially prepared labels for this purpose. Figure 20-3 shows an IV bag with timing tape for visualizing the amount infused each hour. The tape should indicate the start and finish times. When the IV is on a pump, the nurse does not usually mark the IV bag. Volume absorbed and volume to be absorbed may be monitored on the pump system itself.

Administration of Medications by Intravenous Push

Injection ports on IV tubing can be used for direct injection of medication with a syringe, which is called an *IV push*. When using the primary line, the medication should be administered through the port closest to the patient. An IV push medication can also be administered using a saline or heparin lock, which can be attached to the IV catheter. A saline lock indicates that saline is used to flush or maintain IV catheter patency, whereas a heparin lock indicates that heparin is used to maintain the IV catheter patency. Medications can be administered with an IV push by attaching the syringe to the lock and pushing in the medication. The lock is usually flushed after administration of the medication.

When medication is administered by IV push, the patient experiences rapid results from the medication. Direct IV administration is used to deliver diluted or undiluted medication over a brief period (seconds or minutes). Medication literature and institutional guidelines provide the acceptable flow rate for IV push medication administration. Because of the rapidity of action, an error in calculation can result in a serious outcome. Medications can be administered by IV push by registered nurses (RNs) who have been specially trained in this practice at some institutions. Nursing students, RNs, and registered practical nurses (RPNs) who do not practise in a **critical care setting** are unlikely to administer a medication by IV push. Instead, they administer medication via secondary line or IVPB. An *IV*

Figure 20-3 IV solution with time taping. (From Potter, P. A., Perry, A. G., Stockert, P. A., et al. (2011). *Basic nursing* (7th ed.). St. Louis: Mosby.)

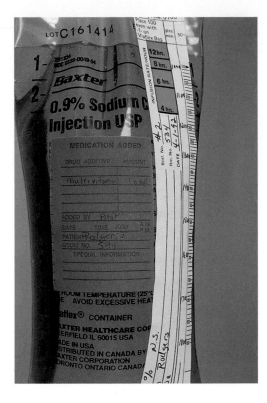

bolus indicates that a volume of IV fluid is infused over a specific period of time through an IV administration set.

Most IV push medications should be administered over a period of 1 to 5 minutes (or longer). The volume of the prescribed medication should be calculated in increments of 15 to 30 seconds. The use of a watch during IV push medications helps to provide accurate administration. The actual administration of IV push medications is beyond the scope of this text. For a detailed description of the technique, consult a clinical skills textbook.

> **SAFETY ALERT!**
>
> Never infuse IV medications more rapidly than recommended. Carefully read the literature for instructions on dilution and time for administration. IV medications are potent and rapid acting.

 CLINICAL **REASONING**

1. **Scenario:** An older adult patient has an order for 1 000 mL D5W at 100 mL per hour. The nurse assigned to the patient attached IV tubing to the IV with a drop factor of 10 gtt per mL without checking the package of IV tubing. As a habit from a previous institution where she worked, the IV flow rate was calculated based on the drop factor of 20 gtt per mL. At the beginning of the next shift, the nurse making rounds noticed that the patient was having difficulty breathing and seemed restless. When the nurse checked the IV flow rate, she discovered that it was 33 gtt per min instead of 17 gtt per min.

    a. What factors contributed to the error? _____

    b. How did the IV flow rate contribute to the problem and why? _____

    c. What should have been the action of the nurse who attached the IV tubing in relation to IV administration? _____

Answers on page 559.

CHAPTER REVIEW

Calculate the flow rate in drops per minute for the following IV administrations.

1. 1 000 mL D5RL to infuse in 8 h.
   Drop factor: 20 gtt/mL.   _____

2. 2 500 mL D5NS to infuse in 24 h.
   Drop factor: 10 gtt/mL.   _____

3. 500 mL D5W to infuse in 4 h.
   Drop factor: 15 gtt/mL.   _____

4. 300 mL NS to infuse in 6 h.
   Drop factor: 60 gtt/mL.   _____

5. 1 000 mL D5W for 24 h KVO (keep
   vein open). Drop factor: 60 gtt/mL.   _____

Calculate the flow rate in millilitres per hour for the following IV administrations.

6. 1 500 mL D5W in 8 h.   _____

7. 3 000 mL RL in 24 h.   _____

8. Infuse 2 L RL in 24 h.   _____

9. 500 mL D5W in 4 h.   _____

10. 1 000 mL D5 0.45% NS in 6 h.   _____

11. Infuse an IV medication with a
    volume of 50 mL in 45 min.   _____

12. Infuse 90 mL/h of NS.   _____

13. Infuse an IV medication in 50 mL
    of 0.9% NS in 40 min.   _____

14. Infuse an IV medication in 100 mL D5W
    in 30 min.   _____

15. Infuse vancomycin 1 g IVPB in
    150 mL D5W in 1.5 h.   _____

16. An IV of D5W 500 mL was to infuse
    over 10 h at 50 mL/h. After 3 hours,
    you notice that 300 mL of IV solution is left.
    Recalculate the flow rate in mL per hour for
    the remaining solution.   _____ mL per hour
    Determine the percentage of change in IV
    flow rate, and state your course of action.   _____ %

17. A patient is receiving 1 000 mL of D5W
    at 100 mL/h. How many hours will it take
    for the IV to infuse?   _____

18. 10 mmol of potassium chloride is placed
    in 500 mL of D5W to be administered at
    the rate of 2 mmol/h. At what flow rate
    in mL per hour should the IV be infused?   _____

19. 25 mmol of potassium chloride is added to
    1 000 mL of D5W to be administered at the
    rate of 4 mmol/h. At what flow rate in mL
    per hour should the IV be infused?   _____

20. Order: Humulin Regular 7 units/h.
    The IV solution contains 50 units of
    Humulin Regular insulin in 250 mL
    of 0.9% NS. At what flow rate in mL
    per hour should the IV be infused?   _____

21. Order: Humulin Regular 18 units/h.
    The IV solution contains 100 units of
    Humulin Regular insulin in 250 mL of
    0.9% NS. At what flow rate in mL per
    hour should the IV be infused?   _____

22. A volume of 150 mL of NS is
    to infuse at 25 mL/h.   _____

    a. Calculate the infusion time.   _____

    b. The IV was started at 3:10 AM.
       What time will the IV be completed?
       State the time in traditional and military time.   _____

23. Order: Lasix 120 mg IV stat.
    Available: 10 mg per mL. The literature states IV
    not to exceed 40 mg/min.

    a. How many mL will you prepare?   _____

    b. Calculate the time required to
       administer the medication ordered.   _____

24. Order: Levaquin 500 mg IVPB in
    100 mL 0.9% NS q12h over 1 h.
    Determine the flow rate in mL per hour.   _____

25. 500 mL D5W with 30 000 units of
    heparin to infuse at 1 500 units/h.
    Determine the flow rate in mL per hour.   _____

26. Order: Humulin Regular 15 units/h.
    The IV solution contains 100 units of
    Humulin Regular in 250 mL of 0.9% NS.
    At what flow rate in mL per hour should the
    IV be infused?   _____

Answers on pages 559–561.

evolve

For additional practice
problems, refer to the
Advanced Calculations
section of the Drug
Calculations Companion,
Version 5 on Evolve.

✳ ANSWERS

Answers to Practice Problems

1. $x \, \text{mL/h} = \dfrac{1\,800 \, \text{mL}}{24 \, \text{h}} \, ; x = 75 \, \text{mL/h}$

2. $x \, \text{mL/h} = \dfrac{2\,400 \, \text{mL}}{24 \, \text{h}} \, ; x = 83.3 = 83 \, \text{mL/h}$

3. $x \, \text{mL/h} = \dfrac{500 \, \text{mL}}{12 \, \text{h}} \, ; x = 41.6 = 42 \, \text{mL/h}$

4. *Remember:* when infusion time is less than an hour, use a ratio and proportion or the formula method to determine the flow rate in mL per h.

    $100 \, \text{mL} : 45 \, \text{min} = x \, \text{mL} : 60 \, \text{min}$

    $$\dfrac{45x}{45} = \dfrac{6\,000}{45} \, ; x = 133.3 \, ; x = 133 \, \text{mL/h}$$

    or

    $$x \, \text{mL/h} = \dfrac{100 \, \text{mL}}{\overset{}{\underset{3}{\cancel{45} \, \cancel{\text{min}}}}} \times \dfrac{\overset{4}{\cancel{60} \, \cancel{\text{min}} \, / \text{h}}}{1}$$

    $$x = \dfrac{400}{3} = x = 133.3 = 133 \, \text{mL/h}$$

5. $x \, \text{mL/h} = \dfrac{1\,500 \, \text{mL}}{24 \, \text{h}} \, ; x = 62.5 = 63 \, \text{mL/h}$

6. $x \, \text{mL/h} = \dfrac{750 \, \text{mL}}{16 \, \text{h}} \, ; x = 46.8 = 47 \, \text{mL/h}$

7. *Remember:* use only the information that is required in the formula. Do not get confused with the mg of medication. You are concerned with the **mL (volume)** that contains the amount (mg, g, mcg etc.) of medication.

    $30 \, \text{mL} : 20 \, \text{min} = x \, \text{mL} : 60 \, \text{min}$

    $$\dfrac{20x}{20} = \dfrac{1\,800}{20} = 90 \, ; x = 90 \, \text{mL/h}$$

    or

    $$x \, \text{mL/h} = \dfrac{30 \, \text{mL}}{\overset{}{\underset{1}{\cancel{20} \, \cancel{\text{min}}}}} \times \dfrac{\overset{3}{\cancel{60} \, \cancel{\text{min}} \, / \text{h}}}{1}$$

    $$x = \dfrac{90}{1} = x = 90 \, \text{mL/h}$$

8. $x \dfrac{\text{mL}}{\text{h}} = \dfrac{50 \, \text{mL}}{15 \, \text{min}} \times 60 \, \text{min/h} = 200 \, \text{mL/h}$

9. This problem could be solved mentally without calculation by just restating 100 mL per hour. However, let's use the formula method to calculate

    $$x \dfrac{\text{mL}}{\text{h}} = \dfrac{100 \, \text{mL}}{60 \, \text{min}} \times 60 \, \text{min/h} = 100 \, \text{mL/h}$$

10. $x \dfrac{\text{mL}}{\text{h}} = \dfrac{50 \, \text{mL}}{15 \, \text{min}} \times 60 \, \text{min/h} = 200 \, \text{mL/h}$

11. 10 gtt/mL

12. 60 gtt/mL

13. 20 gtt/mL

14. 15 gtt/mL

15. $x \, \text{gtt/min} = \dfrac{75 \, \text{mL} \times 10 \, \text{gtt/mL}}{60 \, \text{min}} =$

    $$\dfrac{75 \times 10}{60} = \dfrac{75 \times 1}{6} = \dfrac{75}{6}$$

    $$x = \dfrac{75}{6} \, ; x = 12.5 = 13 \, \text{gtt/min}$$

    Answer: 13 gtt per min

16. $x \, \text{gtt/min} = \dfrac{30 \, \text{mL} \times 60 \, \text{gtt/mL}}{60 \, \text{min}} =$

    $$\dfrac{30 \times 60}{60} = \dfrac{30 \times 1}{1} = \dfrac{30}{1}$$

    $$x = \dfrac{30}{1} \, ; x = 30 \, \text{gtt/min}$$

    Answer: 30 gtt per min

17. $x \, \text{gtt/min} = \dfrac{125 \, \text{mL} \times 15 \, \text{gtt/mL}}{60 \, \text{min}} =$

    $$\dfrac{125 \times 15}{60} = \dfrac{125 \times 1}{4} = \dfrac{125}{4}$$

    $$x = \dfrac{125}{4} \, ; x = 31.2 = 31 \, \text{gtt/min}$$

    Answer: 31 gtt per min

18. Step 1: Calculate mL/h.

$$x\text{ mL/h} = \frac{1\,000\text{ mL}}{6\text{ h}}; x = 166.6 = 167\text{ mL/h}$$

Step 2: Calculate gtt/min

$$x\text{ gtt/min} = \frac{167\text{ mL} \times 15\text{ gtt/mL}}{60\text{ min}} =$$

$$\frac{167 \times 15}{60} = \frac{167 \times 1}{4} = \frac{167}{4}$$

$$x = \frac{167}{4}; x = 41.7 = 42\text{ gtt/min}$$

Answer: 42 gtt per min

19. $x\text{ gtt/min} = \dfrac{60\text{ mL} \times 60\text{ gtt/mL}}{45\text{ min}} =$

$$\frac{60 \times 60}{45} = \frac{60 \times 4}{3} = \frac{240}{3}$$

$$x = \frac{240}{3}; x = 80\text{ gtt/min}$$

Answer: 80 gtt per min

NOTE

These problems could also be done by first determining the flow rate in millilitres per minute to be administered and then calculating the flow rate in drops per minute or by using dimensional analysis.

20. Step 1: Calculate mL per hour.

$$x\text{ mL/h} = \frac{1\,000\text{ mL}}{16\text{ h}}; x = 62.5 = 63\text{ mL/h}$$

Step 2: Calculate gtt per min.

$$x\text{ gtt/min} = \frac{60\text{ mL} \times 15\text{ gtt/mL}}{60\text{ min}} =$$

$$\frac{63 \times 15}{60} = \frac{63 \times 1}{4} = \frac{63}{4}$$

$$x = \frac{63}{4}; x = 15.7 = 16\text{ gtt/min}$$

Answer: 16 gtt per min

21. Step 1: Calculate mL per hour.

$$x\text{ mL/h} = \frac{150\text{ mL}}{2\text{ h}}; x = 75\text{ mL/h}$$

Step 2: Calculate gtt per min.

$$x\text{ gtt/min} = \frac{75\text{ mL} \times 20\text{ gtt/mL}}{60\text{ min}} =$$

$$\frac{75 \times 20}{60} = \frac{75 \times 1}{3} = \frac{75}{3}$$

$$x = \frac{75}{3}; x = 25\text{ gtt/min}$$

Answer: 25 gtt per min

22. Step 1: Calculate mL per hour.

$$x\text{ mL/h} = \frac{3\,000\text{ mL}}{24\text{ h}}; x = 125\text{ mL/h}$$

Step 2: Calculate gtt per min.

$$x\text{ gtt/min} = \frac{125\text{ mL} \times 10\text{ gtt/mL}}{60\text{ min}} =$$

$$\frac{125 \times 10}{60} = \frac{125 \times 1}{6} = \frac{125}{6}$$

$$x = \frac{125}{6}; x = 20.8 = 21\text{ gtt/min}$$

Answer: 21 gtt per min

23. Step 1: Calculate mL per hour.

$$x\text{ mL/h} = \frac{2\,000\text{ mL}}{12\text{ h}}; x = 166.6 = 167\text{ mL/h}$$

Step 2: Calculate gtt per min.

$$x\text{ gtt/min} = \frac{167\text{ mL} \times 15\text{ gtt/mL}}{60\text{ min}} =$$

$$\frac{167 \times 15}{60} = \frac{167 \times 1}{4} = \frac{167}{4}$$

$$x = \frac{167}{4}; x = 41.7 = 42\text{ gtt/min}$$

Answer: 42 gtt per min

24. $x\text{ gtt/min} = \dfrac{60\text{ mL} \times 60\text{ gtt/mL}}{30\text{ min}} =$

$$\frac{60 \times 60}{30} = \frac{60 \times 2}{1} = \frac{120}{1}$$

$$x = \frac{120}{1}; x = 120\text{ gtt/min}$$

Answer: 120 gtt per min

25. 20 gtt/mL

$$\frac{60}{20}$$

Answer: 3

26. 10 gtt/mL

$$\frac{60}{10}$$

Answer: 6

27. 60 gtt/mL

$$\frac{60}{60}$$

Answer: 1

28. Step 1: Determine the drop factor constant.

$60 \div 10 = 6$

Step 2: Calculate gtt per min.

$x \text{ gtt/min } = \dfrac{200 \text{ mL/h}}{1}$; $x = 33.3 = 33$ gtt/min

Answer: 33 gtt per min

29. Step 1: Determine the drop factor constant.

$60 \div 15 = 4$

Step 2: Calculate gtt per min.

$x \text{ gtt/min } = \dfrac{50 \text{ mL/h}}{4}$; $x = 12.5 = 13$ gtt/min

Answer: 13 gtt per min

30. Step 1: Determine the drop factor constant.

$60 \div 60 = 1$

Step 2: Calculate gtt per min.

$x \text{ gtt/min } = \dfrac{80 \text{ mL/h}}{1}$; $x = 80$ gtt/min

Answer: 80 gtt per min

31. Step 1: Determine the drop factor constant.

$60 \div 20 = 3$

Step 2: Calculate gtt per min.

$x \text{ gtt/min } = \dfrac{140 \text{ mL/h}}{3}$; $x = 46.6 = 47$ gtt/min

Answer: 47 gtt per min

32. Step 1: Determine mL per hour.

$x \text{ mL/h } = \dfrac{1\,000 \text{ mL}}{10 \text{ h}}$; $x = 100$ mL/h

Step 2: Determine the drop factor constant.

$60 \div 10 = 6$

Step 3: Calculate gtt per min.

$x \text{ gtt/min } = \dfrac{100 \text{ mL/h}}{6}$; $x = 16.6 = 17$ gtt/min

Answer: 17 gtt per min

33. Step 1: Determine mL per hour.

$x \text{ mL/h } = \dfrac{1\,500 \text{ mL/h}}{12 \text{ h}}$; $x = 125$ mL/h

Step 2: Determine the drop factor constant.

$60 \div 15 = 4$

Step 3: Calculate gtt per min.

$x \text{ gtt/min } = \dfrac{125 \text{ mL/h}}{4}$; $x = 31.2 = 31$ gtt/min

Answer: 31 gtt per min

34. *Remember:* small volumes are multiplied and expressed in mL per hour.

Step 1: Determine mL per hour.

40 mL/20 min = 40×3 (3×20 min) = 120 mL/h

Step 2: Determine the drop factor constant.

$60 \div 10 = 6$

Step 3: Calculate gtt per min.

$x \text{ gtt/min } = \dfrac{120 \text{ mL/h}}{6}$; $x = 20$ gtt/min

Answer: 20 gtt per min

35. $x \text{ gtt/min} = \dfrac{125 \text{ mL} \times 15 \text{ gtt/mL}}{60 \text{ min}} =$

$$\dfrac{125 \times 15}{60} = \dfrac{125 \times 1}{4} = \dfrac{125}{4}$$

$x = \dfrac{125}{4}; x = 31.2 = 31 \text{ gtt/min}$

Answer: 31 gtt per min

36. $x \text{ gtt/min} = \dfrac{100 \text{ mL} \times 60 \text{ gtt/mL}}{60 \text{ min}} =$

$$\dfrac{100 \times 60}{60} = \dfrac{100 \times 1}{1} = \dfrac{100}{1}$$

$x = \dfrac{100}{1}; x = 100 \text{ gtt/min}$

Answer: 100 gtt per min

NOTE

Practice Problems 32–35 could also have been done by using the shortcut method (determining drop factor constant and then calculating drops per minute). This method would give the same answers.

37. $x \text{ mL/h} = \dfrac{100 \text{ mL}}{60 \text{ min}} \times 60 \text{ min/h} = 100 \text{ mL/h}$

Answer: 100 mL per hour

38. $x \text{ gtt/min} = \dfrac{250 \text{ mL} \times 10 \text{ gtt/mL}}{60 \text{ min}} =$

$$\dfrac{250 \times 10}{60} = \dfrac{250 \times 1}{6} = \dfrac{250}{6}$$

$x = \dfrac{250}{6}; x = 41.6 = 42 \text{ gtt/min}$

Answer: 42 gtt per min

39. a. $x \text{ mL} = \dfrac{50 + 10}{45} = \dfrac{60}{45} \times 60 \text{ min/h} = 80 \text{ mL/h}$

Answer: 80 mL per hour

b. $x \text{ gtt/min} = \dfrac{60 \text{ mL} \times 10 \text{ gtt/mL}}{45 \text{ min}} =$

$$\dfrac{60 \times 10}{45} = \dfrac{60 \times 2}{9} = \dfrac{120}{9}$$

$x = \dfrac{120}{9}; x = 13.3 = 13 \text{ gtt/min}$

Answer: 13 gtt per min

40. a. $150 \text{ mg}:1 \text{ mL} = 900 \text{ mg}:x \text{ mL}$

or

$\dfrac{900 \text{ mg}}{150 \text{ mg}} \times 1 \text{ mL} = x \text{ mL}$

Answer: 6 mL. The dosage ordered is more than the available strength; therefore, more than 1 mL is needed to administer the dosage ordered.

b. $x \text{ mL} = \dfrac{75 \text{ mL}}{30 \text{ min}} \times \dfrac{60 \text{ min}}{1 \text{ h}} = 150 \text{ mL/h}$

Answer: 150 mL per hour

41. a. $300 \text{ mg}:2 \text{ mL} = 300 \text{ mg}:x \text{ mL}$

or

$\dfrac{300 \text{ mg}}{300 \text{ mg}} \times 2 \text{ mL} = x \text{ mL}$

Answer: 2 mL. The dosage ordered is contained in a volume of 2 mL. The label indicates 300 mg per 2 mL.

b. $x \text{ mL} = \dfrac{50 \text{ mL}}{30 \text{ min}} \times \dfrac{60 \text{ min}}{1 \text{ h}} = 100 \text{ mL/h}$

Answer: 100 mL per hour

42. a. $x \dfrac{\text{mL}}{\text{h}} = \dfrac{110 \text{ mL} + 10 \text{ mL}}{60 \text{ min}} \times \dfrac{60 \text{ min}}{1 \text{ h}} = 110 \text{ mL/h}$

Answer: 110 mL per hour

b. $x \text{ gtt/min} = \dfrac{110 \text{ mL} \times 15 \text{ gtt/mL}}{60 \text{ min}} =$

$$\dfrac{110 \times 15}{60} = \dfrac{110 \times 1}{4} = \dfrac{110}{4}$$

$x = \dfrac{110}{4}; x = 27.5 = 28 \text{ gtt/min}$

Answer: 28 gtt per min

43. a. $x\dfrac{mL}{h} = \dfrac{300\,mL}{6\,h} = 50\,mL/h$

   Answer: 50 mL per hour

   b. $x\,gtt/min = \dfrac{50\,mL \times 60\,gtt/mL}{60\,min} =$

   $$\dfrac{50 \times 60}{60} = \dfrac{50 \times 1}{1} = \dfrac{50}{1}$$

   $x = \dfrac{50}{1}$; $x = 50\,gtt/min$

   Answer: 50 gtt per min

44. a. $16\,mg:1\,mL = 300\,mg:x\,mL$

   or

   $\dfrac{300\,mg}{16\,mg} \times 1\,mL = x\,mL$

   Answer: 18.8 mL (18.75 mL rounded to the nearest tenth). The dosage ordered is more than the available strength; therefore, you will need more than 1 mL to administer the dosage ordered.

   b. $x\,gtt/min = \dfrac{318.8\,mL \times 10\,gtt/mL}{60\,min} =$

   $$\dfrac{318.8 \times 10}{60} = \dfrac{318.8 \times 1}{6} = \dfrac{318.8}{6}$$

   $x = \dfrac{318.8}{6}$; $x = 53.1 = 53\,gtt/min$

   Answer: 53 gtt per min

45. The available solution indicates each millilitre contains 10 mg of the medication. To administer the dose ordered, you will need to add 10 mL of medication to the IV volume. 100 mL of IV fluid and medication volume gives a total of 110 mL.

   $x\,mL/h = \dfrac{110\,mL}{60\,min} \times \dfrac{60\,min}{1\,h} = 110\,mL/h$

   Answer: 110 mL per hour

46. $\dfrac{Total\ volume}{mL/h} = \dfrac{150\,mL}{60\,mL/h} = 2.5 = 2\dfrac{1}{2}\,h$

47. Total hours $\times$ mL/h = 5 h $\times$ 140 mL/h = 700 mL

48. $\dfrac{180\,mL}{180\,mL/h} = 1\,h$

   Answer: 1 h

49. 180 mL $\times$ 8 h = 1 440 mL

   Answer: 1 440 mL

50. $\dfrac{90\,mL}{60\,mL/h} = 1.5\,h$ or $1\dfrac{1}{2}\,h$

   Answer: $1\dfrac{1}{2}\,h$

51. Step 1: Determine mL per hour for the remaining solution.

   a. $x\,mL/h = \dfrac{250\,mL}{3\,h}$; $x = 83.3 = 83\,mL/h$

   b. Determine the percentage of change.

   $$\dfrac{83 - 63}{63} = \dfrac{20}{63} = 0.317 = 32\%$$

   c. Percentage of change is greater than 25%. Assess patient. Consult prescriber; order may need to be revised.

52. Step 1: Determine mL per hour for the remaining solution.

   a. $x\,mL/h = \dfrac{200\,mL}{1.5\,h}$; $x = 133.3 = 133\,mL/h$

   b. Determine the percentage of change.

   $$\dfrac{133 - 83}{83} = \dfrac{50}{83} = 0.602 = 60\%$$

   c. Percentage of change is greater than 25%. Assess patient. Consult prescriber; order may need to be revised.

53. Step 1: Determine mL per hour for the remaining solution.

   a. $x\,mL/h = \dfrac{850\,mL}{6\,h}$; $x = 141.6 = 142\,mL/h$

   b. Determine the percentage of change.

   $$\dfrac{142\,mL - 125\,mL}{125\,mL} = \dfrac{17}{125} = 0.136 = 14\%$$

   c. The percentage of change is 14%. This is an acceptable increase. Assess whether patient can tolerate adjustment in flow rate. Check if allowed by institution policy.

54. Step 1: Determine mL per hour for the remaining solution.

a. $x \text{ mL/h} = \dfrac{750 \text{ mL}}{8 \text{ h}}; x = 93.7 = 94 \text{ mL/h}$

b. Determine the percentage of change.

$\dfrac{94 \text{ mL} - 83 \text{ mL}}{83 \text{ mL}} = \dfrac{11}{83} = 0.132 = 13\%$

c. The percentage of change is 13%. This is an acceptable increase. Assess whether patient can tolerate adjustment in flow rate. Check if allowed by institution policy.

Answers to Clinical Reasoning Questions

1. a. The nurse was accustomed to using 20 gtt per mL and calculated the IV flow rate using 20 gtt per mL. The tubing used at the institution delivered 10 gtt per mL, and the nurse did not check the drop factor on the package of IV tubing. Failure to check the drop factor of the IV tubing resulted in an incorrect IV flow rate.
   b. Because of the excessive IV flow rate, the patient developed signs of fluid overload and could have developed heart failure.

Answers to Chapter Review

> **NOTE**
> Many of the IV problems involving drops per minute could also be solved using the shortcut method or dimensional analysis.

> **NOTE**
> Some answers in the Chapter Review reflect the number of drops rounded to the nearest whole number and the flow rate in millilitres per hour.

1. a. Determine mL per hour.

$x \text{ mL/h} = \dfrac{1\,000 \text{ mL}}{8 \text{ h}}; x = 125 \text{ mL/h}$

b. Calculate gtt per min.

$x \text{ gtt/min} = \dfrac{125 \text{ mL} \times 20 \text{ gtt/mL}}{60 \text{ min}}$

$x = 42 \text{ gtt/min}$

55. Step 1: Determine mL per hour for the remaining solution.

a. $x \text{ mL/h} = \dfrac{250 \text{ mL}}{3 \text{ h}}; x = 83.3 = 83 \text{ mL/h}$

b. Determine the percentage of change.

$\dfrac{83 - 100}{100} = \dfrac{-17}{100} = -0.17 = -17\%$

c. The percentage of change is −17%. This is an acceptable decrease. Assess whether patient can tolerate adjustment in flow rate. Check if allowed by institution policy.

c. The nurse should never assume what the drop factor for IV tubing is for macrodrop administration sets because they can vary. The nurse should have checked the IV tubing package for the drop factor; the drop factor is printed on the package.

2. a. Determine mL per hour.

$x \text{ mL/h} = \dfrac{2\,500 \text{ mL}}{24 \text{ h}}; x = 104 \text{ mL/h}$

b. Calculate gtt per min.

$x \text{ gtt/min} = \dfrac{104 \text{ mL} \times 10 \text{ gtt/mL}}{60 \text{ min}}$

$x = 17 \text{ gtt/min}$

3. a. Determine mL per hour.

$x \text{ mL/h} = \dfrac{500 \text{ mL}}{4 \text{ h}}; x = 125 \text{ mL/h}$

b. Calculate gtt per min.

$x \text{ gtt/min} = \dfrac{125 \text{ mL} \times 15 \text{ gtt/mL}}{60 \text{ min}}$

$x = 31 \text{ gtt/min}$

4. a. Determine mL per hour.

$$x \text{ mL/h} = \frac{300 \text{ mL}}{6 \text{ h}}; x = 50 \text{ mL/h}$$

b. Calculate gtt per min.

$$x \text{ gtt/min} = \frac{50 \text{ mL} \times 60 \text{ gtt/mL}}{60 \text{ min}}$$

$$x = 50 \text{ gtt/min}$$

5. a. Determine mL per hour.

$$x \text{ mL/h} = \frac{1\,000 \text{ mL}}{24 \text{ h}}; x = 41.6 = 42 \text{ mL/h}$$

b. Calculate gtt per min.

$$x \text{ gtt/min} = \frac{42 \text{ mL} \times 60 \text{ gtt/mL}}{60 \text{ min}}$$

$$x = 42 \text{ gtt/min}$$

6. $x \text{ mL/h} = \dfrac{1\,500 \text{ mL}}{8 \text{ h}}; x = 188 \text{ mL/h}$

7. $x \text{ mL/h} = \dfrac{3\,000 \text{ mL}}{24 \text{ h}}; x = 125 \text{ mL/h}$

8. $1 \text{ L} = 1\,000 \text{ mL}$

$2 \text{ L} = 2\,000 \text{ mL}$

Therefore:

$$x \text{ mL/h} = \frac{2\,000 \text{ mL}}{24 \text{ h}}; x = 83 \text{ mL/h}$$

9. $x \text{ mL/h} = \dfrac{500 \text{ mL}}{4 \text{ h}}; x = 125 \text{ mL/h}$

10. $x \text{ mL/h} = \dfrac{1\,000 \text{ mL}}{6 \text{ h}}; x = 167 \text{ mL/h}$

11. $x \text{ mL/h} = \dfrac{50 \text{ mL}}{45 \text{ min}} \times \dfrac{60 \text{ min}}{1 \text{ h}}; x = 67 \text{ mL/h}$

12. $x \text{ mL/h} = \dfrac{90 \text{ mL}}{60 \text{ min}} \times \dfrac{60 \text{ min}}{1 \text{ h}}; x = 90 \text{ mL/h}$

13. $x \text{ mL/h} = \dfrac{50 \text{ mL}}{40 \text{ min}} \times \dfrac{60 \text{ min}}{1 \text{ h}}; x = 75 \text{ mL/h}$

14. $x \text{ mL/h} = \dfrac{100 \text{ mL}}{30 \text{ min}} \times \dfrac{60 \text{ min}}{1 \text{ h}}; x = 200 \text{ mL/h}$

15. $x \text{ mL/h} = \dfrac{150 \text{ mL}}{1.5 \text{ h}}; x = 100 \text{ mL/h}$

16. Time remaining = 7 h

Volume remaining = 300 mL

a. Determine mL per hour for the remaining solution.

$$x \text{ mL/h} = \frac{300 \text{ mL}}{7 \text{ h}}; x = 43 \text{ mL/h}$$

b. Determine the percentage change.

$$\frac{43 - 50}{50} = \frac{7}{50} = -0.14 = -14\%$$

The −14% is within the acceptable 25% variation. Assess whether patient can tolerate adjustment in flow rate.
A negative percentage of variation (−14%) indicates the adjusted flow rate will be decreased. Assess patient, check the institution's policy, and continue to assess patient during flow rate change.

17. $\dfrac{1\,000 \text{ mL}}{100 \text{ mL/h}} = 10 \text{ h}$

18. 10 mmol : 500 mL = 2 mmol : x mL

$$10x = 500 \times 2$$

$$\frac{10x}{10} = \frac{1\,000}{10}$$

$$x = 100 \text{ mL/h}$$

Answer: 100 mL per hour of fluid would be needed to administer 2 mmol of potassium chloride.

19. 25 mmol : 1\,000 mL = 4 mmol : x mL

$$\frac{25x}{25} = \frac{4\,000}{25} = 160$$

$$x = 160 \text{ mL/h}$$

Answer: 160 mL per hour would deliver 4 mmol of potassium chloride.

20. 50 units : 250 mL = 7 units : x mL

$$\frac{50x}{50} = \frac{1\,750}{50}; x = 35 \text{ mL/h}$$

Answer: 35 mL per hour

21. 100 units : 250 mL = 18 units : x mL

$$\frac{100x}{100} = \frac{4\,500}{100}; x = 45 \text{ mL/h}$$

Answer: 45 mL per hour

22. $\dfrac{150 \cancel{\text{ mL}}}{25 \cancel{\text{ mL}}/\text{h}} = 6\,\text{h}$

a. 6 h = infusion time

b. (3:10 AM + 6 h = 9:10 AM). IV will be completed at 9:10 AM; military time: 0910.

23. a. 10 mg : 1 mL = 120 mg : x mL

$$\frac{10x}{10} = \frac{120}{10}; x = 12 \text{ mL}$$

or

$$\frac{120 \text{ mg}}{10 \text{ mg}} \times 1 \text{ mL} = x \text{ mL}$$

Answer: 12 mL. The dosage ordered is more than the available strength; therefore, more than 1 mL would be required to administer the dosage ordered.

b. 40 mg : 1 min = 120 mg : x min

$$\frac{40x}{40} = \frac{120}{40}; x = 3 \text{ min}$$

Answer: 3 min

24. x mL/h $= \dfrac{100 \text{ mL}}{60 \text{ min}} \times 60 \text{ min/h}$

$$x = 100 \text{ mL/h}$$

Answer: 100 mL/h

25. 30 000 units : 500 mL = 1 500 units : x mL

$$\frac{30\,000x}{30\,000} = \frac{750\,000}{30\,000}$$

$$x = \frac{750\,000}{30\,000}; x = 25 \text{ mL/h}$$

Answer: 25 mL per hour

26. 100 units : 250 mL = 15 units : x mL

$$\frac{100x}{100} = \frac{3\,750}{100}; x = 37.5 = 38 \text{ mL/h}$$

Answer: 38 mL per hour

CHAPTER 21
Heparin Calculations

Objectives

After reviewing this chapter, you should be able to:

1. State the importance of calculating heparin dosages accurately
2. Identify errors that have occurred with heparin administration
3. Calculate subcutaneous heparin dosages
4. Calculate intravenous heparin dosages (mL/h, units/h)
5. Calculate safe heparin dosages based on weight

Heparin Errors

Heparin, like insulin, is classified as a **high-alert** medication because it carries a significant risk of causing serious injuries or death to a patient if misused. Heparin is one of the most commonly reported medications involved in errors that have caused harm to patients. Many errors associated with heparin have occurred during the medication administration phase. The majority of heparin errors have occurred with preparation, dispensing, and dosing.

High-profile incidents have raised public interest in heparin errors: the near death of the newborn twins of actor Dennis Quaid and his wife in 2007 as well as the deaths of three infants in Indiana in 2006. In these incidents, "all [infants] had received inadvertent overdoses of heparin during the flushing of IV catheters" (MacKinnon & David, 2008, p. 348). The packaging of the medication was cited as a contributing factor to these errors (i.e., similar vial size and label colours for different dosages).

Despite the identification of heparin as a high-alert medication and the publicizing of heparin dosage errors, heparin dosage errors continue to occur. The reasons for these errors are the same as the reasons for medication errors mentioned in previous chapters. An additional source of errors is the use of the abbreviation "U" for *units* despite the recommendation by the Institute for Safe Medication Practices Canada (and all other patient safety organizations) that the word *units* be written out (ISMP Canada, 2006a). ISMP Canada lists heparin as one of the top five medications most frequently involved in medication incidents resulting in death or harm in Canada (MacKinnon & Koczmara, 2008).

Because of the increase in the frequency of errors that have occurred with anticoagulants, ISMP Canada and other organizations recently conducted a national Anticoagulant Safety Survey. Recommendations to minimize risk of harm with unfractionated heparin have since been published (ISMP Canada, 2008).

In response to concerns regarding the higher risk of heparin errors, new labelling for heparin sodium injection was launched by pharmaceutical companies. Some of the changes to the new labelling include the following:

- Bolder and larger typeface on all strengths
- Notations of total unit strength and volume to clearly differentiate heparin sodium injection USP from other products, including heparin lock flush solution USP

- A simplified upright text, with an increased focus on a horizontal read of information
- Additional label enhancements to ensure heparin sodium injection's differentiation from heparin lock flush solution USP; for example, "Not for lock flush" labelling on the caps of every vial of heparin sodium injection.

Labels on heparin solutions will be discussed further in this chapter. **Despite the changes in labels, it is essential for the nurse to correctly identify label dosage strengths and to understand that failure to do so will result in continual errors.** Strategies to reduce the risk of harm to patients will also be discussed throughout the chapter.

Heparin is a potent anticoagulant that prevents clot formation and blood coagulation. Heparin dosages are expressed in units. The therapeutic range for heparin is determined individually by monitoring the patient's blood clotting value, activated partial thromboplastin time (aPTT or PTT) measured in seconds. Heparin is considered to be most therapeutically effective when based on weight in kilograms (kg). Recommendations to decrease heparin errors include the use of weight-based heparin infusion charts or nomograms to determine bolus dosages and infusion rates. This concept will be discussed later in the chapter.

Heparin can be administered intravenously or subcutaneously. It is never administered intramuscularly because of the danger of hematoma (a collection of extravasated blood trapped in tissues of skin or in an organ). When administered intravenously, heparin is ordered in units per hour (units/h) or millilitres per hour (mL/h). Usually, however, heparin is ordered in units per hour when ordered intravenously. This amount is converted to millilitres per hour and administered by an electronic infusion device such as an intravenous (IV) pump. When a patient is receiving IV heparin via infusion pump, the keypad of the pump should be kept locked for added safety.

Heparin Dosage Strengths

Heparin is available in a variety of strengths, ranging from 10 to 50 000 units per mL. Heparin comes in single-dose and multidose vials as well as commercially prepared IV solutions and prepackaged syringes. Enoxaparin (Lovenox) and dalteparin sodium (Fragmin) are examples of low molecular weight heparin prescribed for the prevention and treatment of deep vein thrombosis (DVT) following abdominal surgery, hip or knee replacement, unstable angina, and acute coronary syndromes. (See the labels in Figure 21-1.)

Heparin sodium injection is available in several strengths (e.g., 1 000 units per mL; 5 000 units per mL; 20 000 units per mL). Heparin lock flush solution, which is used for flushing (e.g., med-locks, specialized IV lines), is available in 10 and 100 units per mL. Heparin lock flush solution is a different concentration of heparin than what is administered subcutaneously or intravenously.

> ⚠️ **SAFETY ALERT!**
>
> The average heparin lock flush solution dosage strength is 10 units per mL and never exceeds 100 units per mL. Heparin sodium injection and heparin lock flush solution can never be used interchangeably.

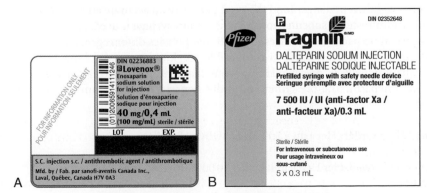

Figure 21-1 A, Lovenox label. **B,** Fragmin label.

Reading Heparin Labels

Heparin labels must always be read carefully to ensure that you have the correct concentrations. As discussed, in an attempt to decrease errors, new labelling for heparin sodium injection was launched in 2008. The following are now commonly seen:

- Bolder and larger typeface
- Simplified upright text, with increased focus on a horizontal read of information
- The statement "Not for lock flush" on the cap as well as the vial

Remember that a number of vial dosage strengths are available. Figure 21-2 shows sample labels of the various dosage strengths. The patient requires continuous monitoring while receiving heparin because of the risk of hemorrhage or clots with an incorrect dosage.

> **SAFETY ALERT!**
> The nurse's primary responsibility is to administer the correct dosage of heparin and to ensure that the dosage being administered is safe. When in doubt regarding a dosage a patient is to receive, check with the prescriber before administering it. To avoid misinterpretation when orders are handwritten or entered in a computer, the word *units* should not be abbreviated.

> **SAFETY ALERT!**
> Heparin is available in different strengths; read the label carefully before administering heparin to ensure the patient's safety. Verify the dosage, vial, and amount to be given. Obtain **independent verification** of the dosage to ensure accuracy. Heparin is a high-alert medication and must be **double-checked** by another nurse.

Commercially prepared IV solutions are also available from pharmaceutical companies in several strengths. The dosage written in red is intended to attract attention to the fact that the bag contains heparin. The use of premixed standardized bags of IV fluid with heparin assists in the prevention of some dosage errors with heparin. In some institutions, heparin for IV use is prepared in the pharmacy in various dosage strengths. If the desired dosage is not available in a commercially prepared solution or from the pharmacy, the nurse is responsible for preparing the solution.

> **SAFETY ALERT!**
> Always carefully read heparin labels (three times) and the prescribed dosage. Adherence to the rights of medication administration (see Chapter 8) is critical in preventing dosing errors with heparin.

Calculating Subcutaneous Heparin Dosages

Because of its inherent dangers and the need to ensure an accurate and exact dosage, when heparin is administered subcutaneously, a tuberculin syringe is used. Heparin is also available for use in prepackaged syringes. Institutional policies differ regarding the administration of heparin, and the nurse is responsible for knowing and following the policies. The calculation methods presented in previous chapters are used to calculate subcutaneous (SUBCUT) heparin. The prescriber will order heparin for subcutaneous administration in *units*.

Example: Order: Heparin 7 500 units SUBCUT daily.

Available: Heparin labelled 10 000 units per mL

How many millilitres will you administer to the patient?

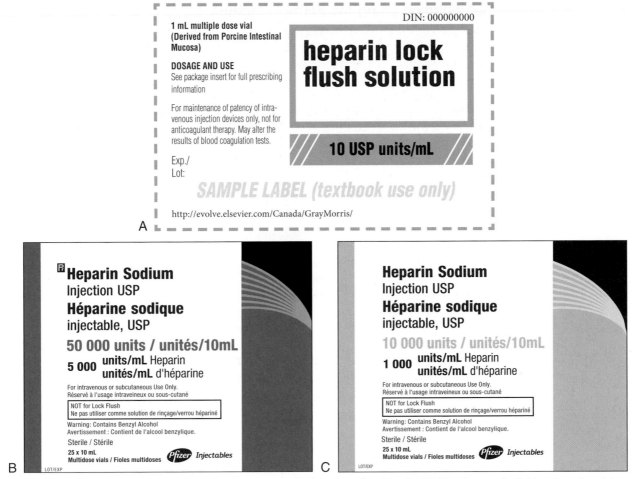

Figure 21-2 A, Heparin lock flush solution, 10 units per mL. **B,** Heparin sodium injection 5 000 units per mL. **C,** Heparin sodium injection 10 000 units per mL. Notice the statement "Not for lock flush" on the labels for 5 000 units per mL and 1 000 units per mL.

✅ PROBLEM SETUP

1. Note that no conversion is necessary. No conversion exists for units.
2. Think: What would be a logical dosage?
3. Set up the problem using the ratio and proportion method, the formula method, or the dimensional analysis method and solve.

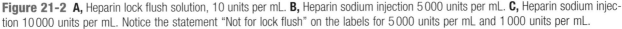

✅ Solution Using Ratio and Proportion

$$10\,000 \text{ units} : 1 \text{ mL} = 7\,500 \text{ units} : x \text{ mL}$$

or

$$\frac{10\,000 \text{ units}}{1 \text{ mL}} = \frac{7\,500 \text{ units}}{x \text{ mL}}$$

$$\frac{10\,000x}{10\,000} = \frac{7\,500}{10\,000}$$

$$x = \frac{7\,5\cancel{00}}{10\,0\cancel{00}}$$

$$x = 0.75 \text{ mL}$$

✔ Solution Using the Formula Method

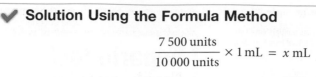

$$\frac{7\,500 \text{ units}}{10\,000 \text{ units}} \times 1\,\text{mL} = x\,\text{mL}$$

$$x = 0.75\,\text{mL}$$

✔ Solution Using Dimensional Analysis

$$x\,\text{mL} = \frac{1\,\text{mL}}{10\,000\,\cancel{\text{units}}} \times \frac{7\,500\,\cancel{\text{units}}}{1}$$

$$x = \frac{7\,5\cancel{00}}{10\,0\cancel{00}}$$

$$x = 0.75\,\text{mL}$$

The dosage of 0.75 mL is reasonable, because the dosage ordered is less than what is available. Therefore, less than 1 mL will be needed to administer the dosage. This dosage can be measured accurately only with a tuberculin syringe (calibrated in tenths and hundredths of a millilitre). This dosage would not be rounded to the nearest tenth of a millilitre. A tuberculin syringe illustrating the dosage to be administered is shown in Figure 21-3.

Calculating Intravenous Heparin Dosages
Using Ratio and Proportion to Calculate Units per Hour

Calculating the rate in units per hour can be done by using the ratio and proportion method or the dimensional analysis method.

Example: Order: Heparin 20 000 units per 1 000 mL D5W to infuse at 30 mL/h. What is the IV heparin dosage in units per hour?

Set up the proportion:

$$20\,000 \text{ units} : 1\,000\,\text{mL} = x \text{ units} : 30\,\text{mL}$$

or

$$\frac{20\,000 \text{ units}}{1\,000\,\text{mL}} = \frac{x \text{ units}}{30\,\text{mL}}$$

$$1\,000x = 20\,000 \times 30$$

$$\frac{1\,000x}{1\,000} = \frac{600\,\cancel{000}}{1\,\cancel{000}}$$

$$x = 600 \text{ units/h}$$

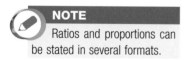

> **NOTE**
> Ratios and proportions can be stated in several formats.

Using Dimensional Analysis to Calculate Units per Hour
Steps:
- Isolate the units per hour being calculated on the left side of the equation.
- Write 20 000 units per 1 000 mL as the starting fraction, placing units in the numerator (to match the units in the numerator being calculated).

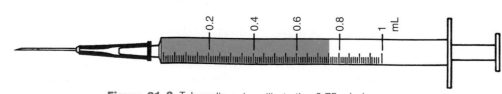

Figure 21-3 Tuberculin syringe illustrating 0.75 mL drawn up.

- Place the 30 mL per hour rate with 30 mL as the numerator; notice that the unit of measurement in this numerator matches the unit of measurement in the starting fraction denominator.
- Cancel "mL" to obtain the desired unit (units/h).
- Reduce if possible, and perform the necessary math operations.

$$\frac{x \text{ units}}{h} = \frac{20\,000 \text{ units}}{1\,000 \text{ mL}} \times \frac{30 \text{ mL}}{1 \text{ h}}$$

$$x = \frac{20 \times 30}{1}$$

$$x = \frac{600}{1}$$

$$x = 600 \text{ units/h}$$

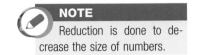

NOTE
Reduction is done to decrease the size of numbers.

Calculating Millilitres per Hour from Units per Hour

Because IV heparin is ordered in units per hour and infused with an electronic infusion device that is programmed in millilitres per hour, it is necessary to do calculations in millilitres per hour.

> **! SAFETY ALERT!**
> An infusion pump is required for the safe administration of all IV heparin drips.

Example 1: Order: Infuse heparin 850 units/h from a solution strength of 25 000 units in 500 mL D5W. At what rate (mL/h) will you set the electronic infusion device?

✔ Solution Using Ratio and Proportion

$$25\,000 \text{ units} : 500 \text{ mL} = 850 \text{ units} : x \text{ mL}$$

or

$$\frac{25\,000 \text{ units}}{500 \text{ mL}} = \frac{850 \text{ units}}{x \text{ mL}}$$

Solve:

$$25\,000x = 500 \times 850$$

$$\frac{25\,000x}{25\,000} = \frac{425\,000}{25\,000}$$

$$x = \frac{425}{25}$$

$$x = 17 \text{ mL/h}$$

✔ Solution Using Dimensional Analysis

Steps:
- Isolate the millilitres per hour being calculated on the left side of the equation.
- Write 25 000 units per 500 mL as the starting fraction, placing mL in the numerator (to match the mL in the numerator being calculated).
- Place the 850 units per hour rate ordered with 850 units as the numerator; notice that the unit of measurement in this numerator matches the unit of measurement in the starting fraction denominator.

- Cancel "units" to obtain the desired unit (mL/h).
- Reduce if possible, and perform the necessary math operations.

$$\frac{x \text{ mL}}{h} = \frac{\overset{1}{\cancel{500}} \text{ mL}}{\underset{50}{\cancel{25\,000}} \text{ \cancel{units}}} \times \frac{850 \text{ \cancel{units}}}{1 \text{ h}}$$

$$x = \frac{85\cancel{0}}{5\cancel{0}}$$

$$x = \frac{85}{5}$$

$$x = 17 \text{ mL/h}$$

Example 2: Order: Infuse heparin 1 200 units/h from a solution strength of 20 000 units in 250 mL D5W. At what rate (mL/h) will you set the electronic infusion device?

✔ Solution Using Ratio and Proportion

$$20\,000 \text{ units} : 250 \text{ mL} = 1\,200 \text{ units} : x \text{ mL}$$

or

Solve:

$$20\,000x = 1\,200 \times 250$$

$$\frac{20\,000x}{20\,000} = \frac{300\cancel{000}}{20\cancel{000}}$$

$$x = \frac{30}{2}$$

$$x = 15 \text{ mL/h}$$

✔ Solution Using Dimensional Analysis

Follow the same steps outlined in Example 1.

$$\frac{x \text{ mL}}{h} = \frac{\overset{1}{\cancel{250}} \text{ mL}}{\underset{80}{\cancel{20\,000}} \text{ \cancel{units}}} \times \frac{1\,200 \text{ \cancel{units}}}{1 \text{ h}}$$

$$x = \frac{1\,20\cancel{0}}{8\cancel{0}}$$

$$x = 15 \text{ mL/h}$$

Calculating Heparin Dosages Based on Weight

To prevent dosage and administration errors with heparin, many hospitals have established **heparin protocols** to guide the administration of IV heparin dosages. The dosages of heparin are individualized based on the patient's weight. Heparin protocols are based on the patient's weight in kilograms and the patient's PTT, a blood clotting value measured in seconds. PTT results are used as the criterion to titrate the dosage, and adjustments are made accordingly (see the sample protocol in Table 21-1). Heparin protocols consist of the following:

- The bolus or loading dosage, which is the initial bolus based on the patient's weight in kilograms
- The initial infusion rate based on the patient's weight in kilograms
- Directions on what additional bolus and rate alterations must be made based on PTT results

Heparin protocols consist of **three steps** in the administration process in the following sequence: (1) **bolus,** (2) **continuous infusion,** and (3) **rebolus and/or adjust infusion rate** (increase, decrease, or discontinue).

It is incumbent upon nurses to be familiar with the protocol at the institution where they work. The bolus and infusion rate can vary among institutions. According to Clayton

TABLE 21-1 Sample Heparin Weight-Based Protocol

Weight-Based Heparin Protocol
Goal of Therapy = PTT of 46–70 Seconds

1. Heparin 80 units/kg IV bolus
2. Initiate IV heparin infusion at 18 units/kg/h from a solution of 25 000 units in 250 mL D5W or a concentration of 100 units/mL
3. PTT 6 hours after rate change and then daily at 7 AM
4. Adjust heparin daily based on PTT results as follows:

PTT (Seconds)	IV Bolus	Stop Infusion	Rate Change (mL/h)	Next PTT
Less than 35	80 units/kg	No	Increase rate by 4 units/kg/h	4 hours after rate increased
35–45	40 units/kg	No	Increase rate by 2 units/kg/h	6 hours after rate increased
46–70 (Target Range)	**None**	**No**	**No Change**	**Next Morning**
71–90	None	No	Decrease rate by 2 units/kg/h	Next morning
Greater than 90	None	For 1 hour	Decrease rate by 3 units/kg/h	6 hours after rate decreased

Note: This protocol is for calculation purposes only. *PTT,* activated partial thromboplastin time.

and Willihnganz (2013), a bolus dosage is about 70 to 100 units per kg, and the infusion rate is usually 15 to 25 units per kg per hour. These values can be different, depending on the institution. Moreover, at some institutions, the weight of the patient is recorded differently; it may be to the nearest tenth of a kilogram or the exact number of kilograms. **Always be familiar with the values and protocol used for heparin administration at the institution to prevent errors and to ensure the safe administration of heparin.**

! SAFETY ALERT!

In order for heparin to be therapeutically effective, the dosage **must** be accurate. A larger dosage than required can cause a patient to hemorrhage, and an underdosage may cause deep vein thrombosis, leading to pulmonary embolism and ultimately death. Any questionable dosages should be verified with the prescriber. Also, some physicians may omit the bolus dosage of heparin, depending on the time the last subcutaneous heparin or low molecular heparin was administered. Be sure to read the protocol correctly.

Remember, IV heparin is administered by infusion pump. Some pumps are capable of delivering IV fluids in tenths of a millilitre, as discussed in Chapter 19. Always check the equipment available at the institution before rounding IV flow rates to whole millilitres per hour. In this text, for the purpose of calculating, round millilitres per hour to a whole number unless provided information to do otherwise.

Let's work through sample problems on calculating heparin dosages based on weight. In these sample problems, the patient's weight will be rounded to the nearest tenth of a kilogram. If the weight is provided in pounds, it must be converted to kilograms.

Example: Order: Heparin 80 units/kg IV bolus. The patient weighs 160 lb. How many units will you give?

Step 1: Calculate the patient's weight in kilograms.

Conversion factor: 1 kg = 2.2 lb

$$160 \text{ lb} \div 2.2 = 72.72 = 72.7 \text{ kg}$$

Step 2: Calculate the heparin bolus dosage.

$$80 \text{ units}/\cancel{kg} \times 72.7 \cancel{kg} = 5816 \text{ units}$$

The patient should receive 5 816 units IV heparin bolus.

Example: Order: Heparin 80 units/kg bolus. Then initiate a drip at 18 units/kg/h from a heparin concentration of 25 000 units in 1 000 mL 0.9% sodium chloride. The patient weighs 75 kg. What is the heparin bolus dosage? What is the IV heparin dosage in units per hour? What is the rate in millilitres per hour at which you will set the electronic infusion device?

Step 1: Calculate the heparin bolus dosage.

$$80 \text{ units}/\cancel{kg} \times 75 \cancel{kg} = 6000 \text{ units}$$

The patient should receive 6 000 units IV heparin as a bolus.

Step 2: Calculate the IV heparin dosage in units per hour.

$$18 \text{ units}/\cancel{kg}/h \times 75 \cancel{kg} = 1350 \text{ units}/h$$

Step 3: Determine the rate in millilitres per hour at which to set the electronic infusion device.

$$1000 \text{ mL} : 25000 \text{ units} = x \text{ mL} : 1350 \text{ units}$$
$$25000x = 1350 \times 1000$$
$$\frac{25000x}{25000} = \frac{1350\ \cancel{000}}{25\ \cancel{000}}$$
$$x = 54 \text{ mL/h}$$

or

The following formula could be used:

$$\frac{D}{H} \times Q = x$$

$$\frac{1350 \text{ units}/h}{25000 \text{ units}} \times 1000 \text{ mL} = x \text{ mL/h}$$

$$x = 54 \text{ mL/h}$$

Now let's do a sample problem going through the steps of calculating the bolus, continuous infusion, rebolus and/or adjust infusion rate using the protocol in Table 21-1 for a patient who weighs 90 kg. Round the weight to the nearest tenth as indicated.

Step 1: Calculate the heparin bolus dosage.

$$80 \text{ units}/\cancel{kg} \times 90 \cancel{kg} = 7200 \text{ units}.$$ The patient should receive 7 200 units IV heparin as a bolus.

To determine the volume (mL) the patient would receive, remember that the concentration of heparin was indicated as 100 units per mL. This calculation can be done using the ratio and proportion method or the dimensional analysis method.

$$100 \text{ units} : 1 \text{ mL} = 7200 \text{ units} : x \text{ mL}$$
$$\frac{100x}{100} = \frac{7200}{100}$$
$$x = 72 \text{ mL (bolus is 72 mL)}$$

Step 2: Calculate the IV heparin infusion rate in units per hour according to the protocol (18 units/kg/h).

$$18 \text{ units}/\cancel{\text{kg}}/\text{h} \times 90 \cancel{\text{kg}} = 1620 \text{ units}/\text{h}$$

Step 3: Determine the rate in millilitres per hour at which to set the infusion device (based on the concentration of 100 units per mL).

$$100 \text{ units}:1 \text{ mL} = 1620 \text{ units}:x \text{ mL}$$

$$\frac{100x}{100} = \frac{1620}{100}$$

$$x = 16.2 = 16 \text{ mL/h}$$

The patient's PTT after 6 hours is reported as 43 seconds. According to the protocol, rebolus with 40 units per kg and increase the rate by 2 units per kg per hour.

Step 4: Calculate the dosage (units/h) of the continuous infusion increase based on the protocol using the patient's weight in kilograms. Then, calculate the dosage (units) of heparin rebolus.

$$40 \text{ units}/\cancel{\text{kg}} \times 90 \cancel{\text{kg}} = 3600 \text{ units}$$

Determine the volume (mL) to administer 3600 units.

$$100 \text{ units}:1 \text{ mL} = 3600 \text{ units}:x \text{ mL}$$

$$\frac{100x}{100} = \frac{3600}{100}$$

$$x = 36 \text{ mL bolus}$$

Now determine the infusion rate increase (2 units/kg/h × kg).

$$2 \text{ units}/\cancel{\text{kg}}/\text{h} \times 90 \cancel{\text{kg}} = 180 \text{ units/h}$$

The infusion rate should be increased by 180 units per hour.

Calculate the adjustment in the hourly infusion rate (mL/h).

$$100 \text{ units}:1 \text{ mL} = 180 \text{ units}:x \text{ mL}$$

$$\frac{100x}{100} = \frac{180}{100}$$

$$x = 1.8 \text{ mL/h}$$

Increase rate:

$$
\begin{array}{r}
16 \text{ mL/h (current rate)} \\
+ \quad 1.8 \text{ mL/h (increase)} \\
\hline
17.8 = 18 \text{ mL/h (new rate)}
\end{array}
$$

Increase the rate on the pump to 18 mL per hour.

> **NOTE**
> Any of the sample problems presented could be solved by using dimensional analysis, ratio and proportion, or the following formula method:
> $$\frac{D}{H} \times Q = x$$

Remember to get another nurse to independently verify the adjusted rate.
Note: The rate in millilitres per hour has been rounded to the nearest whole millilitre. If the pump is programmed to infuse in tenths, express answers in tenths; if not, round to the nearest whole millilitre.

PRACTICE **PROBLEMS**

Solve the following problems in the units of measurement indicated. Use the calculation method that you are most comfortable with.

1. Order: Infuse heparin 1 000 units/h
   from a solution of 25 000 units
   of heparin in 1 000 mL 0.45% NS.
   Calculate the rate in mL per hour.

   _____

2. Order: Infuse heparin 35 mL/h from
   a solution of 25 000 units of heparin
   in 1 000 mL D5 0.9% NS.
   Calculate the dosage in units per hour.

   _____

3. Order: Infuse heparin 25 mL/h from a
   solution of 30 000 units of heparin in 750 mL D5W.
   Calculate the dosage in units per hour.

   _____

4. Order: Infuse heparin 100 mL/h from
   a solution of 25 000 units of heparin
   in 1 000 mL D5W.
   Calculate the dosage in units per hour.

   _____

5. Order: Administer heparin 80 units/kg IV bolus, then initiate a drip at 18 units/kg/h from a solution of 20 000 units in 1 000 mL 0.9% sodium chloride. The patient weighs 176 lb. Calculate the following, rounding weight to the nearest tenth as indicated.

   a. Bolus dosage (units)

   _____

   b. Infusion rate (units/h)

   _____

   c. Infusion rate (mL/h)

   _____

6. A patient who presented to the emergency department with a swollen right leg was diagnosed with deep vein thrombosis (DVT). The patient weighs 61 kg. The patient is prescribed heparin therapy according to the weight-based protocol that follows. (Round weight to the nearest tenth as indicated; the IV pump is calibrated in whole millilitres per hour.)

Weight-Based Heparin Protocol Goal of Therapy = PTT of 46–70 Seconds				

1. Heparin 80 units/kg IV bolus
2. Initiate IV heparin infusion at 18 units/kg/h from a solution of 25 000 units in 500 mL D5W for 50 units/mL
3. Adjust heparin based on PTT results as follows:

PTT (Seconds)	IV Bolus	Stop Infusion	Rate Change (mL/h)	Next PTT
Less than 35	80 units/kg	No	Increase rate by 4 units/kg/h	4 hours after rate increased
35–45	40 units/kg	No	Increase rate by 2 units/kg/h	6 hours after rate increased
46–70 (Target Range)	None	No	No Change	Next Morning
71–90	None	No	Decrease rate by 2 units/kg/h	Next morning
Greater than 90	None	For 1 hour	Decrease rate by 3 units/kg/h	6 hours after rate decreased

Note: This protocol is for calculation purposes only.

a. Calculate the heparin bolus dosage in units.   _____

b. Calculate the initial infusion rate in units per hour.   _____

c. Calculate the initial infusion rate in millilitres per hour.   _____

d. Adjust the hourly infusion rate up or down based on subsequent PTT results. The current PTT result is 31 seconds, 4 hours after heparin therapy was initiated. What should the nurse do now?   _____

Answers on page 583.

POINTS TO REMEMBER

- Heparin is a potent anticoagulant; it is often administered intravenously but can be administered subcutaneously.
- Heparin is measured in units. When orders are written, the word *units* is spelled out to prevent misinterpretation.
- Heparin dosages must be accurately calculated to prevent inherent dangers associated with the medication. Discrepancies in dosage should be verified with the prescriber.
- The heparin order, dosage, vial, and the amount to give should be checked by another nurse before heparin is administered to a patient.
- When heparin is administered subcutaneously, a tuberculin syringe is used (calibrated in tenths and hundredths of a millilitre). Answers are expressed in hundredths.
- Heparin labels must be read carefully because heparin comes in several strengths.
- IV heparin calculations are done in units per hour and mL per hour.
- Heparin is commonly ordered in units per hour, and it is infused with an electronic infusion device in mL per hour.
- Heparin sodium injection and heparin lock flush solution cannot be used interchangeably.
- Heparin dosages are individualized according to the weight of the patient in kilograms and adjusted based on the PTT.
- Protocols for IV heparin vary from institution to institution; always know and follow the institution's policy. Heparin protocols consist of three steps in the administration process in the following sequence: (1) bolus, (2) continuous infusion, and (3) rebolus and/or adjust infusion rate (increase, decrease, or discontinue).
- Monitoring a patient's PTT while he or she is receiving heparin is a **must.**
- Heparin is a high-alert medication that must be independently verified by two nurses.
- Infusion pumps should be locked for added safety when heparin is being infused.

CLINICAL REASONING

1. **Scenario:** A patient has an order for heparin 3 500 units in 500 mL D5W to infuse at a rate of 40 mL per hour. The nurse prepares the IV using a heparin vial labelled 100 units per mL and adds 35 mL of heparin to the IV.

   a. What error occurred in the preparation of the IV solution and why? _____

   _____

   b. What preventive measures should the nurse have taken? _____

Answers on page 584.

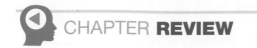

CHAPTER **REVIEW**

For problems 1 to 12, calculate the dosage of heparin you will administer, and shade in the dosage on the syringe provided. For problems 13 to 47, calculate the units as indicated by the problem. Use labels where provided to calculate dosages.

1. Order: Heparin 3 500 units SUBCUT daily.

   Available:

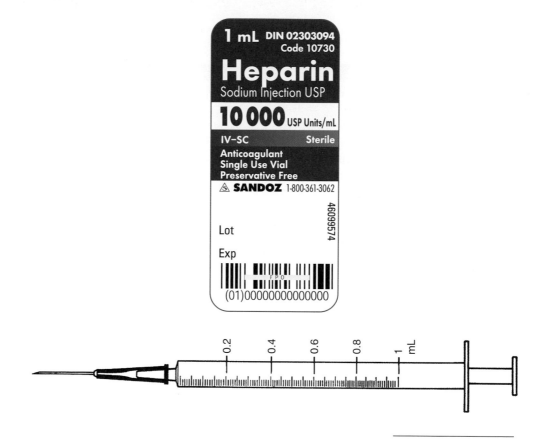

2. Order: Heparin 16 000 units SUBCUT stat.

   Available: Heparin labelled 20 000 units per mL

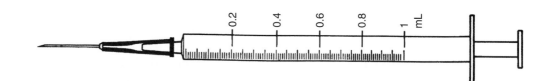

3. Order: Heparin 2 000 units SUBCUT daily.

   Available: Heparin labelled 2 500 units per mL

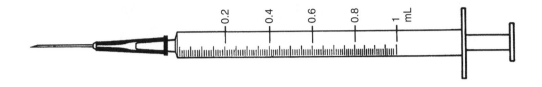

4. Order: Heparin 2 000 units SUBCUT daily.

   Available:

Heparin Sodium
Injection USP
Héparine sodique
injectable, USP

50 000 units / unités/10mL
5 000 **units/mL** Heparin
unités/mL d'héparine

For intravenous or subcutaneous Use Only.
Réservé à l'usage intraveineux ou sous-cutané

NOT for Lock Flush
Ne pas utiliser comme solution de rinçage/verrou hépariné

Warning: Contains Benzyl Alcohol
Avertissement : Contient de l'alcool benzylique.

Sterile / Stérile

25 x 10 mL
Multidose vials / Fioles multidoses   *Pfizer* Injectables

LOT/EXP

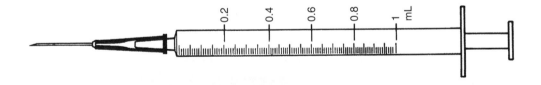

5. Order: Heparin 500 units SUBCUT q4h.

Available:

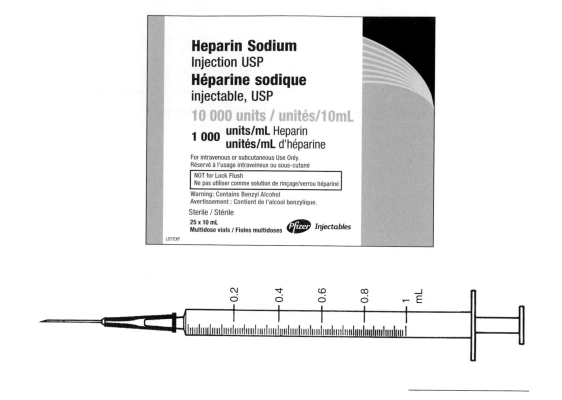

6. Order: Heparin lock flush solution 10 units every shift to flush a heparin lock.

Available:

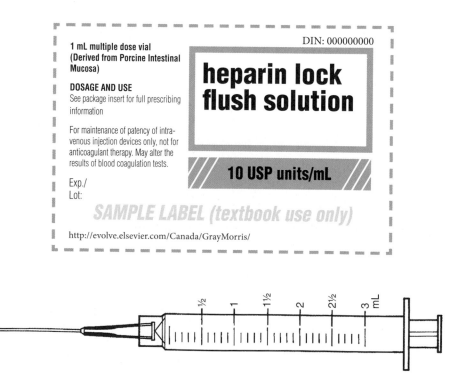

7. Order: Heparin 50 000 units IV in 500 mL D5W.

   Available: 10 000 units per mL

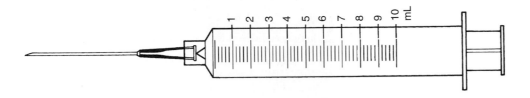

_____

8. Order: Heparin 15 000 units SUBCUT daily.

   Available: Heparin labelled 20 000 units per mL

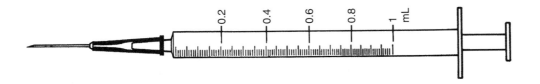

_____

9. Order: 3 000 units of heparin to 1 L of IV solution.

   Available: 2 500 units per mL

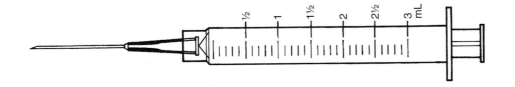

_____

10. Order: Heparin 17 000 units SUBCUT daily.

    Available: Heparin labelled 20 000 units per mL

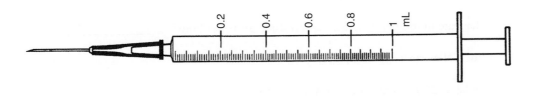

_____

11. Order: Heparin bolus of 8 500 units IV stat.

Available:

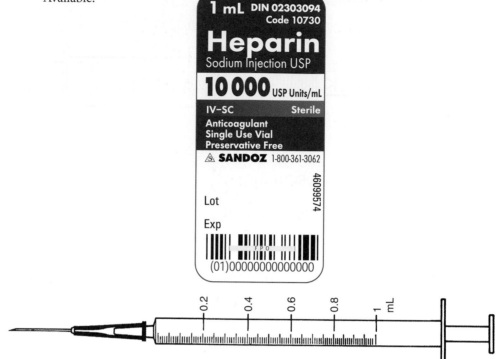

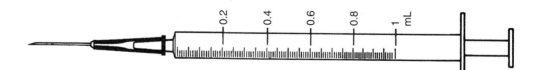

12. Order: Heparin 2 500 units SUBCUT q12h.

Available: Heparin labelled 10 000 units per mL

13. Order: Heparin 2 000 units/h IV.

Available: 25 000 units of heparin in 1 000 mL 0.9% NS

What rate in mL per hour will deliver 2 000 units per hour? _____

14. Order: Heparin 1 500 units/h IV.

Available: 25 000 units of heparin in 500 mL D5W

What rate in mL per hour will deliver 1 500 units per hour? _____

15. Order: Heparin 1 800 units/h IV.

Available: 25 000 units of heparin in 250 mL D5W

What rate in mL per hour will deliver 1 800 units per hour? _____

16. Order: 40 000 units of heparin in 1 L 0.9% NaCl to infuse at 25 mL/h.

    Calculate the heparin dosage in units per hour. _____

17. Order: Heparin 25 000 units in 250 mL D5W to infuse at 11 mL/h.

    Calculate the heparin dosage in units per hour. _____

18. Order: Heparin 40 000 units in 500 mL D5W to infuse at 30 mL/h.

    Calculate the heparin dosage in units per hour. _____

19. Order: Heparin 20 000 units in 500 mL D5W to infuse at 12 mL/h.

    Calculate the heparin dosage in units per hour. _____

20. Order: Heparin 25 000 units in 500 mL D5W to infuse at 15 mL/h.

    Calculate the heparin dosage in units per hour. _____

21. Order: Infuse 40 000 units of heparin in 1 L of 0.9% NS over 24 h. Calculate the following:

    a. The rate in mL per hour _____

    b. The dosage in units per hour _____

22. Order: Infuse 15 000 units of heparin in 1 L D5W over 10 h. Calculate the following:

    a. The rate in mL per hour _____

    b. The dosage in units per hour _____

23. Order: Infuse 35 000 units of heparin in 1 L D5W at 20 mL/h.

    Calculate the heparin dosage in units per hour. _____

24. Order: Infuse 10 000 units of heparin in 500 mL 0.9% NS at 120 mL/h.

    Calculate the heparin dosage in units per hour. _____

25. Order: Infuse 25 000 units of heparin in 500 mL D5W at 25 mL/h.

    Calculate the heparin dosage in units per hour. _____

26. Order: Infuse 20 000 units of heparin in 500 mL D5W at 40 mL/h.

    Calculate the heparin dosage in units per hour. _____

27. Order: Infuse 1 400 units/h of IV heparin.

    Available: Heparin 40 000 units in 1 000 mL D5W

    Calculate the rate in mL per hour. _____

28. Order: Heparin 40 000 units IV in 1 L 0.9% NS at 1 000 units/h.

    Calculate the rate in mL per hour. _____

29. Order: Administer 2 000 units IV heparin every hour. Solution available is 25 000 units of heparin in 1 L 0.9% NS.

    Calculate the rate in mL per hour. _____

30. Order: 50 000 units of heparin in 1 000 mL D5W to infuse at 60 mL/h.

    Calculate the heparin dosage in units per hour. _____

31. Order: 25 000 units of heparin in 500 mL 0.45% NS to infuse at 20 mL/h.

    Calculate the heparin dosage in units per hour. _____

32. Order: 20 000 units of heparin in 500 mL D5W to infuse at 20 mL/h.

    Calculate the heparin dosage in units per hour. _____

33. Order: 25 000 units of heparin in 1 L D5W to infuse at 56 mL/h.

    Calculate the heparin dosage in units per hour. _____

34. Order: 20 000 units of heparin in 1 000 mL D5W to infuse at 45 mL/h.

    Calculate the heparin dosage in units per hour. _____

35. Order: 30 000 units of heparin in 500 mL D5W to infuse at 25 mL/h.

    Calculate the heparin dosage in units per hour. _____

36. Order: 20 000 units of heparin in 1 L D5W to infuse at 40 mL/h.

    Calculate the heparin dosage in units per hour. _____

37. Order: 40 000 units of heparin in 500 mL 0.45% NS to infuse at 25 mL/h.

    Calculate the heparin dosage in units per hour. _____

38. Order: 35 000 units of heparin in 1 L D5W to infuse at 20 mL/h.

    Calculate the heparin dosage in units per hour. _____

39. Order: 25 000 units of heparin in 1 L D5W to infuse at 30 mL/h.

    Calculate the heparin dosage in units per hour. _____

40. Order: 40 000 units of heparin in 1 L D5W to infuse at 30 mL/h.

    Calculate the heparin dosage in units per hour. _____

41. Order: 20 000 units of heparin in 1 L D5W to infuse at 80 mL/h.

    Calculate the heparin dosage in units per hour. _____

42. Order: 50 000 units of heparin in 1 L D5W to infuse at 10 mL/h.

    Calculate the heparin dosage in units per hour. _____

43. Order: 20 000 units of heparin in 500 mL 0.45% NS to infuse at 30 mL/h.

    Calculate the heparin dosage in units per hour.   _____

44. Order: 30 000 units of heparin in 1 L D5W at 25 mL/h.

    Calculate the heparin dosage in units per hour.   _____

45. A central venous line requires flushing with heparin. Which of the two labels shown is appropriate for a heparin flush?

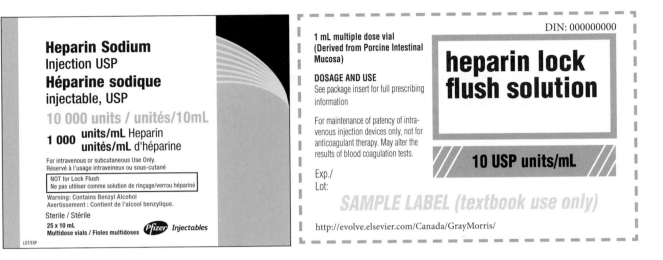

    _____

For problems 46 to 50, round the weight to the nearest tenth where applicable.

46. Order: IV heparin drip at 18 units/kg/h.

    Available: 25 000 units of heparin in 1 000 mL D5W

    The patient weighs 80 kg. At what rate
    will you set the infusion pump?   _____

47. Order: Administer a bolus of heparin IV at
    80 units/kg. The patient weighs 200 lb.
    How many units will you administer?   _____

48. Order: Administer a bolus of heparin sodium at 80 units/kg, IV rounded to the nearest 100 units, then initiate a drip at 14 units/kg/h. Heparin infusion: heparin 25 000 units in 1 000 mL 0.9% NS. The patient weighs 210 lb. Calculate the following:

    a. Bolus dosage (units)   _____

    b. Infusion rate for the IV drip (units/h rounded
       to the nearest 100 units)   _____

    c. The rate at which you will set the infusion pump (mL/h)   _____

49. The hospital heparin protocol is 18 units
    per kg per hour. A patient weighs 50 kg.
    How many units per hour will the patient receive?   _____

50. Heparin infusion: heparin 20 000 units in 1 000 mL D5W. The hospital heparin protocol is to give a bolus to the patient with 80 units per kg and start the drip at 14 units per kg per hour. The patient weighs 70 kg.

    Calculate the following:

    a. Bolus dosage (units)   _____

    b. Infusion rate for the IV drip (units/h)   _____

    c. The rate at which you will set the infusion pump (mL/h)   _____

51. A patient who is admitted to a medical unit with DVT in the left calf weighs 100 kg. The patient is prescribed heparin therapy according to the weight-based protocol that follows.

Weight-Based Heparin Protocol Goal of Therapy = PTT of 46–70 Seconds				
1. Heparin 80 units/kg IV bolus				
2. Initiate IV heparin infusion at 18 units/kg/h from a solution of 25 000 units in 250 mL D5W for 100 units/mL				
3. Adjust heparin based on PTT results as follows:				
PTT (Seconds)	**IV Bolus**	**Stop Infusion**	**Rate Change (mL/h)**	**Next PTT**
Less than 35	80 units/kg	No	Increase rate by 4 units/kg/h	4 hours after rate increased
35–45	40 units/kg	No	Increase rate by 2 units/kg/h	6 hours after rate increased
46–70 (Target Range)	**None**	**No**	**No Change**	**Next Morning**
71–90	None	No	Decrease rate by 2 units/kg/h	Next morning
Greater than 90	None	For 1 hour	Decrease rate by 3 units/kg/h	6 hours after rate decreased

Note: This protocol is for calculation purposes only.

    a. Calculate the heparin bolus dosage in units.   _____

    b. Calculate the initial infusion rate in units per hour. _____

    c. Calculate the initial infusion rate in mL per hour.   _____

    d. Adjust the hourly infusion rate up or down based on subsequent PTT results, which is now 71 seconds, 4 hours after heparin therapy was initiated. What should the nurse do now?   _____

Answers on pages 584–589.

For additional practice problems, refer to the Advanced Calculations section of the Drug Calculations Companion, Version 5 on Evolve.

✳ ANSWERS

Answers to Practice Problems

1. $25\,000$ units : $1\,000$ mL $= 1\,000$ units : x mL

or

$$\frac{25\,000 \text{ units}}{1\,000 \text{ mL}} = \frac{1\,000 \text{ units}}{x \text{ mL}}$$

$$25\,000x = 1\,000 \times 1\,000$$

$$\frac{25\,000x}{25\,000} = \frac{1\,000\,000}{25\,000}$$

$$x = 40 \text{ mL/h}$$

2. $25\,000$ units : $1\,000$ mL $= x$ units : 35 mL

$$\frac{1\,000x}{1\,000} = \frac{875\,000}{1\,000}$$

$$x = 875 \text{ units/h}$$

3. $30\,000$ units : 750 mL $= x$ units : 25 mL

$$\frac{750x}{750} = \frac{750\,000}{750}$$

$$x = 1\,000 \text{ units/h}$$

4. $1\,000$ mL : $25\,000$ units $= 100$ mL : x units

$$\frac{1\,000x}{1\,000} = \frac{2\,500\,\cancel{000}}{1\,\cancel{000}}$$

$$x = \frac{2\,500}{1}$$

$$x = 2\,500 \text{ units/h}$$

5. Convert weight in lb to kg (2.2 lb $= 1$ kg).

176 lb $\div 2.2 = 80$ kg

a. Calculate the bolus dosage.

80 units/ $\cancel{kg}$ $\times 80$ $\cancel{kg}$ $= 6\,400$ units

b. Calculate the infusion rate for the IV drip (initial).

18 units/ $\cancel{kg}$ /h $\times 80$ $\cancel{kg}$ $= 1\,440$ units/h

c. Determine the rate at which to set the infusion pump.

$1\,000$ mL : $20\,000$ units $= x$ mL : 1440 units

$$\frac{20\,000x}{20\,000} = \frac{1\,440\,\cancel{000}}{20\,\cancel{000}}$$

$$x = \frac{144}{2}$$

$$x = 72 \text{ mL/h}$$

6. a. Calculate the heparin bolus dosage in units.
80 units/ $\cancel{kg}$ $\times 61$ $\cancel{kg}$ $= 4\,880$ units. The patient should receive $4\,880$ units IV heparin as a bolus.

b. Calculate the initial infusion rate based on the protocol (18 units/kg/h).
18 units/ $\cancel{kg}$ /h $\times 61$ $\cancel{kg}$ $= 1\,098$ units/h

c. Calculate the initial infusion rate in mL per hour based on the protocol (50 units per mL).

50 units : 1 mL $= 1\,098$ units : x mL

$$\frac{50x}{50} = \frac{1\,098}{50}$$

$$x = \frac{1\,098}{50}$$

$$x = 21.9 = 22 \text{ mL/h}$$

d. The patient's PTT is 31 seconds. According to the heparin protocol, the nurse should rebolus the patient with 80 units per kg and increase the rate by 4 units per kg per hour.

Step 1: Calculate the dosage (units) of heparin rebolus.
80 units/ $\cancel{kg}$ $\times 61$ $\cancel{kg}$ $= 4\,880$ units

Step 2: Now calculate the infusion rate (units/h) increase for this patient according to the protocol.
4 units/ $\cancel{kg}$ /h $\times 61$ $\cancel{kg}$ $= 244$ units/h
The infusion rate should be increased by 244 units per hour.

Step 3: Calculate the adjustment in the hourly infusion rate (mL/h).

50 units : 1 mL $= 244$ units : x mL

$$\frac{50x}{50} = \frac{244}{50}$$

$$x = \frac{244}{50}$$

$$x = 4.8 = 5 \text{ mL/h}$$

Therefore, the new heparin infusion rate is as follows:

$$22 \text{ mL/h (current rate)}$$
$$+ \quad\quad 5 \text{ mL/h (increase)}$$
$$\overline{27 \text{ mL/h (new infusion rate)}}$$

Increase the rate on the pump to 27 mL per hour.
Note: This problem could also be solved using the dimensional analysis method or the formula method.

Answers to Clinical Reasoning Questions

1. a. The nurse used the incorrect concentration of heparin to prepare the IV solution. Heparin concentration of 100 units per mL is used for maintaining the patency of a line and for flushing.

   b. The nurse should have read the label carefully because heparin comes in a variety of concentrations. Heparin lock flush solution is available in 10 and 100 units per mL. Heparin lock flush solution is never used interchangeably with heparin for injection.

Answers to Chapter Review

1. $10\,000 \text{ units}:1 \text{ mL} = 3\,500 \text{ units}:x \text{ mL}$

   or

   $$\frac{3\,500 \text{ units}}{10\,000 \text{ units}} \times 1 \text{ mL} = x \text{ mL}$$

   $x = 0.35$ mL. The dosage ordered is less than the available strength; therefore, you will need less than 1 mL to administer the dosage.

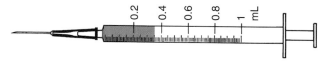

2. $20\,000 \text{ units}:1 \text{ mL} = 16\,000 \text{ units}:x \text{ mL}$

   or

   $$\frac{16\,000 \text{ units}}{20\,000 \text{ units}} \times 1 \text{ mL} = x \text{ mL}$$

   Answer: 0.8 mL. The dosage ordered is less than the available strength; therefore, you will need less than 1 mL to administer the dosage.

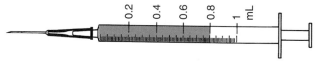

3. $2\,500 \text{ units}:1 \text{ mL} = 2\,000 \text{ units}:x \text{ mL}$

   or

   $$\frac{2\,000 \text{ units}}{2\,500 \text{ units}} \times 1 \text{ mL} = x \text{ mL}$$

   Answer: 0.8 mL. The dosage ordered is less than the available strength; therefore, you will need less than 1 mL to administer the dosage.

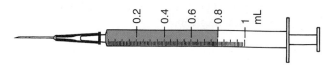

4. $5\,000 \text{ units}:1 \text{ mL} = 2\,000 \text{ units}:x \text{ mL}$

   or

   $$\frac{2\,000 \text{ units}}{5\,000 \text{ units}} \times 1 \text{ mL} = x \text{ mL}$$

   Answer: 0.4 mL. The dosage ordered is less than the available strength; therefore, you will need less than 1 mL to administer the dosage.

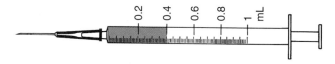

5. $1\,000 \text{ units}:1 \text{ mL} = 500 \text{ units}:x \text{ mL}$

   or

   $$\frac{500 \text{ units}}{1\,000 \text{ units}} \times 1 \text{ mL} = x \text{ mL}$$

   Answer: 0.5 mL. The dosage ordered is less than the available strength; therefore, you will need less than 1 mL to administer the dosage.

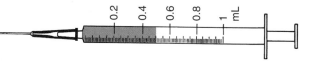

6. $10 \text{ units}:1 \text{ mL} = 10 \text{ units}:x \text{ mL}$

   or

   $$\frac{10 \text{ units}}{10 \text{ units}} \times 1 \text{ mL} = x \text{ mL}$$

   Answer: 1 mL contains 10 units, so you will need 1 mL to flush the heparin lock.

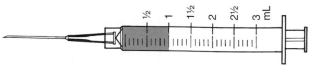

7. $10\,000\text{ units}:1\text{ mL} = 50\,000\text{ units}:x\text{ mL}$

or

$$\frac{50\,000\text{ units}}{10\,000\text{ units}} \times 1\text{ mL} = x\text{ mL}$$

Answer: 5 mL. The dosage ordered is more than the available strength; therefore, you will need more than 1 mL to administer the dosage.

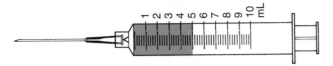

8. $20\,000\text{ units}:1\text{ mL} = 15\,000\text{ units}:x\text{ mL}$

or

$$\frac{15\,000\text{ units}}{20\,000\text{ units}} \times 1\text{ mL} = x\text{ mL}$$

Answer: 0.75 mL. The dosage ordered is less than the available strength; therefore, you will need less than 1 mL to administer the dosage.

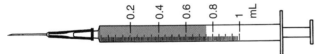

9. $2\,500\text{ units}:1\text{ mL} = 3\,000\text{ units}:x\text{ mL}$

or

$$\frac{3\,000\text{ units}}{2\,500\text{ units}} \times 1\text{ mL} = x\text{ mL}$$

Answer: 1.2 mL. The dosage ordered is more than the available strength; therefore, you will need more than 1 mL to administer the dosage.

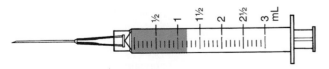

10. $20\,000\text{ units}:1\text{ mL} = 17\,000\text{ units}:x\text{ mL}$

or

$$\frac{17\,000\text{ units}}{20\,000\text{ units}} \times 1\text{ mL} = x\text{ mL}$$

Answer: 0.85 mL. The dosage ordered is less than the available strength; therefore, you will need less than 1 mL to administer the dosage.

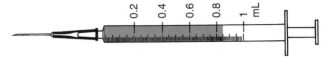

11. $10\,000\text{ units}:1\text{ mL} = 8\,500\text{ units}:x\text{ mL}$

or

$$\frac{8\,500\text{ units}}{10\,000\text{ units}} \times 1\text{ mL} = x\text{ mL}$$

Answer: 0.85 mL. The dosage ordered is less than the available strength; therefore, you will need less than 1 mL to administer the dosage.

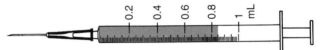

12. $10\,000\text{ units}:1\text{ mL} = 2\,500\text{ units}:x\text{ mL}$

or

$$\frac{2\,500\text{ units}}{10\,000\text{ units}} \times 1\text{ mL} = x\text{ mL}$$

Answer: 0.25 mL. The dosage ordered is less than the available strength; therefore, you will need less than 1 mL to administer the dosage.

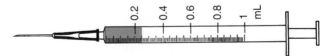

13. $25\,000\text{ units}:1\,000\text{ mL} = 2\,000\text{ units}:x\text{ mL}$

$$\frac{25\,000x}{25\,000} = \frac{2\,000\,000}{25\,000}$$

$$x = 80\text{ mL/h}$$

To administer 2 000 units of heparin per hour, 80 mL per hour must be given.

14. $25\,000\text{ units}:500\text{ mL}=1\,500\text{ units}:x\text{ mL}$

$$\frac{25\,000x}{25\,000}=\frac{750\,000}{25\,000}$$

$$x=\frac{750\,000}{25\,000}$$

$$x=30\text{ mL/h}$$

To administer 1 500 units of heparin per hour, 30 mL per hour must be given.

15. $25\,000\text{ units}:250\text{ mL}=1\,800\text{ units}:x\text{ mL}$

$$\frac{25\,000x}{25\,000}=\frac{450\,000}{25\,000}$$

$$x=18\text{ mL/h}$$

To administer 1 800 units of heparin per hour, 18 mL per hour must be given.

16. $1\text{ L}=1\,000\text{ mL}$

$40\,000\text{ units}:1\,000\text{ mL}=x\text{ units}:25\text{ mL}$

$$\frac{1\,000x}{1\,000}=\frac{1\,000\,000}{1\,000}$$

$$x=\frac{1\,000\,000}{1\,000}$$

$$x=1\,000\text{ units/h}$$

17. $25\,000\text{ units}:250\text{ mL}=x\text{ units}:11\text{ mL}$

$$\frac{250x}{250}=\frac{1\,200\,000}{500}$$

$$x=1\,100\text{ units/h}$$

18. $40\,000\text{ units}:500\text{ mL}=x\text{ units}:30\text{ mL}$

$$\frac{500x}{500}=\frac{1\,200\,000}{500}$$

$$x=2\,400\text{ units/h}$$

19. $20\,000\text{ units}:500\text{ mL}=x\text{ units}:12\text{ mL}$

$$\frac{500x}{500}=\frac{240\,000}{500}$$

$$x=480\text{ units/h}$$

20. $25\,000\text{ units}:500\text{ mL}=x\text{ units}:15\text{ mL}$

$$\frac{500x}{500}=\frac{375\,000}{500}$$

$$x=750\text{ units/h}$$

21. $1\text{ L}=1\,000\text{ mL}$
    a. Calculate mL per hour.

$$\frac{1\,000\text{ mL}}{24\text{ h}}=41.6=42\text{ mL/h}$$

    b. Calculate units per hour.

$40\,000\text{ units}:1\,000\text{ mL}=x\text{ units}:42\text{ mL}$

$$\frac{1\,000x}{1\,000}=\frac{1\,680\,000}{1\,000}$$

$$x=\frac{1\,680\,000}{1\,000}$$

$$x=1\,680\text{ units/h}$$

22. $1\text{ L}=1\,000\text{ mL}$
    a. Calculate mL per hour.

$$\frac{1\,000\text{ mL}}{10\text{ h}}=100\text{ mL/h}$$

    b. Calculate units per hour.

$15\,000\text{ units}:1\,000\text{ mL}=x\text{ units}:100\text{ mL}$

$$\frac{1\,000x}{1\,000}=\frac{1\,500\,000}{1\,000}$$

$$x=\frac{1\,500\,000}{1\,000}$$

$$x=1\,500\text{ units/h}$$

23. $1\text{ L}=1\,000\text{ mL}$

$35\,000\text{ units}:1\,000\text{ mL}=x\text{ units}:20\text{ mL}$

$$\frac{1\,000x}{1\,000}=\frac{700\,000}{1\,000}$$

$$x=\frac{700\,000}{1\,000}$$

$$x=700\text{ units/h}$$

24. $10\,000\text{ units}:500\text{ mL}=x\text{ units}:120\text{ mL}$

$$\frac{500x}{500}=\frac{1\,200\,000}{500}$$

$$x=\frac{1\,200\,000}{500}$$

$$x=2\,400\text{ units/h}$$

25. $25\,000\text{ units}:500\text{ mL}=x\text{ units}:25\text{ mL}$

$$\frac{500x}{500}=\frac{625\,000}{500}$$

$$x=1\,250\text{ units/h}$$

26. 20 000 units : 500 mL = x units : 40 mL

$$\frac{500x}{500} = \frac{800\,000}{500}$$

$$x = 1\,600 \text{ units/h}$$

27. 40 000 units : 1 000 mL = 1 400 units : x mL

$$\frac{40\,000x}{40\,000} = \frac{1\,400\,000}{40\,000}$$

$$x = 35 \text{ mL/h}$$

28. 1 L = 1 000 mL

40 000 units : 1 000 mL = 1 000 units : x mL

$$\frac{40\,000x}{40\,000} = \frac{1\,000\,000}{40\,000}$$

$$x = \frac{1\,000\,000}{40\,000}$$

$$x = 25 \text{ mL/h}$$

29. 1 L = 1 000 mL

25 000 units : 1 000 mL = 2 000 units : x mL

$$\frac{25\,000x}{25\,000} = \frac{2\,000\,000}{25\,000}$$

$$x = \frac{2\,000\,000}{25\,000}$$

$$x = 80 \text{ mL/h}$$

30. 50 000 units : 1 000 mL = x units : 60 mL

$$\frac{1\,000x}{1\,000} = \frac{3\,000\,000}{1\,000}$$

$$x = \frac{3\,000\,000}{1\,000}$$

$$x = 3\,000 \text{ units/h}$$

31. 25 000 units : 500 mL = x units : 20 mL

$$\frac{500x}{500} = \frac{500\,000}{500}$$

$$x = \frac{500\,000}{500}$$

$$x = 1\,000 \text{ units/h}$$

32. 20 000 units : 500 mL = x units : 20 mL

$$\frac{500x}{500} = \frac{400\,000}{500}$$

$$x = \frac{400\,000}{500}$$

$$x = 800 \text{ units/h}$$

33. 1 L = 1 000 mL

25 000 units : 1 000 mL = x units : 56 mL

$$\frac{1\,000x}{1\,000} = \frac{1\,400\,000}{1\,000}$$

$$x = \frac{1\,400\,000}{1\,000}$$

$$x = 1\,400 \text{ units/h}$$

34. 20 000 units : 1 000 mL = x units : 45 mL

$$\frac{1\,000x}{1\,000} = \frac{900\,000}{1\,000}$$

$$x = \frac{900\,000}{1\,000}$$

$$x = 900 \text{ units/h}$$

35. 30 000 units : 500 mL = x units : 25 mL

$$\frac{500x}{500} = \frac{750\,000}{500}$$

$$x = \frac{750\,000}{500}$$

$$x = 1\,500 \text{ units/h}$$

36. 1 L = 1 000 mL

20 000 units : 1 000 mL = x units : 40 mL

$$\frac{1\,000x}{1\,000} = \frac{800\,000}{1\,000}$$

$$x = \frac{800\,000}{1\,000}$$

$$x = 800 \text{ units/h}$$

37. 40 000 units : 500 mL = x units : 25 mL

$$\frac{500x}{500} = \frac{1\,000\,000}{500}$$

$$x = \frac{1\,000\,000}{500}$$

$$x = 2\,000 \text{ units/h}$$

38. 1 L = 1 000 mL

35 000 units : 1 000 mL = x units : 20 mL

$$\frac{1\,000x}{1\,000} = \frac{700\,000}{1\,000}$$

$$x = \frac{700\,000}{1\,000}$$

$$x = 700 \text{ units/h}$$

39. $1 \text{ L} = 1\,000 \text{ mL}$

$25\,000 \text{ units} : 1\,000 \text{ mL} = x \text{ units} : 30 \text{ mL}$

$$\frac{1\,000x}{1\,000} = \frac{750\,000}{1\,000}$$

$$x = \frac{750\,000}{1\,000}$$

$$x = 750 \text{ units/h}$$

40. $1 \text{ L} = 1\,000 \text{ mL}$

$40\,000 \text{ units} : 1\,000 \text{ mL} = x \text{ units} : 30 \text{ mL}$

$$\frac{1\,000x}{1\,000} = \frac{1\,200\,000}{1\,000}$$

$$x = \frac{1\,200\,000}{1\,000}$$

$$x = 1\,200 \text{ units/h}$$

41. $1 \text{ L} = 1\,000 \text{ mL}$

$20\,000 \text{ units} : 1\,000 \text{ mL} = x \text{ units} : 80 \text{ mL}$

$$\frac{1\,000x}{1\,000} = \frac{1\,600\,000}{1\,000}$$

$$x = \frac{1\,600\,000}{1\,000}$$

$$x = 1\,600 \text{ units/h}$$

42. $1 \text{ L} = 1\,000 \text{ mL}$

$50\,000 \text{ units} : 1\,000 \text{ mL} = x \text{ units} : 10 \text{ mL}$

$$\frac{1\,000x}{1\,000} = \frac{500\,000}{1\,000}$$

$$x = \frac{500\,000}{1\,000}$$

$$x = 500 \text{ units/h}$$

43. $1 \text{ L} = 1\,000 \text{ mL}$

$20\,000 \text{ units} : 500 \text{ mL} = x \text{ units} : 30 \text{ mL}$

$$\frac{500x}{500} = \frac{600\,000}{500}$$

$$x = \frac{600\,000}{500}$$

$$x = 1\,200 \text{ units/h}$$

44. $1 \text{ L} = 1\,000 \text{ mL}$

$30\,000 \text{ units} : 1\,000 \text{ mL} = x \text{ units} : 25 \text{ mL}$

$$\frac{1\,000x}{1\,000} = \frac{750\,000}{1\,000}$$

$$x = \frac{750\,000}{1\,000}$$

$$x = 750 \text{ units/h}$$

45. 10 units per mL is appropriate for a heparin flush. Heparin for injection cannot be interchanged with heparin flush lock solution. Check the order with the prescriber.

46. a. First determine units per kg the patient should receive.

$18 \text{ units/kg/h} \times 80 \text{ kg} = 1\,440 \text{ units/h}$

b. $1\,000 \text{ mL} : 25\,000 \text{ units} = x \text{ mL} : 1\,440 \text{ units/h}$

$$\frac{25\,000x}{25\,000} = \frac{1\,440\,000}{25\,000}$$

$$x = \frac{1\,440}{25}$$

$$x = 57.6 = 58 \text{ mL/h}$$

47. a. Convert weight in lb to kg (2.2 lb = 1 kg).

$200 \text{ lb} \div 2.2 = 90.9 \text{ kg}$

b. Calculate the bolus dosage.

$80 \text{ units/kg} \times 90.9 \text{ kg} = 7\,272 \text{ units}$

48. Convert weight in lb to kg (2.2 lb = 1 kg).

$210 \text{ lb} \div 2.2 = 95.45 \text{ kg} = 95.5 \text{ kg}$

a. Calculate the bolus dosage.

$80 \text{ units/kg} \times 95.5 \text{ kg} = 7\,600 \text{ units}$

b. Calculate the infusion rate for the IV drip.

$14 \text{ units/kg/h} \times 95.5 \text{ kg} = 1\,300 \text{ units/h}$

c. Calculate the rate at which to set the infusion pump.

$1\,000 \text{ mL} : 25\,000 \text{ units} = x \text{ mL} : 1\,300 \text{ units/h}$

$$\frac{25\,000x}{25\,000} = \frac{1\,300\,000}{25\,000}$$

$$x = \frac{1\,300}{25}$$

$$x = 52 \text{ mL/h}$$

49. 18 units/ k̶g̶ /h × 50 k̶g̶ = 900 units

50. a. Calculate the bolus dosage.

$$80 \text{ units/ } \cancel{kg} \times 70 \text{ } \cancel{kg} = 5\,600 \text{ units}$$

b. Calculate the infusion rate for the IV drip.

$$14 \text{ units/ } \cancel{kg} /h \times 70 \text{ } \cancel{kg} = 980 \text{ units/h}$$

c. Calculate the rate at which to set the infusion pump.

$$1\,000 \text{ mL} : 20\,000 \text{ units} = x \text{ mL} : 980 \text{ units}$$

$$\frac{20\,000x}{20\,000} = \frac{980\,\cancel{000}}{20\,\cancel{000}}$$

$$x = \frac{98}{2}$$

$$x = 49 \text{ mL/h}$$

51. a. Calculate the heparin bolus dosage in units.
80 units/ k̶g̶ × 100 k̶g̶ = 8 000 units. The patient should receive 8 000 units IV heparin as a bolus.

b. Calculate the initial infusion rate based on the protocol (18 units/kg/h).

$$18 \text{ units/ } \cancel{kg} /h \times 100 \text{ } \cancel{kg} = 1\,800 \text{ units/h}$$

c. Calculate the initial infusion rate in mL per hour based on the protocol (100 units per mL).

$$100 \text{ units} : 1 \text{ mL} = 1\,800 \text{ units} : x \text{ mL}$$

$$\frac{100x}{100} = \frac{1\,800}{100}$$

$$x = \frac{1\,800}{100}$$

$$x = 18 \text{ mL/h}$$

d. The patient's PTT is 71 seconds. According to the heparin protocol, the nurse should decrease the rate by 2 units per kg per h; there is no rebolus.

Step 1: Determine the infusion decrease rate (units/h) for this patient according to the protocol. 2 units/ k̶g̶ /h × 100 k̶g̶ = 200 units/h. The infusion rate should be decreased by 200 units per hour.

Step 2: Calculate the adjustment in the hourly infusion rate (mL/h).

$$100 \text{ units} : 1 \text{ mL} = 200 \text{ units} : x \text{ mL}$$

$$\frac{100x}{100} = \frac{200}{100}$$

$$x = \frac{200}{100}$$

$$x = 2 \text{ mL/h}$$

Therefore, the new heparin infusion rate is as follows:

$$18 \text{ mL/h (current rate)}$$

$$- \quad 2 \text{ mL/h (decrease)}$$

$$\overline{16 \text{ mL/h (new infusion rate)}}$$

Decrease the rate on the pump to 16 mL per hour.

Note: This problem could also be solved using the dimensional analysis method or the formula method.

CHAPTER 22
Pediatric and Adult Dosage Calculations Based on Weight

Objectives

After reviewing this chapter, you should be able to:

1. Calculate dosages based on weight
2. Determine whether a dosage is safe
3. Determine body surface area (BSA) using the West nomogram
4. Calculate BSA using a formula
5. Calculate dosages based on BSA
6. Calculate fluid resuscitation for burn patients
7. Calculate the flow rates for pediatric intravenous (IV) therapy
8. Calculate daily IV maintenance fluid for pediatric patients
9. Calculate safe dosage ranges and determine whether a dosage for IV administration in pediatrics is within normal range

Accuracy in dosage calculation becomes an even greater priority when calculating and administering medications to infants and children. Cohen (2010) indicates that the rate of actual, potential, and preventable adverse drug events is three times higher for pediatric patients. The reasons for adverse drug events in pediatric patients are the same as those for adults. Moreover, confusion can result between adult and pediatric formulations and among the multiple concentrations of oral liquid forms of a medication.

Before administering medications to children, the nurse should know whether the dosage ordered is safe. Accuracy is always important when calculating medication dosages. For infants and children, exact and careful mathematics takes on even greater importance. A miscalculation, even a small discrepancy, may be dangerous because of the size, weight, and body surface area (BSA) of the infant or child. In addition, infants' and children's physiological capabilities (e.g., a lessened ability to metabolize medications, immaturity of systems, differences in rate of medication absorption and excretion) differ from those of adults. Therefore, it is vital that the nurse adhere to pediatric protocols and guidelines and always use a reliable drug reference to verify medication orders to ensure that medication dosages are correct.

Body weight is an important factor used to calculate medication dosages for children and adults, although it is used more frequently with children. Medications may be prescribed based on body weight or BSA.

The safe administration of medications to infants and children requires knowledge of the methods used in calculating dosages. It also requires knowledge of the principles of dosage calculation specific to pediatric patients. Nurses are responsible for educating the families of pediatric patients regarding medication administration.

Dosages for infants and children are based on their unique physiological differences. The prescriber must consider the weight, height, BSA, age, and condition of the child when

590

Copyright © 2017 by Elsevier, Canada. All rights reserved.

ordering dosages. Pediatric dosages are calculated according to body weight (e.g., milligram per kilogram [mg/kg]) or according to BSA (measured in square metres [m²]). The body weight method is more common in pediatrics. Both methods are used in this chapter. The BSA method is based on both height and weight. Both body weight and BSA methods are used to calculate dosages for adults as well, especially in critical care, and the calculation methods used are the same.

Although the prescriber is responsible for ordering the medication and dosage, **the nurse remains responsible for verifying the dosage to be sure it is correct and safe for administration.**

SAFETY ALERT!

As the nurse administering medications to children, you are accountable for recognizing incorrect and unsafe dosages and for alerting the prescriber about them.

If a dosage is higher than normal, it may be unsafe. If a dosage is lower than normal, it may not have the desired therapeutic effect, which makes it unsafe. It is imperative that the nurse check medication labels or package inserts for specific dosage details. Other references that may be consulted for more in-depth information on a medication are drug formularies at the institution, the *Compendium of Pharmaceuticals and Specialities (CPS): The Canadian Drug Reference for Health Professionals*, other drug references, and the hospital pharmacy. Various pocket-size pediatric medication handbooks are also available.

SAFETY ALERT!

To ensure safe practice, when in doubt, consult a reliable source. Always double-check dosages by comparing the prescribed dosage with the recommended safe dosage.

Determining medication dosages according to body weight and BSA is a means of individualizing medication therapy. Although body weight and BSA are common determinants for medication dosing in children, they are also used to calculate dosages for adults, as mentioned, particularly adults who are very old or grossly underweight. Body weight and BSA are also used in the calculation of cancer medication dosages.

Principles of Pediatric Dosage Calculation

Before calculating dosages for the child or infant, it is helpful to know the following principles:

1. The calculation of pediatric dosages, as with adult dosages, involves the use of the ratio and proportion method, the formula method, or the dimensional analysis method to determine the amount of medication to administer.
2. Pediatric dosages are much smaller than those for an adult. Micrograms (mcg) are often used. The tuberculin syringe (1-mL capacity) is used to administer very small dosages.
3. Intramuscular (IM) dosages are usually not more than 1 mL for small children and older infants; however, the amount can vary with the size of the child. The recommended IM dosage for small infants is not more than 0.5 mL.
4. The recommended subcutaneous (SUBCUT) dosage for children is not more than 0.5 mL.
5. Dosages that are less than 1 mL may be measured in tenths of a millilitre or with a tuberculin syringe in hundredths of a millilitre.
6. Medications in pediatrics are not generally rounded off to the nearest tenth and may be administered with a tuberculin syringe (measured in hundredths) to ensure accuracy.
7. All dosage answers must be labelled.
8. The nurse must know the institution's policy on the rounding of pediatric dosages.

Calculating Dosages Based on Body Weight

Infants 0 to 4 weeks old (neonates) and premature infants do get ill and may require medications. An infant's weight may be measured in grams (g) by the scale, or it may be reported to the nurse in grams. Because most dosage recommendations are given in kilograms, the nurse may need to convert the infant patient's weight in grams to kilograms.

As noted in Chapter 6, 1 kg = 1 000 g; therefore, to convert grams to kilograms, divide by 1 000 or move the decimal point three places to the left.

> **RULE**
>
> To convert grams to kilograms, use the conversion factor 1 kg = 1 000 g. Divide the number of grams by 1 000, or move the decimal point three places to the left. Round kilograms to the nearest tenth.

Converting Grams to Kilograms

Example: Convert an infant's weight of 3 000 g to kilograms.

$$1 \text{ kg} = 1\,000 \text{ g} \qquad\qquad \text{(conversion factor)}$$

✔ Solution Using Ratio and Proportion

$$1 \text{ kg} : 1\,000 \text{ g} = x \text{ kg} : 3\,000 \text{ g}$$

$$\frac{1\,000x}{1\,000} = \frac{3\,000}{1\,000}$$

$$x = 3 \text{ kg}$$

Infant's weight = 3 kg

Decimal movement: 3 000 = 3 kg

✔ Solution Using Dimensional Analysis

$$x \text{ kg} = \frac{1 \text{ kg}}{1\,000 \text{ g}} \times \frac{3\,000 \text{ g}}{1}$$

$$x = \frac{3\,000}{1\,000}$$

$$x = 3 \text{ kg}$$

Infant's weight = 3 kg

Example: Convert an infant's weight of 1 350 g to kilograms.

$$1 \text{ kg} = 1\,000 \text{ g} \qquad\qquad \text{(conversion factor)}$$

✔ Solution Using Ratio and Proportion

$$1 \text{ kg} : 1\,000 \text{ g} = x \text{ kg} : 1\,350 \text{ g}$$

$$\frac{1\,000x}{1\,000} = \frac{1\,350}{1\,000}$$

$$x = 1.35 \text{ kg} = 1.4 \text{ kg} \quad \text{(rounded to the nearest tenth)}$$

Infant's weight = 1.4 kg

Decimal movement: 1 350 = 1.35 kg = 1.4 kg   (rounded to the nearest tenth)

✔ Solution Using Dimensional Analysis

$$x \, kg = \frac{1 \, kg}{1000 \, \cancel{g}} \times \frac{1350 \, \cancel{g}}{1}$$

$$x = \frac{135\cancel{0}}{100\cancel{0}}$$

$$x = 1.35 \, kg = 1.4 \, kg \quad \text{(rounded to the nearest tenth)}$$

Infant's weight $= 1.4 \, kg$

Example: Convert an infant's weight of 2700 g to kilograms.

$$1 \, kg = 1000 \, g \qquad \text{(conversion factor)}$$

✔ Solution Using Ratio and Proportion

$$1 \, kg : 1000 \, g = x \, kg : 2700 \, g$$

$$\frac{1000x}{1000} = \frac{27\cancel{00}}{10\cancel{00}}$$

Infant's weight $= 2.7 \, kg$

Decimal movement: $2700 = 2.7 \, kg$

✔ Solution Using Dimensional Analysis

$$x \, kg = \frac{1 \, kg}{1000 \, \cancel{g}} \times \frac{2700 \, \cancel{g}}{\cancel{1}}$$

$$x = \frac{27\cancel{00}}{10\cancel{00}}$$

$$x = 2.7 \, kg$$

Infant's weight $= 2.7 \, kg$

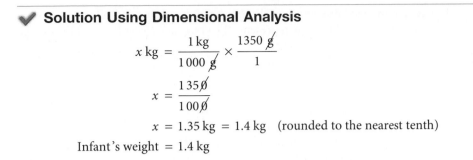 PRACTICE **PROBLEMS**

Convert the following weights in grams to kilograms. Round your answer to the nearest tenth.

1. 4000 g = _____ kg   4. 3600 g = _____ kg

2. 1450 g = _____ kg   5. 1875 g = _____ kg

3. 2900 g = _____ kg

Answers on page 639.

Key Terms and Concepts

Before beginning to calculate dosages based on weight, let's review some key terms and concepts you will encounter.

- **Recommended dosage (also referred to as the *safe dosage*)**—This information comes from the CPS, the medication label, or the package insert. Recommended dosages may also be indicated on the medication label under children's dosages. Dosages are usually expressed in milligrams per kilogram (mg/kg) for a 24-hour period to be given in one or more divided doses. They may also be expressed in micrograms per kilogram (mcg/kg). Recommended dosages may also be stated as a range and referred to as the safe dosage range (SDR). This range represents the upper and lower limits of the dosage as stated by an approved drug reference.

- **Total daily dosage**—This dosage is obtained by multiplying the child's weight after it is converted to kilograms. Multiply the child's weight in kilograms by the dosage (e.g., mg/kg).
- **Divided dosage (also referred to as the *single dose*)**—This dosage represents the amount a child should receive each time the medication is administered. The recommended daily dosage may be stated as milligrams per kilograms per day (mg/kg/day) to be divided into a certain number of individual doses, such as "three divided doses," which means that the total daily dosage is divided equally and administered three times a day or every 8 hours (q8h). The dosage over 24 hours is divided by the frequency, or the number of times the child will receive the medication.
- **Deciding whether the dosage is safe**—This decision is made by comparing the dosage ordered with the recommended dosage. In other words, the safety of a dosage is decided by comparing and evaluating the 24-hour ordered amount with the recommended dosage.

As stated, pediatric dosages are most commonly prescribed according to the child's body weight in kilograms. Therefore, if a child's weight is given in a unit of measurement other than kilograms, it is important to be able to convert the child's weight correctly.

It is essential to follow a systematic approach when verifying the safety of pediatric dosages based on body weight:

1. Convert the child's weight to kilograms if needed (rounded to tenths).
2. Calculate the safe dosage by multiplying the child's weight (kg) by the recommended dosage (mg/kg) based on a reputable drug reference (and round the answer to tenths).
3. Compare the dosage ordered with the recommended dosage, and determine whether the dosage is safe.
4. If the dosage is safe, calculate the amount to give the patient and administer it. If the dosage is unsafe, notify the prescriber and do not administer the medication until a safe dosage is determined.

NOTE

The dosage per kilogram may be milligrams per kilogram (mg/kg), micrograms per kilogram (mcg/kg), and so on.

SAFETY ALERT!

Before administering any medication to a child, always ask yourself whether the dosage is safe. When in doubt, contact the prescriber before administering.

Let's look at examples that consider whether a dosage ordered for a pediatric patient is safe.

Single-Dose Medications

Sometimes medications are ordered as a single dose (mg/kg/dose). Single doses are usually intended for one-time administration or when necessary (prn). The dosage ordered is based on milligrams per kilogram per dose; it is calculated by multiplying the recommended dosage in kilograms by the child's weight in kilograms for each dose.

Example: The prescriber orders naloxone (Narcan) 1.2 mg IV stat for a child who weighs 12 kg.

The recommended dosage is 0.1 mg per kg per dose, based on a drug reference (e.g., the CPS).

Is the dosage ordered safe?

1. Note that no conversion is necessary because the child's weight is in kilograms.
2. Calculate the recommended safe dosage.
   - Multiply mg per kg per dose by the child's weight in kg.

$$0.1 \text{ mg/} \cancel{kg} \text{/dose} \times 12 \cancel{kg} = 1.2 \text{ mg/dose}$$

The calculation of the safe dosage could also be done by the using the ratio and proportion method or the dimensional analysis method.

✔ Solution Using Ratio and Proportion

$$0.1\,\text{mg} : 1\,\text{kg} = x\,\text{mg} : 12\,\text{kg}$$

$$x = 1.2\,\text{mg/dose}$$

Remember that a ratio and a proportion can be written in different formats.

✔ Solution Using Dimensional Analysis

The recommended dosage is the starting fraction (in this case, $\dfrac{0.1\,\text{mg}}{\text{kg/dose}}$).

$$\frac{x\,\text{mg}}{\text{dose}} = \frac{0.1\,\text{mg}}{\cancel{\text{kg}}/\text{dose}} \times \frac{12\,\cancel{\text{kg}}}{1}$$

$$x = 0.1 \times 12$$

$$x = 1.2\,\text{mg/dose}$$

3. Determine whether the dosage is safe by comparing the dosage ordered with the recommended dosage. For this child's weight, 1.2 mg per dose is the recommended dosage, and 1.2 mg is the dosage ordered. Yes, the dosage ordered is safe.
4. Calculate the dosage. Use the ratio and proportion method, the formula method, or the dimensional analysis method to determine the number of millilitres to administer.

   Order: Naloxone (Narcan) 1.2 mg IV stat.

   Available:

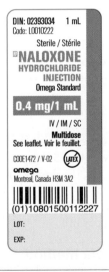

✔ Solution Using Ratio and Proportion

$$0.4\,\text{mg} : 1\,\text{mL} = 1.2\,\text{mg} : x\,\text{mL} \qquad \text{OR} \qquad \frac{0.4\,\text{mg}}{1\,\text{mL}} = \frac{1.2\,\text{mg}}{x\,\text{mL}}$$

$$\frac{0.4x}{0.4} = \frac{1.2}{0.4} \qquad\qquad\qquad\qquad x = 3\,\text{mL}$$

$$x = 3\,\text{mL}$$

✔ Solution Using the Formula Method

$$\frac{1.2\,\text{mg}}{0.4\,\text{mg}} \times 1\,\text{mL} = x\,\text{mL}$$

$$x = 3\,\text{mL}$$

✔ Solution Using Dimensional Analysis

$$x \text{ mL} = \frac{1 \text{ mL}}{0.4 \text{ mg}} \times \frac{1.2 \text{ mg}}{1}$$

$$x = \frac{1.2}{0.4}$$

$$x = 3 \text{ mL}$$

Measure the dose using a 5-mL syringe.

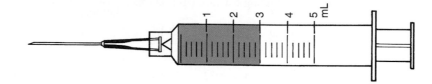

Single-Dose Range Medications

Some single-dose medications indicate a minimum and maximum range.

Example: The prescriber orders dimenhydrinate 25 mg IM q6h prn for nausea. The child weighs 20 kg.

The recommended dosage is 1.25 mg per kg four times a day. Maximum: 300 mg per day.

Is the dosage ordered safe?

1. Note that no conversion is necessary because the child's weight is in kilograms.
2. Calculate the recommended safe dosage.
   - Multiply mg per kg per dose by the child's weight in kg.

   $$1.25 \text{ mg/kg/dose} \times 20 \text{ kg} = 25 \text{ mg/dose}$$

3. Determine whether the dosage is safe by comparing the dosage ordered with the recommended dosage. For this child's weight, 25 mg per dose is the recommended dosage, and 25 mg is the dosage ordered. Yes, the dosage ordered is within the range and safe.
4. Calculate the dosage.
   Order: Dimenhydrinate 25 mg IM q6h prn for nausea.
   Available: Dimenhydrinate 50 mg per mL

✔ Solution Using the Formula Method

$$\frac{25 \text{ mg}}{50 \text{ mg}} \times 1 \text{ mL} = 0.5 \text{ mL}$$

Measure the dose using a 1-mL syringe.

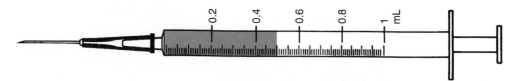

Now let's look at dosages that are around the clock and determine their safety. They are recommended as a total daily dosage (mg/kg/day) and divided into a number of doses per day; for example, "divided doses every 8 hours," "three divided doses," and so on. "Three divided doses" means that the total daily dosage of the medication is divided equally and administered three times a day (TID), or every 8 hours (q8h). "Four divided doses" means that the total daily dosage of the medication is divided equally and administered four times a day (QID), or every 6 hours (q6h). Certain medications are more therapeutic if administered by hours instead of *times per day*. For example, antibiotics better maintain their therapeutic effects if the dosing is q6h rather than QID. As you will see, some medications may specify that the dosage should be divided equally and administered q6h. Attention to time intervals for the day is important in determining whether a dosage is safe.

Example:	The prescriber orders acetaminophen (Tylenol) 700 mg IV q6h for pain for a child who weighs 43 kg.
	Available: Acetaminophen (Tylenol) 10 mg per mL
	The recommended dosage for a child (age 2 to 12 years) or adolescent/adult weighing less than 50 kg is 15 mg per kg per dose q6h, or 12.5 mg per kg per dose q4h IV, up to a maximum of 75 mg per kg per 24 hours.
	Is the dosage ordered safe? If the dosage ordered is safe, calculate the number of millilitres of the medication that need to be added to the IV.
Step 1:	Calculate the recommended dosage. Note that the recommended dosage you will be using is for q6h and for a weight of less than 50 kg. Multiply the mg per kg per dose × the child's weight in kg.

$$15 \text{ mg/ kg /dose} \times 43 \text{ kg } = 645 \text{ mg/dose}$$

Step 2:	Decide whether the dosage is safe by comparing the dosage ordered with the recommended dosage. For this child's weight, 645 mg per dose is the recommended dosage. The dosage is not safe because the dosage ordered of 700 mg q6h exceeds the recommended dosage. Remember that there may be factors that warrant a larger dosage; call the prescriber to verify the dosage.
	Because the dosage ordered is not safe, we will not calculate the number of millilitres to add to the IV.
	When dosages are compared for safety, it may be easiest to calculate how many total milligrams or micrograms are ordered. Doing so usually involves multiplication rather than division. It requires only one calculation, as opposed to two, and may decrease the chance of errors because fewer errors are usually made with multiplication than with division.
Example:	Order: Gentamicin 50 mg IV q8h for a child weighing 18.2 kg.
	The recommended dosage for a child is 6 to 7.5 mg per kg per day divided q8h.
	Is the dosage ordered safe?
Step 1:	Calculate the safe dosage. You must calculate and obtain a range. (The recommended dosage is 6 to 7.5 mg/kg/day.)
	Therefore, calculate the lower (minimum total daily dosage) and upper (maximum total daily dosage) range:

> **NOTE**
> "Per day" could also be stated as "daily" or "every 24 hours."

Minimum total daily dosage: 6 mg/ kg /day × 18.2 kg = 109.2 mg/day

Maximum total daily dosage: 7.5 mg/ ~~kg~~ /day × 18.2 ~~kg~~ = 136.5 mg/day

The safe dosage range for a child weighing 18.2 kg is 109.2 to 136.5 mg per day.

Step 2: Now divide the total daily dosage by the number of times the medication will be given in a day.

$$q8h = 24 \div 8 = 3 \text{ doses/day}$$

$$109.2 \text{ mg} \div 3 = 36.4 \text{ mg/dose}$$

$$136.5 \text{ mg} \div 3 = 45.5 \text{ mg/dose}$$

The dosage range is 36.4 to 45.5 mg per dose q8h. The dosage ordered of 50 mg q8h exceeds the dosage range of 109.2 to 136.5 mg total dosage for 24 hours:

$$50 \text{ mg q8h} = 50 \text{ mg} \times 3 = 150 \text{ mg}$$

Remember that factors such as the child's medical condition might warrant a larger dosage. Because the dosage ordered exceeds the dosage range, the nurse must call the prescriber to verify the dosage.

Example: Order: Penicillin V potassium 100 mg PO q6h for a 3-year-old child weighing 16.4 kg. According to *Mosby's 2016 Nursing Drug Reference*, the recommended dosage of penicillin V potassium PO for a child less than 12 years old is 25 to 50 mg per kg per day in divided doses q6h to q8h.

Is the dosage ordered safe? If the dosage is safe, calculate the number of millilitres required to administer the dosage.

Step 1: Calculate the safe dosage for this child. You must calculate and obtain a range. (The recommended dosage range is 25 to 50 mg per kg per day.)

Therefore, calculate the lower and upper range.

Minimum total daily dosage: 25 mg/ ~~kg~~ /day × 16.4 ~~kg~~ = 410 mg/day

Maximum total daily dosage: 50 mg/ ~~kg~~ /day × 16.4 ~~kg~~ = 820 mg/day

The safe dosage range for a child weighing 16.4 kg is 410 to 820 mg per day.

If 100 mg is ordered q6h, is this a safe dosage?

$$q6h = 24 \text{ h} \div 6 \text{ h} = 4 \text{ doses/day}$$

$$100 \text{ mg} \times 4 \text{ doses} = 400 \text{ mg/day}$$

The dosage ordered is not safe; it is below the recommended dosage. The ordered daily dosage is 400 mg (100 mg × 4 doses = 400 mg/day). The safe daily dosage is 410 to 820 mg per day.

Although the dosage ordered is below the recommended dosage, it would not be considered safe. It is important to realize that even when a small discrepancy exists between the safe dosage and what is ordered (e.g., in this problem, the safe minimum dosage is 410 mg, and the child would receive 400 mg), the difference, although small, can be significant. The dosage ordered may not be sufficient to achieve the therapeutic effect. The prescriber should be notified. Underdosage of an antibiotic may cause a superinfection.

Step 2:   Calculate the amount of medication needed to administer the dosage ordered.

Penicillin V potassium oral solution is available in a dosage strength of 125 mg per 5 mL.

Because the dosage ordered is not safe, we will not calculate the dosage in this problem.

⚠ SAFETY ALERT!
Remember that to avoid medication errors, it is vital to calculate a safe dosage for a child and compare it with the dosage ordered. Question dosages that are significantly low and unusually high before proceeding to administer them. Remember that the nurse is accountable for any medication administered.

When information concerning a pediatric dosage is not present on the medication label, refer to the package insert or a drug reference.

Calculating Adult Dosages Based on Body Weight

The information that has been provided regarding the calculation of dosages for children based on weight can also be applied to adults. Let's look at an example. Refer to the partial ticarcillin package insert.

> **Ticarcillin sodium**
> **For Intramuscular or Intravenous Administration**
>
> **Dosage and Administration**
> Clinical experience indicates that in serious urinary tract and systemic infections, intravenous therapy in the higher doses should be used. Intramuscular injections should not exceed 2 grams per injection.
>
> **Adults:**
> Bacterial septecemia — 200 to 300 mg/kg/day by IV infusion in divided doses for every 4 or 6 hours
>
> Respiratory tract infections / Skin and soft tissue infections / Intra-abdominal infections / Infections of the female pelvis and genital tract — (The usual dose is 3 grams given every 4 hours (18 grams/day) or 4 grams given every 6 hours (16 grams/day) depending on weight and the severity of the infection.)
>
> Urinary tract infections
> Complicated: — 150 to 200 mg/kg/day by IV infusion in divided doses every 4 or 6 hours. (Usual recommended dosage for average (70 kg) adults: 3 g qid.)
> Uncomplicated: — 1 gram IM or direct IV every 6 hours

Example: Order: Ticarcillin 4 g IV q6h for a patient with a respiratory tract infection. The patient weighs 79.5 kg.

The recommended dosage stated in the package insert for a respiratory tract infection is 200 to 300 mg per kg per day q4h to q6h.

Is the dosage ordered safe?

Step 1:   Calculate the recommended dosage.

$$200 \text{ mg/kg/day} \times 79.5 \text{ kg} = 15\,900 \text{ mg/day}$$

$$300 \text{ mg/kg/day} \times 79.5 \text{ kg} = 23\,850 \text{ mg/day}$$

15 900 to 23 850 mg per day is the recommended dosage.

NOTE The same steps used to determine a child's dosage based on weight can be applied to determine an adult's dosage based on weight.

Step 2:   Determine the number of milligrams allowed per dose.

$$15\,900 \text{ mg} \div 4 = 3\,975 \text{ mg/dose}$$
$$23\,850 \div 4 = 5\,962.5 \text{ mg/dose}$$

3 975 to 5 962.5 mg per dose is allowed.

Step 3:   Determine whether the dosage is safe.

Conversion factor: $1\,000 \text{ mg} = 1 \text{ g}$

$$4 \text{ g} = 4\,000 \text{ mg} (4 \times 1\,000) = 4\,000 \text{ mg}$$

$$4\,000 \text{ mg} \times 4 \text{ doses} = 16\,000 \text{ mg/day}$$

The dosage ordered of ticarcillin 4 g q6h is within the range of 15 900 to 23 850 mg per day and is safe.

PRACTICE **PROBLEMS**

Solve the following problems. Round weights and dosages to the nearest tenth as indicated. Use labels where provided to answer the questions.

6. A child weighs 15.9 kg and has an order for cephalexin 150 mg PO q6h.

Available:

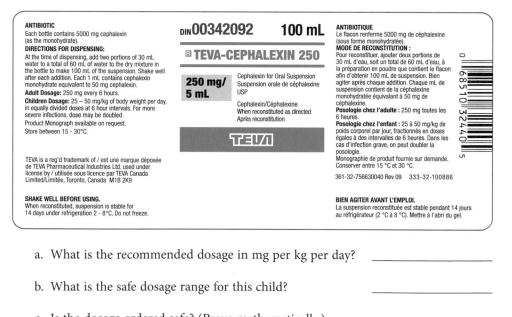

a. What is the recommended dosage in mg per kg per day?   _____

b. What is the safe dosage range for this child?   _____

c. Is the dosage ordered safe? (Prove mathematically.)   _____

d. How many mL will you administer for each dose?   _____

7. Kanamycin 200 mg IV q8h is ordered for a child weighing 35 kg. The recommended dosage of Kanamycin IV for a child is 15 to 30 mg per kg per day divided q8h to q12h.

a. What is the safe dosage for this child for 24 hours?   _____

b. What is the divided dosage?   _____

c. Is the dosage ordered safe? (Prove mathematically.)   _____

8. The recommended dosage of clindamycin oral solution is 10–30 mg per kg per 24 hours divided q6h–q8h. The child weighs 40 kg. (Base calculations on the medication being administered q6h.)

   a. What is the maximum dosage for this child in 24 hours? _____

   b. What is the divided dosage range? _____

9. Phenobarbital 10 mg PO q12h is ordered for a child weighing 4.1 kg. The recommended maintenance dosage is 3 to 5 mg per kg per day q12h.

   a. What is the safe dosage range for this child? _____

   b. Is the dosage ordered safe? (Prove mathematically.) _____

   c. Phenobarbital elixir is available in a dosage strength of 20 mg per 5 mL. What will you administer for one dose? Calculate the dosage if it is safe. _____

10. Morphine sulphate 7.5 mg SUBCUT q4h prn is ordered for a child weighing 38.2 kg. The recommended dosage range for a child is 0.1 to 0.2 mg per kg per dose.

    Available:

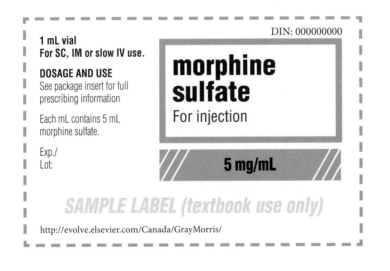

1 mL vial
For SC, IM or slow IV use.

DOSAGE AND USE
See package insert for full prescribing information

Each mL contains 5 mL morphine sulfate.

Exp./
Lot:

DIN: 000000000

morphine sulfate
For injection

5 mg/mL

SAMPLE LABEL (textbook use only)

http://evolve.elsevier.com/Canada/GrayMorris/

   a. What is the safe dosage range for this child? _____

   b. Is the dosage ordered safe? (Prove mathematically.) _____

   c. How many mL will you administer for one dose? _____

11. The recommended dosage of Dilantin is 4 to 8 mg per kg per day q12h. Dilantin 15 mg PO q12h is ordered for a child weighing 5 kg.

Available:

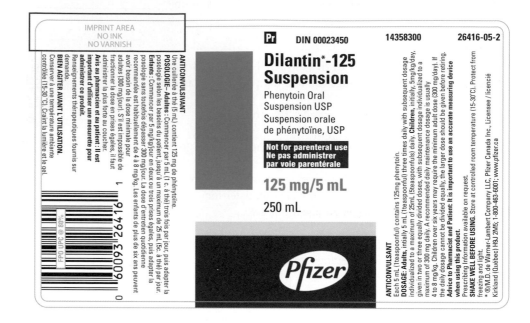

a. What is the safe dosage range for this child? _____

b. Is the dosage ordered safe? (Prove mathematically.) _____

c. How many mL will you administer for one dose? _____

12. The recommended initial dosage of mercaptopurine is 2.5 to 5 mg per kg per day PO. The child weighs 20 kg.

What is the initial safe daily dosage range for this child? _____

13. For a child, the recommended dosage of IV vancomycin is 40 mg per kg per day. Vancomycin 200 mg IV q6h is ordered for a child weighing 17.3 kg.

a. What is the safe dosage for this child for 24 hours? _____

b. What is the divided dosage? _____

c. Is the dosage ordered safe? (Prove mathematically.) _____

14. A 7.3-kg child has an order for amoxicillin 125 mg PO q8h.

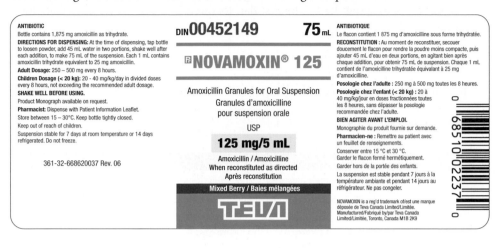

ANTIBIOTIC

Bottle contains 1,875 mg amoxicillin as trihydrate.

DIRECTIONS FOR DISPENSING: At the time of dispensing, tap bottle to loosen powder, add 45 mL water in two portions, shake well after each addition, to make 75 mL of the suspension. Each 1 mL contains amoxicillin trihydrate equivalent to 25 mg amoxicillin.

Adult Dosage: 250 – 500 mg every 8 hours.

Children Dosage (< 20 kg): 20 - 40 mg/kg/day in divided doses every 8 hours, not exceeding the recommended adult dosage.

SHAKE WELL BEFORE USING.

Product Monograph available on request.

Pharmacist: Dispense with Patient Information Leaflet.

Store between 15 – 30°C. Keep bottle tightly closed.

Keep out of reach of children.

Suspension stable for 7 days at room temperature or 14 days refrigerated. Do not freeze.

361-32-668620037 Rev. 06

DIN 00452149   **75** mL

℞ **NOVAMOXIN® 125**

Amoxicillin Granules for Oral Suspension

Granules d'amoxicilline pour suspension orale

USP

125 mg/5 mL

Amoxicillin / Amoxicilline

When reconstituted as directed

Après reconstitution

Mixed Berry / Baies mélangées

TEVA

ANTIBIOTIQUE

Le flacon contient 1 875 mg d'amoxicilline sous forme trihydratée.

RECONSTITUTION : Au moment de reconstituer, secouer doucement le flacon pour rendre la poudre moins compacte, puis ajouter 45 mL d'eau en deux portions, en agitant bien après chaque addition, pour obtenir 75 mL de suspension. Chaque 1 mL contient de l'amoxicilline trihydratée équivalent à 25 mg d'amoxicilline.

Posologie chez l'adulte : 250 mg à 500 mg toutes les 8 heures.

Posologie chez l'enfant (< 20 kg) : 20 à 40 mg/kg/jour en doses fractionnées toutes les 8 heures, sans dépasser la posologie recommandée chez l'adulte.

BIEN AGITER AVANT L'EMPLOI.

Monographie du produit fournie sur demande.

Pharmacien-ne : Remettre au patient avec un feuillet de renseignements.

Conserver entre 15 °C et 30 °C.

Garder le flacon fermé hermétiquement.

Garder hors de la portée des enfants.

La suspension est stable pendant 7 jours à la température ambiante et pendant 14 jours au réfrigérateur. Ne pas congeler.

NOVAMOXIN is a reg'd trademark of/est une marque déposée de Teva Canada Limited/Limitée.

Manufactured/Fabriqué by/par Teva Canada Limited/Limitée, Toronto, Canada M1B 2K9

a. What is the recommended dosage in mg per kg per day? _____

b. What is the safe range of dosage for this child for 24 hours? _____

c. Is the dosage ordered safe? _____

15. A 44-lb child has an order for erythromycin oral suspension 250 mg PO q6h. The usual dosage for children under 22.7 kg is 30 to 50 mg per kg per day in divided dosages q6h.

a. What is the safe range of dosage for this child for 24 hours? _____

b. Is the dosage ordered safe? (Prove mathematically.) _____

16. Refer to the amphotericin B insert to calculate the dosage for an adult weighing 66.3 kg with good cardio-renal function. _____

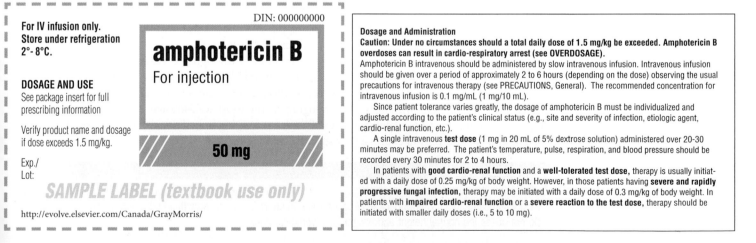

For IV infusion only.

Store under refrigeration 2°- 8°C.

amphotericin B

For injection

DOSAGE AND USE

See package insert for full prescribing information

Verify product name and dosage if dose exceeds 1.5 mg/kg.

Exp./

Lot:

50 mg

SAMPLE LABEL (textbook use only)

http://evolve.elsevier.com/Canada/GrayMorris/

DIN: 000000000

Dosage and Administration

Caution: Under no circumstances should a total daily dose of 1.5 mg/kg be exceeded. Amphotericin B overdoses can result in cardio-respiratory arrest (see OVERDOSAGE).

Amphotericin B intravenous should be administered by slow intravenous infusion. Intravenous infusion should be given over a period of approximately 2 to 6 hours (depending on the dose) observing the usual precautions for intravenous therapy (see PRECAUTIONS, General). The recommended concentration for intravenous infusion is 0.1 mg/mL (1 mg/10 mL).

Since patient tolerance varies greatly, the dosage of amphotericin B must be individualized and adjusted according to the patient's clinical status (e.g., site and severity of infection, etiologic agent, cardio-renal function, etc.).

A single intravenous **test dose** (1 mg in 20 mL of 5% dextrose solution) administered over 20-30 minutes may be preferred. The patient's temperature, pulse, respiration, and blood pressure should be recorded every 30 minutes for 2 to 4 hours.

In patients with **good cardio-renal function** and a **well-tolerated test dose,** therapy is usually initiated with a daily dose of 0.25 mg/kg of body weight. However, in those patients having **severe and rapidly progressive fungal infection,** therapy may be initiated with a daily dose of 0.3 mg/kg of body weight. In patients with **impaired cardio-renal function** or a **severe reaction to the test dose,** therapy should be initiated with smaller daily doses (i.e., 5 to 10 mg).

17. A 90.9 kg adult is to be treated with Ticar for a complicated urinary tract infection. The recommended dosage is 150 to 200 mg per kg per day IV in divided dosages every 4 or 6 hours.

What is the daily dosage range in grams for this patient? _____

18. A child with esophageal candidiasis weighs 5.6 kg. The recommended dosage of IV fluconazole is 6 mg per kg on the first day, followed by 3 mg per kg once daily for 2 weeks.

   a. What is the dosage for this child on the first day? _____

   b. What is the subsequent daily dosage for this child? _____

Answers on pages 639–642.

POINTS TO REMEMBER

- To convert grams to kilograms, divide by 1 000; round to the nearest tenth as indicated.
- If weight is provided in pounds, convert to kilograms. To calculate a dosage, the weight must be in kilograms.
- To calculate the dosage based on weight, do the following:
  1. Determine the weight in kilograms if needed.
  2. Multiply the weight in kilograms by the recommended dosage.
  3. Divide the total daily dosage by the number of doses needed to administer the medication.
  4. Calculate the number of tablets or the volume to administer for each dose using the ratio and proportion method, the formula method, or the dimensional analysis method.
- When the recommended dosage is given as a range, calculate the lower and upper values for the dosage range.
- Question any discrepancies in dosages ordered and remember that factors such as age, weight, and medical condition can cause the differences. Ask the prescriber to clarify the order when a discrepancy exists. A small discrepancy can be significant. A dosage that exceeds the recommended dosage is not safe, and a dosage that is less than recommended is also unsafe because it may not achieve the intended therapeutic effect.
- Use appropriate resources to determine the safe range for a child's dosage. Compare the safe dosage with the dosage ordered to decide whether the dosage is safe.

Calculating Pediatric Dosages Using Body Surface Area

BSA is used to calculate dosages for infants and children. BSA can be determined with the use of a chart, referred to as a *nomogram,* which estimates the BSA. BSA can also be determined by a formula calculation that we will discuss.

BSA is determined from the height and weight of a child and the use of a West nomogram (Figure 22-1). The resulting BSA is then applied to a formula for dosage calculation. Remember that all children are not the same size at the same age. The West nomogram can be used to determine the BSA of a particular child. Although the West nomogram is not easy to use, it is still employed in some institutions. The nomogram can be used to calculate the BSA for both children and adults who are up to 240 cm (95 inches) tall and weigh up to 80 kg (180 lb). The West nomogram is the most well-known BSA chart (see Figure 22-1). It is possible to determine the BSA from weight alone if the child is of normal height and weight. BSA is expressed in square metres (m^2).

SAFETY ALERT!

To use the normal column on the West nomogram, you must be familiar with the normal height and weight standards for children. Check reliable resources such as a pediatric growth and development chart. Do not guess the normal height and weight for a particular age.

Reading the West Nomogram Chart

Refer to Figure 22-1. Notice that the increments of measurement and the spaces on the BSA nomogram are not consistent. **Always read the numbers to determine what the calibrations are measuring.** For example, refer to the column for children of normal height and weight (second column from left); the calibrations between 15 and 20 lb are 1-lb

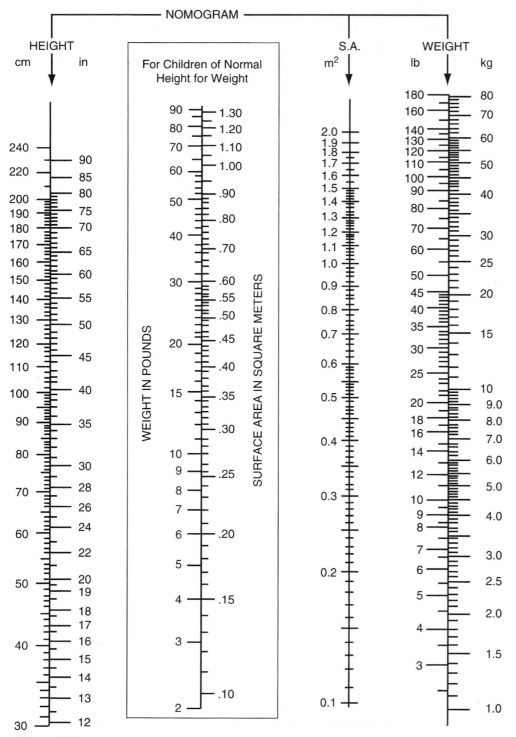

Figure 22-1 West nomogram for estimation of body surface area. (From Kliegman, R. M., Stanton, B. F., St. Geme, J. W., et al. (2011). *Nelson textbook of pediatrics* (19th ed.). Philadelphia: Saunders.)

increments. However, if you look at the bottom of the scale representing surface area in square metres, there are four calibrations between 0.10 and 0.15. Each of these lines, therefore, is read as 0.11, 0.12, 0.13, and 0.14. If the child is of a normal height and weight for his or her age, BSA can be determined from weight alone. Notice the boxed column listing weight on the left and surface in square metres on the right; this column is used when a child is of normal height for his or her weight. For example, a child weighing 70 lb has a BSA of 1.10 m². If you look on the nomogram for a child who weighs 10 lb and use the nomogram column of normal height for weight, you will see that a 10-lb child has a BSA of 0.27 m². Using the nomogram for a child weighing 70 lb and having a normal height for weight reveals that this child would have a BSA of 1.10 m².

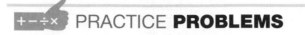

SAFETY ALERT!

The increments and the spaces on the BSA nomogram are not consistent. Be certain that you read the numbers and the calibration values between them correctly.

PRACTICE **PROBLEMS**

Refer to the West nomogram in Figure 22-1 and determine the BSA (expressed in square metres) for the following children of normal height and weight.

19. A child weighing 30 lb   _____

20. A child weighing 42 lb   _____

21. A child weighing 52 lb   _____

22. A child weighing 44 lb   _____

23. A child weighing 11 lb   _____

24. A child weighing 20 lb   _____

Answers on page 642.

Answers on page 642.

> **NOTE**
> Remember that if the ruler is slightly off the height or weight, the BSA will be incorrect.

In addition to being determined based on weight, the BSA can also be calculated by using both height and weight. In the West nomogram chart in Figure 22-1, you will notice the columns for height and weight. This chart includes weight in both pounds and kilograms and height in both centimetres and inches.

For children who are not of normal height for their weight, the scales at the far left (height) and far right (weight) are used. Notice that both of these scales have two measurements: centimetres and inches for height and pounds and kilograms for weight. To find the BSA, place a ruler extending from the height column on the left to the weight column on the far right. The estimated BSA for the child is where the line intersects the SA (surface area) column. For example, by using the far right and left scales, you will find that a child who weighs 50 lb and is 36 inches tall has a BSA of 0.8 m².

PRACTICE **PROBLEMS**

Using the West nomogram in Figure 22-1, calculate the BSA for the following patients.

25. A child who is 90 cm long and weighs 23 kg   _____

26. A child who is 60 cm long and weighs 4.5 kg   _____

27. A child who is 100 cm long and weighs 10 kg   _____

28. A child who is 77 cm long and weighs 9 kg   _____

29. A child who weighs 27 kg and is 100 cm tall   _____

30. A baby who weighs 5.9 kg and is 48 cm long   _____

31. A child who weighs 13.6 kg and is 83 cm tall   _____

32. A child who weighs 13 kg and is 65 cm tall   _____

33. A child who is 90 cm long and weighs 18.2 kg   _____

34. A child who is 49 cm long and weighs 2.3 kg   _____

Answers on page 642.

Calculating Body Surface Area Using a Formula

BSA is used in calculating dosages for children and adults, often to determine dosages for medications such as chemotherapeutic agents that are used in the treatment of cancer. As already shown, a patient's BSA can be determined using a West nomogram. However, this tool requires practice and can result in an error if the ruler used to determine BSA is just slightly off the line.

The BSA of patients (adults and children) can also be calculated with the following two tools:
1. Calculator
2. Formula

Calculators are increasingly being used to determine dosages in critical care and in pediatric units, where extensive calculations may be required. It has been determined that the safest way to calculate BSA is to use a formula and a calculator that can perform square roots ($\sqrt{}$). The formula used is based on the units in which the weight and height measurements are obtained (e.g., kilograms and centimetres, pounds and inches).

Formula for Calculating Body Surface Area From Kilograms and Centimetres

Steps:
1. Multiply the weight in kilograms by the height in centimetres.
2. Divide the product obtained in Step 1 by 3 600.
3. Enter the square root sign into the calculator.
4. Round the final BSA in square metres to the nearest hundredth.

Formula

$$\text{Metric BSA (m}^2) = \sqrt{\frac{\text{Weight (kg)} \times \text{Height (cm)}}{3\,600}}$$

> **NOTE**
> This formula uses metric measures. The constant denominator is 3 600.

Example: Calculate the BSA for a child who weighs 23 kg and whose height is 128 cm. Express the BSA to the nearest hundredth.

$$\sqrt{\frac{23\,(\text{kg}) \times 128\,(\text{cm})}{3\,600}} = \sqrt{0.817}$$

$$\sqrt{0.817} = 0.903 = 0.9\,\text{m}^2$$

The BSA was calculated as follows: $23 \times 128 \div 3\,600 = 0.817$, then the square root ($\sqrt{}$) was entered. The final BSA in square metres was rounded to the nearest hundredth.

Example: Calculate the BSA for an adult who weighs 100 kg and whose height is 180 cm. Express the BSA to the nearest hundredth.

$$\sqrt{\frac{100\,(\text{kg}) \times 180\,(\text{cm})}{3\,600}} = \sqrt{5}$$

$$\sqrt{5} = 2.236 = 2.24\,\text{m}^2$$

Formula for Calculating Body Surface Area From Pounds and Inches

The formula is the same with the exception of the number used in the denominator, which is 3131, and the measurements used are household units.

Formula

$$\text{Household BSA (m}^2\text{)} = \sqrt{\frac{\text{Weight (lb)} \times \text{Height (in)}}{3131}}$$

Example: Calculate the BSA for a child who weighs 25 lb and is 32 inches tall. Express the BSA to the nearest hundredth.

$$\sqrt{\frac{25\,\text{(lb)} \times 32\,\text{(in)}}{3131}} = \sqrt{0.255}$$

$$\sqrt{0.255} = 0.504 = 0.5\,\text{m}^2$$

Technological Advances

Computer technology is often used to calculate BSA. Applications that calculate BSA are available online and can be downloaded onto devices such as smartphones. Examples of applications that calculate BSA include the following:

- PASI BSA Calculator App: Available for Android and Apple devices
- Body Surface Area Calculator for Medication Doses: http://www.halls.md/body-surface-area/bsa.htm
- Evidence-Based Medicine Consult—Adult BMI, Ideal Body Weight, and BSA Calculator: http://www.pharmacologyweekly.com/app/medical-calculators/body-mass-index-bmi-weight-bsa-calculator

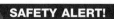 PRACTICE **PROBLEMS**

Determine the BSA for the following patients using a formula. Express the BSA to the nearest hundredth.

35. An adult whose weight is 95.5 kg and height is 180 cm _____

36. A child whose weight is 10 kg and height is 70 cm _____

37. A child whose weight is 4.8 lb and height is 21 inches _____

38. A child whose weight is 24 kg and height is 92 cm _____

Answers on page 642.

> (!) **SAFETY ALERT!**
> Always check a dosage ordered based on BSA (in m²) against the recommended dosage based on BSA (in m²) using appropriate resources (e.g., a package insert or a pediatric medication handbook).

Medications, particularly chemotherapy agents, often provide the recommended dosage according to BSA in square metres.

Example: Cisplatin is an antineoplastic agent. The recommended pediatric/adult IV dosage for bladder cancer is 50 to 70 mg per m² every 3 to 4 weeks. For carmustine, which is used to treat Hodgkin disease and brain tumours, the recommended IV dosage for an adult is 150 to 200 mg per m².

POINTS TO REMEMBER

- BSA is determined with the West nomogram by using the child's height and weight and is expressed in square metres.
- The normal height and weight column on the West nomogram is used only when the child's height and weight are within normal limits.
- The numbers and the calibration values between them on the West nomogram must be read carefully.
- The formula method to calculate BSA is more accurate than the nomogram method.
- The formulas used to calculate BSA are as follows:

$$\text{Metric BSA (m}^2) = \sqrt{\frac{\text{Weight (kg)} \times \text{Height (cm)}}{3\,600}}$$

$$\text{Household BSA (m}^2) = \sqrt{\frac{\text{Weight (lb)} \times \text{Height (in)}}{3\,131}}$$

- **Determining BSA with a formula requires a calculator:**
  - Multiply height × weight (cm × kg, or lb × inches).
  - Divide by 3 600 or 3 131, depending on the units of measurement (divide by 3 600 if measurements are in metric units [cm, kg] and by 3 131 if measurements are in household units [inches, lb]).
  - Enter the $\sqrt{\ }$ (square root sign) to arrive at BSA in square metres.
  - Round square metres to hundredths (two decimal places).
- Applications that calculate BSA are available online and can be downloaded.

Calculating Dosages Based on Body Surface Area

If you know a child's BSA, the dosage is calculated by multiplying the recommended dosage by the child's BSA (m^2).

Example: The recommended dosage is 3 mg per m^2. The child has a BSA of 1.2 m^2. What is the dosage?

$$1.2 \text{ m}^2 \times \frac{3 \text{ mg}}{\text{m}^2} = 3.6 \text{ mg}$$

✔ Solution Using Dimensional Analysis

$$x \text{ mg} = \frac{3 \text{ mg}}{\text{m}^2} \times \frac{1.2 \text{ m}^2}{1}$$
$$x = 1.2 \times 3$$
$$x = 3.6 \text{ mg}$$

Example: The recommended dosage is 30 mg per m^2. The child has a BSA of 0.75 m^2. What is the dosage?

$$0.75 \text{ m}^2 \times \frac{30 \text{ mg}}{\text{m}^2} = 22.5 \text{ mg}$$

✔ Solution Using Dimensional Analysis

$$x \text{ mg} = \frac{30 \text{ mg}}{\text{m}^2} \times \frac{0.75 \text{ m}^2}{1}$$
$$x = 30 \times 0.75$$
$$x = 22.5 \text{ mg}$$

To do the calculation with dimensional analysis, use the recommended dosage given to convert the BSA to dosage in milligrams, as the first fraction.

Formula for Calculating Pediatric Dosages Based on Body Surface Area

A child's BSA is expressed in square metres and inserted into the formula that follows.

Formula

$$\frac{\text{BSA of child (m}^2)}{1.7 \text{ (m}^2)} \times \text{Adult dosage} = \text{Estimated child's dosage}$$

> **RULE**
>
> If only the recommended dosage for an adult is cited, then a formula is used to calculate the child's dosage. The formula uses the average adult dosage, the average adult BSA (1.7 m²), and the child's BSA in square metres.

Example: The prescriber has ordered a medication for which the average adult dosage is 125 mg. What will the dosage be for a child with a BSA of 1.4 m²?

$$\frac{1.4 \text{ m}^2}{1.7 \text{ m}^2} \times 125 \text{ mg} = 102.94 \text{ mg} = 102.9 \text{ mg (round to the nearest tenth)}$$

Example: The adult dosage for a medication is 100 to 300 mg. What will the dosage range be for a child with a BSA of 0.5 m²?

$$\frac{0.5 \text{ m}^2}{1.7 \text{ m}^2} \times 100 = 29.41 \text{ mg} = 29.4 \text{ mg (rounded to nearest tenth)}$$

$$\frac{0.5 \text{ m}^2}{1.7 \text{ m}^2} \times 300 = 88.23 \text{ mg} = 88.2 \text{ mg (rounded to nearest tenth)}$$

The dosage range is 29.4 to 88.2 mg.

+−÷× PRACTICE **PROBLEMS**

Using the West nomogram (see Figure 22-1) where indicated, calculate the child's dosage for the following medications. Express your answer to the nearest tenth.

39. The child's height is 32 inches and weight is 25 lb. The recommended adult dosage is 25 mg.

    a. What is the child's BSA? _____

    b. What is the child's dosage? _____

40. The child's height is 100 cm and weight is 10 kg. The adult dosage is 200 to 400 mg.

    a. What is the child's BSA? _____

    b. What is the child's dosage range? _____

41. The normal adult dosage of a medication is
    5 to 15 mg. What will the dosage range be for a
    child whose BSA is 1.5 m²?   _____

42. 5 mg of a medication is ordered for a
    child with a BSA of 0.8 m². The average
    adult dosage is 20 mg. Is this dosage correct?
    (Prove mathematically.)   _____

43. 7 mg of a medication is ordered for a
    child with a BSA of 0.9 m². The average
    adult dosage is 25 mg. Is this dosage correct?
    (Prove mathematically.)   _____

44. An antibiotic for which the average adult
    dosage is 250 mg is ordered for a
    child with a BSA of 1.5 m².
    What will the child's dosage be?   _____

45. The recommended adult dosage of a
    medication is 20 to 30 mg. The child has
    a BSA of 0.74 m². What will the child's
    dosage range be?   _____

46. 8 mg of a medication is ordered for a
    child who has a BSA of 0.67 m².
    The average adult dosage is 20 mg. Is this
    dosage correct? (Prove mathematically.)   _____

47. The child has a BSA of 0.94 m².
    The recommended adult dosage of a
    medication is 10 to 20 mg. What will the
    child's dosage range be?   _____

48. The child's weight is 20 lb and height is 30 inches. The adult dosage of a medication
    is 500 mg.

    a. What is the child's BSA?   _____

    b. What is the child's dosage?   _____

49. The recommended adult dosage for an
    antibiotic is 500 mg four times a day.
    The child's BSA is 1.3 m². What will the
    child's dosage be?   _____

50. The child's weight is 30 lb and height is 28 inches. The adult dosage of a medication
    is 25 mg.

    a. What is the child's BSA?   _____

    b. What is the child's dosage?   _____

51. The child's BSA is 0.52 m².
    The average adult dosage for a medication
    is 15 mg. What will the child's
    dosage be?   _____

52. The recommended adult dosage for a
medication is 150 mg. The child's BSA is 1.1 m². _____
What will the child's dosage be?

Answers on pages 642–643.

⚙ POINTS TO REMEMBER

- When you know a child's BSA, the dosage is determined by multiplying the BSA by the recommended dosage. (This calculation is used when the recommended dosage is written by using the average dosage per square metre.) Dimensional analysis can also be used with the recommended dosage as the equivalent fraction.
- To determine whether a child's dosage is safe, a comparison must be made between the dosage ordered and the calculated dosage based on the BSA.
- To calculate a child's dosage when only the average adult dosage is available, use this formula:

$$\frac{\text{BSA of child (m}^2)}{1.7\ (\text{m}^2)} \times \text{Adult dosage} = \text{Estimated child's dosage}$$

- If a dosage seems unsafe, consult the prescriber before administering the dosage.

<table><tr><td>✎ **NOTE**

The fluid resuscitation formula for infants who are burned is not the same as that for children and adults. Infant fluid resuscitation will not be discussed in this chapter.</td></tr></table>

Fluid Resuscitation After a Burn Injury

Fluid management is central to treating burn patients during the first 24 to 48 hours after the event. A sufficient volume of fluid is necessary to avert shock as a result of comprehensive burn injuries. The aim of fluid resuscitation is to restore and maintain adequate oxygen delivery to all tissues of the body following the loss of sodium, water, and protein. Burns of more than 15% of BSA in adults and 10% in children warrant formal resuscitation (Williams, 2008).

The Parkland Formula

The formula most commonly used to determine the amount of IV fluid (Ringer's lactate; RL) required by a burn patient in the first 24 hours is the Parkland formula. It is used for both adults and children older than 10. Children usually receive daily maintenance fluids in addition to resuscitation fluids. Calculating daily maintenance fluids for children will be discussed later in this chapter.

Advocates of the Parkland formula find it user-friendly. Moreover, the large volume of fluid replacement it results in leads to fewer respiratory complications. At the same time, general edema in the patient during initial stages of fluid resuscitation because of the increased fluid volume is not uncommon. The formula calculates the fluid requirement from the time of the burn injury until the end of the first 24 hours after the burn occurred (Box 22-1). It estimates fluid replacement to be 4 mL per kilogram of body weight per percentage of BSA burned.

The Post–24-Hour Formula

For the second 24 hours (hours 25 to 48) after a burn, the amount of IV fluid (D5W; dextrose 5% solution) to be administered is based on maintaining a **minimum urine output**

BOX 22-1	**The Parkland Formula for Total Fluid Replacement in the First 24 Hours After a Burn**

4 mL × Weight (kg) × % BSA burned = Total volume (mL)
- 50% of fluids are given in the first 8 hours
- 50% of fluids are given in the next 16 hours

Adapted from Williams, C. (2008). Fluid resuscitation in burn patients 1: Using formulas. *Nursing Times, 104*(14), 28–29. Retrieved from http://www.nursingtimes.net/nursing-practice/clinical-zones/accident-and-emergency/fluid-resuscitation-in-burns-patients-1-using-formulas/1060595.article

in the patient. Typically, minimum urine output is 0.5 to 1.0 mL per kg per hour for adults and 1.0 to 1.5 mL per kg per hour for children under 30 kg (Macklin, Chernecky, & Infortuna, 2011; Williams, 2008). Fluid replacement in the post–24-hour period based on urine output is calculated using the formula that follows.

Formula

> 1 mL × kg × % BSA burned = Total volume (mL)

To calculate the fluids needed for resuscitation, review the patient's chart to find the information necessary for accurate calculation: weight, time of burn, time of admission, and percentage of BSA estimated to have been burned.

Calculating Fluid Replacement for Burn Patients

Let's use the Parkland formula and the post–24-hour formula based on urine output to work out sample problems on fluid resuscitation over the first 48 hours after a burn. Remember that in the first 24 hours, 50% of replacement fluid is given in the first 8 hours and the remaining 50% is given in the following 16 hours. We will also determine the infusion rate (mL/h) for the IV during both parts of the first 24-hour period as well as the next 25- to 48-hour period. Answers will be rounded to the nearest whole number.

Example: An adult who weighs 88 kg has 40% of total BSA burned in a car accident.

Order: IV RL to infuse as per Parkland formula × 24 h. IV D5W infusion based on the post–24-hour formula for 25 to 48 hours post-burn.

Step 1: Determine the first 24-hour Ringer's lactate solution to be infused.

(constant)　(kg)　(% BSA burned)　(Total volume)

4 mL　×　88　×　40　=　14 080 mL

Step 2: Determine the first 8-hour volume (50% of total 24-hour volume).

Convert 50% to a decimal: 0.5

14 080 mL × 0.5 = 7 040 mL

Step 3: Determine the first 8-hour infusion rate (mL/h).

7 040 mL ÷ 8 h = 880 mL/h

Step 4: Determine the next 16-hour volume (50% of total 24-hour volume).

14 080 mL − 7 040 mL = 7 040 mL

Step 5: Determine the infusion rate for this 16-hour volume (mL/h).

7 040 mL ÷ 16 h = 440 mL/h

Step 6: Determine the D5W fluid replacement for hours 25 to 48 post-burn.

(constant)　(kg)　(% BSA burned)　(Total volume)

1 mL　×　88　×　40　=　3 520 mL

Step 7: Determine the infusion rate for hours 25 to 48.

3 520 mL ÷ 24 h = 146.6 = 147 mL/h

Example: A child who weighs 29 kg has 35% of total BSA burned in a house fire.

Order: IV RL to infuse as per Parkland formula × 24 h. IV D5W infusion based on post–24-hour formula for hours 25 to 48 post-burn.

Step 1: Determine the first 24-hour Ringer's lactate solution to be infused.

(constant)   (kg)   (% BSA burned)   (Total volume)

4 mL × 29 × 35 = 4 060 mL

Step 2: Determine the first 8-hour volume (50% of total 24-hour volume).

Convert 50% to a decimal: 0.5

4 060 mL × 0.5 = 2 030 mL

Step 3: Determine the first 8-hour infusion rate (mL/h).

2 030 mL ÷ 8 h = 253.75 = 254 mL/h

Step 4: Determine the next 16-hour volume (50% of total 24-hour volume).

4 060 mL − 2 030 mL = 2 030 mL

Step 5: Determine the infusion rate for this 16-hour volume (mL/h).

2 030 mL ÷ 16 = 126.8 = 127 mL/h

Step 6: Determine the D5W fluid replacement for hours 25 to 48 post-burn.

(constant)   (kg)   (% BSA burned)   (Total volume)

1 mL × 29 × 35 = 1 015 mL

Step 7: Determine the infusion rate for hours 25 to 48.

1 015 mL ÷ 24 h = 42.2 = 42 mL/h

(!) SAFETY ALERT!

The fluid resuscitation of patients with burns requires a substantial amount of IV fluids. Select the proper IV site and monitor it. Also monitor the patient closely for fluid overload and respiratory complications. Multiple lines or a central line with multiple ports may be an option for the IV.

POINTS TO REMEMBER

- Use the Parkland formula to determine fluid resuscitation for adults and children older than 10 in the first 24 hours after a burn injury.
- Check your institution's policy regarding fluid replacement for different medical conditions, including burns, for the first 24 hours and after.
- Choose the appropriate IV site to manage the large amount of infusion.
- Note that children usually receive maintenance fluids in addition to resuscitation fluids.
- Apply the Parkland formula from the time of the burn injury and not from the time that the patient is assessed.
- Over the 25 to 48 hours that follow a burn injury, calculate the amount of fluid replacement needed based on the patient's minimum urine output.

╋━➗✕ PRACTICE **PROBLEMS**

Complete the following problems on fluid resuscitation using the Parkland formula and the post–24-hour formula based on urine output. The infusing solutions are Ringer's lactate for the first 24 hours and D5W for the next 25 to 48 hours.

Parkland formula: 4 mL × kg × % BSA burned = Total volume (mL)

Post–24-hour formula based on urine output: 1 mL × kg × % BSA burned = Total volume (mL)

Round your answers to whole numbers as required.

53. Patient Profile: An adult patient arrived at the emergency department with 60% of BSA burned from a work explosion. He weighs 110 kg.

    a. What is the 24-hour total IV fluid replacement?　　　_____

    b. What is the first 8-hour total IV fluid replacement?　　　_____

    c. What is the first 8-hour infusion rate in mL per hour?　　　_____

    d. What is the next 16-hour total IV fluid replacement?　　　_____

    e. What is the infusion rate for this 16-hour
       volume in mL per hour?　　　_____

    f. What is the total IV fluid replacement for
       hours 25 to 48 post-burn?　　　_____

    g. What is the infusion rate for hours 25 to 48 post-burn
       in mL per hour?　　　_____

54. Patient Profile: An adult patient sustained burns to 45% of BSA in a house fire. He weighs 98.5 kg.

    a. What is the 24-hour total IV fluid replacement?　　　_____

    b. What is the first 8-hour total IV fluid replacement?　　　_____

    c. What is the first 8-hour infusion rate in mL per hour?　　　_____

    d. What is the next 16-hour total IV fluid replacement?　　　_____

    e. What is the infusion rate for this 16-hour
       volume in mL per hour?　　　_____

    f. What is the total IV fluid replacement
       for hours 25 to 48 post-burn?　　　_____

    g. What is the infusion rate for hours 25 to 48
       post-burn in mL per hour?　　　_____

55. Patient Profile: An 11-year-old has 30% of BSA burned as a result of a backyard barbecue grill blow-up. She weighs 36.3 kg.

    a. What is the 24-hour total IV fluid replacement?　　　_____

    b. What is the first 8-hour total IV fluid replacement?　　　_____

    c. What is the first 8-hour infusion rate in mL per hour? _____

    d. What is the next 16-hour total IV fluid replacement? _____

    e. What is the infusion rate for this 16-hour
       volume in mL per hour? _____

    f. What is the total IV fluid replacement
      for hours 25 to 48 post-burn? _____

    g. What is the infusion rate for hours 25 to 48
      post-burn in mL per hour? _____

56. Patient Profile: An adult patient has 65% BSA burned from a highway traffic accident. She weighs 90 kg.

    a. What is the 24-hour total IV fluid replacement? _____

    b. What is the first 8-hour total IV fluid replacement? _____

    c. What is the first 8-hour infusion rate in mL per hour? _____

    d. What is the next 16-hour total IV fluid replacement? _____

    e. What is the infusion rate for this 16-hour
       volume in mL per hour? _____

    f. What is the total IV fluid replacement
      for hours 25 to 48 post-burn? _____

    g. What is the infusion rate for hours 25 to 48
      post-burn in mL per hour? _____

Answers on pages 643–644.

Intravenous Therapy and Children
Pediatric Intravenous Administration

The administration of IV fluids to children is very specific because of their physiological development. Microdrop sets are used for infants and small children; electronic devices are used to control the rate of delivery. The rate of infusion for infants and children must be carefully monitored. The IV drop rate must be slow for small children to prevent complications such as cardiac failure because of fluid overload. Various IV devices decrease the size of the drop to "mini" or "micro" drop or 1/60 mL, thus delivering 60 minidrops or microdrops per millilitre. IV medications may be administered to a child over a period of time (several hours) or on an intermittent basis. For intermittent medication administration, several methods of delivery are used, including the following:

- **Small-volume IV bags**—These may be used if the child has a primary IV line in place. A secondary tubing set is attached to a small-volume IV bag, and the piggyback method is used.
- **Calibrated burettes**—These are often referred to by their trade names: Buretrol, Volutrol, or Soluset. (Figure 22-2 shows a typical system that consists of a calibrated chamber that can hold 100 to 150 mL of fluid.) The burette is calibrated in small increments that allow exact measurements of small volumes. Medication is added to the IV fluid in the chamber for a prescribed dilution of volume.

An electronic controller or pump may also be used with a Buretrol to administer intermittent IV medications. When used together for added patient safety, the tubing of the

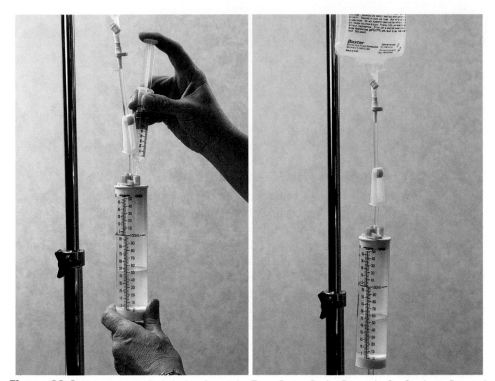

Figure 22-2 Volume-controlled device (burette). (From Potter P. A., Perry, A. G., Stockert, P., et al. (2013). *Fundamentals of nursing* (8th ed.). St. Louis: Mosby.)

Buretrol is threaded through the electronic pump, which sounds an alarm when the Buretrol chamber is empty. Understand that if an electronic pump is added, there is no need to count or calibrate drops per minute (gtt/min) because the pump is programmed to infuse in millilitres per hour (mL/h). In this case, the roller clamp of the Buretrol is left open to allow the medication or other IV fluid to flow from the Buretrol via the pump until infusion is complete and the alarm is activated. Buretrols may also be used in the adult setting for patients with fluid restrictions.

! SAFETY ALERT!

IV infusions should be monitored as frequently as every 30 minutes to 1 hour. A solution to flush the IV tubing is administered after medication is administered.

Regardless of the method used for medication administration in children, **a solution to flush the IV tubing is administered after the medication.** The purpose of the flush is to make sure the medication has cleared the tubing and the total dosage has been administered. Most institutions flush with normal saline (NS) solution. The amount of fluid used varies according to the length of the tubing from the medication source to the infusion site. **When IV medications are diluted for administration, the policy for including medication volume as part of the volume specified for dilution varies from institution to institution, as does the amount of flush. When flow rates (gtt/min, mL/h) are calculated, whether the flush is included varies from institution to institution. The nurse is responsible for checking the protocol at the institution to ensure that the correct procedure is followed.**

! SAFETY ALERT!

An excessively high concentration of an IV medication can cause vein irritation and potentially life-threatening effects.

BOX 22-2	Holliday-Segar Method for Calculating Maintenance Fluid Requirements in Children	
	Holliday-Segar Method	**Holliday-Segar Estimate**
First 10 kg	100 mL/kg/day	4 mL/kg/h
Second 10 kg	50 mL/kg/day	2 mL/kg/h
Every kg thereafter	20 mL/kg/day	1 mL/kg/h

From Meyers, Rachel S. (2009). Pediatric fluid and electrolyte therapy. *Journal of Pediatric Pharmacology and Therapeutics, 14*(4), 204–211. Table 2. Retrieved from http://www.ncbi.nlm.nih.gov/pmc/articles/PMC3460795/pdf/i1551-6776-14-4-204.pdf

Calculating Pediatric Intravenous Fluid Maintenance

Fluid therapy is a vital part of hospitalized care delivery for pediatric patients. Many factors may contribute to the fluid requirements of children encompassing the three categories of maintenance, deficit, and replacement. In this section, we will briefly discuss fluid maintenance.

Usually a physician calculates and orders the daily fluid requirement for a child admitted to hospital. However, before implementing the order, the nurse is responsible for checking its accuracy and safety for that child, considering the child's overall medical condition. All institutions have fluid maintenance policies and procedures. However, the Holliday-Segar formula remains the standard method for calculating the daily volume for maintenance fluids in children. In fact, the Holliday-Segar formula is the method of choice in children's hospitals in North America, including the world-renowned Hospital for Sick Children in Toronto.

Box 22-2 shows the Holliday-Segar method for calculating maintenance fluid requirements in children (Meyers, 2009).

The choice of fluid for maintenance depends on the patient's condition and needs, which is further dependent on the patient's physiological changes from day to day. For example, children admitted to hospital for fever, burn injury, asthma exacerbation, and any hypermetabolic state will need increased fluid and electrolyte therapy. Different concentrations of NS or dextrose with potassium chloride may be ordered. Large volumes of 5% dextrose should be avoided because they could predispose a child to hyponatremia, which can lead to neurological deficits.

When a physician prescribes daily fluid maintenance, the child's weight and medical condition is paramount to the selection and concentration of IV fluids. For the purposes of our calculations, only the child's weight will be provided. Let's look at a few examples. You will need the formula in Box 22-2 to work through them. To increase the accuracy of fluid and medication infusion, all IVs are connected to an IV pump with or without a Buretrol. The pumps are calibrated to deliver whole numbers as well as tenths of a millilitre of fluid. Answers with hourly rates are rounded to the nearest tenth of a millilitre.

Example: Calculate the daily maintenance fluid volume and the hourly infusion rate for a child who weighs 9.5 kg.

Step 1: Calculate the daily maintenance fluid volume.

100 mL/kg/day × 9.5 kg = 950 mL/day (24 hours) (first 10 kg)

Note: There is no need to use the other lines in the formula because the child is under 10 kg.

Step 2: Calculate the hourly infusion rate.

950 mL/24 h = 39.58 mL = 39.6 mL/h

Note that the rate of infusion could have been calculated directly by using the "4-2-1" rule or formula in the Holliday-Segar estimate (see Box 22-2), which would yield a similar result.

4 mL/kg/h × 9.5 kg/h = 38 mL/h (first 10 kg)

Example: Calculate the daily maintenance fluid volume and the hourly infusion rate for a child who weighs 32 kg.

Step 1:   Calculate the daily maintenance fluid volume.

100 mL/kg/day × 10 kg = 1 000 mL/day

50 mL/kg/day × 10 kg = 500 mL/day

20 mL/kg/day × 12 kg = 240 mL/day

Total: 1 000 mL/day + 500 mL/day + 240 mL/day = 1 740 mL/day

Step 2:   Calculate the hourly infusion rate.

1 740 mL/24 h = 72.5 mL/h

Example: Calculate the hourly infusion rate for a child who weighs 33 kg.

For this calculation, you can use the 4-2-1 rule, because the formula is in mL per kg per hour.

4 mL/kg/h × 10 kg/h = 40 mL/h

2 mL/kg/h × 10 kg/h = 20 mL/h

1 mL/kg/h × 13 kg/h = 13 mL/h

Total: 40 mL/h + 20 mL/h + 13 mL/h = 73 mL/h

PRACTICE **PROBLEMS**

Using the Holliday-Segar method or estimate for calculating pediatric fluid maintenance, answer the following questions.

57. Calculate the total daily maintenance fluid volume and hourly infusion rate for a child who weighs 26 kg.

a. Daily maintenance fluid volume   _____

b. Hourly infusion rate   _____

58. Calculate the hourly infusion rate for a child who weighs 15 kg.   _____

Answers on page 644.

Calculating Intravenous Medications by Burette

A calibrated burette can be used to administer medications by using a roller clamp rather than a pump. In this case, it is necessary to use the formula presented in Chapter 20 or dimensional analysis and calculate drops per minute (gtt/min). Remember, burettes are volume control devices and have a drop factor of 60 gtt per mL.

> **NOTE**
> When calculating drops per minute for a burette, the total volume will include the medication + the diluent.

$$x\,gtt/min = \frac{Total\ volume\ (mL) \times Drop\ factor\ (gtt/mL)}{Time\ (min)}$$

Example: An antibiotic dose of 100 mg in 2 mL is to be diluted in 20 mL of D5W to infuse over 30 minutes. A 15-mL flush follows. The administration set is a microdrop (burette).

Step 1: Read the medication label, and determine what volume the 100 mg is contained in. The label states that this is 2 mL.

Step 2: Allow 18 mL of D5W to run into the burette, and then add the 2 mL containing the 100 mg of medication. Roll the burette between your hands to allow the medication to mix thoroughly. (2 mL + 18 mL = 20 mL for volume)

Step 3: Determine the flow rate necessary to deliver the medication plus the flush in 30 minutes.

Total volume is 20 mL. Infusion time is 30 minutes.

$$x\,\text{gtt/min} = \frac{20\,\text{mL (diluted medication)} \times 60\,\text{gtt/mL}}{30\,\text{min}}$$

$$x = \frac{20 \times \overset{2}{\cancel{60}}}{\underset{1}{\cancel{30}}} = 40\,\text{gtt/min}$$

$$x = 40\,\text{gtt/min}$$

✔ Solution Using Dimensional Analysis

To calculate drops per minute, refer to the steps in Chapter 20, if necessary:

$$\frac{x\,\text{gtt}}{\text{min}} = \frac{\overset{20}{\cancel{60}}\,\text{gtt}}{1\,\cancel{\text{mL}}} \times \frac{\overset{2}{\cancel{20}}\,\cancel{\text{mL}}}{\underset{\underset{1}{\cancel{3}}}{\cancel{30}}\,\text{min}}$$

$$x = \frac{40}{1}$$

$$x = 40\,\text{gtt/min};\ 40\,\text{microgtt/min}$$

Step 4: Adjust the IV flow rate to deliver 40 microgtt per min (40 gtt/min).

Step 5: Label the burette with the medication name, dosage, and medication infusing label.

Step 6: When administration of the medication is completed, add the 15-mL flush and continue to infuse at 40 microgtt per min. Replace the label with a "flush infusing" label.

Step 7: When the flush is completed, restart the primary line and remove the flush infusing label. Document the medication according to institution policy on the medication administration record (MAR) (handwritten or in the computer) and the volume of fluid on the intake and output (I&O) flow sheet according to institution policy.

> ### ⓘ TIPS FOR CLINICAL PRACTICE
>
> To express the volume of drops per minute in millilitres per hour, remember that a microdrop administration set delivers 60 gtt per mL; therefore, gtt/min = mL/h. In this case, if the gtt/min = 40, then the mL/h = 40.

As already mentioned, the burette can be used with an electronic controller or pump. Note that an electronic infusion device will sound an alarm each time the burette empties. Let's examine the calculation necessary when the burette is used with an electronic controller or pump. When the burette is used with an electronic controller or pump, calculations are done in millilitres per hour. Let's use the same example shown previously to illustrate the difference in calculation steps.

Example: An antibiotic dose of 100 mg in 2 mL is to be diluted in 20 mL of D5W to infuse over 30 minutes. A 15-mL flush follows. An infusion controller is used, and the tubing is a microdrop burette.

The same Steps 1 and 2 as shown in the previous example for burette only are followed.

Step 1:   Calculate the flow rate for this microdrop.

Total volume is 20 mL; the flush is not considered in the volume.

Step 2:   Total volume is 20 mL. Infusion time is 30 minutes. Use the ratio and proportion method or the dimensional analysis method to calculate the rate in millilitres per hour.

> **NOTE**
> When medication has infused, add the 15 mL-flush and continue to infuse at 40 mL per hour; replace the label with a "flush infusing" label. Once the flush is finished, restart the primary IV or disconnect it from lock. Remove the "flush infusing" label. Document the medication according to institution policy on the MAR (handwritten or in the computer) and on the I&O flow sheet according to institution policy.

✔ Solution Using Ratio and Proportion

$$20\,\text{mL} : 30\,\text{minutes} = x\,\text{mL} : 60\,\text{minutes}$$
$$30x = 60 \times 20$$
$$\frac{30x}{30} = \frac{120\cancel{0}}{3\cancel{0}} = 40\,\text{mL/h}$$
$$x = 40\,\text{mL/h}$$

✔ Solution Using Dimensional Analysis

To calculate millilitres per hour, refer to the steps in Chapter 20, if necessary.

$$\frac{x\,\text{mL}}{\text{h}} = \frac{20\,\text{mL}}{\underset{1}{\cancel{30}\,\cancel{\text{min}}}} \times \frac{\overset{2}{\cancel{60}\,\cancel{\text{min}}}}{1\,\text{h}}$$
$$x = \frac{40}{1}$$
$$x = 40\,\text{mL/h}$$

> **NOTE**
> As shown in Chapter 20, the shortcut method using the drop factor constant could be used. Ratio and proportion can be stated by using several formats.

Example: An antibiotic dose of 150 mg in 1 mL is to be diluted in 35 mL NS to infuse over 45 minutes. A 15-mL flush follows. A volumetric pump will be used.

Total volume is 35 mL. Infusion time is 45 minutes. Calculate the infusion rate (mL/h).

$$35\,\text{mL} : 45\,\text{minutes} = x\,\text{mL} : 60\,\text{minutes}$$
$$45x = 35 \times 60$$
$$\frac{45x}{45} = \frac{2100}{45} = 46.6 = 47\,\text{mL/h}$$
$$x = 47\,\text{mL/h}$$

✔ Solution Using Dimensional Analysis

$$\frac{x \text{ mL}}{\text{h}} = \frac{35 \text{ mL}}{\overset{}{\underset{3}{\cancel{45} \text{ min}}}} \times \frac{\overset{4}{\cancel{60}} \text{ min}}{1 \text{ h}}$$

$$x = \frac{140}{3} = 46.6 = 47 \text{ mL}$$

$$x = 47 \text{ mL/h}$$

➕➖➗✖ PRACTICE **PROBLEMS**

Determine the volume of solution that must be added to the burette in the following problems. Then determine the flow rate in drops per minute for each IV using a microdrop, and indicate the infusion rate for a controller (mL/h).

59. An IV medication dosage of 500 mg is ordered to be diluted to 30 mL and infuse over 50 minutes with a 15-mL flush to follow. The dosage of medication is contained in 3 mL. Determine the following:

    a. Dilution volume   _____

    b. Flow rate in gtt per min   _____

    c. Flow rate in mL per hour   _____

60. The volume of a 20 mg dosage of medication is 2 mL. Dilute to 15 mL, and administer over 45 minutes with a 15-mL flush to follow. Determine the following:

    a. Dilution volume   _____

    b. Flow rate in gtt per min   _____

    c. Flow rate in mL per hour   _____

Answers on page 644.

Determining Whether a Pediatric Intravenous Dosage Is Safe

As seen earlier in this chapter, medications can be calculated based on milligrams per kilogram (mg/kg) or BSA. IV dosages for children are calculated on that basis as well. An IV medication can be assessed to determine whether it is within normal range as well. The safe daily dosage is calculated and then compared with the dosage ordered.

To determine whether an IV dosage for a child is safe, consult an appropriate drug reference for the recommended dosage. Remember to carefully read the reference to determine whether the medication is calculated according to BSA in square metres (common with chemotherapy medications), micrograms, units per day, or units per hour. When a dosage is within normal range, calculate and administer the dosage. If a dosage is not within normal range, consult the prescriber before administering the medication. *Note:* If the order is based on the child's BSA and the BSA is not known, you will need to use the West nomogram or the formula presented in this chapter to calculate the BSA. Let's look at some examples.

Example: A child's BSA is 0.8 m², and the order is for 1.8 mg of a medication in 100 mL D5W at 10:00 AM. The recommended dosage is 2 mg per m².

Step 1:   As previously shown in this chapter, if BSA is known, calculate the dosage for the child by multiplying the recommended dosage by the BSA. The recommended dosage is 2 mg per m², and the child's BSA is 0.8 m².

$$0.8 \, \cancel{m^2} \times 2 \, mg/\cancel{m^2} = 1.6 \, mg$$

Step 2:   Determine whether the dosage is within normal range.

The safe dosage is 1.6 mg for this child, but 1.8 mg is ordered. Notify the prescriber before administering the dosage. *Note:* The dosage in this example can also be determined by using the dimensional analysis method.

✔ Solution Using Dimensional Analysis

$$x \, mg = \frac{2 \, mg}{\cancel{m^2}} \times \frac{0.8 \, \cancel{m^2}}{1}$$
$$x = 1.6 \, mg$$

Example: A child weighing 10 kg has an order for IV Solu-Medrol 125 mg IV q6h for 48 hours. The recommended dosage is 30 mg per kg per day IV and can be replicated q4h to q6h for 48 hours.

Step 1:   Determine the dosage for the child.

$$10 \, \cancel{kg} \times 30 \, mg/\cancel{kg}/day = 300 \, mg/day$$

Step 2:   Determine whether the dosage ordered is within normal range.

The dosage: 125 mg q6h (4 doses).

$$125 \, mg \times 4 = 500 \, mg/day$$

Check with the prescriber; the dosage is more than what the child should receive. *Note:* The dosage in this example can also be determined by using the dimensional analysis method.

✔ Solution Using Dimensional Analysis

$$\frac{x \, mg}{kg} = \frac{30 \, mg}{1 \, \cancel{kg}/day} \times \frac{10 \, \cancel{kg}}{1}$$
$$x = 300 \, mg/day$$

+−÷× PRACTICE **PROBLEMS**

Determine the normal dosage range for the following problems to the nearest tenth. State your course of action.

61. A child weighing 17 kg has an order for an IV of 250 mL D5W containing 2 500 units of medication, which is to infuse at 50 mL per hour. The recommended dosage for the medication is 10 to 25 units per kg per hour.

Determine whether the dosage ordered is within normal range, and state your course of action.   _____

62. A child with a BSA of 0.75 m² has an order for an IV of 84 mg of a medication in 100 mL D5W q12h. The recommended dosage is 100 to 250 mg per m² per day in two divided doses. Determine whether the dosage ordered is within normal range, and state your course of action. _____

Answers on page 644.

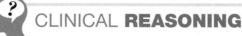 **POINTS** TO **REMEMBER**

- Pediatric IV medications are diluted for administration. It is important to know the institution's policy as to whether the medication volume is included as part of the total dilution volume.
- A flush is used after administration of IV medications in children. The volume of the flush will vary, depending on the length of the IV tubing from the medication source.
- The institution's policy on whether the volume of the flush is added to the diluted medication volume should be checked.
- Pediatric medication administration requires frequent assessment.
- A reputable drug reference should be used to calculate the normal dosage range for IV administration. The dosage ordered should be compared with the normal dosage range to determine whether the dosage ordered is safe.

Pediatric Oral and Parenteral Medications

Several methods have been presented to determine dosages for children in this chapter. It is important, however, to bear in mind that although the dosage may be determined according to weight, BSA, and so on, the dosage to administer is calculated using the same methods used to calculate adult dosages (ratio and proportion, the formula method, or dimensional analysis). It is important to remember the following differences with children's dosages.

Remember

- Dosages are smaller for children than for adults.
- Most oral medications for infants and small children come in liquid form to facilitate swallowing.
- The oral route is preferred; however, when necessary, medications are administered by the parenteral route.
- Not more than 1 mL is injected IM for small children and older infants; small infants should not receive more than 0.5 mL by IM injection.
- Parenteral dosages are frequently administered with a tuberculin syringe.

! **SAFETY ALERT!**

When in doubt, always double-check pediatric dosages with another person to decrease the chance of an error. Never assume! Think before administering.

? CLINICAL **REASONING**

1. **Scenario:** According to *Mosby's 2016 Nursing Drug Reference*, the recommended dosage for a child 5 months to 12 years old for ibuprofen as an antipyretic is 5 to 10 mg per kg per dose q6h to q8h PO. The 7-month-old weighs $18\frac{1}{2}$ lb. The prescriber ordered 20 mg PO q6h for a temperature above 39.2°C. The infant's temperature is 39.3°C, and the nurse is preparing to administer the medication. The nurse believes the dosage is low but administers the medication based on the dosage being safe because it is below the safe dosage range. Several hours have passed, and the infant's temperature continues to increase.

a. What is the required single dose
for this infant?   _____

b. What should the nurse's actions have been and why?   _____

c. What preventive measures could have been
taken by the nurse in this situation?   _____

Answers on page 645.

CHAPTER **REVIEW**

Read the dosage information or label provided for the following problems. Express body
weight conversion to the nearest tenth as indicated and dosages to the nearest tenth.

1. Lasix 10 mg IV stat is ordered for a child
weighing 10 kg. The recommended dosage
is 1 to 2 mg per kg per dose. Is the dosage
ordered safe? (Prove mathematically.)   _____

2. Amoxicillin 150 mg PO q8h is ordered for an infant weighing 10.5 kg.

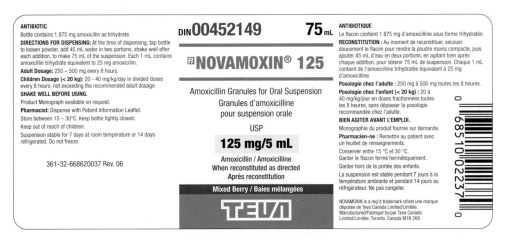

a. What is the recommended dosage range?   _____

b. What is the divided dosage range?   _____

c. Is the dosage ordered safe? (Prove mathematically.)   _____

3. Furadantin oral suspension 25 mg PO q6h is ordered for a child weighing 17 kg. The
recommended dosage is 5 to 7 mg per kg per 24 hour divided q6h.

Available: Furadantin oral suspension 25 mg per 5 mL

a. What is the dosage range for this child?   _____

b. Is the dosage ordered safe? (Prove mathematically.)   _____

c. How many mL must be given per dose to
administer the dosage ordered? Calculate
the dosage if the order is safe.   _____

4. Cefaclor 225 mg PO q8h is ordered for a child weighing 35 kg.

   Available:

   100 mL when mixed.
   Shake well before using.
   Store at 20°-25°C.

   DOSAGE AND USE
   See package insert for full prescribing information

   Usual Dosage: Children, 20 mg/kg a day (40 mg/kg in otitis media) in three divided doses.

   Exp./
   Lot:

   DIN: 000000000

   # cefaclor
   For oral suspension

   187 mg per 5 mL

   SAMPLE LABEL (textbook use only)

   http://evolve.elsevier.com/Canada/GrayMorris/

   Is the dosage ordered safe? (Prove mathematically) _____

5. Vibramycin 50 mg PO q12h is ordered for a child weighing 13.6 kg. The recommended dosage is 2.2 to 4.4 mg per kg per day in two divided doses. Is the dosage ordered safe? (Prove mathematically.) _____

6. Oxacillin oral solution 250 mg PO q6h is ordered for a child weighing 19.1 kg. The recommended dosage is 50 to 100 mg per kg per day in equally divided dosages q6h. Is the dosage ordered safe? (Prove mathematically.) _____

7. Cleocin suspension 150 mg PO q8h is ordered for a child weighing 16.4 kg. The recommended dosage is 10 to 30 mg per kg per day divided q6h to q8h. Is the dosage ordered safe? (Prove mathematically.) _____

8. Cephalexin (Keflex) suspension 250 mg PO q6h is ordered for a child weighing 30 kg. The usual pediatric dosage is 25 to 50 mg per kg per day in four divided doses.

   Available: Keflex suspension 250 mg per 5 mL

   a. Is the dosage ordered safe? (Prove mathematically.) _____

   b. How many mL would you need to administer one dose? Calculate the dosage if the order is safe. _____

9. Streptomycin sulphate 400 mg IM daily is ordered for a child weighing 35 kg. The recommended dosage is 20 to 40 mg per kg per day once daily.

   a. Is the dosage ordered safe? (Prove mathematically.) _____

b. A 1 g vial of streptomycin sulphate is available in powdered form with the following instructions: Dilution with 1.8 mL of sterile water will yield 400 mg per mL. How many mL will you need to administer the dosage ordered? Calculate the dosage if the order is safe.   _____

10. A child weighing 20.9 kg has an order for ranitidine (Zantac) 20 mg IV q8h. Is the dosage ordered safe? (Prove mathematically.)

Available:

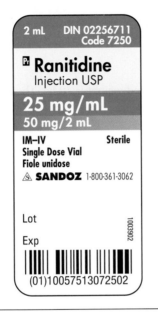

Pediatric Use
While limited data exist on the administration of IV ranitidine to children, the recommended dose in pediatric patients is for a total daily dose of 2 to 4 mg/kg, to be divided and administered every 6 to 8 hours, up to a maximum of 50 mg given every 6 to 8 hours. This recommendation is derived from adult clinical studies and pharmacokinetic data in pediatric patients. Limited data in neonatal patients (less than one month of age) receiving ECMO have shown that a dose of 2 mg/kg is usually sufficient to increase gastric pH to >4 for at least 15 hours. Therefore, doses of 2 mg/kg given every 12 to 24 hours or as a continuous infusion should be considered.

11. The recommended dosage for neonates receiving ceftazidime (Tazicef) is 30 mg per kg q12h. The neonate weighs 3 500 g.

a. What is the neonate's weight in kg to the nearest tenth?   _____

b. What is the safe dosage for this neonate?   _____

12. An 18.2-kg child who is 5 years old has an order for midazolam 1.5 mg IV stat. The recommended dosage for a child 6 months to 5 years is 0.05 to 0.1 mg per kg per dose. Is the dosage ordered safe?   _____

13. The recommended dosage for Mithracin for the treatment of testicular tumours is 25 to 30 mcg per kg. A patient weighs 86.4 kg. What is the dosage range in mg for this patient? (Round to the nearest tenth.)   _____

Using the West nomogram in Figure 22-1, determine the BSA and calculate each child's dosage by using the formula. Express dosages to the nearest tenth.

14. The child's height is 30 inches, and weight is 20 lb. The adult dosage of an antibiotic is 500 mg.

    a. What is the BSA? _____

    b. What is the child's dosage? _____

15. The child's height is 32 inches, and weight is 27 lb. The adult dosage for a medication is 25 mg.

    a. What is the BSA? _____

    b. What is the child's dosage? _____

16. The child's height is 120 cm, and weight is 40 kg. The adult dosage for a medication is 250 mg.

    a. What is the BSA? _____

    b. What is the child's dosage? _____

17. The child's height is 50 inches, and weight is 75 lb. The adult dosage for a medication is 30 mg.

    a. What is the BSA? _____

    b. What is the child's dosage? _____

18. The child's height is 50 inches, and weight is 70 lb. The adult dosage for a medication is 150 mg.

    a. What is the BSA? _____

    b. What is the child's dosage? _____

Determine the child's dosage for the following medications. Express your answers to the nearest tenth.

19. The adult dosage of a medication is 50 mg.
    What is the dosage for a child with a BSA of 0.7 m²? _____

20. The adult dosage of a medication is 10 to 20 mg.
    What is the dosage range for a child
    with a BSA of 0.66 m²? _____

21. The adult dosage of a medication is 2 000 units.
    What is the dosage for a child
    with a BSA of 0.55 m²? _____

22. The adult dosage of a medication is 200 to 250 mg.
    What is the dosage range for a child with a BSA of 0.55 m²? _____

23. The adult dosage of a medication is 150 mg.
    What is the dosage for a child with a BSA of 0.22 m²? _____

Calculate the child's dosage in the following problems. Determine whether the prescriber's order is correct. If the order is incorrect, give the correct dosage. Express your answers to the nearest tenth.

24. A child with a BSA of 0.49 m^2
    has an order for 25 mg of a medication.
    The adult dosage is 60 mg.   _____

25. A child with a BSA of 0.32 m^2 has an order
    for 4 mg of a medication.
    The adult dosage is 10 mg.   _____

26. A child with a BSA of 0.68 m^2 has an order
    for 50 mg of a medication.
    The adult dosage is 125 to 150 mg.   _____

27. A child with a BSA of 0.55 m^2
    has an order for 5 mg of a medication.
    The adult dosage is 25 mg.   _____

28. A child with a BSA of 1.2 m^2 has an
    order for 60 mg of a medication.
    The adult dosage is 75 to 100 mg.   _____

Using the formula method for calculating BSA, determine the BSA in the following patients, and express your answers to the nearest hundredth.

29. A 15-year-old who weighs 100 lb and is 55 inches tall   _____

30. An adult who weighs 60.9 kg and is 130 cm tall   _____

31. A child who weighs 55 lb and is 45 inches tall   _____

32. A child who weighs 60 lb and is 35 inches tall   _____

33. An adult who weighs 65 kg and is 132 cm tall   _____

34. A child who weighs 24 lb and is 28 inches tall   _____

35. An infant who weighs 6 kg and is 55 cm long   _____

36. A child who weighs 42 lb and is 45 inches tall   _____

37. An infant who weighs 8 kg and is 70 cm long   _____

38. An adult who weighs 74 kg and is 160 cm tall   _____

Calculate the following dosages using the labels or the information provided.

39. Order: Azidothymidine 7 mg PO q6h.

    Available: Azidothymidine 10 mg per mL   _____

40. Order: Epivir 150 mg PO BID.

    Available: Epivir oral solution labelled 10 mg per mL   _____

41. Order: Digoxin 0.1 mg PO daily.

    Available:

    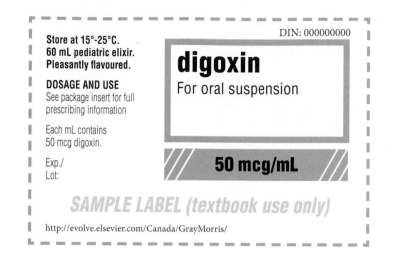

    _____

42. Order: Retrovir 80 mg PO q8h.

    Available: Retrovir syrup labelled 50 mg per 5 mL   _____

43. Order: Amoxicillin/clavulanate potassium 250 mg PO q6h.

    Available:

    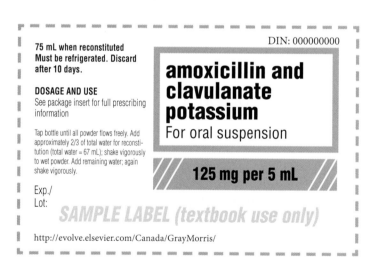

    _____

44. Order: Carbamazepime 0.25 g PO TID.

    Available:

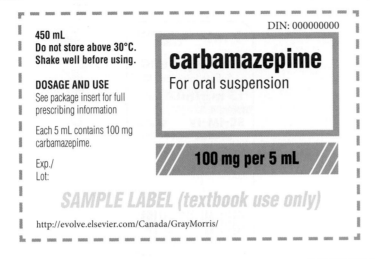

450 mL
Do not store above 30°C.
Shake well before using.

DOSAGE AND USE
See package insert for full prescribing information

Each 5 mL contains 100 mg carbamazepime.

Exp./
Lot:

DIN: 000000000

carbamazepime
For oral suspension

100 mg per 5 mL

SAMPLE LABEL (textbook use only)

http://evolve.elsevier.com/Canada/GrayMorris/

_____

45. Order: Amoxicillin 100 mg PO TID.

    Available: Amoxicillin oral suspension
    labelled 250 mg per 5 mL   _____

Calculate the following dosages using the labels or the information provided. Express your answers to the nearest hundredth as indicated.

46. Order: Gentamicin 7.3 mg IM q12h.

    Available: 20 mg per 2 mL

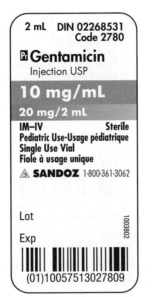

2 mL   DIN 02268531
        Code 2780

℞ **Gentamicin**
Injection USP

10 mg/mL
20 mg/2 mL

IM–IV   Sterile
Pediatric Use-Usage pédiatrique
Single Use Vial
Fiole à usage unique
⚠ **SANDOZ** 1-800-361-3062

Lot

Exp

1003802

(01)10057513027809

_____

47. Order: Atropine 0.1 mg SUBCUT stat.

    Available: Atropine 400 mcg per mL   _____

48. Order: Ampicillin 160 mg IM q12h.

    Available: Ampicillin 250 mg per mL   _____

49. Order: Morphine 3.5 mg SUBCUT q6h prn for pain.

    Available:

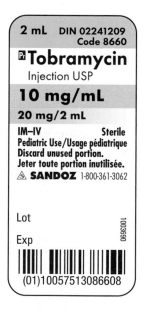

50. Order: Tobramycin 60 mg IV q8h.

    Available:

Calculate the following dosages using the labels or the information provided. Express your answers to the nearest tenth as indicated (express answers in millilitres).

51. Order: Tylenol 0.4 g PO q4h prn for temp greater than 38.3°C.

    Available: Tylenol elixir labelled 160 mg per 5 mL

52. Order: Methotrexate 35 mg IM daily once a week (on Tuesdays).

    Available:

20 mL DIN 02398427 Code 44037415	Antimetabolite and antirheumatic IM, IV, IA only Not for intrathecal administration Multidose Vial • Sterile Store between 15-25°C. Protect from light.		Sandoz Canada Inc. 1-800-361-3062
℞**Methotrexate** Injection USP 25 mg/mL **500 mg/20 mL** CONTAINS BENZYL ALCOHOL AS PRESER-VATIVE • AVEC ALCOOL BENZYLIQUE COMME AGENT DE CONSERVATION △ **SANDOZ**	Antimétabolite et antirhumatismal IM, IV, IA seulement Pas pour administration intrathécale Fiole multidose • Stérile Conserver entre 15-25 °C. Protéger de la lumière. 46073553	C CYTOTOXIC CYTOTOXIQUE	Lot: XXXXXX EXP: XXXXXX

————————————

53. Order: Clindamycin 100 mg IV q6h.

    Available: Clindamycin labelled 150 mg per mL   ————————————

54. Order: Procaine penicillin 150 000 units IM q12h.

    Available: Procaine penicillin 300 000 units per mL   ————————————

55. Order: Amikacin 150 mg IV q8h.

    Available:

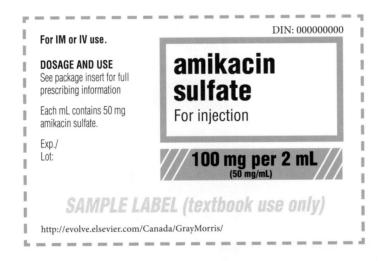

For IM or IV use.

DOSAGE AND USE
See package insert for full prescribing information

Each mL contains 50 mg amikacin sulfate.

Exp./
Lot:

DIN: 000000000

**amikacin
sulfate**
For injection

100 mg per 2 mL
(50 mg/mL)

SAMPLE LABEL (textbook use only)

http://evolve.elsevier.com/Canada/GrayMorris/

————————————

56. Order: Dilantin 62.5 mg PO BID.

    Available: Dilantin oral suspension labelled
    125 mg per 5 mL   ————————————

57. Order: Meperidine (Demerol) 20 mg IM q4h prn.

    Available: Meperidine labelled 25 mg per mL   ————————————

58. Order: Erythromycin 300 mg PO q6h.

    Available:

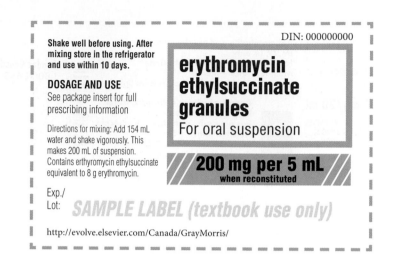

Shake well before using. After mixing store in the refrigerator and use within 10 days.

DOSAGE AND USE
See package insert for full prescribing information

Directions for mixing: Add 154 mL water and shake vigorously. This makes 200 mL of suspension. Contains erthyromycin ethylsuccinate equivalent to 8 g erythromycin.

Exp./
Lot:

DIN: 000000000

erythromycin ethylsuccinate granules
For oral suspension

200 mg per 5 mL
when reconstituted

SAMPLE LABEL (textbook use only)

http://evolve.elsevier.com/Canada/GrayMorris/

_____

59. Order: Albuterol 3 mg PO BID.

    Available:

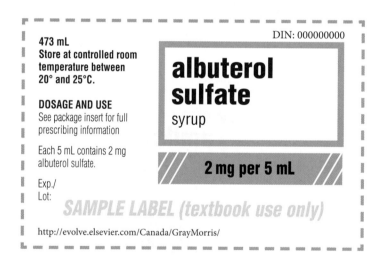

473 mL
Store at controlled room temperature between 20° and 25°C.

DOSAGE AND USE
See package insert for full prescribing information

Each 5 mL contains 2 mg albuterol sulfate.

Exp./
Lot:

DIN: 000000000

albuterol sulfate
syrup

2 mg per 5 mL

SAMPLE LABEL (textbook use only)

http://evolve.elsevier.com/Canada/GrayMorris/

_____

60. Order: Tetracycline 250 mg PO q6h.

    Available: Tetracycline oral suspension labelled 125 mg per 5 mL

    _____

61. Order: Theophylline 40 mg PO BID.

    Available: Theophylline elixir labelled 80 mg per 15 mL

    _____

62. Order: Ferrous sulphate 45 mg PO daily.

    Available: Ferrous sulphate drops 15 mg per 0.6 mL

    _____

63. Order: Methylprednisolone 14 mg IV q6h.

    Available:

DIN 02231893   Sterile/Stérile

℞ methyl**PREDNIS**olone
SODIUM SUCCINATE
FOR INJECTION, USP

40 mg

methyl**PREDNIS**olone per vial
Glucocorticoid /
Glucocorticoïde
Anti-inflammatory /
Anti-inflammatoire
IM or IV Use Only /
Usage IM ou IV seulement

Reconstitute (dilute) before use.
Discard unused portion.
RECONSTITUTION: Add 1 mL Sterile Water for Injection and use within 24 hours or 1 mL Bacteriostatic Water for Injection and use within 48 hours. Each reconstituted vial contains approximately 1 mL. Each mL contains 40 mg methyl**PREDNIS**olone. Store powder at 15°C- 25°C. Protect from light. See enclosed package insert.
Reconstituer (diluer) avant l'emploi.
Jeter toute portion inutilisée.
RECONSTITUTION: Pour le mode de reconstitution, voir le dépliant de conditionnement ci-joint. Conserver la poudre à 15 °C - 25 °C. Protéger de la lumière.

(01)00068510933010

Novopharm Limited/Limitée,
Toronto, Canada M1B 2K9
361-32-765710101 Rev 07

1-29114850/C

LOT

EXP.

_____

64. Order: Famotidine 20 mg PO BID.

    Available: Famotidine 8 mg per mL   _____

65. Order: Furosemide 75 mg IV BID.

    Available:

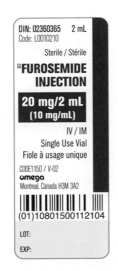

DIN: 02360365   2 mL
Code: L0010210

Sterile / Stérile

℞**FUROSEMIDE**
INJECTION

20 mg/2 mL
(10 mg/mL)

IV / IM
Single Use Vial
Fiole à usage unique

C0OE1150 / V-02
omega
Montreal, Canada H3M 3A2

(01)10801500112104

LOT:

EXP:

_____

Solve the following problems in the units of measurement indicated. Round answers to the nearest tenth as indicated.

66. Order: Cefaclor 180 mg PO q8h. The infant weighs 4.5 kg. The recommended dosage is 20 mg per kg per day in three divided doses.

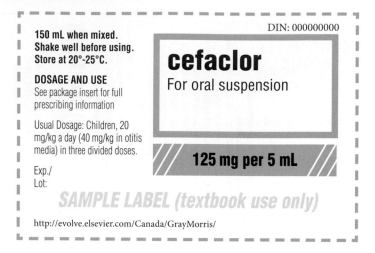

150 mL when mixed.
Shake well before using.
Store at 20°-25°C.

DOSAGE AND USE
See package insert for full prescribing information

Usual Dosage: Children, 20 mg/kg a day (40 mg/kg in otitis media) in three divided doses.

Exp./
Lot:

DIN: 000000000

cefaclor
For oral suspension

125 mg per 5 mL

SAMPLE LABEL (textbook use only)

http://evolve.elsevier.com/Canada/GrayMorris/

a. Is the dosage ordered safe? _____

b. How many mL will you need to administer the dosage? Calculate the dosage to administer if the dosage is safe. _____

67. Order: Clarithromycin 200 mg PO q12h for a child weighing 45 lb.

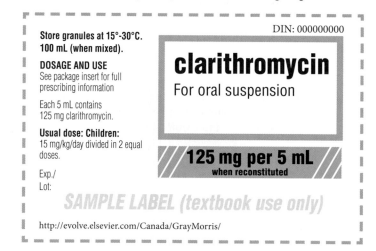

Store granules at 15°-30°C.
100 mL (when mixed).

DOSAGE AND USE
See package insert for full prescribing information

Each 5 mL contains 125 mg clarithromycin.

Usual dose: Children:
15 mg/kg/day divided in 2 equal doses.

Exp./
Lot:

DIN: 000000000

clarithromycin
For oral suspension

125 mg per 5 mL
when reconstituted

SAMPLE LABEL (textbook use only)

http://evolve.elsevier.com/Canada/GrayMorris/

Is the dosage ordered safe? _____

68. Order: Amprenavir 650 mg PO TID for a child weighing 30 kg. The recommended dosage is 22.5 mg per kg up to three times a day.

Is the dosage ordered safe? _____

69. Acetaminophen (Tylenol) 525 mg IV q4h is ordered for a child weighing 42 kg. According to *Mosby's 2016 Nursing Drug Reference,* the dosage for a child who is greater than or equal to 2 years old and weighs less than 50 kg is 15 mg per kg per dose q6h, or 12.5 mg per kg per dose q4h IV up to a maximum of 75 mg per kg per day.

a. What is the safe dosage for this child? _____

b. Is the dosage ordered safe? _____

70. Order: Minoxidil for a child weighing 31 lb. The recommended dosage range is 0.25 to 1 mg per kg per day.

   What is the safe dosage range for this child? _____

Determine the dosage or dosage range in the following problems. Round dosages to the nearest tenth as indicated.

71. The recommended dosage for vincristine (Oncovin) is 2 mg per m². The child has a BSA of 0.8 m². _____

72. The recommended dosage for acyclovir is 250 mg per m². The child has a BSA of 0.82 m². _____

73. The recommended dosage for bleomycin in an adult with Hodgkin disease is 10 to 20 units per m². The adult has a BSA of 1.83 m². _____

Determine the flow rate in drops per minute for each IV using a microdrip, then indicate the millilitres per hour infusion rate for a controller. (Consider the medication volume as part of the total dilution volume as shown in the chapter.)

74. A child is to receive 10 units of a medication. The dosage of 10 units is contained in 1 mL. Dilute to 30 mL, and infuse in 20 minutes. A 15-mL flush is to follow. Medication is placed in a burette. Determine the flow rate in the following:

   a. gtt per min _____

   b. mL per hour _____

75. A child is to receive 80 mg of a medication. The dosage of 80 mg is contained in 2 mL. Dilute to 80 mL, and infuse in 60 minutes. A 15-mL flush is to follow. Medication is placed in a burette. Determine the flow rate in the following:

   a. gtt per min _____

   b. mL per hour _____

76. A dosage of 250 mg in 5 mL has been ordered diluted to 40 mL and infused in 45 minutes. A 15-mL flush follows. Medication is placed in a burette. Determine the flow rate in the following:

   a. gtt per min _____

   b. mL per hour _____

Determine the normal dosage range for the following problems to the nearest tenth. State your course of action.

77. A child weighing 23 kg has an order for 500 mg of a medication in 100 mL D5W q12h. The normal dosage range is 40 to 50 mg per kg per day. Determine whether the dosage ordered is within normal range, and state your course of action. _____

78. A child weighing 20 kg has an order for 2 mg of a medication in 100 mL D5W at 10:00 AM. The normal daily dosage is 0.05 mg per kg. Determine whether the dosage ordered is within normal range, and state your course of action.

_____

79. A child weighing 15 kg has an order for 55 mcg of a medication IV q12h. The dosage range is 6 to 8 mcg per kg per day q12h. Determine whether the dosage ordered is within normal range, and state your course of action.

_____

80. A patient presents to the emergency department after a fire explosion at work. On assessment, the physician concludes that 37% of his total BSA is burned. He weighs 81 kg. Use the Parkland formula or the post–24-hour formula based on urine output to determine the fluid replacement of RL and D5W as indicated.

_____

Parkland formula: 4 mL × kg × % BSA burned = Total volume (mL)
Post–24-hour formula based on urine output: 1 mL × kg × % BSA burned = Total volume (mL)

a. What is the 24-hour total amount of RL IV fluid replacement that the patient should receive?

_____

b. What is the first 8-hour total amount of RL IV fluid replacement that the patient should receive?

_____

c. What is the first 8-hour infusion rate of RL IV fluid replacement in mL per hour?

_____

d. What is the next 16-hour total amount of RL IV fluid replacement that the patient should receive?

_____

e. What is the infusion rate for this 16-hour volume in mL per hour?

_____

f. What is the total amount of D5W IV fluid replacement for hours 25 to 48 post-burn?

_____

g. What is the infusion rate of D5W IV fluid replacement for hours 25 to 48 post-burn in mL per hour?

_____

Refer to the pediatric daily fluid guidelines in Box 22-2 to answer the following questions.

81. A child who weighs 35 kg was admitted to a medical unit with diarrhea. The child was ordered NS as daily maintenance IV fluid according to protocol. What is the child's hourly IV rate?

_____

82. A child who weighs 19 kg was admitted to hospital with asthma and is receiving IV NS according to daily maintenance guidelines.

    a. What is the 24-hour total maintenance IV fluid for this child? _____

    b. What is the infusion rate of the maintenance IV fluid? _____

Answers on pages 645–652.

✳ ANSWERS

Answers to Practice Problems

1. 4 kg

2. 1.5 kg

3. 2.9 kg

4. 3.6 kg

5. 1.9 kg

NOTE

Any of the methods presented in Chapter 20 can be used to calculate dosages; not all methods are shown in the Answer Key.

6. a. 25 to 50 mg per kg per day

   $25 \text{ mg}:1 \text{ kg} = x \text{ mg}:15.9 \text{ kg}$

   $x = 397.5 \text{ mg/day}$

   $50 \text{ mg}:1 \text{ kg} = x \text{ mg}:15.9 \text{ kg}$

   $x = 795 \text{ mg/day}$

   or

   $25 \text{ mg/kg/day} \times 15.9 \text{ kg} = 397.5 \text{ mg/day}$

   $50 \text{ mg/kg/day} \times 15.9 \text{ kg} = 795 \text{ mg/day}$

   b. The safe dosage range is 397.5 to 795 mg per day.
   c. The dosage ordered falls within the range that is safe (150 mg × 4 = 600 mg). 600 mg per day falls within the 397.5 to 795 mg per day range.

d. $250 \text{ mg}:5 \text{ mL} = 150 \text{ mg}:x \text{ mL}$

   or

   $\dfrac{150 \text{ mg}}{250 \text{ mg}} \times 5 \text{ mL} = x \text{ mL}$

   $x = 3 \text{ mL}$

7. a. $15 \text{ mg}:1 \text{ kg} = x \text{ mg}:35 \text{ kg}$

   $x = 525 \text{ mg/day}$

   $30 \text{ mg}:1 \text{ kg} = x \text{ mg}:35 \text{ kg}$

   $x = 1050 \text{ mg/day}$

   or

   $15 \text{ mg/kg/day} \times 35 \text{ kg} = 525 \text{ mg/day}$

   $30 \text{ mg/kg/day} \times 35 \text{ kg} = 1050 \text{ mg/day}$

   The safe dosage range for the child is 525 to 1050 mg per day.

   b. $\dfrac{525 \text{ mg}}{3} = 175 \text{ mg q8h}$

   $\dfrac{1050 \text{ mg}}{3} = 350 \text{ mg q8h}$

   The divided dosage range is 175 to 350 mg q8h.
   c. The dosage ordered is safe. 200 mg × 3 = 600 mg. 600 mg per day falls within the range of 525 to 1050 mg per day. Also, the dosage q8h falls within the divided dosage range of 175 to 350 mg q8h.

evolve

For additional practice problems, refer to the Pediatric Calculations section of the Drug Calculations Companion, Version 5 on Evolve.

8. a.

$$10 \text{ mg} : 1 \text{ kg} = x \text{ mg} : 40 \text{ kg}$$

$$x = 400 \text{ mg/day}$$

or

$$10 \text{ mg/kg/day} \times 40 \text{ kg} = 320 \text{ mg/day}$$

$$30 \text{ mg} : 1 \text{ kg} = x \text{ mg} : 40 \text{ kg}$$

$$x = 1\,200 \text{ mg/day}$$

or

$$30 \text{ mg/kg/day} \times 40 \text{ kg} = 1\,200 \text{ mg/day}$$

Answer: 1 200 mg per day is the maximum dosage.
b. q6h = 24 ÷ 4 = 4 doses/day
400 mg ÷ 4 = 100 mg q6h
1 200 mg ÷ 4 = 300 mg q6h
Answer: 100 to 300 mg q6h is the divided dosage range (300 mg q6h is the maximum divided dose).

9. a.

$$3 \text{ mg} : 1 \text{ kg} = x \text{ mg} : 4.1 \text{ kg}$$

$$x = 12.3 \text{ mg/day}$$

or

$$3 \text{ mg/kg/day} \times 4.1 \text{ kg} = 12.3 \text{ mg/day}$$

$$5 \text{ mg} : 1 \text{ kg} = x \text{ mg} : 4.1 \text{ kg}$$

$$x = 20.5 \text{ mg/day}$$

or

$$5 \text{ mg/kg/day} \times 4.1 \text{ kg} = 20.5 \text{ mg/day}$$

The safe dosage range for the child is
12.3 to 20.5 mg per day.
b. The dosage ordered is safe.
10 mg × 2 = 20 mg/day. The maximum dosage per day is 20.5 mg.
c.

$$20 \text{ mg} : 5 \text{ mL} = 10 \text{ mg} : x \text{ mL}$$

or

$$\frac{10 \text{ mg}}{20 \text{ mg}} \times 5 \text{ mL} = x \text{ mL}$$

$$x = 2.5 \text{ mL}$$

You need to give 2.5 mL to administer the dosage ordered of 10 mg.

10. a.

$$0.1 \text{ mg} : 1 \text{ kg} = x \text{ mg} : 38.2 \text{ kg}$$

$$x = 3.8 \text{ mg/dose}$$

or

$$38.2 \text{ kg} \times 0.1 \text{ mg/kg/dose} = 3.82 \text{ mg} = 3.8 \text{ mg/dose}$$

or

$$0.2 \text{ mg} : 1 \text{ kg} = x \text{ mg} : 38.2 \text{ kg}$$

$$x = 7.6 \text{ mg/dose}$$

$$38.2 \text{ kg} \times 0.2 \text{ mg/kg/dose} = 7.64 \text{ mg} = 7.6 \text{ mg/dose}$$

The safe dosage range for the child is 3.8 to 7.6 mg per dose.
b. The dosage ordered is safe. 7.5 mg is less than 7.6 mg.
c.

$$5 \text{ mg} : 1 \text{ mL} = 7.5 \text{ mg} : x \text{ mL}$$

or

$$\frac{7.5 \text{ mg}}{5 \text{ mg}} \times 1 \text{ mL} = x \text{ mL}$$

$$x = 1.5 \text{ mL}$$

You would administer 1.5 mL for one dose.

11. a.

$$4 \text{ mg} : 1 \text{ kg} = x \text{ mg} : 5 \text{ kg}$$

$$x = 20 \text{ mg/day}$$

or

$$4 \text{ mg/kg/day} \times 5 \text{ kg} = 20 \text{ mg/day}$$

$$8 \text{ mg} : 1 \text{ kg} = x \text{ mg} : 5 \text{ kg}$$

$$x = 40 \text{ mg/day}$$

or

$$8 \text{ mg/kg/day} \times 5 \text{ kg} = 40 \text{ mg/day}$$

The safe dosage range for the child is 20 to 40 mg per day.
b. The dosage that is ordered is safe. It falls within the safe range. 15 mg × 2 = 30 mg/day.
c.

$$125 \text{ mg} : 5 \text{ mL} = 15 \text{ mg} : x \text{ mL}$$

or

$$\frac{15 \text{ mg}}{125 \text{ mg}} \times 5 \text{ mL} = x \text{ mL}$$

You would administer 0.6 mL for one dose.

12. $$2.5 \text{ mg}:1 \text{ kg} = x \text{ mg}:20 \text{ kg}$$

$$x = 50 \text{ mg/day}$$

or

$$5 \text{ mg}:1 \text{ kg} = x \text{ mg}:20 \text{ kg}$$

$$x = 100 \text{ mg/day}$$

or

$$5 \text{ mg/} \cancel{kg} \text{/day} \times 20 \cancel{kg} = 100 \text{ mg/day}$$

The initial safe dosage range for the child is 50 to 100 mg per day.

13. a. $$40 \text{ mg}:1 \text{ kg} = x \text{ mg}:17.3 \text{ kg}$$

$$x = 692 \text{ mg/day}$$

or

$$40 \text{ mg/} \cancel{kg} \text{/day} \times 17.3 \cancel{kg} = 692 \text{ mg/day}$$

b. $$\frac{692 \text{ mg}}{4} = 173 \text{ mg/dose}$$

c. The dosage ordered is not safe. 200 mg × 4 = 800 mg/day. 800 mg per day is greater than 692 mg per day. It also exceeds the dose that should be given q6h. Check with the prescriber.

14. a. 20 to 40 mg per kg per day

$$20 \text{ mg}:1 \text{ kg} = x \text{ mg}:7.3 \text{ kg}$$

$$x = 146 \text{ mg/day}$$

or

$$20 \text{ mg/} \cancel{kg} \text{/day} \times 7.3 \cancel{kg} = 146 \text{ mg/day}$$

$$40 \text{ mg}:1 \text{ kg} = x \text{ mg}:7.3 \text{ kg}$$

$$x = 292 \text{ mg/day}$$

or

$$40 \text{ mg/} \cancel{kg} \text{/day} \times 7.3 \cancel{kg} = 292 \text{ mg/day}$$

b. The safe dosage range for the child is 146 to 292 mg per day.
c. The dosage ordered is not safe. 125 mg × 3 = 375 mg/day. 375 mg per day is greater than 146 to 292 mg per day. Check with the prescriber.

15. Convert weight (2.2 lb = 1 kg).

$$44 \text{ lb} \div 2.2 = 20 \text{ kg}$$

$$30 \text{ mg}:1 \text{ kg} = x \text{ mg}:20 \text{ kg}$$

$$x = 600 \text{ mg/day}$$

or

$$30 \text{ mg/} \cancel{kg} \text{/day} \times 20 \cancel{kg} = 600 \text{ mg/day}$$

$$50 \text{ mg}:1 \text{ kg} = x \text{ mg}:20 \text{ kg}$$

$$x = 1000 \text{ mg/day}$$

or

$$50 \text{ mg/} \cancel{kg} \text{/day} \times 20 \cancel{kg} = 1000 \text{ mg/day}$$

a. The safe dosage range is 600 to 1000 mg per day.
b. The dosage ordered is safe. 250 mg × 4 = 1000 mg. 1000 mg falls within the safe range.

16. $$0.25 \text{ mg}:1 \text{ kg} = x \text{ mg}:66.3 \text{ kg}$$

$$x = 16.57 = 16.6 \text{ mg}$$

or

$$0.25 \text{ mg/} \cancel{kg} \times 66.3 \cancel{kg} = 16.57 = 16.6 \text{ mg}$$

Answer: 16.6 mg is the dosage for the adult.

17. $$150 \text{ mg}:1 \text{ kg} = x \text{ mg}:90.9 \text{ kg}$$

$$x = 13635 \text{ mg/day}$$

or

$$150 \text{ mg/} \cancel{kg} \text{/day} \times 90.9 \cancel{kg} = 13635 \text{ mg/day}$$

$$200 \text{ mg}:1 \text{ kg} = x \text{ mg}:90.9 \text{ kg}$$

$$x = 18180 \text{ mg/day}$$

or

$$200 \text{ mg/} \cancel{kg} \text{/day} \times 90.9 \cancel{kg} = 18180 \text{ mg/day}$$

To determine the number of grams, convert the mg obtained to grams (1000 mg = 1 g).

13635 mg ÷ 1000 = 13.63 g (13.6 g to nearest tenth)

18180 mg ÷ 1000 = 18.18 g (18.2 g to nearest tenth)

The daily dosage range in grams is 13.6 to 18.2 g per day.

18. a.

$$6 \text{ mg} : 1 \text{ kg} = x \text{ mg} : 5.6 \text{ kg}$$

$$x = 33.6 \text{ mg}$$

or

$$6 \text{ mg}/\cancel{kg} \times 5.6 \cancel{kg} = 33.6 \text{ mg}$$

Answer: 33.6 mg for the first day.

b.

$$3 \text{ mg} : 1 \text{ kg} = x \text{ mg} : 5.6 \text{ kg}$$

$$x = 16.8 \text{ mg}$$

or

$$3 \text{ mg}/\cancel{kg} \times 5.6 \cancel{kg} = 16.8 \text{ mg}$$

Answer: 16.8 mg daily for the subsequent dosage.

35.

$$\sqrt{\dfrac{95.5 \,(\text{kg}) \times 180 \,(\text{cm})}{3\,600}}$$

$$\sqrt{4.775} = 2.185 = 2.19 \text{ m}^2$$

Answer: 2.19 m²

36.

$$\sqrt{\dfrac{10 \,(\text{kg}) \times 70 \,(\text{cm})}{3\,600}}$$

$$\sqrt{0.194} = 0.44 \text{ m}^2$$

Answer: 0.44 m²

37.

$$\sqrt{\dfrac{4.8 \,(\text{lb}) \times 21 \,(\text{in})}{3\,131}}$$

$$\sqrt{0.032} = 0.178 = 0.18 \text{ m}^2$$

Answer: 0.18 m²

38.

$$\sqrt{\dfrac{24 \,(\text{kg}) \times 92 \,(\text{cm})}{3\,600}}$$

$$\sqrt{0.613} = 0.783 = 0.78 \text{ m}^2$$

Answer: 0.78 m²

39. a. 0.52 m²

b. $\dfrac{0.52 \cancel{m^2}}{1.7 \cancel{m^2}} \times 25 \text{ mg} = \dfrac{0.52 \times 25}{1.7} = \dfrac{13}{1.7} = 7.64$

Answer: 7.6 mg

19. 0.6 m²

20. 0.78 m²

21. 0.9 m²

22. 0.8 m²

23. 0.28 m²

24. 0.44 m²

25. 0.8 m²

26. 0.28 m²

27. 0.52 m²

28. 0.45 m²

29. 0.9 m²

30. 0.3 m²

31. 0.58 m²

32. 0.51 m²

33. 0.68 m²

34. 0.18 m²

40. a. 0.53 m²

b. $\dfrac{0.53 \cancel{m^2}}{1.7 \cancel{m^2}} \times 200 \text{ mg} = \dfrac{0.53 \times 200}{1.7} = \dfrac{106}{1.7}$

$$\dfrac{106}{1.7} = 62.35 = 62.4 \text{ mg}$$

$$\dfrac{0.53 \cancel{m^2}}{1.7 \cancel{m^2}} \times 400 \text{ mg} = \dfrac{212}{1.7} = 124.7$$

Answer: The child's dosage range is 62.4 to 124.7 mg.

41. $\dfrac{1.5 \cancel{m^2}}{1.7 \cancel{m^2}} \times 5 \text{ mg} = \dfrac{1.5 \times 5}{1.7} = \dfrac{7.5}{1.7}$

$$\dfrac{7.5}{1.7} = 4.41 \text{ mg} = 4.4 \text{ mg}$$

$$\dfrac{1.5 \cancel{m^2}}{1.7 \cancel{m^2}} \times 15 \text{ mg} = \dfrac{22.5}{1.7} = 13.23$$

$$13.23 \text{ mg} = 13.2 \text{ mg}$$

Answer: 4.4 to 13.2 mg

42. $\dfrac{0.8 \cancel{m^2}}{1.7 \cancel{m^2}} \times 20 \text{ mg} = \dfrac{0.8 \times 20}{1.7} = \dfrac{16}{1.7}$

$$\dfrac{16}{1.7} = 9.41 \text{ mg} = 9.4 \text{ mg}$$

Answer: The dosage is incorrect. The correct dosage is 9.4 mg.

43. $\dfrac{0.9 \text{ m}^2}{1.7 \text{ m}^2} \times 25 \text{ mg} = \dfrac{0.9 \times 25}{1.7} = \dfrac{22.5}{1.7}$

$$\dfrac{22.5}{1.7} = 13.23 \text{ mg} = 13.2 \text{ mg}$$

Answer: The dosage is incorrect. The correct dosage is 13.2 mg.

44. $\dfrac{1.5 \text{ m}^2}{1.7 \text{ m}^2} \times 250 \text{ mg} = \dfrac{1.5 \times 250}{1.7} = \dfrac{375}{1.7}$

$$\dfrac{375}{1.7} = 220.58 = 220.6 \text{ mg}$$

Answer: The child's dosage is 220.6 mg.

45. $\dfrac{0.74 \text{ m}^2}{1.7 \text{ m}^2} \times 20 \text{ mg} = \dfrac{0.74 \times 20}{1.7} = \dfrac{14.8}{1.7}$

$$\dfrac{14.8}{1.7} = 8.7 \text{ mg}$$

$\dfrac{0.74 \text{ m}^2}{1.7 \text{ m}^2} \times 30 \text{ mg} = \dfrac{0.74 \times 30}{1.7} = \dfrac{22.2}{1.7}$

$$\dfrac{22.2}{1.7} = 13.05 = 13.1 \text{ mg}$$

Answer: The child's dosage range is 8.7 to 13.1 mg.

46. $\dfrac{0.67 \text{ m}^2}{1.7 \text{ m}^2} \times 20 \text{ mg} = \dfrac{13.4}{1.7} = 7.88 \text{ mg} = 7.9 \text{ mg}.$

Answer: The dosage is correct.

47. $\dfrac{0.94 \text{ m}^2}{1.7 \text{ m}^2} \times 10 \text{ mg} = 5.5 \text{ mg}$

$\dfrac{0.94 \text{ m}^2}{1.7 \text{ m}^2} \times 20 \text{ mg} = 11.1 \text{ mg}$

Answer: The child's dosage range is 5.5 to 11.1 mg.

48. a. 0.44 m²

b. $\dfrac{0.44 \text{ m}^2}{1.7 \text{ m}^2} \times 500 \text{ mg} = \dfrac{220}{1.7} = 129.41$

Answer: The child's dosage is 129.4 mg.

49. $\dfrac{1.3 \text{ m}^2}{1.7 \text{ m}^2} \times 500 \text{ mg} = \dfrac{1.3 \times 500}{1.7} = \dfrac{650}{1.7} = 382.35$

Answer: The child's dosage is 382.4 mg.

50. a. 0.52 m²

b. $\dfrac{0.52 \text{ m}^2}{1.7 \text{ m}^2} \times 25 \text{ mg} = \dfrac{0.52 \times 25}{1.7} = \dfrac{13}{1.7}$

$$\dfrac{13}{1.7} = 7.64 = 7.6 \text{ mg}$$

Answer: The child's dosage is 7.6 mg.

51. $\dfrac{0.52 \text{ m}^2}{1.7 \text{ m}^2} \times 15 \text{ mg} = \dfrac{0.52 \times 15}{1.7}$

$$= \dfrac{7.8}{1.7} = 4.58 = 4.6 \text{ mg}$$

Answer: The child's dosage is 4.6 mg.

52. $\dfrac{1.1 \text{ m}^2}{1.7 \text{ m}^2} \times 150 \text{ mg} = \dfrac{1.1 \times 150}{1.7}$

$$= \dfrac{165}{1.7} = 97.05 = 97.1 \text{ mg}$$

Answer: The child's dosage is 97.1 mg.

53. a. 4 mL × 110 kg × 60 = 26 400 mL (24-h total)
   b. 26 400 mL × 0.5 = 13 200 mL (first 8-h total)
   c. 13 200 mL/8 h = 1 650 mL/h (8-h infusion rate)
   d. 26 400 mL − 13 200 mL = 13 200 mL (next 16-h total)
   e. 13 200 mL/16 h = 825 mL/h (16-h infusion rate)
   f. 1 mL × 110 kg × 60 = 6 600 mL (post–24-h total)
   g. 6 600 mL × 24 h = 275 mL/h

54. a. 4 mL × 98.5 kg × 45 = 17 730 mL (24-h total)
   b. 17 730 mL × 0.5 = 8 865 mL (first 8-h total)
   c. 8 865 mL/8 h = 1 108 mL/h (8-h infusion rate)
   d. 17 730 mL − 8 865 mL = 8 865 mL (next 16-h total)
   e. 8 865 mL/16 h = 554 mL/h (16-h infusion rate)
   f. 1 mL × 98.5 kg × 45 = 4 433 mL (post–24-h total)
   g. 4 433 mL × 24 h = 185 mL/h

55. a. 4 mL × 36.3 kg × 30 = 4 356 mL (24-h total)
   b. 4 356 mL × 0.5 = 2 178 mL (first 8-h total)
   c. 2 178 mL/8 h = 272 mL/h (8-h infusion rate)
   d. 4 356 mL − 2 178 mL = 2 178 mL (next 16-h total)
   e. 2 178 mL/16 h = 136 mL/h (16-h infusion rate)
   f. 1 mL × 36.3 kg × 30 = 1 089 mL (post–24-h total)
   g. 1 089 mL × 24 h = 45 mL/h

56. a. 4 mL × 90 kg × 65 = 23 400 mL (24-h total)
    b. 23 400 mL × 0.5 = 11 700 mL (first 8-h total)
    c. 11 700 mL/8 h = 1 463 mL/h (8-h infusion rate)
    d. 23 400 mL − 11 700 mL = 11 700 mL (next 16-h total)
    e. 11 700 mL/16 h = 731 mL/h (16-h infusion rate)
    f. 1 mL × 90 kg × 65 = 5 850 mL (post–24-h total)
    g. 5 850 mL × 24 h = 244 mL/h

57. a. Formula: 100 mL/kg/day × 10 kg = 1 000 mL (first 10 kg)
    50 mL/kg/day × 10 kg = 500 mL (second 10 kg)
    20 mL/kg/day × 6 kg = 120 mL (remaining kg)
    Total: 1 000 mL/day + 5 000 mL/day + 120 mL/day = 1 620 mL/day
    b. Hourly infusion rate: 1 620 mL/24 h = 67.5 = 68 mL/h

58. Use the 4-2-1 formula:
    4 mL/kg/h × 10 kg = 40 mL/h (first 10 kg)
    2 mL/kg/h × 5 kg = 10 mL/h (only 5 kg remaining)
    Add for total: 40 mL/h + 10 mL/h = 50 mL/h

59. a. Dilution volume: 27 mL
    b. $x \text{ gtt/min} = \dfrac{30 \text{ mL (diluted medication)} \times 60 \text{ gtt/mL}}{50 \text{ min}}$

    $x = \dfrac{30 \times 60}{50} = \dfrac{1\,800}{50} = 36 \text{ gtt/min}$

    or

    Use ratio and proportion to determine mL per hour first. Remember that with a burette when a pump or controller is not used, mL/h = gtt/min.

    30 mL : 50 min = x mL : 60 min

    or

    $\dfrac{30 \text{ mL}}{50 \text{ min}} = \dfrac{x \text{ mL}}{60 \text{ mnin}}$

    Answer: x = 36 gtt/min; 36 microgtt/min
    c. 36 mL per hour

60. a. Dilution volume: 13 mL
    b. $x \text{ gtt/min} = \dfrac{15 \text{ mL (diluted medication)} \times 60 \text{ gtt/mL}}{45 \text{ min}}$

    $x = \dfrac{15 \times 60}{45} = \dfrac{900}{45} = 20 \text{ gtt/min}$

    or

    Use ratio and proportion to determine mL per hour first.

    15 mL : 45 min = x mL : 60 min

    or

    $\dfrac{15 \text{ mL}}{45 \text{ min}} = \dfrac{x \text{ mL}}{60 \text{ min}}$

    Answer: x = 20 gtt/min; 20 microgtt/min
    c. 20 mL per hour

61. Step 1: Determine the dosage range per hour.
    10 units/kg/h × 17 kg = 170 units/h
    25 units/kg/h × 17 kg = 425 units/h
    Step 2: Determine the dosage infusing per hour.
    2 500 units : 250 mL = x units : 50 mL
    $250x = 2\,500 \times 50$

    $\dfrac{250x}{250} = \dfrac{125\,000}{250} = 500$

    $x = 500 \text{ units/h}$
    Step 3: Compare the dosage ordered to see if it is within the safe range.
    The IV is infusing at 50 mL per hour, which is 500 units per hour. The normal dosage range is 170 to 425 units per hour. 500 units per hour is greater than the dosage range. Check with the prescriber before administering.

62. Step 1: Determine the dosage range.
    0.75 m² × 100 mg/m²/day = 75 mg/day
    0.75 m² × 250 mg/m²/day = 187.5 mg/day
    The dosage range is 75 to 187.5 mg per day.
    Step 2: Determine the dosage the child is receiving.
    84 mg q12h (2 dosages)
    84 mg × 2 = 168 mg/day
    Step 3: Determine whether the dosage is within the safe range. The 84 mg q12h (84 mg × 2 = 168 mg/day) is within the safe range of 75 to 187.5 mg per day, so administer the medication.

Answers to Clinical Reasoning Questions

1. a. 42 to 84 mg per dose
   b. Contact the prescriber; the dosage is too low. The dosage is not safe because it is below the recommended therapeutic dose to decrease the child's temperature.
   c. The nurse should have notified the prescriber immediately so that the order could be revised. The child's temperature indicates an underdosage that is not safe. Do not assume that a dosage is safe because it is lower than the recommended dosage.

Answers to Chapter Review

> **NOTE**
> Problems 1 to 13 in the Chapter Review could be solved using alternative methods, such as the ratio and proportion method and the dimensional analysis method. These methods are shown in the examples in Chapter 20. Refer to them if necessary.

1. $1 \, \text{mg}/\text{kg} \times 10 \, \text{kg} = 10 \, \text{mg/dose}$
   $2 \, \text{mg}/\text{kg} \times 10 \, \text{kg} = 20 \, \text{mg/dose}$
   The dosage ordered for this child is safe. 10 mg falls within the range of 10 to 20 mg per dose.

2. a. $20 \, \text{mg}/\text{kg}/\text{day} \times 10.5 \, \text{kg} = 210 \, \text{mg/day}$
   $40 \, \text{mg}/\text{kg}/\text{day} \times 10.5 \, \text{kg} = 420 \, \text{mg/day}$
   The safe dosage range for the infant is 210 to 420 mg per day.
   b. The medication is given in divided dosages q8h.
   $\text{q8h} = 24 \div 8 = 3 \, \text{doses/day}$
   $210 \, \text{mg} \div 3 = 70 \, \text{mg/dose}$
   $420 \, \text{mg} \div 3 = 140 \, \text{mg/dose}$
   The divided dosage range is 70 to 140 mg per dose q8h.
   c. The dosage ordered is not safe; $150 \, \text{mg} \times 3 = 450 \, \text{mg/day}$. 450 mg per day is greater than 420 mg per day. Also, the dose to be given q8h exceeds the dose recommended. Notify the prescriber and question the order.

3. a. The dosage range is 5 to 7 mg per 24 hours (day).
   $5 \, \text{mg}/\text{kg}/24 \, \text{h} \times 17 \, \text{kg} = 85 \, \text{mg}/24 \, \text{h}$
   $7 \, \text{mg}/\text{kg}/24 \, \text{h} \times 17 \, \text{kg} = 119 \, \text{mg}/24 \, \text{h}$
   Answer: The dosage range is 85 to 119 mg per day.
   b. $\text{q6h} = 24 \div 6 = 4 \, \text{doses/day}$
   $85 \, \text{mg} \div 4 = 21.25 \, \text{mg} = 21.3 \, \text{mg/dose}$
   $119 \, \text{mg} \div 4 = 29.75 \, \text{mg} = 29.8 \, \text{mg/dose}$
   The divided dosage range is 21.3 to 29.8 mg per dose q6h. The dosage ordered is 25 mg q6h. The dosage ordered is safe because 25 mg × 4 doses = 100 mg/day. It falls within the range of 85 to 119 mg per day. The dosage q6h also falls within the divided dosage range of 21.3 to 29.8 mg q6h.

   c. $25 \, \text{mg} : 5 \, \text{mL} = 25 \, \text{mg} : x \, \text{mL}$

   or

   $$\frac{25 \, \text{mg}}{25 \, \text{mg}} \times 5 \, \text{mL} = x \, \text{mL}$$
   $$x = 5 \, \text{mL}$$
   Answer: Give 5 mL per dose. The dosage ordered is contained in 5 mL.

4. The recommended dosage is 20 mg per kg per day.
   $20 \, \text{mg}/\text{kg}/\text{day} \times 35 \, \text{kg} = 700 \, \text{mg/day}$
   $\text{q8h} = 24 \div 8 = 3 \, \text{doses/day}$
   $700 \, \text{mg} \div 3 = 233.33 = 233.3 \, \text{mg per dose}$
   The dosage ordered is not safe. $225 \, \text{mg} \times 3 = 675 \, \text{mg/day}$. 675 mg per day is less than 700 mg per day. Also, the dose to be given q6h is less than 233.3 mg. Check with the prescriber. The dose may be too low to be effective.

5. The recommended dosage is 2.2 to 4.4 mg per kg per day.
   $2.2 \, \text{mg}/\text{kg}/\text{day} \times 13.6 \, \text{kg} = 29.9 \, \text{mg/day}$.
   $4.4 \, \text{mg}/\text{kg}/\text{day} \times 13.6 \, \text{kg} = 59.8 \, \text{mg/day}$.
   $\text{q12h} = 24 \div 2 = 2 \, \text{doses/day}$
   $29.9 \, \text{mg} \div 2 = 15 \, \text{mg/dose}$
   $59.8 \, \text{mg} \div 2 = 29.9 \, \text{mg/dose}$
   $50 \, \text{mg} \times 2 = 100 \, \text{mg/day}$
   The dosage is too high; notify the prescriber. 100 mg per day is greater than 29.9 to 59.8 mg per day. Also, the dose to be given q12h exceeds the recommended dosage.

6. The recommended dosage is 50 to 100 mg per kg per day.
   $50 \, \text{mg}/\text{kg}/\text{day} \times 19.1 \, \text{kg} = 955 \, \text{mg/day}$
   $100 \, \text{mg}/\text{kg}/\text{day} \times 19.1 \, \text{kg} = 1\,910 \, \text{mg/day}$
   $955 \, \text{mg} \div 4 = 238.8 \, \text{mg/dose}$
   $1\,910 \, \text{mg} \div 4 = 477.5 \, \text{mg/dose}$
   The dosage ordered is safe because $250 \, \text{mg} \times 4 = 1\,000 \, \text{mg/day}$.
   1 000 mg per day falls within the range of 955 to 1 910 mg per day.
   Also, the dose to be given q6h falls within the recommended dosage.

7. The recommended dosage is 10 to 30 mg per kg per day.
   10 mg/kg/day × 16.4 kg = 164 mg/day
   30 mg/kg/day × 16.4 kg = 492 mg/day
   The medication is given q6h to q8h. The dosage in this problem is ordered q8h.
   q8h = 24 ÷ 8 = 3 doses/day
   164 mg ÷ 3 = 54.7 mg/dose
   492 mg ÷ 3 = 164 mg/dose
   The dosage ordered is 150 mg q8h.
   150 mg × 3 = 450 mg/day
   The dosage is safe. 450 mg per day falls within the range of 164 to 492 mg per day. Also, the dose to be given q8h falls within the range of 54.7 to 164 mg per dose.

8. a. The recommended dosage is 25 to 50 mg per kg per day.
   25 mg/kg/day × 30 kg = 750 mg/day
   50 mg/kg/day × 30 kg = 1 500 mg/day
   The safe dosage range is 750 to 1 500 mg per day. The dosage ordered is q6h.
   q6h = 24 ÷ 6 = 4 doses/day
   750 mg ÷ 4 = 187.5 mg/dose
   1 500 mg ÷ 4 = 375 mg/dose
   The divided dosage range is 187.5 to 375 mg per dose q6h. 250 mg × 4 = 1 000 mg/day. This dosage is safe because the total dosage falls within the safe range for 24 hours, and the divided dosage range.
   b. You would give 5 mL for one dose.
   $$250 \text{ mg} : 5 \text{ mL} = 250 \text{ mg} : x \text{ mL}$$

   or

   $$\frac{250 \text{ mg}}{250 \text{ mg}} \times 5 \text{ mL} = x \text{ mL}$$

   $$x = 5 \text{ mL}$$

   The dosage ordered is contained in 5 mL; therefore, you will need to administer 5 mL.

9. a. The recommended dosage is 20 to 40 mg per kg per day.
   20 mg/kg/day × 35 kg = 700 mg/day
   40 mg/kg/day × 35 kg = 1 400 mg/day
   The safe dosage range is 700 to 1 400 mg per day. The prescriber ordered 400 mg IM daily. This dosage is not safe. 400 mg daily falls below the safe range for 24 hours. The dosage ordered may not be effective. Contact the prescriber.
   b. The dosage is not calculated; the dosage ordered daily is not safe.

10. The recommended dosage is 2 to 4 mg per kg per day.
    2 mg/kg/day × 20.9 kg = 41.8 mg/day
    4 mg/kg/day × 20.9 kg = 83.6 mg/day
    The safe dosage range is 41.8 to 83.6 mg per day. The dosage is ordered q8h.
    q8h = 24 ÷ 8 = 3 doses/day
    41.8 mg ÷ 3 = 13.9 mg/dose
    83.6 mg ÷ 3 = 27.9 mg/dose
    The dose ordered is safe. 20 mg × 3 = 60 mg/day. 60 mg per day falls within the range of 41.8 to 83.6 mg per day. The dose to be given q8h also falls within the range of 13.9 to 27.9 mg per dose.

11. Convert the neonate's weight in grams to kg (1 000 g = 1 kg).
    a. 3 500 g = 3.5 kg
    b. 30 mg/kg × 3.5 kg = 105 mg
       The safe dosage for the neonate is 105 mg q12h.

12. The recommended dosage is 0.05 to 0.1 mg per kg per dose.
    0.05 mg/kg/dose × 18.2 kg = 0.9 mg per dose
    0.1 mg/kg/dose × 18.2 kg = 1.8 mg per dose
    The dosage range for the child is 0.9 to 1.8 mg per dose. The dosage ordered is safe. 1.5 mg falls within the range of 0.9 to 1.8 mg per dose.

13. 86.4 kg × 25 mcg/kg = 2 160 mcg
    86.4 kg × 30 mcg/kg = 2 592 mcg
    To determine the number of mg, convert the mcg obtained to mg (1 000 mcg = 1 mg).
    2 160 mcg ÷ 1 000 = 2.16 mg (2.2 mg, to the nearest tenth)
    2 592 mcg ÷ 1 000 = 2.59 mg (2.6 mg, to the nearest tenth)
    The daily dosage range is 2.2 to 2.6 mg.

14. a. 0.45 m²
    b. $\dfrac{0.45 \text{ m}^2}{1.7 \text{ m}^2} \times 500 \text{ mg} = 132.35 = 132.4 \text{ mg}$

15. a. 0.53 m²
    b. $\dfrac{0.53 \text{ m}^2}{1.7 \text{ m}^2} \times 25 \text{ mg} = 7.79 = 7.8 \text{ mg}$

16. a. 1.2 m²
    b. $\dfrac{1.2 \text{ m}^2}{1.7 \text{ m}^2} \times 250 \text{ mg} = 176.5 \text{ mg}$

17. a. 1.1 m²
    b. $\dfrac{1.1 \text{ m}^2}{1.7 \text{ m}^2} \times 30 \text{ mg} = 19.4 \text{ mg}$

18. a. $1.06 \, m^2$

b. $\dfrac{1.06 \, m^2}{1.7 \, m^2} \times 150 \, mg = 93.52 = 93.5 \, mg$

19. $\dfrac{0.7 \, m^2}{1.7 \, m^2} \times 50 \, mg = 20.6 \, mg$

20. $\dfrac{0.66 \, m^2}{1.7 \, m^2} \times 10 \, mg = 3.9 \, mg$

$\dfrac{0.66 \, m^2}{1.7 \, m^2} \times 20 \, mg = 7.8 \, mg$

The dosage range is 3.9 to 7.8 mg.

21. $\dfrac{0.55 \, m^2}{1.7 \, m^2} \times 2\,000 \, units = 647.1 \, units$

22. $\dfrac{0.55 \, m^2}{1.7 \, m^2} \times 200 \, mg = 64.7 \, mg$

$\dfrac{0.55 \, m^2}{1.7 \, m^2} \times 250 \, mg = 80.9 \, mg$

The dosage range is 64.7 to 80.9 mg.

23. $\dfrac{0.22 \, m^2}{1.7 \, m^2} \times 150 \, mg = 19.4 \, mg$

24. The dosage is incorrect; the child's dosage is 17.3 mg.

$\dfrac{0.49 \, m^2}{1.7 \, m^2} \times 60 \, mg = 17.3 \, mg$

The dosage of 25 mg is too high.

25. $\dfrac{0.32 \, m^2}{1.7 \, m^2} \times 10 \, mg = 1.9 \, mg$

The dosage of 4 mg is too high.

26. The dosage is correct.

$\dfrac{0.68 \, m^2}{1.7 \, m^2} \times 125 \, mg = 50 \, mg$

$\dfrac{0.68 \, m^2}{1.7 \, m^2} \times 150 \, mg = 60 \, mg$

The dosage of 50 mg falls within the range of 50 to 60 mg.

27. The dosage is incorrect.

$\dfrac{0.55 \, m^2}{1.7 \, m^2} \times 25 \, mg = 8.1 \, mg$

The dosage of 5 mg is too low.

28. The dosage is correct.

$\dfrac{1.2 \, m^2}{1.7 \, m^2} \times 75 \, mg = 52.9 \, mg$

$\dfrac{1.2 \, m^2}{1.7 \, m^2} \times 100 \, mg = 70.6 \, mg$

The dosage ordered is 60 mg, which falls within the dosage range of 52.9 to 70.6 mg.

29. $\sqrt{\dfrac{100 \, (lb) \times 55 \, (in)}{3\,131}} = \sqrt{\dfrac{5\,500}{3\,131}} = \sqrt{1.756}$

$\sqrt{1.756} = 1.325$

Answer: $1.33 \, m^2$

30. $\sqrt{\dfrac{60.9 \, (kg) \times 130 \, (cm)}{3\,600}} = \sqrt{\dfrac{7\,917}{3\,600}} = \sqrt{2.199}$

$\sqrt{2.199} = 1.482$

Answer: $1.48 \, m^2$

31. $\sqrt{\dfrac{55 \, (lb) \times 45 \, (in)}{3\,131}} = \sqrt{\dfrac{2\,475}{3\,131}} = \sqrt{0.790}$

$\sqrt{0.790} = 0.888$

Answer: $0.89 \, m^2$

32. $\sqrt{\dfrac{60 \, (lb) \times 35 \, (in)}{3\,131}} = \sqrt{\dfrac{2\,100}{3\,131}} = \sqrt{0.670}$

$\sqrt{0.670} = 0.818$

Answer: $0.82 \, m^2$

33. $\sqrt{\dfrac{65\,(\text{kg}) \times 132\,(\text{cm})}{3\,600}} = \sqrt{\dfrac{8\,580}{3\,600}} = \sqrt{2.383}$

$$\sqrt{2.383} = 1.543$$

Answer: 1.54 m²

34. $\dfrac{\sqrt{24\,(\text{lb}) \times 28\,(\text{in})}}{3\,131} = \sqrt{\dfrac{672}{3\,131}} = \sqrt{0.214}$

$$\sqrt{0.214} = 0.462$$

Answer: 0.46 m²

35. $\sqrt{\dfrac{6\,(\text{kg}) \times 55\,(\text{cm})}{3\,600}} = \sqrt{\dfrac{330}{3\,600}} = \sqrt{0.091}$

$$\sqrt{0.091} = 0.301$$

Answer: 0.3 m²

36. $\sqrt{\dfrac{42\,(\text{lb}) \times 45\,(\text{in})}{3\,131}} = \sqrt{\dfrac{1\,890}{3\,131}} = \sqrt{0.603}$

$$\sqrt{0.603} = 0.776$$

Answer: 0.78 m²

37. $\sqrt{\dfrac{8\,(\text{kg}) \times 70\,(\text{cm})}{3\,600}} = \sqrt{\dfrac{560}{3\,600}} = \sqrt{0.155}$

$$\sqrt{0.155} = 0.393$$

Answer: 0.39 m²

38. $\sqrt{\dfrac{74\,(\text{kg}) \times 160\,(\text{cm})}{3\,600}} = \sqrt{\dfrac{11\,840}{3\,600}} = \sqrt{3.288}$

$$\sqrt{3.288} = 1.813$$

Answer: 1.81 m²

39. $\qquad 10\ \text{mg} : 1\ \text{mL} = 7\ \text{mg} : x\ \text{mL}$

or

$$\dfrac{7\ \text{mg}}{10\ \text{mg}} \times 1\ \text{mL} = x\ \text{mL}$$

Answer: 0.7 mL. The dosage ordered is less than the available strength; therefore, you will need less than 1 mL to administer the dosage.

40. $\qquad 10\ \text{mg} : 1\ \text{mL} = 150\ \text{mg} : x\ \text{mL}$

or

$$\dfrac{150\ \text{mg}}{10\ \text{mg}} \times 1\ \text{mL} = x\ \text{mL}$$

Answer: 15 mL. The dosage ordered is more than the available strength; therefore, you will need more than 1 mL to administer the dosage.

41. $\qquad 0.05\ \text{mg} : 1\ \text{mL} = 0.1\ \text{mg} : x\ \text{mL}$

or

$$\dfrac{0.1\ \text{mg}}{0.05\ \text{mg}} \times 1\ \text{mL} = x\ \text{mL}$$

Answer: 2 mL. The dosage ordered is more than the available strength; therefore, you will need more than 1 mL to administer the dosage.

42. $\qquad 50\ \text{mg} : 5\ \text{mL} = 80\ \text{mg} : x\ \text{mL}$

or

$$\dfrac{80\ \text{mg}}{50\ \text{mg}} \times 5\ \text{mL} = x\ \text{mL}$$

Answer: 8 mL. The dosage ordered is greater than the available strength; therefore, you will need more than 5 mL to administer the dosage.

43. $\qquad 125\ \text{mg} : 5\ \text{mL} = 250\ \text{mg} : x\ \text{mL}$

or

$$\dfrac{250\ \text{mg}}{125\ \text{mg}} \times 5\ \text{mL} = x\ \text{mL}$$

Answer: 10 mL. The dosage ordered is greater than the available strength; therefore, you will need more than 5 mL to administer the dosage.

44. Conversion is required. Conversion factor: 1 000 mg = 1 g. Therefore, 0.25 g = 250 mg.

$$100 \text{ mg}:5 \text{ mL} = 250 \text{ mg}:x \text{ mL}$$

or

$$\frac{250 \text{ mg}}{100 \text{ mg}} \times 5 \text{ mL} = x \text{ mL}$$

Answer: 12.5 mL. The dosage ordered is greater than the available strength; therefore, you will need more than 5 mL to administer the dosage.

45. $$250 \text{ mg}:5 \text{ mL} = 100 \text{ mg}:x \text{ mL}$$

or

$$\frac{100 \text{ mg}}{250 \text{ mg}} \times 5 \text{ mL} = x \text{ mL}$$

Answer: 2 mL. The dosage ordered is less than the available strength; therefore, you will need less than 5 mL to administer the dosage.

46. $$20 \text{ mg}:2 \text{ mL} = 7.3 \text{ mg}:x \text{ mL}$$

or

$$\frac{7.3 \text{ mg}}{20 \text{ mg}} \times 2 \text{ mL} = x \text{ mL}$$

Answer: 0.73 mL. The dosage ordered is less than the available strength; therefore, you will need less than 2 mL to administer the dosage.

47. Conversion is required. Conversion factor: 1 000 mcg = 1 mg. Therefore, 0.1 mg = 100 mcg.

$$400 \text{ mcg}:1 \text{ mL} = 100 \text{ mcg}:x \text{ mL}$$

or

$$\frac{100 \text{ mcg}}{400 \text{ mcg}} \times 1 \text{ mL} = x \text{ mL}$$

Answer: 0.25 mL. The dosage ordered is less than the available strength; therefore, you will need less than 1 mL to administer the dosage.

48. $$250 \text{ mg}:1 \text{ mL} = 160 \text{ mg}:x \text{ mL}$$

or

$$\frac{160 \text{ mg}}{250 \text{ mg}} \times 1 \text{ mL} = x \text{ mL}$$

Answer: 0.64 mL. The dosage ordered is less than the available strength; therefore, you will need less than 1 mL to administer the dosage.

49. $$15 \text{ mg}:1 \text{ mL} = 3.5 \text{ mg}:x \text{ mL}$$

or

$$\frac{3.5 \text{ mg}}{15 \text{ mg}} \times 1 \text{ mL} = x \text{ mL}$$

Answer: 0.23 mL. The dosage ordered is less than the available strength; therefore, you will need less than 1 mL to administer the dosage.

50. $$20 \text{ mg}:2 \text{ mL} = 60 \text{ mg}:x \text{ mL}$$

or

$$\frac{60 \text{ mg}}{20 \text{ mg}} \times 2 \text{ mL} = x \text{ mL}$$

Answer: 6 mL. The dosage ordered is more than the available strength; therefore, you will need more than 2 mL to administer the dosage.

51. Conversion is required. Conversion factor: 1 000 mg = 1 g. Therefore, 0.4 g = 400 mg.

$$160 \text{ mg}:5 \text{ mL} = 400 \text{ mg}:x \text{ mL}$$

or

$$\frac{400 \text{ mg}}{160 \text{ mg}} \times 5 \text{ mL} = x \text{ mL}$$

Answer: 12.5 mL. The dosage ordered is more than the available strength; therefore, you will need more than 5 mL to administer the dosage.

52. $$25 \text{ mg}:1 \text{ mL} = 35 \text{ mg}:x \text{ mL}$$

or

$$\frac{35 \text{ mg}}{25 \text{ mg}} \times 1 \text{ mL} = x \text{ mL}$$

Answer: 1.4 mL. The dosage ordered is more than the available strength; therefore, you will need more than 1 mL to administer the dosage.

53.   150 mg:1 mL = 100 mg:x mL

or

$$\frac{100 \text{ mg}}{150 \text{ mg}} \times 1 \text{ mL} = x \text{ mL}$$

Answer: 0.66 = 0.7 mL. The dosage ordered is less than the available strength; therefore, you will need less than 1 mL to administer the dosage.

54.   300 000 units:1 mL = 150 000 units:x mL

or

$$\frac{150\,000 \text{ units}}{300\,000 \text{ units}} \times 1 \text{ mL} = x \text{ mL}$$

Answer: 0.5 mL. The dosage ordered is less than the available strength; therefore, you will need less than 1 mL to administer the dosage.

55.   100 mg:2 mL = 150 mg:x mL

or

$$\frac{150 \text{ mg}}{100 \text{ mg}} \times 2 \text{ mL} = x \text{ mL}$$

Answer: 3 mL. The dosage ordered is more than the available strength; therefore, you will need more than 2 mL to administer the dosage.

56.   125 mg:5 mL = 62.5 mg:x mL

or

$$\frac{62.5 \text{ mg}}{125 \text{ mg}} \times 5 \text{ mL} = x \text{ mL}$$

Answer: 2.5 mL. The dosage ordered is less than the available strength; therefore, you will need less than 5 mL to administer the dosage.

57.   25 mg:1 mL = 20 mg:x mL

or

$$\frac{20 \text{ mg}}{25 \text{ mg}} \times 1 \text{ mL} = x \text{ mL}$$

Answer: 0.8 mL. The dosage ordered is less than the available strength; therefore, you will need less than 1 mL to administer the dosage.

58.   200 mg:5 mL = 300 mg:x mL

or

$$\frac{300 \text{ mg}}{2\,000 \text{ mg}} \times 5 \text{ mL} = x \text{ mL}$$

Answer: 7.5 mL. The dosage ordered is more than the available strength; therefore, you will need more than 5 mL to administer the dosage.

59.   2 mg:5 mL = 3 mg:x mL

or

$$\frac{3 \text{ mg}}{2 \text{ mg}} \times 5 \text{ mL} = x \text{ mL}$$

Answer: 7.5 mL. The dosage ordered is more than the available strength; therefore, you will need more than 5 mL to administer the dosage.

60.   125 mg:5 mL = 250 mg:x mL

or

$$\frac{250 \text{ mg}}{125 \text{ mg}} \times 5 \text{ mL} = x \text{ mL}$$

Answer: 10 mL. The dosage ordered is more than the available strength; therefore, you will need more than 5 mL to administer the dosage.

61.   80 mg:15 mL = 40 mg:x mL

or

$$\frac{40 \text{ mg}}{80 \text{ mg}} \times 15 \text{ mL} = x \text{ mL}$$

Answer: 7.5 mL. The dosage ordered is less than the available strength; therefore, you will need less than 15 mL to administer the dosage.

62.   15 mg:0.6 mL = 45 mg:x mL

or

$$\frac{45 \text{ mg}}{15 \text{ mg}} \times 0.6 \text{ mL} = x \text{ mL}$$

Answer: 1.8 mL. The dosage ordered is greater than the available strength; therefore, you will need more than 0.6 mL to administer the dosage.

63. $40 \text{ mg} : 1 \text{ mL} = 14 \text{ mg} : x \text{ mL}$

or

$$\frac{14 \text{ mg}}{40 \text{ mg}} \times 1 \text{ mL} = x \text{ mL}$$

Answer: 0.35 = 0.4 mL rounded to the nearest tenth. The dosage ordered is less than the available strength; therefore, you will need less than 1 mL to administer the dosage.

64. $8 \text{ mg} : 1 \text{ mL} = 20 \text{ mg} : x \text{ mL}$

or

$$\frac{20 \text{ mg}}{8 \text{ mg}} \times 1 \text{ mL} = x \text{ mL}$$

Answer: 2.5 mL. The dosage ordered is more than the available strength; therefore, you will need more than 1 mL to administer the dosage.

65. $10 \text{ mg} : 1 \text{ mL} = 75 \text{ mg} : x \text{ mL}$

or

$$\frac{75 \text{ mg}}{10 \text{ mg}} \times 1 \text{ mL} = x \text{ mL}$$

Answer: 7.5 mL. The dosage ordered is greater than the available strength; therefore, you will need more than 1 mL to administer the dosage.

66. a. The recommended dosage is 20 mg per kg per day.
     20 mg/kg/day × 4.5 kg = 90 mg/day
     The dosage for the child is ordered q8h.
     q8h = 24 ÷ 8 = 3 doses/day
     90 mg ÷ 3 = 30 mg/dose
     180 mg × 3 = 540 mg/day
     Notify the prescriber; the dosage is too high and therefore not safe.
     The dosage ordered of 540 mg per day is greater than the recommended dosage of 90 mg per day. Also, the dose the child is to receive q8h exceeds the dose recommended.
   b. The volume to be administered is not calculated because the dosage ordered is not safe.

67. Convert the child's weight in lb to kg (2.2 lb = 1 kg). The recommended dosage is 15 mg per kg per day.
    45 lb = 45 ÷ 2.2 = 20.5 kg
    15 mg/kg/day × 20.5 kg = 307.5 mg/day
    The medication is given in divided doses q12h.
    q12h = 24 ÷ 12 = 2 doses/day
    307.5 mg ÷ 2 = 153.8 mg/dose
    200 mg × 2 = 400 mg/day
    Notify the prescriber; the dosage is high and therefore not safe. 400 mg per day is greater than 307.5 mg per day. Also, the dose the child is to receive q12h is higher than the dose recommended.

68. The recommended dosage is 22.5 mg per kg.
    22.5 mg/kg × 30 kg = 675 mg/dose
    The medication is given up to three times a day. The dosage for the child is ordered TID. The dosage ordered is not safe. The child is to receive 650 mg per dose, which is less than the recommended dosage and may not be effective. Notify the prescriber.

69. a. The recommended dosage is ordered q4h. The dosage is determined using 12.5 mg per kg per dose.
     12.5 mg/kg/dose × 42 kg = 525 mg/dose
     The safe dosage for this child is 525 mg per dose.
   b. The dosage ordered for the child is safe. For this child's weight, 525 mg per dose is the recommended dosage, and 525 mg is the dosage ordered.

70. Convert the child's weight in lb to kg (2.2 lb = 1 kg). The recommended dosage is 0.25 to 1 mg per kg.
    31 lb = 31 ÷ 2.2 = 14.1 kg
    0.25 mg/kg/day × 14.1 kg = 3.5 mg/day
    1 mg/kg/day × 14.1 kg = 14.1 mg/day
    The safe dosage range for the child is 3.5 to 14.1 mg per day.

71. $0.8 \text{ m}^2 \times \dfrac{2 \text{ mg}}{\text{m}^2} = 1.6 \text{ mg}$

72. $0.82 \text{ m}^2 \times \dfrac{250 \text{ mg}}{\text{m}^2} = 205 \text{ mg}$

73. $1.83 \text{ m}^2 \times \dfrac{10 \text{ units}}{\text{m}^2} = 18.3 \text{ units}$

$1.83 \text{ m}^2 \times \dfrac{20 \text{ units}}{\text{m}^2} = 36.6 \text{ units}$

The dosage range is 18.3–36.6 units.

NOTE

For problems 74 to 76, a ratio and proportion could be set up and mL per hour determined first, which, when a burette is used without a pump or controller, is the same as gtt per min. If gtt per min is determined first, remember that it is the same as mL per hour.

74. $x \text{ gtt/min} = \dfrac{30 \text{ mL} \times 60 \text{ gtt/mL}}{20 \text{ min}}$

$x = \dfrac{1\,800}{20}; x = 90 \text{ gtt/min}$

or

mL per hour determined with ratio and proportion:
30 mL : 20 min = x mL : 60 min

or

$\dfrac{30 \text{ mL}}{20 \text{ min}} = \dfrac{x \text{ mL}}{60 \text{ min}}$

a. 90 gtt per min; 90 microgtt per min
b. 90 mL per hour

75. $x \text{ gtt/min} = \dfrac{80 \text{ mL} \times 60 \text{ gtt/mL}}{60 \text{ min}}$

$x = \dfrac{4\,800}{60}; x = 80 \text{ gtt/min}$

or

Determine mL per hour.
80 mL : 60 min = x mL : 60 min

$\dfrac{80 \text{ mL}}{60 \text{ min}} = \dfrac{x \text{ mL}}{60 \text{ min}}$

a. 80 gtt per min; 80 microgtt per min
b. 80 mL per hour

76. $x \text{ gtt/min} = \dfrac{40 \text{ mL} \times 60 \text{ gtt/mL}}{45 \text{ min}}$

$\dfrac{2\,400}{45} = 53 \text{ gtt/min}$

or

Determine mL per hour.
40 mL : 45 min = x mL : 60 min

$\dfrac{40 \text{ mL}}{45 \text{ min}} = \dfrac{x \text{ mL}}{60 \text{ min}}$

a. 53 gtt per min; 53 microgtt per min
b. 53 mL per hour

77. Step 1: Calculate the safe dosage range for the child.
23 kg × 40 mg/kg = 920 mg
23 kg × 50 mg/kg = 1150 mg
Step 2: Calculate the dosage the child receives in 24 h.
500 mg q12h (2 doses) 500 × 2 = 1 000 mg
Step 3: Compare the dosage ordered with the safe dosage range.
The dosage ordered is 1 000 mg per day; it is within the safe dosage range of 920 to 1 150 mg per day.

78. Step 1: Calculate the safe dosage range for the child.
20 kg × 0.05 mg/kg = 1 mg
Step 2: The child is to receive 2 mg of medication at 10:00 AM.
Step 3: The dosage ordered is 2 mg. Since the safe dosage is 1 mg, notify the prescriber that 2 mg is not a safe dose.

79. Step 1: Calculate the safe dosage range for the child.
15 kg × 6 mcg/kg/day = 90 mcg/day
15 kg × 8 mcg/kg/day = 120 mcg/day
Step 2: 55 mcg q12h (2 doses); 55 mcg × 2 = 110 mcg/day
Step 3: The dosage ordered is 110 mcg per day; it is within the safe range of 90 to 120 mcg per day. Administer the dose as ordered.

80. a. 4 mL × 81 kg × 37 = 11 988 mL
b. 11 988 mL × 0.5 = 5 994 mL
c. 5 994 mL ÷ 8 h = 749.25 or 749 mL/h
d. 11 988 mL × 0.5 = 5 994 mL
e. 5 994 mL ÷ 16 h = 374.6 or 375 mL/h
f. 1 mL × 81 kg × 37 = 2 997 mL
g. 2 997 mL ÷ 24 h = 124.8 or 125 mL/h

81. The 4-2-1 rule may be used for hourly rate calculations. The child weighs 35 kg.
First 10 kg = 4 mL × 10 kg/h = 40 mL
Second 10 kg = 2 mL × 10 kg/h = 20 mL
Remaining 15 kg = 1 mL × 15 kg = 15 mL
40 mL + 20 mL + 15 mL = 75 mL/h

82. a. Since the 24-hour total volume is required, use the longer formula. The child weighs 19 kg.
First 10 kg = 100 mL × 10 kg/day = 1 000 mL/day
Remaining 9 kg = 50 mL × 9 kg = 450 mL/day
1 000 mL + 450 mL = 1 450 mL/day
b. 1 450 mL/24 h = 60.4 or 60 mL/h

CHAPTER 23

Critical Care Calculations

Objectives

After reviewing this chapter, you should be able to:

1. Calculate dosages in micrograms per minute, micrograms per hour, and milligrams per minute
2. Calculate dosages in milligrams per kilogram per hour, milligrams per kilogram per minute, and micrograms per kilogram per minute
3. Calculate dosages in units per millilitre, units per hour, and millilitres per hour

The content in this chapter may not be required as part of the nursing curriculum. It is included as a reference for nurses working in specialty areas.

This chapter provides basic information on medicated IV drips and titration. The care of patients receiving medications to control vital functions requires continual nursing intervention. In the critical care setting, the medications administered to patients are often potent and require close monitoring. They may include medications to maintain the patient's blood pressure (BP) within normal range and antiarrhythmic medications to regulate the patient's heart rate and/or rhythm. When these medications are administered, the nurse continuously monitors the patient's vital signs (BP and pulse) to titrate (adjust) the dosage of medications in response to the patient's vital signs.

Because of the potency of the medications used in critical care and the tendency of these medications to induce changes in BP and heart rate, accurate calculation of dosages is essential. These medications may be administered at a constant rate, or the rate of the IV may be titrated to patient response.

Medications used in critical care can be ordered in millilitres per hour (mL/h), drops per minute (gtt/min) using a microdrop set, micrograms per kilogram per minute (mcg/kg/min), or milligrams per hour (mg/h). Infusion pumps and volume control devices are usually used to administer these medications. Examples of medicated IV drips that require titration include dopamine, isoproterenol, and epinephrine.

Titrated medications are added to a specific volume of fluid and then adjusted to infuse at the rate at which the desired effect is obtained. **The medications that are titrated are potent antiarrhythmic, vasopressor, and vasodilator medications; they must be monitored very carefully by the nurse.** Because of the potency of these medications, minute changes in the infusion can cause an effect on the patient. Infusion pumps are used for titration; when one is not available, a microdrip set calibrated at 60 gtt per mL must be used.

An example of an order that involves titration of medication is as follows: "Titrate dopamine to maintain systolic blood pressure greater than 90 mm Hg." The nurse may start, for example, at 3 mcg per kg per min, and then gradually increase the IV flow rate until the systolic BP is maintained above 90 mm Hg. Each time there is a change in flow rate, the dosage of medication the patient receives is changed; therefore, it is essential that the dosage be recalculated each time the nurse changes the flow rate. Dosages are adjusted until the desired effect is achieved.

> **(!) SAFETY ALERT!**
>
> Electronic infusion devices are routinely used to administer medications that are potent and require close monitoring. If an electronic infusion device, such as a volumetric pump or syringe pump, is not available, a microdrip set calibrated at 60 gtt per mL must be used.

Calculating the Intravenous Flow Rate in Millilitres per Hour

Calculating the IV flow rate in millilitres per hour from a medication dosage ordered for IV administration is one of the most common calculations the nurse will encounter. Let's look at some examples illustrating this calculation before getting into other types of calculation.

Example: A solution of labetalol (Apo-Labetalol) 100 mg in 100 mL D5W is to infuse at a rate of 25 mg per hour. Calculate the IV flow rate in millilitres per hour using the solution strength available.

✔ Solution Using Ratio and Proportion

$$100 \, \text{mg} : 100 \, \text{mL} = 25 \, \text{mg} : x \, \text{mL}$$
$$100x = 100 \times 25$$
$$\frac{100x}{100} = \frac{2\,500}{100}$$
$$x = 25 \, \text{mL/h}$$

✔ Solution Using the Formula Method

$$\frac{25 \, \text{mg}}{100 \, \text{mg}} \times 100 \, \text{mL} = x \, \text{mL/h}$$
$$x = 25 \, \text{mL/h}$$

To infuse 25 mg per hour, set the IV flow rate at 25 mL per hour.

✔ Solution Using Dimensional Analysis

- As shown in previous chapters involving medications in solution, set up the dimensional analysis equation by first isolating what is being calculated. In this example, it is millilitres per hour; therefore, millilitres per hour is placed on the left side of the equation.
- Note that the starting fraction will be the information in the problem containing millilitres (millilitres is placed in the numerator).
- Set up each fraction after the starting fraction to match the previous denominator.
- Cancel the units, reduce if possible, and perform the mathematical operations.

The equation is as follows:

$$\frac{x \, \text{mL}}{\text{h}} = \frac{100 \, \text{mL}}{\overset{}{\underset{4}{\cancel{100} \, \cancel{\text{mg}}}}} \times \frac{\overset{1}{\cancel{25} \, \cancel{\text{mg}}}}{1 \, \text{h}}$$
$$x = \frac{100}{4}$$
$$x = 25 \, \text{mL/h}$$

Example: A solution of Apo-Isoproterenol 2 mg in 250 mL D5W is to infuse at a rate of 5 mcg per min. Calculate the IV flow rate in millilitres per hour.

1. Calculate the dosage per hour (60 min = 1 h).

$$5 \text{ mcg/min} \times 60 \text{ min/h} = 300 \text{ mcg/h}$$

2. Convert 300 mcg to milligrams to match the available strength.

$$\text{Conversion factor: } 1\,000 \text{ mcg} = 1 \text{ mg}$$
$$\text{Therefore, } 300 \text{ mcg} = 0.3 \text{ mg}$$

3. Calculate the IV flow rate in millilitres per hour.

$$2 \text{ mg} : 250 \text{ mL} = 0.3 \text{ mg} : x \text{ mL}$$
$$2x = 250 \times 0.3$$
$$\frac{2x}{2} = \frac{75}{2}$$
$$x = 37.5 = 38 \text{ mL/h}$$

To infuse 5 mcg per min, set the IV flow rate at 38 mL per hour.

NOTE

Conversions may be made from the solution strength to the dosage ordered, or the opposite.

✔ Solution Using Dimensional Analysis

Note: In this equation, you will need two conversion factors: 60 min = 1 h and 1 000 mcg = 1 mg.

$$\frac{x \text{ mL}}{h} = \frac{\overset{125}{\cancel{250} \text{ mL}}}{\underset{1}{\cancel{2} \text{ mg}}} \times \frac{1 \text{ mg}}{\underset{200}{\cancel{1\,000} \text{ mcg}}} \times \frac{\overset{1}{\cancel{5} \text{ mcg}}}{1 \text{ min}} \times \frac{60 \text{ min}}{1 \text{ h}}$$

$$x = \frac{125 \times 60}{200}$$
$$x = \frac{7\,5\cancel{00}}{2\cancel{00}}$$
$$x = 37.5 = 38 \text{ mL/h}$$

Remember

Ratio and proportion can be set up using several formats.

Now that you have seen examples of how to calculate the IV flow rate in millilitres per hour, let's look at some other types of calculations.

Calculating Critical Care Dosages per Hour or per Minute

Example: Dopamine 400 mg in 500 mL D5W is to infuse at a rate of 30 mL per hour. Calculate the dosage in micrograms per minute and micrograms per hour.

✔ Solution Using Ratio and Proportion

1.
$$400 \text{ mg} : 500 \text{ mL} = x \text{ mg} : 30 \text{ mL}$$
$$\text{(known)} \qquad \text{(unknown)}$$
$$500x = 400 \times 30$$
$$500x = 12\,000$$
$$x = \frac{12\,000}{500}$$
$$x = 24 \text{ mg/h}$$

2. Convert 24 mg to micrograms because the question asked for micrograms per minute and micrograms per hour. Convert milligrams to micrograms by using the conversion factor 1 mg = 1 000 mcg. To convert milligrams to micrograms, multiply by 1 000 or move the decimal point three places to the right.

$$24 \text{ mg/h} = 24\,000 \text{ mcg/h}$$

3. Now that you have the micrograms per hour, change micrograms per hour to micrograms per minute. This is done by dividing the number of micrograms per hour by 60 (60 minutes = 1 hour).

$$24\,000 \text{ mcg/}\cancel{h} \div 60 \text{ min/}\cancel{h} = 400 \text{ mcg/min}$$

(*Note:* This answer is in micrograms per minute; however, dopamine is usually delivered in millilitres per hour by pump, so you would need to take this calculation further. You will see sample problems on changing micrograms per minute to millilitres per hour later in this chapter.)

✔ Solution Using Dimensional Analysis

$$\frac{x \text{ mg}}{h} = \frac{\overset{4}{\cancel{400}} \text{ mg}}{\underset{5}{\cancel{500}} \text{ mL}} \times \frac{30 \text{ mL}}{1 \text{ h}}$$

$$x = \frac{120}{5}$$

$$x = 24 \text{ mg/h}$$

To determine milligrams per minute, 24 mg ÷ 60 min/h = 0.4 mg/min = 400 mcg/min

> (!) **SAFETY ALERT!**
> Accurate math is essential because critical care medications are extremely potent.

Medications Ordered in Milligrams per Minute

Medications such as lidocaine and procainamide are ordered in milligrams per minute.

Example: A patient is receiving procainamide 60 mL per hour. The solution available is procainamide 2 g in 500 mL D5W. Calculate the dosage in milligrams per hour and milligrams per minute.

1. Note that a conversion is necessary; grams must be converted to milligrams, the unit of measurement you are being asked for (mg/min, mg/h).

$$\text{Conversion factor: } 1 \text{ g} = 1\,000 \text{ mg}$$

Therefore, 2 g = 2 000 mg (2 × 1 000), or move the decimal three places to right.

2. Determine the milligrams per hour by setting up a proportion.

$$2\,000 \text{ mg} : 500 \text{ mL} = x \text{ mg} : 60 \text{ mL}$$
$$500x = 2\,000 \times 60$$
$$\frac{500x}{500} = \frac{120\,000}{500}$$
$$x = 240 \text{ mg/h}$$

3. Convert milligrams per hour to milligrams per minute.

$$240 \text{ mg/}\cancel{h} \div 60 \text{ min/}\cancel{h} = 4 \text{ mg/min}$$

✔ Solution Using Dimensional Analysis

(*Note:* Here, the starting fraction is the conversion factor to match the desired numerator, and milligrams per minute is desired; the solution strength is in grams.)

$$\frac{x \text{ mg}}{h} = \frac{\overset{2}{\cancel{1000}} \text{ mg}}{1 \cancel{g}} \times \frac{2 \cancel{g}}{\cancel{500} \cancel{\text{mL}}} \times \frac{60 \cancel{\text{mL}}}{1 \text{ h}}$$

$$x = \frac{240}{1}$$

$$x = 240 \text{ mg/h}$$

To determine milligrams per minute, $240 \text{ mg/}\cancel{h} \div 60 \text{ min/}\cancel{h} = 4 \text{ mg/min}$

Calculating Dosages Based on Micrograms per Kilogram per Minute

Medications are also ordered for patients based on dosage per kilogram per minute. These medications include nitroprusside, dopamine, and dobutamine. In the following problems, weight will be rounded to the nearest tenth for calculation.

Example: Order: Dopamine 2 mcg/kg/min. The solution available is 400 mg in 250 mL D5W. The patient weighs 150 lb. Calculate the IV flow rate in millilitres per hour.

1. Convert the patient's weight in pounds to kilograms.

   Conversion factor: 2.2 lb = 1 kg

   To convert the patient's weight, divide 150 lb by 2.2.

   $150 \text{ lb} \div 2.2 = 68.18 \text{ kg} = 68.2 \text{ kg}$

   Note that the conversion could also be done using ratio and proportion or dimensional analysis.

2. Now that you have the patient's weight in kilograms, determine the dosage in micrograms per minute.

   $68.2 \cancel{\text{kg}} \times 2 \text{ mcg/}\cancel{\text{kg}}\text{/min} = 136.4 \text{ mcg/min}$

   Converting micrograms per minute to millilitres per hour, then, would be easy using this example.

   a. Convert micrograms per minute to micrograms per hour.

      $136.4 \text{ mcg/}\cancel{\text{min}} \times 60 \cancel{\text{min}}\text{/h} = 8184 \text{ mcg/h}$

   b. Convert micrograms per hour to milligrams per hour.

      Conversion factor: $1000 \text{ mcg} = 1 \text{ mg}$
      $8184 \text{ mcg/h} \div 1000 = 8.18 = 8.2 \text{ mg/h}$

3. Determine the IV flow rate in millilitres per hour.

✔ Solution Using Ratio and Proportion

$$400 \text{ mg} : 250 \text{ mL} = 8.2 \text{ mg} : x \text{ mL}$$

$$400x = 250 \times 8.2$$

$$\frac{400\,x}{400} = \frac{2\,050}{400}$$

$$x = 5.1 = 5 \text{ mL/h}$$

✔ Solution Using Dimensional Analysis

$$\frac{x \text{ mL}}{\text{h}} = \frac{\overset{5}{\cancel{250}} \text{ mL}}{\underset{8}{\cancel{400}} \text{ mg}} \times \frac{1 \cancel{\text{ mg}}}{1\,000 \cancel{\text{ mcg}}} \times \frac{136.4 \cancel{\text{ mcg}}}{1 \cancel{\text{ min}}} \times \frac{60 \cancel{\text{ min}}}{1 \text{ h}}$$

$$x = \frac{40\,92\cancel{0}}{8\,00\cancel{0}}$$

$$x = 5.1 = 5 \text{ mL/h}$$

Intravenous Flow Rates for Titrated Medications

As already mentioned, critical care medications are ordered within parameters to obtain a desirable response in a patient. When a solution is titrated, the **lowest dosage of the medication is set first and increased or decreased as necessary. The higher dosage should not be exceeded without an order.**

Dosage errors with titrated medications can result in dire consequences. Therefore, the nurse should have knowledge regarding the medication, the proper dosage adjustment, and the frequency of adjustments based on patient assessment and the prescribed parameters. Electronic infusion devices (pumps) are used to administer critical care medications that are titrated. As discussed in Chapter 20, the nurse must know how to calculate millilitres per hour to use electronic infusion devices such as the pump. It is important to remember that there are pumps used in the critical care area that can accept one decimal place. Always check the equipment you are using before deciding to round IV flow rates to whole millilitres per hour. **Because of the consequences associated with titrated medications, it is common practice at many institutions to have double or triple checking of medication dosages and the mathematical computations associated with them.**

> **! SAFETY ALERT!**
> Know the institution's policy regarding the administration of titrated medications. **Never exceed** the prescribed upper dosage limit. Notify the prescriber when the maximum limit is reached for a new order.

Example 1: Nitroprusside (Nipride) has been ordered to titrate at 3 to 6 mcg per kg per min to maintain a patient's systolic BP below 140 mm Hg. The solution contains 50 mg Nipride in 250 mL D5W. The patient weighs 56 kg. Determine the flow rate setting for a volumetric pump.

1. Convert to **like units of measurement before solving the problem.**
   Conversion factor: 1 mg = 1 000 mcg
   Therefore, 50 mg = 50 000 mcg

2. Calculate the concentration of solution in micrograms per millilitre.

$$50\,000 \text{ mcg} : 250 \text{ mL} = x \text{ mcg} : 1 \text{ mL}$$

$$\frac{250x}{250} = \frac{50\,000}{250}$$

$$x = 200 \text{ mcg/mL}$$

The concentration of solution is 200 mcg per mL.

3. Calculate the dosage range using the upper and lower dosages.

$$(\text{Lower dosage}) \ 3 \ \text{mcg/} \cancel{kg}\text{/min} \times 56 \ \cancel{kg} = 168 \ \text{mcg/min}$$

$$(\text{Upper dosage}) \ 6 \ \text{mcg/} \cancel{kg}\text{/min} \times 56 \ \cancel{kg} = 336 \ \text{mcg/min}$$

4. Convert the dosage range to millilitres per minute.

$$(\text{Lower dosage}) \ 200 \ \text{mcg} : 1 \ \text{mL} = 168 \ \text{mcg} : x \ \text{mL}$$

$$\frac{200x}{200} = \frac{168}{200}$$

$$x = 0.84 \ \text{mL/min}$$

$$(\text{Upper dosage}) \ 200 \ \text{mcg} : 1 \ \text{mL} = 336 \ \text{mcg} : x \ \text{mL}$$

$$\frac{200x}{200} = \frac{336}{200}$$

$$x = 1.68 \ \text{mL/min}$$

5. Convert millilitres per minute to millilitres per hour.

$$(\text{Lower dosage}) \ 0.84 \ \text{mL/} \cancel{min} \times 60 \ \cancel{min}\text{/h} = 50.4 = 50 \ \text{mL/h (gtt/min)}$$

$$(\text{Upper dosage}) \ 1.68 \ \text{mL/} \cancel{min} \times 60 \ \cancel{min}\text{/h} = 100.8 = 101 \ \text{mL/h (gtt/min)}$$

A dosage range of 3 to 6 mcg per kg per min is equal to a flow rate of 50 to 101 mL per hour (gtt/min).

The patient's condition has stabilized, and the IV flow rate is now maintained at 60 mL per hour. What dosage will be infusing per minute?

$$200 \ \text{mcg} : 1 \ \text{mL} = x \ \text{mcg} : 60 \ \text{mL}$$

$$x = 12\,000 \ \text{mcg/h}$$

$$12\,000 \ \text{mcg/} \cancel{h} \div 60 \ \text{min/} \cancel{h} = 200 \ \text{mcg/min}$$

✔ Solution Using Dimensional Analysis

1. Calculate the dosage range first.

$$(\text{Lower dosage}) \ 3 \ \text{mcg/} \cancel{kg}\text{/min} \times 56 \ \cancel{kg} = 168 \ \text{mcg/min}$$

$$(\text{Upper dosage}) \ 6 \ \text{mcg/} \cancel{kg}\text{/min} \times 56 \ \cancel{kg} = 336 \ \text{mcg/min}$$

2. Calculate the flow rate in millilitres per hour for the lower dosage.

$$\frac{x \ \text{mL}}{h} = \frac{\overset{250}{\cancel{250} \ \text{mL}}}{\underset{1}{\cancel{50} \ \cancel{mg}}} \times \frac{1 \ \cancel{mg}}{1\,000 \ \cancel{mcg}} \times \frac{168 \ \cancel{mcg}}{1 \ \cancel{min}} \times \frac{60 \ \cancel{min}}{1 \ h}$$

$$x = 50.4 = 50 \ \text{mL/h (gtt/min)}$$

3. Calculate the flow rate in millilitres per hour for the upper dosage.

$$\frac{x \ \text{mL}}{h} = \frac{\overset{5}{\cancel{250} \ \text{mL}}}{\underset{1}{\cancel{50} \ \cancel{mg}}} \times \frac{1 \ \cancel{mg}}{1\,000 \ \cancel{mcg}} \times \frac{336 \ \cancel{mcg}}{1 \ \cancel{min}} \times \frac{60 \ \cancel{min}}{1 \ h}$$

$$x = 100.8 = 101 \ \text{mL/h (gtt/min)}$$

A dosage range of 3 to 6 mcg per kg per min is equal to a flow rate of 50 to 101 mL per hour (gtt/min).

The patient's condition has stabilized, and the IV flow rate is now maintained at 60 mL per hour. What dosage will be infusing per minute?

$$\frac{x \text{ mcg}}{\text{min}} = \frac{\overset{4}{\cancel{1000}} \text{ mcg}}{1 \cancel{\text{ mg}}} \times \frac{50 \cancel{\text{ mg}}}{\underset{1}{\cancel{250}} \cancel{\text{ mL}}} \times \frac{60 \cancel{\text{ mL}}}{1 \cancel{\text{ h}}} \times \frac{1 \cancel{\text{ h}}}{60 \text{ min}}$$

$$x = 200 \text{ mcg/min}$$

Developing a Titration Table

After calculating an initial IV flow rate for a medication being titrated, the patient is monitored. If the desired response is not achieved, the dosage may have to be increased. This will require the nurse to find the corresponding IV flow rate in millilitres per hour for the new dosage. Any time the dosage is changed, recalculation of the corresponding IV flow rate is required. Rather than performing calculations each time a dosage is modified, the nurse can develop a titration table to provide the IV flow rate for any possible change in the medication dosage. To help minimize waste due to concentration changes and reduce the chance of medication errors, some institutions have adopted a standard drip rate chart for many critical care medications (e.g., dopamine, nitroprusside) in common concentrations. If the ordered concentration chart for a particular medication is not available, then the nurse does the dosage calculation accordingly.

Let's look at the previous example (Example 1) and develop a titration table to increase the dosage by 1 mcg per min up to 6 mcg per min. Set up a ratio proportion to develop the titration table; use the minimum rate required to deliver 3 mcg per min to find the incremental IV flow rate that provides a dosage rate change of 1 mcg per min.

The proportion is as follows:

$$\frac{3 \text{ mcg/min}}{50 \text{ mL/h}} = \frac{1 \text{ mcg/min}}{x \text{ mL/h}}$$

$$\frac{3x}{3} = \frac{50}{3}$$

$$x = 16.6 = 17 \text{ mL/h}$$

Therefore, for each change of 1 mcg per min, the incremental IV flow rate is 17 mL per hour.

Titration Table	
Dosage Rate (mcg/min)	**IV Flow Rate (mL/h)**
3 mcg/min **(minimum)**	50 mL/h
4 mcg/min	67 mL/h
5 mcg/min	84 mL/h
6 mcg/min **(maximum)**	101 mL/h

Notice in this problem that millilitres per hour were rounded to the nearest whole number. Remember: there are pumps used in the critical care area that can accept one decimal place.

Example 2: Nitroglycerine has been ordered to titrate at 10 to 60 mcg per min, and the rate should be increased by 10 mcg per min every 3 to 5 min for chest pain. The solution contains 50 mg nitroglycerine in 250 mL D5W. Determine the incremental IV flow rate and develop a titration table.

1. Calculate the dosage per hour using the upper and lower dosages.

$$10 \text{ mcg/} \cancel{\text{min}} \times 60 \cancel{\text{ min}} /h = 600 \text{ mcg/h}$$

$$60 \text{ mcg/} \cancel{\text{min}} \times 60 \cancel{\text{ min}} /h = 3\,600 \text{ mcg/h}$$

2. Convert micrograms to milligrams to match the available strength.

$$\text{Conversion factor: } 1\,000\text{ mcg} = 1\text{ mg}$$
$$600\text{ mcg} = 0.6\text{ mg}$$
$$3\,600\text{ mcg} = 3.6\text{ mg}$$

3. Calculate the IV flow rate in millilitres per hour.

$$50\text{ mg}:250\text{ mL} = 0.6\text{ mg}:x\text{ mL}$$
$$50x = 250 \times 0.6$$
$$\frac{50x}{50} = \frac{150}{50}$$
$$x = 3\text{ mL/h}$$

To infuse 10 mcg per min, set the IV flow rate at 3 mL per hour (minimum).

$$50\text{ mg}:250\text{ mL} = 3.6\text{ mg}:x\text{ mL}$$
$$50x = 250 \times 3.6$$
$$\frac{50x}{50} = \frac{900}{50}$$
$$x = 18\text{ mL/h}$$

To infuse 60 mcg per min, set the IV flow rate at 18 mL per hour (maximum). A dosage range of 10 to 60 mcg per min is equal to a flow rate of 3 to 18 mL per hour.

Dimensional Analysis Setup

Calculate the lower dosage.

$$\frac{x\text{ mL}}{\text{h}} = \frac{\overset{5}{\cancel{250}}\text{ mL}}{\underset{1}{\cancel{50}}\text{ mg}} \times \frac{1\text{ }\cancel{mg}}{1\,000\text{ }\cancel{mcg}} \times \frac{10\text{ }\cancel{mcg}}{1\text{ }\cancel{min}} \times \frac{60\text{ }\cancel{min}}{1\text{ h}}$$
$$x = 3\text{ mL/h}$$

Calculate the upper dosage.

$$\frac{x\text{ mL}}{\text{h}} = \frac{\overset{5}{\cancel{250}}\text{ mL}}{\underset{1}{\cancel{50}}\text{ mg}} \times \frac{1\text{ }\cancel{mg}}{1\,000\text{ }\cancel{mcg}} \times \frac{60\text{ }\cancel{mcg}}{1\text{ }\cancel{min}} \times \frac{60\text{ }\cancel{min}}{1\text{ h}}$$
$$x = 18\text{ mL/h}$$

A dosage range of 10 to 60 mcg per min is equal to an IV flow rate of 3 to 18 mL per hour.

The titration table will be based on 10 mcg increments. Set up the proportion using the minimum to determine the dosage change of 10 mcg per min.

$$\frac{10\text{ mcg/min}}{3\text{ mL/h}} = \frac{10\text{ mcg/min}}{x\text{ mL/h}}$$
$$\frac{10x}{10} = \frac{30}{10}$$
$$x = 3\text{ mL/h}$$

Therefore, for each change of 10 mcg per min, the incremental IV flow rate is 3 mL per hour.

Titration Table

Dosage Rate (mcg/min)	IV Flow Rate (mL/h)
10 mcg/min (minimum)	3 mL/h
20 mcg/min	6 mL/h
30 mcg/min	9 mL/h
40 mcg/min	12 mL/h
50 mcg/min	15 mL/h
60 mcg/min (maximum)	18 mL/h

Example 3: Norepinephrine bitartrate (Levophed) has been ordered to titrate at 3 to 10 mcg per min, and the rate should be increased at 1 mcg per min to maintain BP and keep systolic BP greater than 100 mm Hg. The solution contains 2 mg Levophed in 250 mL D_5W. Determine the incremental IV flow rate and develop a titration table at 1 mcg increments. Assume that the pump delivers in tenths.

1. Calculate the dosage per hour using the upper and lower dosages.

$$3 \text{ mcg/min} \times 60 \text{ min/h} = 180 \text{ mcg/h}$$
$$10 \text{ mcg/min} \times 60 \text{ min/h} = 600 \text{ mcg/h}$$

2. Convert micrograms to milligrams to match the available strength.

$$\text{Conversion factor: } 1000 \text{ mcg} = 1 \text{ mg}$$
$$180 \text{ mcg} = 0.18 \text{ mg}$$
$$600 \text{ mcg} = 0.6 \text{ mg}$$

3. Calculate the IV flow rate in millilitres per hour.

$$2 \text{ mg} : 250 \text{ mL} = 0.18 \text{ mg} : x \text{ mL}$$
$$2x = 250 \times 0.18$$
$$\frac{2x}{2} = \frac{45}{2}$$
$$x = 22.5 \text{ mL/h}$$

To infuse 3 mcg per min, set the IV flow rate at 22.5 mL per hour (minimum).

$$2 \text{ mg} : 250 \text{ mL} = 0.6 \text{ mg} : x \text{ mL}$$
$$2x = 250 \times 0.6$$
$$\frac{2x}{2} = \frac{150}{2}$$
$$x = 75 \text{ mL/h}$$

To infuse 10 mcg per min, set the IV flow rate at 75 mL per hour. A dosage range of 3 to 10 mcg per min is equal to a flow rate of 22.5 to 75 mL per hour.

Dimensional Analysis Setup

Calculate the lower dosage.

$$\frac{x \text{ ml}}{h} = \frac{\overset{125}{\cancel{250}} \text{ mL}}{\underset{1}{\cancel{2}} \text{ mg}} \times \frac{1 \text{ mg}}{1000 \text{ mcg}} \times \frac{3 \text{ mcg}}{1 \text{ min}} \times \frac{60 \text{ min}}{1 \text{ h}}$$
$$x = 22.5 \text{ mL/h}$$

Calculate the upper dosage.

$$\frac{x\ \text{ml}}{\text{h}} = \frac{\overset{125}{\cancel{250}}\ \text{mL}}{\underset{1}{\cancel{2}}\ \cancel{\text{mg}}} \times \frac{1\ \cancel{\text{mg}}}{1\,000\ \cancel{\text{mcg}}} \times \frac{10\ \cancel{\text{mcg}}}{1\ \cancel{\text{min}}} \times \frac{60\ \cancel{\text{min}}}{1\ \cancel{\text{h}}}$$

$$x = 75\ \text{mL/h}$$

A dosage range of 3 to 10 mcg per min is equal to an IV flow rate of 22.5 to 75 mL per hour.
   Find the incremental IV flow rate for a dosage rate change of 1 mcg per min by setting up a ratio proportion.
   The proportion is as follows:

$$\frac{3\ \text{mcg/min}}{22.5\ \text{mL/h}} = \frac{1\ \text{mcg/min}}{x\ \text{mL/h}}$$

$$\frac{3x}{3} = \frac{22.5}{3}$$

$$x = 7.5\ \text{mL/h}$$

Therefore, for each change of 1 mcg per min, the incremental IV flow rate is 7.5 mL per hour.

Titration Table

Dosage Rate (mcg/min)	IV Flow Rate (mL/h)
3 mcg/min **(minimum)**	22.5 mL/h
4 mcg/min	30 mL/h
5 mcg/min	37.5 mL/h
6 mcg/min	45 mL/h
7 mcg/min	52.5 mL/h
8 mcg/min	60 mL/h
9 mcg/min	67.5 mL/h
10 mcg/min **(maximum)**	75 mL/h

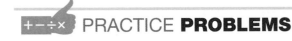 PRACTICE **PROBLEMS**

1. A patient weighing 50 kg is to receive a dobutamine (Dobutrex) solution of 250 mg in 500 mL D5W ordered to titrate between 2.5 and 5 mcg per kg per min.

   a. Determine the flow rate setting for a volumetric pump.   _____

   b. If the flow rate is being maintained at 25 mL per hour after several titrations, what is the dosage infusing per minute?   _____

2. Order: Epinephrine at 30 mL/h. The solution available is 2 mg of epinephrine in 250 mL D5W. Calculate the following:

   a. mg per hour   _____

   b. mcg per hour   _____

   c. mcg per min   _____

3. Aminophylline 0.25 g is added to 500 mL D5W to infuse at 20 mL per hour. Calculate the mg per hour.

    _____

4. Order: Oxytocin (Pitocin) at 15 microgtt/min. The solution contains 10 units of Pitocin in 1 000 mL D5W.

Calculate the number of units per hour the patient is to receive.

    _____

5. Order: 3 mcg/kg/min of nitroprusside (Nipride).

Available: 50 mg of Nipride in 250 mL D5W. The patient's weight is 60 kg.

Calculate the flow rate in mL per hour that will deliver this dosage.

    _____

6. A nitroglycerine drip is infusing at 3 mL per hour. The solution available is 50 mg of nitroglycerine in 250 mL D5W. Calculate the following:

a. mcg per hour

    _____

b. mcg per min

    _____

7. Order: Procainamide to titrate at 2 mg/min to a maximum of 6 mg/min. The solution available is procainamide 2 g in 250 mL D_5W. Develop a titration table in 2 mg per min increments up to the maximum dose.

    _____

Answers on pages 672–673.

POINTS TO REMEMBER

- Note: the safest way to administer potent medications that require frequent monitoring is by an electronic infusion device.
- When calculating dosages to be administered without any type of electronic infusion pump, always use microdrop tubing (60 gtt = 1 mL). This tubing is preferred because the drops are smaller, so more accurate titration is possible.
- Calculate dosages accurately. Double-checking math calculations helps ensure a proper dosage.
- Obtain the accurate weight of your patient.
- Use a calculator whenever possible.
- Use an infusion pump for titration of IV medications in millilitres per hour.
- Know the institution's policy relating to titration.
- Do not exceed the upper dosage limit.

CLINICAL **REASONING**

1. **Scenario:** Apo-Isoproterenol is ordered for a patient at the rate of 3 mcg per min with a solution containing Apo-Isoproterenol 1 mg in 250 mL D5W. The nurse performed the following steps to determine the IV flow rate by pump in millilitres per hour.

Step 1: Calculated the dosage per hour

$$3 \text{ mcg/min} \times 60 \text{ min/h} = 180 \text{ mcg/h}$$

Step 2: Converted 180 mcg to milligrams to match the units in the solution strength

$$180 \text{ mcg} = 0.018 \text{ mg}$$

Step 3: Calculated the flow rate in millilitres per hour

$$1\,mg : 250\,mL = 0.018\,mg : x\,mL$$
$$x = 250 \times 0.018$$
$$x = 4.5 = 5\,mL/h$$

a. What error did the nurse make in her calculations to determine the flow rate in mL per hour?   _____

b. What could be the potential outcome of the error?   _____

c. What should the flow rate be in mL per hour?   _____

d. What preventive measures could have been taken by the nurse?   _____

Answers on page 674.

 CHAPTER **REVIEW**

Calculate the dosages as indicated. Use the labels where provided.

1. The patient is receiving Apo-Isoproterenol at 30 mL per hour. The solution available is 2 mg of Isuprel in 250 mL D5W. Calculate the following:

   a. mg per hour   _____

   b. mcg per hour   _____

   c. mcg per min   _____

2. The patient is receiving epinephrine at 40 mL per hour. The solution available is 4 mg of epinephrine in 500 mL D5W. Calculate the following:

   a. mg per hour   _____

   b. mcg per hour   _____

   c. mcg per min   _____

3. Infuse dopamine 800 mg in 500 mL D5W at 30 mL per hour. Calculate the following:

   a. mcg per hour _____

   b. mcg per min _____

   c. Number of mL you will add to the IV for this dosage _____

   Available:

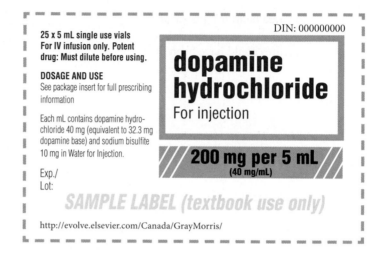

4. Infuse Nipride at 30 mL per hour. The solution available is 50 mg sodium nitroprusside in D5W 250 mL.

   Available:

Calculate the following:

   a. mcg per hour _____

   b. mcg per min _____

   c. Number of mL you will add to the IV for this dosage _____

5. Order: 200 mg dopamine in 250 mL D5W to infuse at 25 mL/h. Calculate the following:

   a. mcg per hour   _____

   b. mcg per min   _____

6. Order: Lidocaine 2 g in 250 mL D5W to infuse at 60 mL/h. Calculate the following:

   a. mg per hour   _____

   b. mg per min   _____

7. Order: Aminophylline 0.25 g to be added to 250 mL of D5W. The order is to infuse over 6 h.

   Available:

   Calculate the following:

   a. Dosage in mg per hour   _____

   b. Number of mL you will add to the IV for this dosage   _____

8. A patient is receiving Apo-Procainamide at 30 mL per hour. The solution available is 2 g Apo-Procainamide in 250 mL D5W. Calculate the following:

   a. mg per hour   _____

   b. mg per min   _____

9. Order: Oxytocin (Pitocin) drip at 45 microgtt/min. The solution available is 20 units of Pitocin in 1 000 mL of D5W. Calculate the following:

   a. units per min   _____

   b. units per hour   _____

10. Order: 30 units oxytocin (Pitocin) in 1 000 mL D5W at 40 mL/h.

    How many units of Pitocin is the patient
    receiving per hour? _____ units per hour

11. A total of 30 units of Pitocin is added to 500 mL D5RL for an induction. The patient is receiving 45 mL per hour.

    How many units of Pitocin is the
    patient receiving per hour? _____ units per hour

12. A patient is receiving bretylium at 30 microgtt per min. The solution available is 2 g bretylium in 500 mL D5W. Calculate the following:

    a. mg per hour _____

    b. mg per min _____

13. A patient is receiving bretylium at 45 microgtt per min. The solution available is 2 g bretylium in 500 mL D5W. Calculate the following:

    a. mg per hour _____

    b. mg per min _____

14. A patient is receiving nitroglycerine 50 mg in 250 mL D5W. The order is to infuse at 500 mcg per min.

    What flow rate in mL per hour would
    be needed to deliver this amount? _____

15. Dopamine has been ordered to maintain a patient's BP; 400 mg dopamine has been placed in 500 mL D5W to infuse at 35 mL per hour.

    How many mg are being administered per hour? _____

16. A patient is receiving isoproterenol (Isuprel) 2 mg in 250 mL D5W. The order is to infuse at 20 mL per hour. Calculate the following:

    a. mg per hour _____

    b. mcg per hour _____

    c. mcg per min _____

17. Order: 1 g of aminophylline in 1 000 mL D5W to infuse over 10 h.

    Calculate the dosage in mg per hour. _____

18. A patient is receiving lidocaine 2 g in 250 mL D5W. The solution is infusing at 22 mL per hour. Calculate the following:

    a. mg per hour _____

    b. mg per min _____

19. Order: Epinephrine 4 mg in 250 mL D5W at 8 mL/h.

    Calculate the dosage in mcg per hour.   _____

20. Order: Esmolol 2.5 g in 250 mL 0.9% NS at 30 mL/h. Calculate the following:

    a. mg per hour   _____

    b. mg per min   _____

21. Order: Dobutamine 500 mg in 500 mL D5W to infuse at 30 mL/h.

    Calculate the following:

    a. mcg per hour   _____

    b. mcg per min   _____

22. Order: 2 g/h of 50% magnesium sulphate. The solution available is 25 g of 50% magnesium sulphate in 300 mL D5W.

    What flow rate in mL per hour would be
    needed to administer the required dosage?   _____

23. Order: Dopamine 400 mg in 500 mL 0.9% NS to infuse at 200 mcg/min. A volumetric pump is being used.

    Calculate the flow rate in mL per hour.   _____

24. Order: Magnesium sulphate 3 g/h.

    Available: 25 g of 50% magnesium sulphate in 300 mL D5W

    What rate in mL per hour would be needed
    to administer the required dosage?   _____

25. A patient with chest pain has an order for nitroglycerine 50 mg in 250 mL D5W at 10 mcg per min.

    Calculate the flow rate in gtt per min for
    a microdrop administration set.   _____

26. Order: Nitroprusside (Nipride) 50 mg in 250 mL D5W to infuse at 2 mcg/kg/min. The patient's weight is 120 lb.

    Calculate the dosage in mcg per min.   _____

27. Order: Dobutamine (Dobutrex) 250 mg in 500 mL of D5W at 3 mcg/kg/min. The patient weighs 80 kg.

    What dosage in mcg per min should the patient receive?   _____

28. Order: Infuse 500 mL D5W with 800 mg theophylline at 0.7 mg/kg/h. The patient weighs 73.5 kg.

    How many mg should this patient receive per hour?   _____

29. Order: Infuse 1 g of aminophylline in 1 000 mL of D5W at 0.7 mg/kg/h. The patient weighs 110 lb.

    a. Calculate the dosage in mg per hour. _____

    b. Calculate the dosage in mg per min. _____

    c. Note that the drug reference states no more than 20 mg per min. Is the dosage ordered safe? _____

30. Norepinephrine (Levophed) 2 to 6 mcg per min has been ordered to maintain a patient's systolic BP at 100 mm Hg. The solution concentration is 2 mg in 500 mL D5W.

    Determine the flow rate setting for a volumetric pump. _____

31. Esmolol is to titrate between 50 and 75 mcg per kg per min. The patient weighs 60 kg. The solution strength is 5 000 mg of esmolol in 500 mL D5W.

    a. Determine the flow rate setting for a volumetric pump. _____

    b. The titration rate is at 24 mL per hour. What is the dosage infusing per min? _____

32. Order: Dobutamine 500 mg in 250 mL D5W to infuse at 10 mcg/kg/min. The patient weighs 65 kg.

    Calculate the flow rate in mL per hour (gtt/min). _____

33. Aminophylline 0.25 g is added to 250 mL D5W. The order is to infuse over 6 hours.

    Calculate the dosage in mg per hour. _____

34. A patient is receiving lidocaine 1 g in 500 mL D5W at a rate of 20 mL per hour. Calculate the following:

    a. mg per hour _____

    b. mg per min _____

35. A patient is receiving Septra 300 mg in 500 mL D5W (based on trimethoprim) at a rate of 15 gtt per min (15 microgtt/min). The tubing is microdrop (60 gtt/mL). Calculate the following:

    a. mg per min _____

    b. mg per hour _____

36. Esmolol 1.5 g in 250 mL D5W has been ordered at a rate of 100 mcg per kg per min for a patient weighing 102.4 kg. Calculate the following:

    a. Dosage in mcg per min _____

    b. Flow rate in mL per hour _____

37. Order: Dopamine 400 mg in 500 mL D5W to infuse at 20 mL/h. Determine the following:

    a. mg per min   _____

    b. mcg per min   _____

38. A patient has an order for inamrinone (previously called amrinone) 250 mg in 250 mL 0.9% NS at 3 mcg per kg per min. The patient's weight is 59.1 kg. Determine the flow rate in mL per hour.   _____

39. Inocor 250 mg in 250 mL of 0.9% NS to infuse at a rate of 5 mcg per kg per min is ordered for a patient weighing 165 lb. Calculate the following:

    a. mcg per min   _____

    b. mcg per hour   _____

    c. mL per hour   _____

40. Order: Diltiazem 125 mg in 100 mL D5W to infuse at 20 mg/h.

    Available:

    a. How many mL will you add to the IV?   _____

    b. Determine the flow rate in mL per hour.
       (Consider the medication in the volume.)   _____

41. Order: 2 g procainamide (Pronestyl) in 500 mL D5W to infuse at 2 mg/min.

    Determine the flow rate in mL per hour.   _____

42. Dopamine is ordered at a rate of 3 mcg per kg per min for a patient weighing 95.9 kg. The solution strength is 400 mg dopamine in 250 mL D$_5$W. Determine the flow rate for an IV pump. The pump is capable of delivering in tenths of a mL.

    _____

43. Infuse dobutamine 250 mg in 500 mL D$_5$W at 5 mcg per kg per min. The patient weighs 143 lb. The concentration of the solution is 500 mcg per mL. How many mcg of dobutamine will be infused per minute? _____ Per hour? _____

44. A medication has been ordered at 3 mcg per min. The solution strength is 1 mg of the medication in 250 mL D$_5$W. Determine the flow rate. _____

45. A medication has been ordered at 2 to 4 mcg per min to maintain a patient's systolic BP greater than 100 mm Hg. The medication being titrated has 8 mg of medication in 250 mL D$_5$W. Determine the flow rate for a 2- to 4-mcg range. Then assume that after several changes in mL per hour have been made, the BP has stabilized at a rate of 5 mL per hour. How many mcg per min is the patient receiving at this rate? The IV pump is capable of delivering in tenths of a mL.

   a. Flow rate for a 2- to 4-mcg range _____

   b. Dosage in mcg per min at 5 mL per hour _____

46. Order: Nitroglycerine is to titrate at 40 mcg per min for chest pain to a maximum of 100 mcg per min. The solution contains 40 mg of nitroglycerine in 250 mL D5W. Develop a titration table from minimum to maximum dosage in 20 mcg per min increments. Assume that the pump can deliver in tenths.

47. Order: Norepinephrine (Levophed) 4 mcg/min to maintain BP systolic greater than 100 mm Hg to a maximum of 12 mcg/min.

   Available: Levophed 4 mg in 500 mL D5W

   Develop a titration table in 2 mcg per min increments.

   Answers on pages 674–681.

⁂ ANSWERS

Answers to Practice Problems

1. a. Step 1: Convert mg to mcg (1 mg = 1 000 mcg).
   250 mg = 250 000 mcg
   Step 2: 250 000 mcg : 500 mL = x mcg : 1 mL
   $$\frac{500x}{500} = \frac{250\,000}{500}; x = 500 \text{ mcg/mL}$$
   The concentration of solution is 500 mcg per mL.
   Step 3: Calculate the dosage range.
   Lower dosage:
   2.5 mcg/kg/min × 50 kg = 125 mcg/min
   Upper dosage:
   5 mcg/kg/min × 50 kg = 250 mcg/min

   Step 4: Convert the dosage range to mL per min.
   Lower dosage:
   500 mcg : 1 mL = 125 mcg : x mL
   $$\frac{500x}{500} = \frac{125}{500}$$
   $$x = 0.25 \text{ mL/min}$$
   Upper dosage:
   500 mcg : 1 mL = 250 mcg : x mL
   $$\frac{500x}{500} = \frac{250}{500}$$
   $$x = 0.5 \text{ mL/min}$$

evolve

Step 5: Convert mL per min to mL per hour.
Lower dosage:
0.25 mL/~~min~~ × 60 ~~min~~ /h = 15 mL/h (gtt/min)
Upper dosage:
0.5 mL/~~min~~ × 60 ~~min~~ /h = 30 mL/h (gtt/min)
A dosage range of 2.5 to 5 mcg per kg per min is equal to a flow rate of 15 to 30 mL per hour (gtt/min).
b. Determine the dosage infusing per min at 25 mL per hour.

$$500 \text{ mcg} : 1 \text{ mL} = x \text{ mcg} : 25 \text{ mL}$$
$$x = 12\,500 \text{ mcg/h}$$
$$12\,500 \text{ mcg} \div 60 \text{ min} = 208.3 \text{ mcg/min}$$

2. a. $2 \text{ mg} : 250 \text{ mL} = x \text{ mg} : 30 \text{ mL}$
$$\frac{250x}{250} = \frac{60}{250}$$
$$x = 0.24 \text{ mg/h}$$
b. Convert mg per hour to mcg per hour (1 mg = 1 000 mcg).
0.24 mg/h × 1 000 = 240 mcg/h
c. Convert mcg per hour to mcg per min.
240 mcg/~~h~~ ÷ 60 min/~~h~~ = 4 mcg/min

3. Step 1: Convert grams to mg (1 g = 1 000 mg). (Note that you were asked to calculate mg per hour.)
0.25 g = 250 mg
Step 2: Calculate mg per hour.
$$250 \text{ mg} : 500 \text{ mL} = x \text{ mg} : 20 \text{ mL}$$
$$\frac{500x}{500} = \frac{5\,000}{500}$$
$$x = 10 \text{ mg/h}$$

4. *Note:* Calculate units per hour only.
Step 1: $60 \text{ gtt} : 1 \text{ mL} = 15 \text{ gtt} : x \text{ mL}$
$$\frac{60x}{60} = \frac{15}{60}$$
$$x = 0.25 \text{ mL/min}$$
Step 2: 0.25 mL/~~min~~ × 60 ~~min~~ /h = 15 mL/h
Step 3: 10 units : 1 000 mL = x units : 15 mL
$$\frac{1\,000x}{1\,000} = \frac{150}{1\,000}; x = 0.15 \text{ units/h}$$

5. Step 1: Determine the dosage in mcg per min.
60 ~~kg~~ × 3 mcg/ ~~kg~~ /min = 180 mcg/min
Step 2: Convert the dosage to mcg per hour.
180 mcg/~~min~~ × 60 ~~min~~ /h = 10 800 mcg/h
Step 3: Convert to like units of measurement (1 000 mcg = 1 mg).
10 800 mcg = 10.8 mg
Step 4: Calculate the flow rate (mL/h).
$$50 \text{ mg} : 250 \text{ mL} = 10.8 \text{ mg} : x \text{ mL}$$
$$50x = 250 × 10.8$$
$$\frac{50x}{50} = \frac{2\,700}{50}$$
$$x = 54 \text{ mL/h}$$

6. a. $50 \text{ mg} : 250 \text{ mL} = x \text{ mg} : 3 \text{ mL}$
$$\frac{250x}{250} = \frac{150}{250}$$
$$x = 0.6 \text{ mg/h}$$
Convert mg per hour to mcg per hour (1 mg = 1 000 mcg).
0.6 mg/h × 1 000 = 600 mcg/h
b. Convert mcg per hour to mcg per min.
600 mcg/~~h~~ ÷ 60 min/~~h~~ = 10 mcg/min

7. Step 1: Calculate the dosage per hour using the lower and upper dosages.
2 mg/~~min~~ × 60 ~~min~~ /h = 120 mg/h
6 mg/~~min~~ × 60 ~~min~~ /h = 360 mg/h
Step 2: Convert mg to grams to match the available strength (1 000 mg = 1 g).
120 mg = 0.12 g
360 mg = 0.36 g
Step 3: Calculate the flow rate (mL/h).
$$2 \text{ g} : 250 \text{ mL} = 0.12 \text{ g} : x \text{ mL}$$
$$2x = 250 × 0.12$$
$$\frac{2x}{2} = \frac{30}{2}$$
$$x = 15 \text{ mL/h}$$
To infuse 2 mg per min, set the IV flow rate at 15 mL per hour (minimum).
$$2 \text{ g} : 250 \text{ mL} = 0.36 \text{ g} : x \text{ mL}$$
$$2x = 250 × 0.36$$
$$\frac{2x}{2} = \frac{90}{2}$$
$$x = 45 \text{ mL/h}$$
To infuse 6 mg per min, set the IV flow rate at 45 mL per hour (maximum).
A dosage range of 2 to 6 mg per min is equal to a flow rate of 15 to 45 mL per hour.
Set up a proportion to determine the dosage of 2 mg per min.
$$\frac{2 \text{ mg/min}}{15 \text{ mL/h}} = \frac{2 \text{ mg/min}}{x \text{ mL/h}}$$
$$\frac{2x}{2} = \frac{30}{2}$$
$$x = 15 \text{ mL/h}$$
Therefore, for a change of 2 mg per min, the incremental IV flow rate is 15 mL per hour.

Titration Table

Dosage Rate (mcg/min)	IV Flow Rate (mL/h)
2 mg/min **(minimum)**	15 mL/h
4 mg/min	30 mL/h
6 mg/min **(maximum)**	45 mL/h

Note: This problem could also be solved using dimensional analysis.

Answers to Clinical Reasoning Questions

1. a. The nurse made the error in Step 2. This error led to the error in the calculation of the IV flow rate in mL per hour (Step 3).

   $180 \text{ mcg} = 0.18 \text{ mg} \ (1\,000 \text{ mcg} = 1 \text{ mg})$

   $180 \text{ mcg} \div 1\,000 = 0.18 \text{ mg}$

   b. The error would result in an incorrect IV flow rate in mL per hour; the answer obtained in Step 2 is used to determine the flow rate in mL per hour. Using 0.018 mg would net an incorrect answer.

   $1 \text{ mg} : 250 \text{ mL} = 0.018 \text{ mg} : x \text{ mL}$

   $$x = 250 \times 0.018$$

   $$x = 4.5 = 5 \text{ mL/h}$$

   c. The flow rate in mL per hour should be 45 mL per hour and not 5 mL per hour.

   $1 \text{ mg} : 250 \text{ mL} = 0.18 \text{ mg} : x \text{ mL}$

   $$x = 250 \times 0.18$$

   $$x = 45 \text{ mL/h}$$

   d. The nurse should have double-checked the math at each step. In addition, having another nurse check the calculation may have helped in recognizing the error in calculation.

Answers to Chapter Review

1. a. Calculate the dosage in mg per hour.

   $2 \text{ mg} : 250 \text{ mL} = x \text{ mg} : 30 \text{ mL}$

   $$\frac{250x}{250} = \frac{60}{250}$$

   $$x = \frac{60}{250}$$

   $$x = 0.24 \text{ mg/h}$$

   b. Convert mg per hour to mcg per hour (1 mg = 1 000 mcg).

   $0.24 \text{ mg/h} \times 1\,000 = 240 \text{ mcg/h}$

   c. Convert mcg per hour to mcg per min.

   $240 \text{ mcg/h} \div 60 \text{ min} = 4 \text{ mcg/min}$

2. a. Calculate the dosage in mg per hour.

   $4 \text{ mg} : 500 \text{ mL} = x \text{ mg} : 40 \text{ mL}$

   $$\frac{500x}{500} = \frac{160}{500}$$

   $$x = \frac{160}{500}$$

   $$x = 0.32 \text{ mg/h}$$

   b. Convert mg per hour to mcg per hour (1 mg = 1 000 mcg).

   $0.32 \text{ mg/h} \times 1\,000 = 320 \text{ mcg/h}$

   c. Convert mcg per hour to mcg per min.

   $320 \text{ mcg/} \cancel{h} \div 60 \text{ min/} \cancel{h} = 5.33 = 5.3 \text{ mcg/min}$

3. a. Step 1: Calculate the dosage in mg per hour.

   $800 \text{ mg} : 500 \text{ mL} = x \text{ mg} : 30 \text{ mL}$

   $$\frac{500x}{500} = \frac{24\,000}{500}$$

   $$x = \frac{24\,000}{500}$$

   $$x = 48 \text{ mg/h}$$

   Step 2: Convert mg per hour to mcg per hour (1 mg = 1 000 mcg).

   $48 \text{ mg/h} \times 1\,000 = 48\,000 \text{ mcg/h}$

   b. Convert mcg per hour to mcg per min.

   $48\,000 \text{ mcg/} \cancel{h} \div 60 \text{ min/} \cancel{h} = 800 \text{ mcg/min}$

   c. $200 \text{ mg} : 5 \text{ mL} = 800 \text{ mg} : x \text{ mL}$

   or

   $$\frac{800 \text{ mg}}{200 \text{ mg}} \times 5 \text{ mL} = x \text{ mL}$$

   Answer: 20 mL. The dosage ordered is more than the available strength; therefore, you will need more than 5 mL to administer the dosage.

4. a. Step 1: Determine the dosage in mg per hour.

   $50 \text{ mg} : 250 \text{ mL} = x \text{ mg} : 30 \text{ mL}$

   $$\frac{250x}{250} = \frac{1\,500}{250}$$

   $$x = \frac{1\,500}{250}$$

   $$x = 6 \text{ mg/h}$$

   Step 2: Convert mg per hour to mcg per hour (1 mg = 1 000 mcg).

   $6 \text{ mg/h} \times 1\,000 = 6\,000 \text{ mcg/h}$

   b. Convert mcg per hour to mcg per min.

   $6\,000 \text{ mcg/} \cancel{h} \div 60 \text{ min/} \cancel{h} = 100 \text{ mcg/min}$

   c. $50 \text{ mg} : 2 \text{ mL} = 50 \text{ mL} : x \text{ mL}$

   $$\frac{50 \text{ mg}}{50 \text{ mg}} \times 2 \text{ mL} = x \text{ mL}$$

   Answer: 2 mL. The dosage ordered is contained in a volume of 2 mL.

   Alternative solution: $25 \text{ mg} : 1 \text{ mL} = 50 \text{ mg} : x \text{ mL}$

   or

   $$\frac{50 \text{ mg}}{25 \text{ mg}} \times 1 \text{ mL} = x \text{ mL}$$

5. a. Step 1: Determine the dosage in mg per hour.
   200 mg : 250 mL $= x$ mg : 25 mL

   $$\frac{250x}{250} = \frac{5\,000}{250}$$
   $$x = \frac{5\,000}{250}$$
   $$x = 20 \text{ mg/h}$$

   Step 2: Convert mg per hour to mcg per hour
   (1 mg = 1 000 mcg).
   20 mg/h × 1 000 = 20 000 mcg/h

   b. Convert mcg per hour to mcg per min.
   20 000 mcg/h ÷ 60 min/h = 333.33 =
   333 mcg/min

6. a. Step 1: Convert the unit of measurement ordered
   (grams) to the unit of measurement requested
   (mg) (1 g = 1 000 mg).
   2 g = 2 000 mg
   Step 2: Calculate mg per hour.
   2 000 mg : 250 mL $= x$ mg : 60 mL

   $$\frac{250x}{250} = \frac{120\,000}{250}$$
   $$x = \frac{120\,000}{250}$$
   $$x = 480 \text{ mg/h}$$

   b. Convert mg per hour to mg per min.
   480 mg/h ÷ 60 min/h = 8 mg/min

7. a. Step 1: Convert grams to mg (1 g = 1 000 mg).
   0.25 g = 250 mg
   Step 2: Calculate the dosage in mg per hour.
   250 mg : 6 h $= x$ mg : 1 h

   $$\frac{6x}{6} = \frac{250}{6}$$
   $$x = \frac{250}{6}$$
   $$x = 41.66 = 41.7 \text{ mg/h}$$

   b.   500 mg : 20 mL = 250 mg : x mL

   or

   $$\frac{250 \text{ mg}}{500 \text{ mg}} \times 20 \text{ mL} = x \text{ mL}$$

   Answer: 10 mL. The dosage ordered is less than the
   available strength; therefore, you will need less
   than 20 mL to administer the dosage.
   Alternative solution: 25 mg : 1 mL = 250 mg : x mL

   or

   $$\frac{250 \text{ mg}}{25 \text{ mg}} \times 1 \text{ mL} = x \text{ mL}$$

8. a. Step 1: Convert grams to mg (1 g = 1 000 mg).
   2 g = 2 000 mg
   Step 2: Calculate mg per hour.
   2 000 mg : 250 mL $= x$ mg : 30 mL

   $$\frac{250x}{250} = \frac{60\,000}{250}$$
   $$x = \frac{60\,000}{250}$$
   $$x = 240 \text{ mg/h}$$

   b. Convert mg per hour to mg per min.
   240 mg/h ÷ 60 min/h = 4 mg/min

9. a. Step 1: Calculate gtt per min to mL per min.
   60 gtt : 1 mL = 45 gtt : x mL

   $$\frac{60x}{60} = \frac{45}{60}$$
   $$x = \frac{45}{60}$$
   $$x = 0.75 \text{ mL/min}$$

   Step 2: Calculate units per min.
   20 units : 1 000 mL = x units : 0.75 mL

   $$\frac{1\,000x}{1\,000} = \frac{15}{1\,000}$$
   $$x = \frac{15}{1\,000}$$
   $$x = 0.015 \text{ units/min}$$

   b. Calculate units per hour.
   0.015 units/min × 60 min/h = 0.9 units/h

10. 30 units : 1 000 mL = x units : 40 mL

   $$\frac{1\,000x}{1\,000} = \frac{1\,200}{1\,000}$$
   $$x = \frac{1\,200}{1\,000}$$
   $$x = 1.2 \text{ units/h}$$

11. 30 units : 500 mL = x units : 45 mL

   $$\frac{500x}{500} = \frac{1\,350}{500}$$
   $$x = \frac{1\,350}{500}$$
   $$x = 2.7 \text{ units/h}$$

12. a. Step 1: Convert the unit of measurement (grams) to the unit of measurement requested (mg) (1 g = 1 000 mg).

2 g = 2 000 mg

Step 2: Calculate mg per hour.

2 000 mg : 500 mL = x mg : 30 mL

$$\frac{500x}{500} = \frac{60\,000}{500}$$

$$x = \frac{60\,000}{500}$$

$$x = 120 \text{ mg/h}$$

b. Convert mg per hour to mg per min.

120 mg/h ÷ 60 min/h = 2 mg/min

13. a. Step 1: Convert the unit of measurement (grams) to the unit of measurement requested (mg) (1 g = 1 000 mg).

2 g = 2 000 mg

Step 2: Calculate mg per hour.

2 000 mg : 500 mL = x mg : 45 mL

$$\frac{500x}{500} = \frac{90\,000}{500}$$

$$x = \frac{90\,000}{500}$$

$$x = 180 \text{ mg/h}$$

b. Convert mg per hour to mg per min.

180 mg/h ÷ 60 min/h = 3 mg/min

14. Step 1: Determine the dosage in mg per hour.

500 mcg/min × 60 min /h = 30 000 mcg/h

Step 2: Convert mcg per hour to mg per hour to match the available strength (1 000 mcg = 1 mg).

30 000 mcg/h ÷ 1 000 = 30 mg/h

Step 3: Calculate the flow rate (mL/h).

50 mg : 250 mL = 30 mg : x mL

$$\frac{50x}{50} = \frac{7\,500}{50}$$

$$x = 150 \text{ mL/h}$$

Set at 150 mL per hour to deliver 500 mcg per min.

15. 400 mg : 500 mL = x mg : 35 mL

$$\frac{500x}{500} = \frac{14\,000}{500}$$

$$x = 28 \text{ mg/h}$$

16. a. Calculate mg per hour.

2 mg : 250 mL = x mg : 20 mL

$$\frac{250x}{250} = \frac{40}{250}$$

$$x = \frac{40}{250}$$

$$x = 0.16 \text{ mg/h}$$

b. Convert mg per hour to mcg per hour (1 mg = 1 000 mcg).

0.16 mg/h × 1 000 = 160 mcg/h

c. Convert mcg per hour to mcg per min.

160 mcg/h ÷ 60 min/h = 2.66 = 2.7 mcg/min

17. Step 1: Convert grams to mg.

1 g = 1 000 mg

Step 2: Calculate mg per hour.

1 000 mg : 10 h = x mg : 1 h

$$\frac{10x}{10} = \frac{1\,000}{10}$$

$$x = 100 \text{ mg/h}$$

18. a. Step 1: Convert grams to mg (1 g = 1 000 mg).

2 g = 2 000 mg

Step 2: Calculate mg per hour.

2 000 mg : 250 mL = x mg : 22 mL

$$\frac{250x}{250} = \frac{44\,000}{250}$$

$$x = \frac{44\,000}{250}$$

$$x = 176 \text{ mg/h}$$

b. Convert mg per hour to mg per min.

176 mg/h ÷ 60 min/h = 2.93 = 2.9 mg/min

19. Step 1: Calculate the dosage in mg per hour.

4 mg : 250 mL = x mg : 8 mL

$$\frac{250x}{250} = \frac{32}{250}$$

$$x = \frac{32}{250}$$

$$x = 0.128 \text{ mg/h}$$

Step 2: Convert mg per hour to mcg per hour (1 mg = 1 000 mcg).

0.128 mg/h × 1 000 = 128 mcg/h

20. a. Step 1: Convert grams to mg (1 g = 1 000 mg).

2.5 g = 2 500 mg

Step 2: Calculate mg per hour.

250 mL : 2 500 mg = 30 mL : x mg

$$\frac{250x}{250} = \frac{75\,000}{250}$$

$$x = \frac{75\,000}{250}$$

$$x = 300 \text{ mg/h}$$

b. Convert mg per hour to mg per min.

300 mg/h ÷ 60 min/h = 5 mg/min

21. a. Step 1: Calculate mg per hour.
    500 mg : 500 mL = x mg : 30 mL

    $$\frac{500x}{500} = \frac{15\,000}{500}$$

    $$x = \frac{15\,000}{500}$$

    $$x = 30 \text{ mg/h}$$

    Step 2: Convert mg per hour to mcg per hour
    (1 mg = 1 000 mcg).
    30 mg/h × 1 000 = 30 000 mcg/h

    b. Convert mcg per hour to mcg per min.
    30 000 mcg/h̸ ÷ 60 min/h̸ = 500 mcg/min

22. 25 g : 300 mL = 2 g : x mL

    $$\frac{25x}{25} = \frac{600}{25}$$

    $$x = \frac{600}{25}$$

    $$x = 24 \text{ mL/h; would administer 2 g/h}$$

23. Step 1: Determine the dosage in mcg per hour.
    200 mcg/min̸ × 60 min̸/h = 12 000 mcg/h
    Step 2: Convert mcg per hour to mg per hour
    (1 000 mcg = 1 mg).
    12 000 mcg/h ÷ 1 000 = 12 mg/h
    Step 3: Calculate the flow rate (mL/h).
    400 mg : 500 mL = 12 mg : x mL

    $$\frac{400x}{400} = \frac{6\,000}{400}$$

    $$x = 15 \text{ mL/h}$$

24. 25 g : 300 mL = 3 g : x mL

    $$\frac{25x}{25} = \frac{900}{25}$$

    $$x = \frac{900}{25}$$

    $$x = 36 \text{ mL/h; would administer 3 g/h}$$

25. Step 1: Convert the dosage per min to dosage
    per hour.
    10 mcg/min̸ × 60 min̸/h = 600 mcg/h
    Step 2: Convert to like units of measurement (mcg to
    mg; 1 000 mcg = 1 mg).
    600 mcg = 0.6 mg
    Step 3: Calculate mL per hour.
    50 mg : 250 mL = 0.6 mg : x mL

    $$\frac{50x}{50} = \frac{150}{50}$$

    $$x = 3 \text{ mL/h}$$

Step 4: Calculate the flow rate in gtt per min.

$$x \text{ gtt/min} = \frac{3 \text{ mL} \times 60 \text{ gtt/mL}}{60 \text{ min}}$$

$$x = 3 \text{ gtt/min; 3 microgtt/min}$$

To deliver 10 mcg per min, the IV is to infuse at 3 gtt
per min (3 microgtt per min).

26. Step 1: Convert the weight from lb to kg
    (2.2 lb = 1 kg).
    120 lb ÷ 2.2 = 54.54 = 54.5 kg
    Step 2: Calculate the dosage in mcg per min.
    54.5 kg̸ × 2 mcg/kg̸/min = 109 mcg/min

27. No conversion of weight is required.
    80 kg̸ × 3 mcg/kg̸/min = 240 mcg/min

28. No conversion of weight is required.
    73.5 kg̸ × 0.7 mg/kg̸/h = 51.45 = 51.5 mg/h

29. a. Step 1: Convert the weight from lb to kg
    (2.2 lb = 1 kg).
    110 lb ÷ 2.2 = 50 kg
    Step 2: Calculate the dosage in mg per hour.
    50 kg̸ × 0.7 mg/kg̸/h = 35 mg/h

    b. Calculate the dosage in mg per min.
    35 mg/h̸ ÷ 60 min/h̸ = 0.58 mg/min = 0.6 mg/min

    c. The dosage is safe; it falls within the safe range.

30. Step 1: Convert to like units of measurement
    (1 mg = 1 000 mcg).
    2 mg = 2 000 mcg
    Step 2: Calculate the concentration of solution in mcg
    per mL.
    2 000 mcg : 500 mL = x mcg : 1 mL

    $$\frac{500x}{500} = \frac{2\,000}{500}$$

    $$x = 4 \text{ mcg/mL}$$

    Lower dosage: 4 mcg : 1 mL = 2 mcg : x mL

    $$\frac{4x}{4} = \frac{2}{4}$$

    $$x = 0.5 \text{ mL/min}$$

    Upper dosage: 4 mcg : 1 mL = 6 mcg : x mL

    $$\frac{4x}{4} = \frac{6}{4}$$

    $$x = 1.5 \text{ mL/min}$$

    Step 3: Convert mL per min to mL per hour.
    Lower dosage:
    0.5 mL/min̸ × 60 min̸/h = 30 mL/h (gtt/min)
    Upper dosage:
    1.5 mL/min̸ × 60 min̸/h = 90 mL/h (gtt/min)
    A dosage range of 2 to 6 mcg per min is equal to a
    flow rate of 30 to 90 mL per hour (gtt/min).

31. a. Step 1: Convert to like units of measurement
(1 mg = 1 000 mcg).
5 000 mg = 5 000 000 mcg
Step 2: Calculate the concentration of solution in mcg per mL.
5 000 000 mcg : 500 mL $= x$ mcg : 1 mL

$$\frac{500x}{500} = \frac{5\,000\,000}{500}$$

$$x = 10\,000 \text{ mcg per mL}$$

The concentration of solution is 10 000 mcg per mL.
Step 3: Calculate the dosage range.
Lower dosage:
50 mcg/ k̶g̶ /min × 60 k̶g̶ = 3 000 mcg/min
Upper dosage:
75 mcg/ k̶g̶ /min × 60 k̶g̶ = 4 500 mcg/min
Step 4: Convert the dosage range to mL per min.
10 000 mcg : 1 mL = 1 000 mcg : x mL
Lower dosage:
10 000 mcg : 1 mL = 3 000 mcg : x mL

$$\frac{10\,000x}{10\,000} = \frac{3\,000}{10\,000}$$

$$x = 0.3 \text{ mL/min}$$

Upper dosage:
10 000 mcg : 1 mL = 4 500 mcg : x mL

$$\frac{10\,000x}{10\,000} = \frac{4\,500}{10\,000}$$

$$x = 0.45 \text{ mL/min}$$

Step 5: Convert mL per min to mL per hour.
Lower dosage:
0.3 mL/ m̶i̶n̶ × 60 m̶i̶n̶ /h = 18 mL/h (gtt/min)
Upper dosage:
0.45 mL/ m̶i̶n̶ × 60 m̶i̶n̶ /h = 27 mL/h (gtt/min)

A dosage range of 50 to 75 mcg is equal to a flow rate of 18 to 27 mL/h (gtt/min).

b. Determine the dosage per min infusing at 24 mL per hour.
10 000 mcg : 1 mL = x mcg : 24 mL
$x = 10\,000 × 24 = 240\,000$ mcg/h
240 000 mcg/ h̶ ÷ 60 min/ h̶ = 4 000 mcg/min

32. Step 1: Calculate the dosage in mcg per min.
65 k̶g̶ × 10 mcg/ k̶g̶ /min = 650 mcg/min
Step 2: Determine the dosage in mcg per hour.
650 mcg/ m̶i̶n̶ × 60 m̶i̶n̶ /h = 39 000 mcg/h
Step 3: Convert to like units of measurement
(1 000 mcg = 1 mg).
39 000 mcg/h = 39 mg/h

Step 4: Calculate the flow rate (mL/h).
500 mg : 250 mL = 39 mg : x mL

$$\frac{500x}{500} = \frac{9\,750}{500}$$

$$x = 19.5 = 20 \text{ mL/h}$$

Answer: To deliver a dosage of 10 mcg per kg per min, set the flow rate at 20 mL per hour (gtt/min).

33. Step 1: Convert grams to mg (1 g = 1 000 mg).
0.25 g = 250 mg
Step 2: Calculate mg per hour.
250 mg ÷ 6 h = 41.6 = 42 mg/h

34. a. Step 1: Convert grams to mg.
1 g = 1 000 mg
Step 2: Calculate mg per hour.
1 000 mg : 500 mL = x mg : 20 mL

$$\frac{500x}{500} = \frac{20\,000}{500}$$

$$x = \frac{20\,000}{500}$$

$$x = 40 \text{ mg/h}$$

b. Convert mg per hour to mg per min.
40 mg/ h̶ ÷ 60 min/ h̶ = 0.66 = 0.7 mg/min
Answer: At the rate of 20 mL per hour, the patient is receiving a dosage of 40 mg per hour or 0.7 mg per min.

35. a. Step 1: Convert gtt per min to mL per min.
60 gtt : 1 mL = 15 gtt : x mL

$$\frac{60x}{60} = \frac{15}{60}$$

$$x = 0.25 = 0.3 \text{ mL/min}$$

Step 2: Determine mg per min.
300 mg : 500 mL = x mg : 0.3 mL

$$\frac{500x}{500} = \frac{90}{500}$$

$$x = 0.18 = 0.2 \text{ mg/min}$$

b. Calculate mg per hour.
0.2 mg/ m̶i̶n̶ × 60 m̶i̶n̶ /h = 12 mg/h
Answer: At 15 gtt per min, the patient is receiving a dosage of 0.2 mg per min and 12 mg per hour.

36. a. Calculate the dosage in mcg per min.

$100 \text{ mcg/ kg /min} \times 102.4 \text{ kg} = 10\,240 \text{ mcg/min}$

b. Calculate the flow rate in mL per hour.

Step 1: Convert mcg per min to mg per min (1 000 mcg = 1 mg).

$10\,240 \text{ mcg/min} \div 1\,000 = 10.24 = 10.2 \text{ mg/min}$

Step 2: Convert mg per min to mg per hour.

$10.2 \text{ mg/ min} \times 60 \text{ min /h} = 612 \text{ mg/h}$

Step 3: Calculate the flow rate.

$1 \text{ g} = 1\,000 \text{ mg}; 1.5 \text{ g} = 1\,500 \text{ mg}$

$1\,500 \text{ mg} : 250 \text{ mL} = 612 \text{ mg} : x \text{ mL}$

$$1\,500x = 250 \times 612$$

$$\frac{1\,500x}{1\,500} = \frac{153\,000}{1\,500}$$

$$x = 102 \text{ mL/h}$$

or

$$\frac{1\,500 \text{ mg}}{250 \text{ mL}} = \frac{612 \text{ mg}}{x \text{ mL}}$$

$$x = 102 \text{ mL/h}$$

37. a. Step 1: Calculate mg per hour.

$500 \text{ mL} : 400 \text{ mg} = 20 \text{ mL} : x \text{ mg}$

or

$$\frac{500 \text{ mL}}{400 \text{ mg}} = \frac{20 \text{ mL}}{x \text{ mg}}$$

$$500x = 400 \times 20$$

$$\frac{500x}{500} = \frac{8\,000}{500}$$

$$x = 16 \text{ mg/h}$$

Step 2: Calculate mg per min.

$16 \text{ mg/ h} \div 60 \text{ min/ h} = 0.266 = 0.27 \text{ mg/min}$

b. Convert mg per min to mcg per min (1 mg = 1 000 mcg).

$0.27 \text{ mg/min} \times 1\,000 = 270 \text{ mcg/min}$

38. Step 1: Calculate the dosage in mcg per min.

$3 \text{ mcg/ kg /min} \times 59.1 \text{ kg} = 177.3 \text{ mcg/min}$

Step 2: Convert mcg per min to mcg per hour.

$177.3 \text{ mcg/ min} \times 60 \text{ min /h} = 10\,638 \text{ mcg/h}$

Step 3: Convert mcg per hour to mg per hour (1 000 mcg = 1 mg).

$10\,638 \text{ mcg/h} \div 1\,000 = 10.63 = 10.6 \text{ mg/h}$

Step 4: Calculate the flow rate (mL/h).

$250 \text{ mg} : 250 \text{ mL} = 10.6 \text{ mg} : x \text{ mL}$

or

$$\frac{250 \text{ mg}}{250 \text{ mL}} = \frac{10.6 \text{ mg}}{x \text{ mL}}$$

$$250x = 250 \times 10.6$$

$$\frac{250x}{250} = \frac{2\,650}{250}$$

$$x = 10.6 = 11 \text{ mL/h}$$

39. a. Step 1: Convert the weight from lb to kg (2.2 lb = 1 kg).

$165 \text{ lb} \div 2.2 = 75 \text{ kg}$

Step 2: Calculate the dosage in mcg per min.

$5 \text{ mcg/ kg /min} \times 75 \text{ kg} = 375 \text{ mcg/min}$

b. Convert mcg per min to mcg per hour.

$375 \text{ mcg/ min} \times 60 \text{ min /h} = 22\,500 \text{ mcg/h}$

c. Step 1: Convert mcg per hour to mg per hour (1 000 mcg = 1 mg).

$22\,500 \text{ mcg/h} \div 1\,000 = 22.5 \text{ mg/h}$

Step 2: Calculate the flow rate (mL/h).

$250 \text{ mg} : 250 \text{ mL} = 22.5 \text{ mg} : x \text{ mL}$

or

$$\frac{250 \text{ mg}}{250 \text{ mL}} = \frac{22.5 \text{ mg}}{x \text{ mL}}$$

$$250x = 250 \times 22.5$$

$$\frac{250x}{250} = \frac{5\,625}{250}$$

$$x = 22.5 = 23 \text{ mL/h}$$

40. a. $5 \text{ mg} : 1 \text{ mL} = 125 \text{ mg} : x \text{ mL}$

or

$$\frac{125 \text{ mg}}{5 \text{ mg}} \times 1 \text{ mL} = x \text{ mL}$$

Answer: 25 mL. The dosage ordered is more than the available strength; therefore, you will need more than 5 mL to administer the dosage.

b. $125 \text{ mg} : 125 \text{ mL} = 20 \text{ mg} : x \text{ mL}$

$$125x = 125 \times 20$$

$$\frac{125x}{125} = \frac{2\,500}{125}$$

$$x = 20 \text{ mL/h}$$

41. Step 1: Calculate the dosage per hour.
    2 mg/min × 60 min/h = 120 mg/h
    Step 2: Convert grams to mg (1 g = 1 000 mg).
    2 g = 2 000 mg
    Step 3: Calculate the flow rate (mL/h).
    2 000 mg : 500 mL = 120 mg : x mL

    $$2\,000x = 500 \times 120$$

    $$\frac{2\,000x}{2\,000} = \frac{60\,000}{2\,000}$$

    $$x = 30 \text{ mL/h}$$

42. Step 1: Calculate the dosage in mcg per min.
    3 mcg/kg/min × 95.9 kg = 287.7 mcg/min
    Step 2: Convert mcg per min to mcg per hour.
    287.7 mcg/min × 60 min/h = 17 262 mcg/h
    Step 3: Convert mcg per hour to mg per hour
    (1 000 mcg = 1 mg).
    17 262 mcg/h ÷ 1 000 = 17.26 = 17.3 mg/h
    Step 4: Calculate the flow rate (mL/h).
    400 mg : 250 mL = 17.3 mg : x mL

    $$400x = 250 \times 17.3$$

    $$\frac{400x}{400} = \frac{4\,325}{400}$$

    $$x = \frac{4\,325}{400}$$

    $$x = 10.81 = 10.8 \text{ mL/h}$$

    To infuse 3 mcg per kg per min, set the rate at
    10.8 mL per hour. The rate is not rounded to 11 mL
    per hour because the IV pump is capable of delivering
    in tenths of a mL.

43. Step 1: Convert the weight from lb to kg
    (2.2 lb = 1 kg).
    143 lb ÷ 2.2 = 65 kg
    Step 2: Find the concentration per minute (mcg/min).
    65 kg × 5 mcg/kg/min = 325 mcg/min
    Step 3: Find the concentration per hour.
    325 mcg/min × 60 min/h = 19 500 mcg/h
    The concentration of dobutamine infused is 325 mcg
    per min and 19 500 mcg per hour.

44. Step 1: Calculate the dosage per hour.
    3 mcg/min × 60 min/h = 180 mcg/h
    Step 2: Convert 180 mcg to mg to match the available
    strength (1 000 mcg = 1 mg).
    180 mcg ÷ 1 000 = 0.18 mg
    Step 3: Calculate the flow rate (mL/h).
    1 mg : 250 mL = 0.18 mg : x mL

    $$x = 250 \times 0.18$$

    $$x = 45 \text{ mL/h}$$

45. a. Step 1: Convert mcg per min to mcg per hour.
    2 mcg/min × 60 min/h = 120 mcg/h
    Step 2: Convert mcg per hour to mg per hour
    (1 000 mcg = 1 mg).
    120 mcg/h ÷ 1 000 = 0.12 mg/h
    Step 3: Calculate the lower flow rate (mL/h).
    8 mg : 250 mL = 0.12 mg : x mL

    $$8x = 250 \times 0.12$$

    $$\frac{8x}{8} = \frac{30}{8}$$

    $$x = \frac{30}{8}$$

    $$x = 3.8 \text{ mL/h}$$

    The flow rate for the lower 2 mcg per min is
    3.8 mL per hour.
    Step 4: Calculate the upper 4 mcg per min
    flow rate.
    Convert mcg per min to mcg per hour.
    4 mcg/min × 60 min/h = 240 mcg/h
    Step 5: Convert mcg per hour to mg per hour
    (1 000 mcg = 1 mg).
    240 mcg/h ÷ 1 000 = 0.24 mg/h
    Step 6: Calculate the upper flow rate (mL/h).
    8 mg : 250 mL = 0.24 mg : x mL

    $$8x = 250 \times 0.24$$

    $$\frac{8x}{8} = \frac{60}{8}$$

    $$x = \frac{60}{8}$$

    $$x = 7.5 \text{ mL/h}$$

    The flow rate for the upper 4 mcg per min is
    7.5 mL per hour.
    The flow rate range to titrate a dosage of
    2 to 4 mcg per min is 3.8 to 7.5 mL per hour
    (mL/h is not rounded; the pump is capable of
    delivering in tenths of a mL).

    b. Step 1: Calculate the dosage infusing at 5 mL per
    hour.
    250 mL : 8 mg = 5 mL : x mg

    $$\frac{250x}{250} = \frac{8 \times 5}{250}$$

    $$x = \frac{40}{250}$$

    $$x = 0.16 \text{ mg/h}$$

    Step 2: Convert mg per hour to mcg per hour
    (1 mg = 1 000 mcg).
    0.16 mg/h × 1 000 = 160 mcg/h
    Step 3: Convert mcg per hour to mcg per min.
    160 mcg/h ÷ 60 min/h = 2.66 = 2.7 mcg/min
    At the flow rate of 5 mL per hour, the patient is
    receiving 2.7 mcg per min.

46. Step 1: Calculate the dosage per hour using the lower and upper dosages.

$40 \text{ mcg}/\text{min} \times 60 \text{ min}/\text{h} = 2\,400 \text{ mcg}/\text{h}$

$100 \text{ mcg}/\text{min} \times 60 \text{ min}/\text{h} = 6\,000 \text{ mcg}/\text{h}$

Step 2: Convert mcg to mg to match the available strength ($1\,000 \text{ mcg} = 1 \text{ mg}$).

$2\,400 \text{ mcg} = 2.4 \text{ mg}$

$6\,000 \text{ mcg} = 6 \text{ mg}$

Step 3: Calculate the flow rate (mL/h).

$40 \text{ mg} : 250 \text{ mL} = 2.4 \text{ mg} : x \text{ mL}$

$$40x = 250 \times 2.4$$

$$\frac{40x}{40} = \frac{600}{40}$$

$$x = 15 \text{ mL}/\text{h}$$

To infuse 40 mcg per min, set the IV flow rate at 15 mL per hour (minimum).

$40 \text{ mg} : 250 \text{ mL} = 6 \text{ mg} : x \text{ mL}$

$$40x = 250 \times 6$$

$$\frac{40x}{40} = \frac{1\,500}{40}$$

$$x = 37.5 \text{ mL}/\text{h}$$

To infuse 100 mcg per min, set the IV flow rate at 37.5 mL per hour (maximum).

A dosage of 40 to 100 mcg per min is equal to 15 to 37.5 mL per hour.

Step 4: Set up a proportion to determine the dosage change of 20 mcg per min.

$$\frac{40 \text{ mcg}/\text{min}}{15 \text{ mL}/\text{h}} = \frac{20 \text{ mcg}/\text{min}}{x \text{ mL}/\text{h}}$$

$$\frac{40x}{40} = \frac{300}{40}$$

$$x = 7.5 \text{ mL}/\text{h}$$

Therefore, for each change of 20 mcg per min, the incremental IV flow rate is 7.5 mL per hour.

Titration Table	
Dosage Rate (mcg/min)	**IV Flow Rate (mL/h)**
40 mcg/min **(minimum)**	15 mL/h
60 mcg/min	22.5 mL/h
80 mcg/min	30 mL/h
100 mcg/min **(maximum)**	37.5 mL/h

47. Step 1: Calculate the dosage per hour using the lower and upper dosages.

$4 \text{ mcg}/\text{min} \times 60 \text{ min}/\text{h} = 240 \text{ mcg}/\text{h}$

$12 \text{ mcg}/\text{min} \times 60 \text{ min}/\text{h} = 720 \text{ mcg}/\text{h}$

Step 2: Convert mcg per hour to mg per hour to match the available strength ($1\,000 \text{ mcg} = 1 \text{ mg}$).

$240 \text{ mcg}/\text{h} \div 1\,000 = 0.24 \text{ mg}/\text{h}$

$720 \text{ mcg}/\text{h} \div 1\,000 = 0.72 \text{ mg}/\text{h}$

Step 3: Calculate the flow rate (mL/h).

$4 \text{ mg} : 500 \text{ mL} = 0.24 \text{ mg} : x \text{ mL}$

$$4x = 500 \times 0.24$$

$$\frac{4x}{4} = \frac{120}{4}$$

$$x = 30 \text{ mL}/\text{h}$$

To infuse 4 mcg per min, set the IV flow rate at 30 mL per hour (minimum).

$4 \text{ mg} : 500 \text{ mL} = 0.72 \text{ mg} : x \text{ mL}$

$$4x = 500 \times 0.72$$

$$\frac{4x}{4} = \frac{360}{4}$$

$$x = 90 \text{ mL}/\text{h}$$

To infuse 12 mcg per min, set the IV flow rate at 90 mL per hour (maximum).

A dosage of 4 to 12 mcg per min is equal to 30 to 90 mL per hour.

Step 4: Set up a proportion to determine the dosage change of 2 mcg per min.

$$\frac{4 \text{ mcg}/\text{min}}{30 \text{ mL}/\text{h}} = \frac{2 \text{ mcg}/\text{min}}{x \text{ mL}/\text{h}}$$

$$\frac{4x}{4} = \frac{60}{4}$$

$$x = 15 \text{ mL}/\text{h}$$

For each change of 2 mcg per min, the incremental IV flow rate is 15 mL per hour.

Titration Table	
Dosage Rate (mcg/min)	**IV Flow Rate (mL/h)**
4 mcg/min **(minimum)**	30 mL/h
6 mcg/min	45 mL/h
8 mcg/min	60 mL/h
10 mcg/min	75 mL/h
12 mcg/min **(maximum)**	90 mL/h

Comprehensive Post-Test

Solve the following calculation problems. Remember to apply the principles relating to dosages learned in the text. Use labels where provided. Shade in the dosage on the syringe where indicated.

1. Order: Amoxicillin and clavulanate potassium 300 mg PO q8h (ordered according to dosage of amoxicillin).

   Available:

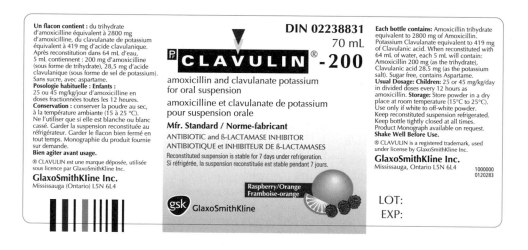

2. Order: Procan SR (procainamide) 1 g PO q6h for a patient with atrial fibrillation.

   Available: Procan SR tablets 500 mg

---

3. Order: Acamprosate calcium 666 mg PO TID.

Available:

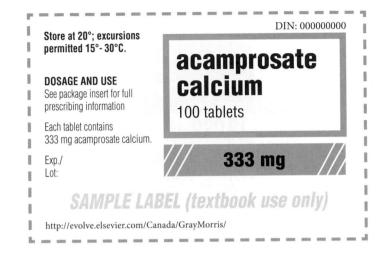

4. Order: Trimethoprim and sulfamethoxazole DS 1 tab PO q12h for 14 days.

Available:

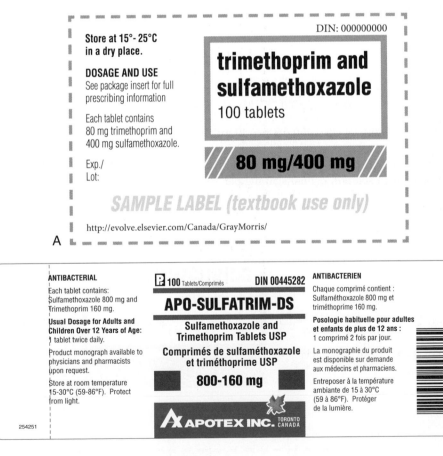

a. Indicate which tablets (A or B) you would choose to administer to the patient based on the order. _____

b. State why. _____

5. Order: Diazepam (Valium) 7 mg IM stat.

    Available: Valium labelled 5 mg per mL   _____

6. Order: Heparin 6 500 units SUBCUT daily. (Express your answer in hundredths.)

    Available:

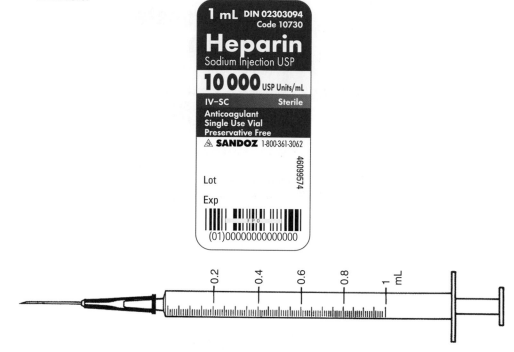

                                                                _____

7. Order: Ciprofloxacin (Cipro) 0.75 g IV q12h for 7 days.

    Available: Cipro labelled 400 mg per 40 mL   _____

8. Order: Amphotericin B 75 mg in 1 000 mL D5W to infuse over 6 hours daily. The reconstituted solution contains 50 mg per 10 mL.

    Available:

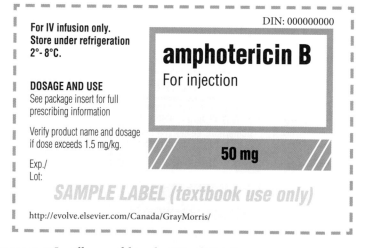

    a. How many mL will you add to the IV solution?   _____

    b. The IV is to infuse in 6 hours. The administration
        set delivers 10 gtt per mL. At what rate in gtt per
        min should the IV infuse?   _____

9. The recommended dose of Retrovir for adults with symptomatic HIV infection is 1 mg per kg infused over 1 hour q4h. Determine the dosage for a patient weighing 110 lb.

_____

10. Order: Epivir 0.3 g PO daily.

   Available: Epivir tablets labelled 150 mg

   How many tablets will you administer?

_____

11. Order: Ceftazidime 0.25 g IV q12h.

   Available:

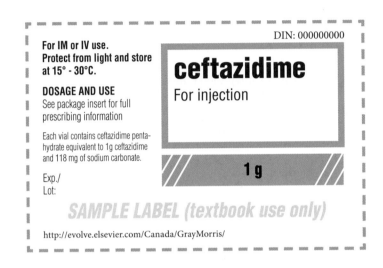

Directions for reconstitution state the following for IV infusion: 1-g vial, add 10 mL sterile water to provide 95 mg per mL; 2-g vial, add 10 mL sterile water to provide 180 mg per mL.

   a. Using the label provided, what concentration will you prepare?

_____

   b. How many mL will you administer?

_____

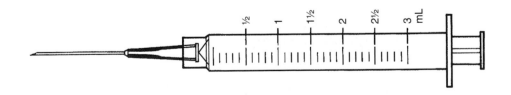

12. Order: GlucoNorm 3 mg PO BID.

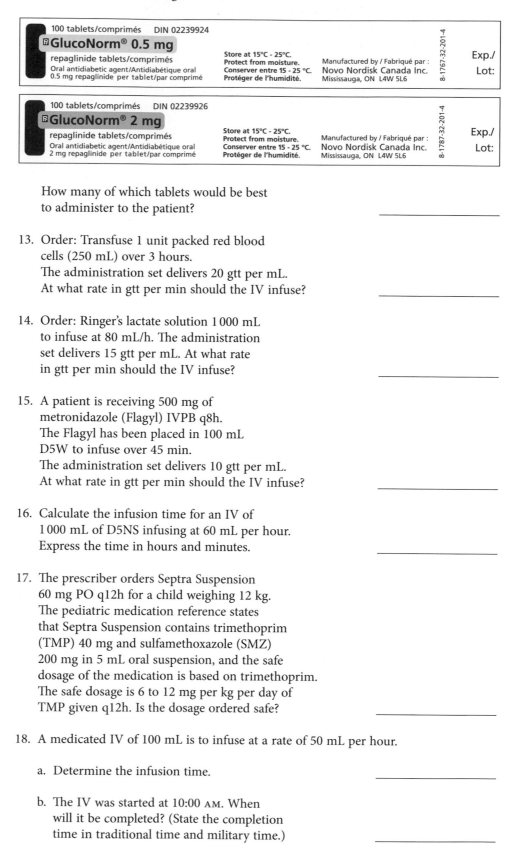

How many of which tablets would be best
to administer to the patient?

_____

13. Order: Transfuse 1 unit packed red blood
cells (250 mL) over 3 hours.
The administration set delivers 20 gtt per mL.
At what rate in gtt per min should the IV infuse?

_____

14. Order: Ringer's lactate solution 1 000 mL
to infuse at 80 mL/h. The administration
set delivers 15 gtt per mL. At what rate
in gtt per min should the IV infuse?

_____

15. A patient is receiving 500 mg of
metronidazole (Flagyl) IVPB q8h.
The Flagyl has been placed in 100 mL
D5W to infuse over 45 min.
The administration set delivers 10 gtt per mL.
At what rate in gtt per min should the IV infuse?

_____

16. Calculate the infusion time for an IV of
1 000 mL of D5NS infusing at 60 mL per hour.
Express the time in hours and minutes.

_____

17. The prescriber orders Septra Suspension
60 mg PO q12h for a child weighing 12 kg.
The pediatric medication reference states
that Septra Suspension contains trimethoprim
(TMP) 40 mg and sulfamethoxazole (SMZ)
200 mg in 5 mL oral suspension, and the safe
dosage of the medication is based on trimethoprim.
The safe dosage is 6 to 12 mg per kg per day of
TMP given q12h. Is the dosage ordered safe?

_____

18. A medicated IV of 100 mL is to infuse at a rate of 50 mL per hour.

a. Determine the infusion time.

_____

b. The IV was started at 10:00 AM. When
will it be completed? (State the completion
time in traditional time and military time.)

_____

19. A patient is to receive 10 mcg per min of nitroglycerine IV. The concentration of solution is 50 mg in 250 mL D5W. What should the IV flow rate be (in mL/h) to deliver 10 mcg per min? _____

20. Order: Novolin Toronto U-100 6 units and Novolin NPH U-100 16 units SUBCUT at 7:30 AM.

    What is the total volume you will administer? _____

10 mL DIN 02024233 100 IU/mL	10 mL DIN 02024225 100 IU/mL
Novolin®ge Toronto	**Novolin®ge NPH**
100 IU/mL	100 IU/mL
Insulin Injection, Human Biosynthetic (Regular) s.c., i.v. Insuline injectable, biosynthétique humaine (Régulière), s.c., i.v.	Insulin Isophane, Human Biosynthetic, s.c. Insuline isophane, biosynthétique humaine, s.c.
Do not freeze. See leaflet. 1 vial of 10 mL contains 1,000 IU **Ne pas congeler.** Voir feuillet. 1 fiole de 10 mL contient 1000 UI HUMAN/HUMAINE	**Shake carefully. Do not freeze.** Directions for use: See leaflet. **Agiter avec soin.** **Ne pas congeler.** Mode d'emploi : Voir feuillet. HUMAN/HUMAINE
Mfr. by / Fabr. par : Novo Nordisk Canada Inc. Mississauga, ON, Canada, L4W 5L6 8-0201-32-210-1	Mfr. by / Fabr. par : Novo Nordisk Canada Inc. Mississauga, ON, Canada, L4W 5L6 8-0227-32-210-1
Exp./ Lot.:	Exp./ Lot.:

21. A dosage of 500 mg in a volume of 3 mL is to be diluted to 55 mL to infuse over 50 minutes. A 20-mL flush is to follow.

    a. What is the dilution volume? _____

    b. At what rate in gtt per min should the IV infuse? (Administration set is a microdrop.) _____

    c. Indicate the rate in mL per hour. _____

22. Order: Zocor 40 mg PO daily.

    Available: Zocor tablets labelled 10 mg and 20 mg

    Which strength of Zocor would you administer and why? _____

23. Calculate the body surface area (BSA), using the formula, for a child who weighs 102 lb and is 51 inches tall. Calculate the BSA to the nearest hundredth. _____

24. Acyclovir IV is to be administered to a child who has herpes simplex encephalitis. The child weighs 13.6 kg and is 60 cm tall. The recommended dosage is 500 mg per m^2. Use the formula to calculate the BSA.

Available:

For IV infusion only. Inject 20 mL sterile water into vial. Shake vial until a clear solution is achieved and use within 12 hours.

DOSAGE AND USE
See package insert for full prescribing information

Each mL contains 1000 mg acyclovir.

Exp./
Lot:

DIN: 000000000

acyclovir
For injection

1000 mg

SAMPLE LABEL (textbook use only)

http://evolve.elsevier.com/Canada/GrayMorris/

a. What is the BSA? (Express your answer to the nearest hundredth.) _____

b. What will the dosage be? _____

c. The reconstituted Zovirax provides 50 mg per mL. Calculate the number of mL to administer. _____

25. Order: Captopril (Capoten) 50 mg PO. Hold if systolic blood pressure is less than 100.

Available: Capoten tablets labelled 25 mg

a. How many tablets will you administer? _____

b. The patient's blood pressure is 90/60. What should the nurse do? _____

26. Prepare the following solution strength: $\frac{2}{5}$-strength Ensure Plus 250 mL. _____

27. Order: 400 mL of Pulmocare over 6 hours by nasogastric tube. The feeding is placed in an enteral infusion pump. Determine the IV flow rate in mL per hour. (Round your answer to the nearest whole number.) _____

28. A medication of 1 g in 4 mL is to be diluted to 70 mL and infused over 50 minutes. A 15-mL flush follows. Medication is placed in a burette. Determine the following:

a. gtt per min _____

b. mL per hour _____

29. A child weighing 21.4 kg has an order for 500 mg of a medication in 100 mL D5W q12h. The normal daily dosage range is 40 to 50 mg per kg. Determine whether the dosage is within normal range, and state your course of action. _____

30. Calculate the amount of dextrose and sodium chloride (NaCl) in 2 L of D5 $\frac{1}{4}$ NS.

    a. Dextrose _____ g

    b. NaCl _____ g

31. 500 mL D5W was to infuse in 3 hours at 28 gtt per min (28 macrogtt per min). The drop factor is 10 gtt per mL. After $1\frac{1}{2}$ hours, you notice 175 mL has infused.

    a. Recalculate the IV flow rate. _____

    b. Determine the percentage of change. _____

    c. State your course of action. _____

32. 1 000 mL D5RL was to infuse in 8 hours at 31 gtt per min (31 macrogtt per min). After 4 hours, you notice 600 mL has infused. The administration set delivers 15 gtt per mL.

    a. Recalculate the IV flow rate. _____

    b. Determine the percentage of change. _____

    c. State your course of action. _____

33. Order: Infuse D5W 500 mL with 20 000 units heparin at 25 mL/h. Determine the following:

    _____ units per hour

34. Order: Promethazine 25 mg IV push before surgery. The literature states the following: Do not give at a rate above 25 mg/min.

    Available:

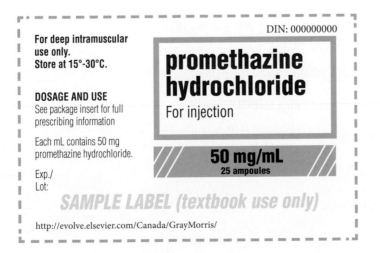

a. How many mL will you prepare? _____

b. For how many minutes should the medication be administered? _____

35. Order: Morphine sulphate 80 mg in 250 mL of IV fluid to infuse at a rate of 20 mL/h.

Determine the dosage in mg per hour the patient is receiving. _____

36. Order: Diltiazem 25 mg IV over 2 minutes.

Available:

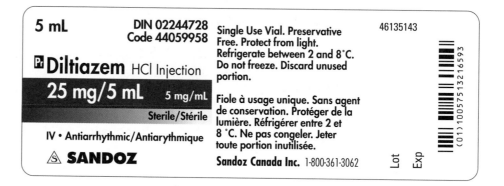

a. How many mL will you add to the IV? _____

b. How many mL will you infuse per minute? _____

37. Order: Ciprofloxacin (Cipro) 0.5 g PO q12h.

Available: Cipro tablets labelled 250 mg

How many tablets will be needed for 10 days of therapy? _____

38. Order: Digoxin (Lanoxin) tablets 0.375 mg PO stat.

Available: Scored tablets labelled 125 mcg, 250 mcg, and 500 mcg

a. Which Lanoxin tablet(s) will you use to prepare the dosage? _____

b. How many tablets should the patient receive? _____

39. Order: Infergen 12 mcg SUBCUT stat.

Available: Infergen 15 mcg per 0.5 mL

How many mL will you administer? _____

40. Order: Digoxin 0.125 mg IV daily for 7 days.

    Available:

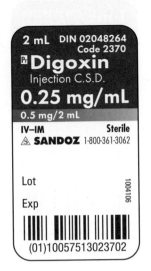

a. How many mL will you administer?   _____

b   Shade in the dosage on the syringe provided.

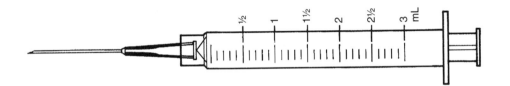

For problems 41 to 43, round the weight to the nearest tenth as indicated.

41. The heparin protocol at an institution is as follows: Bolus patient with 80 units per kg of body weight and start drip at 14 units per kg per hour. Using this heparin protocol, determine the following for a patient weighing 242 lb.

    a. Heparin bolus dosage   _____

    b. Infusion rate for the heparin IV drip   _____

42. Order: 20 units/kg/h heparin IV. The patient weighs 88 kg.

    How many units per hour will the patient receive?   _____

43. Order: 20 000 units heparin IV in 250 mL to infuse at 25 units/kg/h. The patient weighs 184 lb.

    How many units per hour will the patient receive?   _____

44. Order: Digoxin 0.375 mg IV push (infused slowly over 5 minutes).

    Available: Digoxin 0.25 mg per mL

    a. How many mL should you administer?   _____

    b. At what rate in mL per min should the IV infuse?   _____

45. Order: Morphine 8 mg IV q4h prn (infusion not to exceed 10 mg/4 min).

    Available:

    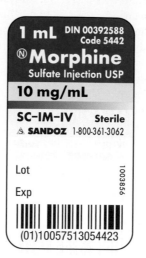

    a. How many mL should you administer? _____

    b. How many minutes will it take for the IV to infuse? _____

46. Refer to the following chart and calculate the patient's fluid intake in millilitres.

Oral Intake	IV Intake
4 oz gelatin	100 mL
2 oz water	
12 oz apple juice	

    What is the patient's fluid intake in mL? _____

47. Refer to the heparin weight-based protocol that follows to answer this question. Determine the bolus dosage of heparin and the initial intravenous rate of heparin for a patient who weighs 187 lb. The patient's PPT is reported as being 43 seconds. Determine the rebolus and adjust the IV flow rate based on the PPT results.

WEIGHT-BASED HEPARIN PROTOCOL
GOAL OF THERAPY = PTT OF 46 to 70 SECONDS

1. Heparin 80 units/kg IV bolus
2. Initiate IV heparin infusion at 18 units/kg/h from a solution of 25 000 units heparin in 250 mL D5W for 1 000 units/mL
3. Adjust heparin daily based on PTT results as follows:

PTT (seconds)	IV Bolus	Stop Infusion	Rate Change (mL/h)	Next PTT
Less than 35	80 units/kg	No	Increase rate by 4 units/kg/h	4 hours after rate increased
35–45	40 units/kg	No	Increase rate by 2 units/kg/h	6 hours after rate increased
46–70 (Target Range)	**None**	**No**	**No Change**	**Next Morning**
71–90	None	No	Decrease rate by 2 units/kg/h	Next morning
Greater than 90	None	For 1 hour	Decrease rate by 3 units/kg/h	6 hours after rate decreased

Note: This protocol is for calculation purposes only.

48. A patient is ordered to begin norepinephrine bitartrate (Levophed) at 4 mcg per min to maintain blood pressure and titrate to maintain systolic blood pressure greater than 100 mm Hg to a maximum of 12 mcg per min. The available solution is Levophed 8 mg in 1 000 mL D5W. Develop a titration table from minimum to maximum dose in 2 mcg per min increments. (The IV pump is calibrated in whole mL.)

49. Midazolam (Versed) 10 mcg per kg IV is ordered for sedation of a patient. The patient weighs 127.2 lb. How many mcg should the patient receive?   _____

50. Order: Penicillin G potassium 500 000 units IV q6h.

    Available:

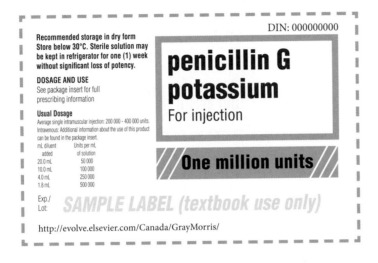

a. Which concentration will you choose and why?   _____

b. How many mL will you add to the IV?   _____

c. Shade in the dosage on the syringe provided.

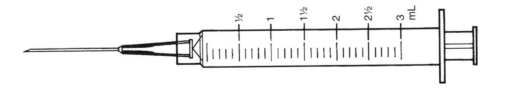

51. Order: Tobramycin 5 mg IV q6h for an infant.

    Available:

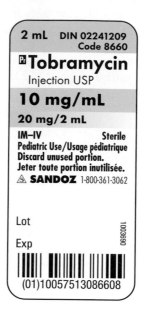

a. How many mL will you add to the IV?

b. Shade in the dosage on the syringe provided.

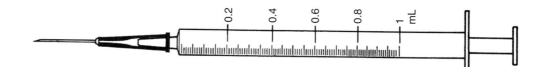

52. Order: Kantrex 32 mg IV q8h for an infant.

    Available: Kantrex labelled 75 mg per 2 mL

    a. How many mL will you add to the IV?

    b. Shade in the dosage on the syringe provided.

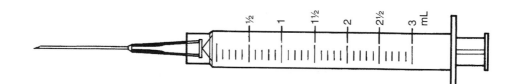

53. Order: Clindamycin 900 mg IV weekly.

    Available:

    | 2 mL | DIN 02230540 |
    | | Code 2050 |

    ℞ Clindamycin
    Injection USP

    150 mg/mL

    300 mg/2 mL

    IM–IV   Sterile
    Discard unused portion.
    Jeter toute portion inutilisée.
    ⚠ **SANDOZ** 1-800-361-3062

    Lot

    Exp

    (01)10057513020503

    How many mL will you add to the IV?   _____

54. A patient has type 2 diabetes and was admitted with sepsis on the medical unit. The patient was on oral antihyperglycemic medication at home, but the physician feels that a basal bolus regimen with correction dose insulin that is rapid acting should be administered to help reduce the patient's blood glucose (BG) while in hospital. The long-acting basal insulin analogue is 20 units at bedtime, and the rapid-acting insulin for bolus at mealtimes is as follows: breakfast = 7 units, lunch = 6 units, and dinner = 7 units. Use the following correction scale to answer the questions.

BG (mmol/L)	Bolus Insulin (Units)
less than 4	Call MD
4.1–10	0
10.1–13	2
13.1–16	4
16.1–19	6
greater than 19	Call MD

    a. If the patient's BG is 13.1 mmol per L before dinner, what is the *total* amount of rapid-acting insulin the patient will receive?   _____

    b. How much supplemental rapid-acting insulin will the patient receive if BG is 8.3 mmol per L before breakfast?   _____

55. Correct the following medication orders according to the Institute for Safe Medication Practices Canada (ISMP Canada) list of error-prone abbreviations, symbols, and dose designations (the "Do Not Use" list, see Table 9-3.)

    a. MS 4 mg sc q4h prn pain   _____

    b. Digoxin .375 mg PO qd   _____

56. An 8-year-old child is admitted to the medical pediatric unit due to a respiratory infection. The physician prescribed cefprozil 375 mg PO q12h. The child weighs 55 lb. Use the medication label to calculate the dosage.

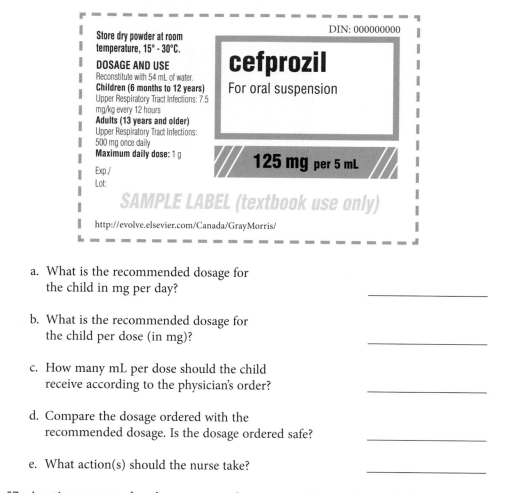

Store dry powder at room temperature, 15° - 30°C.

DOSAGE AND USE
Reconstitute with 54 mL of water.
Children (6 months to 12 years)
Upper Respiratory Tract Infections: 7.5 mg/kg every 12 hours
Adults (13 years and older)
Upper Respiratory Tract Infections: 500 mg once daily
Maximum daily dose: 1 g

Exp./
Lot:

DIN: 000000000

cefprozil
For oral suspension

125 mg per 5 mL

SAMPLE LABEL (textbook use only)

http://evolve.elsevier.com/Canada/GrayMorris/

a. What is the recommended dosage for the child in mg per day?   _____

b. What is the recommended dosage for the child per dose (in mg)?   _____

c. How many mL per dose should the child receive according to the physician's order?   _____

d. Compare the dosage ordered with the recommended dosage. Is the dosage ordered safe?   _____

e. What action(s) should the nurse take?   _____

57. A patient presented to the emergency department with a swollen right leg after a long plane trip. Diagnostic tests reveal deep vein thrombosis (DVT). The physician's order is to administer heparin bolus of 90 units per kg and then initiate heparin infusion at 20 units per kg per hour from a heparin concentration of 25 000 units in 500 mL D5W. The patient weighs 187 lb. Use the heparin label for calculation as necessary.

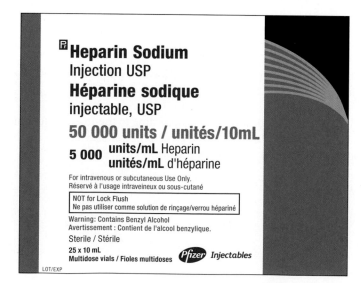

℗**Heparin Sodium**
Injection USP
Héparine sodique
injectable, USP

50 000 units / unités/10mL
5 000 units/mL Heparin
unités/mL d'héparine

For intravenous or subcutaneous Use Only.
Réservé à l'usage intraveineux ou sous-cutané

NOT for Lock Flush
Ne pas utiliser comme solution de rinçage/verrou hépariné

Warning: Contains Benzyl Alcohol
Avertissement : Contient de l'alcool benzylique.

Sterile / Stérile

25 x 10 mL
Multidose vials / Fioles multidoses   *Pfizer* Injectables

LOT/EXP

a. What is the bolus dosage of heparin
   in units for this patient?   _____

b. How many mL of heparin should the nurse add to the 500 mL of D5W to get the
   infusion concentration of 25 000 units per 500 mL?   _____

c. How many units per hour of heparin will the patient receive according to the
   physician's order?   _____

d. At what rate in mL per hour should the nurse program the IV pump for the heparin
   infusion?   _____

58. A patient is receiving an IV infusion of 0.9% sodium chloride 750 mL in 5 hours. The
    nurse is using a microdrip administration set for the infusion. At what rate in gtt per
    min should the IV be regulated?   _____

59. Refer to this case to answer the questions that follow.

> A 22-year-old patient is in diabetic ketoacidosis (DKA). She weighs 50 kg.
>   She continues to have fluid resuscitation with normal saline to correct dehydration. Her serum potassium level has increased to 3.5 mmol per L and her BG is 16.6 mmol per L.
>   The physician's order is as follows: Mix 50 units insulin regular (Humulin R) in 250 mL 0.9% sodium chloride for 0.2 unit/mL. Initiate the insulin infusion at 0.1 unit/kg/h. Check BG according to protocol.

a. What is the rate of the patient's insulin
   infusion in units per hour?   _____

b. What is the rate of the insulin infusion
   in mL per hour?   _____

60. A patient presented to the emergency department with 56% of BSA burned as a result
    of a car explosion. He weighs 95 kg. Use the Parkland formula (4 mL × kg × % BSA
    burned) and the post–24-hour formula based on urine output (1 mL × kg × % BSA
    burned) to answer the following:

a. What is the 24-hour total amount of Ringer's lactate solution (RL) IV fluid
   replacement that the patient should receive?   _____

b. What is the first 8-hour total amount of RL IV fluid replacement that the patient
   should receive?   _____

c. What is the first 8-hour infusion rate of RL IV fluid replacement in mL per hour?

                                                          _____

d. What is the next 16-hour total amount of RL IV fluid replacement that the patient
   should receive?   _____

e. What is the infusion rate for this 16-hour volume in mL per hour?

                                                          _____

f. What is the total amount of D5W IV fluid replacement for hours 25 to
   48 post-burn?   _____

g. What is the infusion rate of D5W IV fluid replacement for hours 25 to 48 post-burn
   in mL per hour?   _____

evolve

For another comprehensive post-test, refer to the Drug Calculations Companion, Version 5 on Evolve.

Answers on pages 698–704.

✳ ANSWERS

NOTE
Calculations may be performed using the ratio and proportion method, the formula method, or the dimensional analysis method.

1. $200 \text{ mg} : 5 \text{ mL} = 300 \text{ mg} : x \text{ mL}$

   or

   $$\frac{300 \text{ mg}}{200 \text{ mg}} \times 5 \text{ mL} = x \text{ mL}$$

   Answer: 7.5 mL

2. Conversion is required. Conversion factor:
   1 g = 1 000 mg.
   $500 \text{ mg} : 1 \text{ tab} = 1 000 \text{ mg} : x \text{ tab}$

   or

   $$\frac{1 000 \text{ mg}}{500 \text{ mg}} \times 1 \text{ tab} = x \text{ tab}$$

   Answer: 2 tabs

3. $333 \text{ mg} : 1 \text{ tab} = 666 \text{ mg} : x \text{ tab}$

   or

   $$\frac{666 \text{ mg}}{333 \text{ mg}} \times 1 \text{ tab} = x \text{ tab}$$

   Answer: 2 tabs

4. a. Tablets B: Septra DS.
   b. The prescriber's order indicates DS, which means double strength; therefore, the patient should be given the tabs that are labelled DS.

5. $5 \text{ mg} : 1 \text{ mL} = 7 \text{ mg} : x \text{ mL}$

   or

   $$\frac{7 \text{ mg}}{5 \text{ mg}} \times 1 \text{ mL} = x \text{ mL}$$

   Answer: 1.4 mL

6. $10 000 \text{ units} : 1 \text{ mL} = 6 500 \text{ units} : x \text{ mL}$

   or

   $$\frac{6 500 \text{ units}}{10 000 \text{ units}} \times 1 \text{ mL} = x \text{ mL}$$

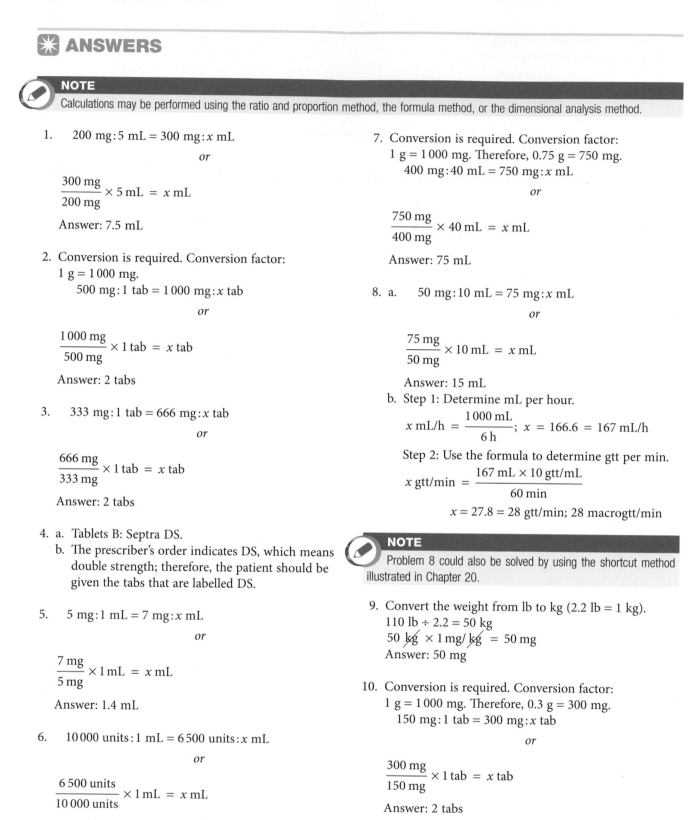

   Answer: 0.65 mL

7. Conversion is required. Conversion factor:
   1 g = 1 000 mg. Therefore, 0.75 g = 750 mg.
   $400 \text{ mg} : 40 \text{ mL} = 750 \text{ mg} : x \text{ mL}$

   or

   $$\frac{750 \text{ mg}}{400 \text{ mg}} \times 40 \text{ mL} = x \text{ mL}$$

   Answer: 75 mL

8. a. $50 \text{ mg} : 10 \text{ mL} = 75 \text{ mg} : x \text{ mL}$

   or

   $$\frac{75 \text{ mg}}{50 \text{ mg}} \times 10 \text{ mL} = x \text{ mL}$$

   Answer: 15 mL

   b. Step 1: Determine mL per hour.
   $$x \text{ mL/h} = \frac{1 000 \text{ mL}}{6 \text{ h}}; \; x = 166.6 = 167 \text{ mL/h}$$

   Step 2: Use the formula to determine gtt per min.
   $$x \text{ gtt/min} = \frac{167 \text{ mL} \times 10 \text{ gtt/mL}}{60 \text{ min}}$$

   $x = 27.8 = 28 \text{ gtt/min}; \; 28 \text{ macrogtt/min}$

NOTE
Problem 8 could also be solved by using the shortcut method illustrated in Chapter 20.

9. Convert the weight from lb to kg (2.2 lb = 1 kg).
   $110 \text{ lb} \div 2.2 = 50 \text{ kg}$
   $50 \text{ kg} \times 1 \text{ mg/kg} = 50 \text{ mg}$
   Answer: 50 mg

10. Conversion is required. Conversion factor:
    1 g = 1 000 mg. Therefore, 0.3 g = 300 mg.
    $150 \text{ mg} : 1 \text{ tab} = 300 \text{ mg} : x \text{ tab}$

    or

    $$\frac{300 \text{ mg}}{150 \text{ mg}} \times 1 \text{ tab} = x \text{ tab}$$

    Answer: 2 tabs

11. a. 95 mg per mL (the vial is 1 g).
    b. Conversion is required. Conversion factor:
       1 g = 1 000 mg. Therefore, 0.25 g = 250 mg.
       $$95 \text{ mg} : 1 \text{ mL} = 250 \text{ mg} : x \text{ mL}$$

       or

       $$\frac{250 \text{ mg}}{95 \text{ mg}} \times 1 \text{ mL} = x \text{ mL}$$

       Answer: 2.63 = 2.6 mL

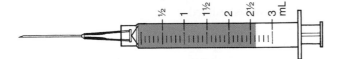

12. Answer: 3 tabs (one 2-mg tab and two 0.5-mg tabs)
    Total = 3 mg (2 mg tab + 1 mg = 3 mg)
    Administer the least number of tablets to the patient.

13. Step 1: Determine mL per hour.

    $$x \text{ mL/h} = \frac{250 \text{ mL}}{3 \text{ h}}; \ x = 83.3 = 83 \text{ mL/h}$$

    Step 2: Calculate gtt per min.

    $$x \text{ gtt/min} = \frac{83 \text{ mL} \times 20 \text{ gtt/mL}}{60 \text{ min}}$$

    $$x = 27.6 = 28 \text{ gtt/min}$$

    Answer: 28 gtt per min; 28 macrogtt per min
    The shortcut method could also have been used to solve this problem.

14. $$x \text{ gtt/min} = \frac{80 \text{ mL} \times 15 \text{ gtt/mL}}{60 \text{ min}}$$

    $$x = 20 \text{ gtt/min}$$
    Answer: 20 gtt per min; 20 macrogtt per min

15. $$x \text{ gtt/min} = \frac{100 \text{ mL} \times 10 \text{ gtt/mL}}{45 \text{ min}}$$

    $$x = 22.2 = 22 \text{ gtt/min}$$
    Answer: 22 gtt per min; 22 macrogtt per min

16. $$\frac{1\,000 \text{ mL}}{60 \text{ mL/h}} = 16.66$$

    60 min = 1 h
    60 min/h × 0.66/h = 39.6 = 40 min
    Answer: 16 h + 40 min

17. No weight conversion required. Weight is stated in kg.
    6 mg/kg/day × 12 kg = 72 mg/day
    12 mg/kg/day × 12 kg = 144 mg/day
    Divided dosage: 72 mg/day ÷ 2 = 36 mg q12h
    144 mg/day ÷ 2 = 72 mg q12h
    The safe dosage range is 72 to 144 mg per day.

The divided dosage is 36 to 72 mg q12h.
Answer: The prescriber ordered 60 mg q12h.
The dosage is safe (60 mg × 2 = 120 mg);
it falls within the safe dosage range.

18. $$\frac{100 \text{ mL}}{50 \text{ mL/h}} = 2 \text{ h}$$

    a. 2 h
    b. 12 noon or 12 PM (10:00 AM and 2 hours); military time: 1200

19. Step 1: Determine the dosage per hour.
    10 mcg/min × 60 min = 600 mcg/h
    Step 2: Convert mcg to mg to match the solution.
    Conversion factor: 1 000 mcg = 1 mg; therefore,
    600 mcg = 0.6 mg.
    Step 3: Calculate mL per hour.
    50 mg : 250 mL = 0.6 mg : x mL

    or

    $$\frac{50 \text{ mg}}{250 \text{ mL}} = \frac{0.6 \text{ mg}}{x \text{ mL}}$$

    $$x = 3 \text{ mL/h}$$

    Answer: To deliver 10 mcg per min, set the flow rate at 3 mL per hour (gtt/min).

20. 22 units (Humulin Regular 6 units + Humulin NPH 16 units)

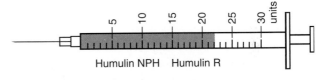

Humulin NPH   Humulin R

21. a. 52 mL
    b. $$x \text{ gtt/min} = \frac{55 \text{ mL} \times 60 \text{ gtt/mL}}{50 \text{ min}}$$

       $$x = 66 \text{ gtt/min}$$
       Answer: 66 gtt per min; 66 microgtt per min
       The shortcut method could also have been used to solve this problem.
    c. 66 mL per hour (gtt/min with a microdrop = mL/h)

22. Administer two 20-mg tablets. The patient should receive the least number of tabs. If 10-mg tabs are used, the patient would require 4 tabs. Generally, the maximum number of tablets that should be administered is three. Remember to question any order requiring more than three tablets.

    1 20-mg tab
    +1 20-mg tab
    ――――――
    40 mg

23. $\sqrt{\dfrac{102\,(\text{lb}) \times 50\,(\text{in})}{3\,131}} = \sqrt{1.66} = 1.288 = 1.29\ \text{m}^2$

    Answer: 1.29 m²

24. a. $\sqrt{\dfrac{13.6\,(\text{kg}) \times 60\,(\text{cm})}{3\,600}} = \sqrt{0.226} = 0.475 = 0.48\ \text{m}^2$

     Answer: 0.48 m²

   b. $0.48\ \cancel{\text{m}^2} \times 500\ \text{mg}/\cancel{\text{m}^2} = 240\ \text{mg}$

     Answer: 240 mg

   c. $50\ \text{mg}:1\ \text{mL} = 240\ \text{mg}:x\ \text{mL}$

             or

    $\dfrac{240\ \text{mg}}{50\ \text{mg}} \times 1\ \text{mL} = x\ \text{mL}$

     Answer: 4.8 mL. The dosage ordered is greater than the available strength; therefore, you will need more than 1 mL to administer the dosage.

25. a. $25\ \text{mg}:1\ \text{tab} = 50\ \text{mg}:x\ \text{tab}$

             or

    $\dfrac{50\ \text{mg}}{25\ \text{mg}} \times 1\ \text{tab} = x\ \text{tab}$

     Answer: 2 tabs

   b. Hold the medication because the systolic blood pressure (top number) is less than 100, and notify the prescriber.

26. $\dfrac{2}{5} \times 250\ \text{mL} = x\ \text{mL}$

       $\dfrac{500}{5} = x$

          $x = 100\ \text{mL of Ensure Plus}$

  250 mL − 100 mL = 150 mL (water)
Therefore, you would add 150 mL of water to 100 mL of Ensure Plus to make 250 mL $\dfrac{2}{5}$-strength Ensure Plus.

27. $x\ \text{mL/h} = \dfrac{400\ \text{mL}}{6\ \text{h}}$

       $x = 66.6 = 67\ \text{mL/h}$
  Answer: 67 mL per hour

28. $x\ \text{gtt/min} = \dfrac{70\ \text{mL} \times 60\ \text{gtt/mL}}{50\ \text{min}}$

        $x = 84\ \text{gtt/min}$

   a. 84 gtt per min; 84 microgtt per min. The shortcut method could also have been used to solve this problem.

   b. 84 mL per hour (gtt/min with a microdrop = mL/h)

29. Step 1: Calculate the normal daily dosage range.
    $40\ \text{mg}/\cancel{\text{kg}}/\text{day} \times 21.4\ \cancel{\text{kg}} = 856\ \text{mg}$
    $50\ \text{mg}/\cancel{\text{kg}}/\text{day} \times 21.4\ \cancel{\text{kg}} = 1\,070\ \text{mg}$
    The safe dosage range is 856 to 1 070 mg per day.
    Step 2: Calculate the dosage infusing in 24 hours.
    500 mg q12h = (2 dosages)
    500 mg × 2 = 1 000 mg in 24 h
    Step 3: Assess the accuracy of the dosage ordered.
    500 mg q12h (1 000 mg) falls within the 856 to 1 070 mg per day dosage range. Administer the medication as ordered.

30. Conversion is required. Conversion factor:
    1 L = 1 000 mL; therefore, 2 L = 2 000 mL.
   a. Dextrose: $5\ \text{g}:100\ \text{mL} = x\ \text{g}:2\,000\ \text{mL}$

        $\dfrac{100x}{100} = \dfrac{10\,000}{100}$

              or

        $\dfrac{5\ \text{g}}{100\ \text{mL}} = \dfrac{x\ \text{g}}{2\,000\ \text{mL}}$

          $x = 100\ \text{g dextrose}$

   b. NaCl: $0.225\ \text{g}:100\ \text{mL} = x\ \text{g}:2\,000\ \text{mL}$

        $\dfrac{100x}{100} = \dfrac{450}{100}$

              or

        $\dfrac{0.225\ \text{g}}{100\ \text{mL}} = \dfrac{x\ \text{g}}{2\,000\ \text{mL}}$

          $x = 4.5\ \text{g NaCl}$

> ✎ **NOTE**
>
> Remember: $\dfrac{1}{4}$ NS (sodium chloride) is written as 0.225.

31. Time remaining: $3\ \text{h} - 1.5\ \text{h} = 1.5\ \text{h}\ (1\tfrac{1}{2}\ \text{h})$

    Volume remaining: 500 mL − 175 mL = 325 mL
   a. Step 1: Calculate mL per hour.
     325 mL ÷ 1.5 h = 216.6 = 217 mL/h
    Step 2: Calculate gtt per min.

     $x\ \text{gtt/min} = \dfrac{217\ \text{mL} \times 10\ \text{gtt/mL}}{60\ \text{min}}$

        $x = \dfrac{217 \times 1}{6} = \dfrac{217}{6}$

       $x = 36\ \text{gtt/min};\ 36\ \text{macrogtt/min}$

    The IV flow rate would have to be changed to 36 gtt per min (36 macrogtt per min).
   b. Determine the percentage of change.

     $\dfrac{36 - 28}{28} = \dfrac{8}{28} = 0.285 = 29\%$

c. State your course of action: Assess the patient and notify the prescriber. This increase is greater than 25%. The order may have to be revised.
Alternative calculation without percentages:
Ordered rate ± (ordered rate ÷ 4) = acceptable IV readjustment rate
28 gtt/min + (28 ÷ 4) = 28 + 7 = 35 gtt/min; 35 macrodrop/min
28 gtt/min − (28 ÷ 4) = 28 − 7 = 21 gtt/min; 21 macrodrop/min
The safe dosage range is 21 to 35 gtt per min (21 to 35 macrogtt per min). Note that 36 gtt per min (36 macrogtt per min) is more than the acceptable range.

32. Time remaining: 8 h − 4 h = 4 h
Volume remaining: 1 000 mL − 600 mL = 400 mL
   a. Step 1: Calculate mL per hour.
   400 mL ÷ 4 h = 100 mL/h
   Step 2: Calculate gtt per min.

   $$x \text{ gtt/min} = \frac{100 \text{ mL} \times 15 \text{ gtt/mL}}{60 \text{ min}}$$

   $$x = \frac{100 \times 1}{4} = \frac{100}{4}$$

   $$x = 25 \text{ gtt/min}; \ 25 \text{ macrogtt/min}$$

   The IV flow rate would have to be changed to 25 gtt per min (25 macrogtt per min).
   b. Determine the percentage of change.

   $$\frac{25 - 31}{31} = \frac{-6}{31} = -0.193 = -19\%$$

   c. State your course of action: Assess the patient and lower the IV flow rate to 25 gtt per min (25 macrogtt per min). This decrease (−19%) is acceptable; it is within the acceptable 25% variation. Also check the institution's policy and continue observation of the patient.
   Alternative calculation without percentages:
   Ordered rate ± (ordered rate ÷ 4) = acceptable IV adjustment rate
   31 gtt/min + (31 ÷ 4) = 31 + 7.75 = 38.75 = 39 gtt/min (39 macrogtt/min)
   31 gtt/min − (31 ÷ 4) = 31 − 7.75 = 23.25 = 23 gtt/min (23 macrogtt/min)
   The safe dosage range is 23 to 39 gtt per min (23 to 39 macrogtt per min). Note that 25 gtt per min (25 macrogtt per min) is within the safe dosage range.

> ✎ **NOTE**
> In problems 31 and 32, gtt per min could also be calculated using the drop factor constant (see Chapter 20).

33. Calculate the units per hour infusing.
500 mL : 20 000 units = 25 mL : x units

$$\frac{500x}{500} = \frac{500\,000}{500}$$

$$x = 1\,000 \text{ units/h}$$

An IV of 500 mL containing 20 000 units of heparin infusing at 25 mL per hour is administering 1 000 units per hour.

34. a.   50 mg : 1 mL = 25 mg : x mL
            or

   $$\frac{25 \text{ mg}}{50 \text{ mg}} \times 1 \text{ mL} = x \text{ mL}$$

   $$x = 0.5 \text{ mL}$$

   b. 25 mg : 1 min = 25 mg : x min

   $$\frac{25x}{25} = \frac{25}{25} = 1$$

   $$x = 1 \text{ min}$$

35. 80 mg : 250 mL = x mg : 20 mL

   $$\frac{250x}{250} = \frac{1\,600}{250} = 6.4$$

   $$x = 6.4 \text{ mg/h}$$

36. a.   5 mg : 1 mL = 25 mg : x mL

   $$\frac{25 \text{ mg}}{5 \text{ mg}} \times 1 \text{ mL} = x \text{ mL}$$

   $$x = 5 \text{ mL}$$

   b. $\dfrac{5 \text{ mL}}{2 \text{ min}} = 2.5 \text{ mL/min}$

37. Conversion is required. Conversion factor:
1 g = 1 000 mg; therefore, 0.5 g = 500 mg.
Answer: 40 tabs (2 tabs per dose × 2 = 4 tabs; 4 tabs × 10 days = 40 tabs)

38. Conversion is required. Conversion factor: 1 mg = 1 000 mcg; therefore, 0.375 mg = 375 mcg.
   a. Give the patient one 250-mcg tab and one 125-mcg tab.

   250-mcg tab
   +125-mcg tab
   ⎯⎯⎯⎯⎯⎯
   375-mcg tab

   b. 2 tabs (one 250-mcg tab and one 125-mcg tab); give the least number of tablets without scoring.

39.   15 mcg : 0.5 mL = 12 mcg : x mL

or

$$\frac{12 \text{ mcg}}{15 \text{ mcg}} \times 0.5 \text{ mL} = x \text{ mL}$$

$$x = 0.4 \text{ mL}$$

40. Conversion is required. Conversion factor: 1 mg = 1 000 mcg. Therefore, 0.125 mg = 125 mcg.
   a.   500 mcg : 2 mL = 125 mcg : x mL

or

$$\frac{125 \text{ mcg}}{500 \text{ mcg}} \times 2 \text{ mL} = x \text{ mL}$$

$$x = 0.5 \text{ mL}$$

b.

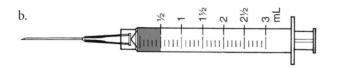

41. Convert the weight from lb to kg (2.2 lb = 1 kg).
   242 lb ÷ 2.2 = 110 kg
   a. 80 units/kg × 110 kg = 8 800 units
   b. 14 units/kg/h × 110 kg = 1 540 units/h

42. 20 units/kg/h × 88 kg = 1 760 units/h

43. Convert the weight from lb to kg (2.2 lb = 1 kg).
   184 lb ÷ 2.2 = 83.63 = 83.6 kg
   25 units/kg/h × 83.6 kg = 2 090 units/h

44. a.   0.25 mg : 1 mL = 0.375 mg : x mL

or

$$\frac{0.375 \text{ mg}}{0.25 \text{ mg}} \times 1 \text{ mL} = x \text{ mL}$$

   Answer: 1.5 mL
   b. 1.5 mL : 5 min = x mL : 1 min

$$5x = 1.5$$

$$x = 0.3 \text{ mL/min}$$

45. a.   10 mg : 1 mL = 8 mg : x mL

or

$$\frac{8 \text{ mg}}{10 \text{ mg}} \times 1 \text{ mL} = x \text{ mL}$$

   Answer: 0.8 mL
   b. 10 mg : 4 min = 8 mg : x min

$$\frac{10x}{10} = \frac{32}{10}$$

$$x = 3.2 \text{ min}$$

46. Conversion is required. Conversion factor:
   1 oz = 30 mL.
   Total oz = 18 oz
   18 oz × 30 = 540 mL
   540 mL (PO) + 100 mL (IV) = 640 mL
   Answer: 640 mL

47. Step 1: Convert the weight from lb to kg
   (2.2 lb = 1 kg).
   187 lb ÷ 2.2 = 85 kg
   Step 2: Calculate the heparin bolus dosage.
   80 units/kg × 85 kg = 6 800 units. The patient
   should receive 6 800 units IV heparin as a bolus.
   Determine the volume (mL) the patient would
   receive. The concentration of heparin is 1 000 units
   per mL.
   1 000 units : 1 mL = 6 800 units : x mL

$$\frac{1\,000x}{1\,000} = \frac{6\,800}{1\,000}$$

$$x = \frac{6\,800}{1\,000}$$

$$x = 6.8 \text{ mL (bolus is 6.8 mL)}$$

Step 3: Calculate the infusion rate (18 units/kg/h).
18 units/kg/h × 85 kg = 1 530 units/h
Determine the rate in mL per hour at which to set the
infusion device using the concentration of 1 000 units
per mL.

1 000 units : 1 mL = 1 530 units : x mL

$$\frac{1\,000x}{1\,000} = \frac{1\,530}{1\,000}$$

$$x = \frac{1\,530}{1\,000}$$

x = 1.53 = 1.5 mL/h (not rounded to a whole
number because pump is capable of delivering in
tenths of a mL)
The patient's PPT is 43 seconds. According to the
protocol, rebolus with 40 units per kg and increase
the rate by 2 units per kg per hour.
Step 4: Calculate the dosage of heparin rebolus and
the continuous infusion increase based on the PPT
according to the protocol.
Calculate the dosage (units) of heparin rebolus.
40 units/kg × 85 kg = 3 400 units
Determine the volume (mL) to administer 3 400 units.
1 000 units : 1 mL = 3 400 units : x mL

$$\frac{1\,000x}{1\,000} = \frac{3\,400}{1\,000}$$

$$x = \frac{3\,400}{1\,000}$$

$$x = 3.4 \text{ mL (bolus)}$$

Now determine the infusion rate increase
(2 units/kg/h × kg).
2 units/kg/h × 85 kg = 170 units/h
The infusion rate should be increased by 170 units per hour.
Calculate the adjustment in the hourly infusion rate (mL/h).
$1\,000\ \text{units} : 1\ \text{mL} = 170\ \text{units} : x\ \text{mL}$

$$\frac{1\,000x}{1\,000} = \frac{170}{1\,000}$$

$$x = \frac{170}{1\,000}$$

$$x = 0.17 = 0.2\ \text{mL/h}$$

The IV flow rate should be increased by 0.2 mL per hour.

Increase rate:

1.5 mL/h (current rate)

+ 0.2 mL/h (increase)

1.7 mL/h (new infusion rate; not rounded to a whole number because pump is capable of delivering in tenths of a mL)

48. Step 1: Calculate the dosage per hour using the upper and lower limits of the dosage.
4 mcg/min × 60 min/h = 240 mcg/h
12 mcg/min × 60 min/h = 720 mcg/h
Step 2: Convert mcg per hour to match the available strength.
Conversion factor: 1 000 mcg = 1 mg
240 mcg = 0.24 mg
720 mcg = 0.72 mg
Step 3: Calculate the rate in mL per hour for the upper and lower dosage.
$8\ \text{mg} : 1\,000\ \text{mL} = 0.24\ \text{mg} : x\ \text{mL}$

$$\frac{8x}{8} = \frac{1\,000 \times 0.24}{8}$$

$$\frac{8x}{8} = \frac{240}{8}$$

$$x = \frac{240}{8}$$

$$x = 30\ \text{mL/h}$$

To infuse 4 mcg per min, set the infusion pump at 30 mL per hour.
$8\ \text{mg} : 1\,000\ \text{mL} = 0.72\ \text{mg} : x\ \text{mL}$

$$\frac{8x}{8} = \frac{1\,000 \times 0.72}{8}$$

$$\frac{8x}{8} = \frac{720}{8}$$

$$x = \frac{720}{8}$$

$$x = 90\ \text{mL/h}$$

To infuse 12 mcg per min, set the infusion pump at 90 mL per hour.
The dosage range of 4 to 12 mcg per min is equal to an IV flow rate of 30 to 90 mL per hour.
Step 4: Set up a proportion to determine the incremental flow rate for a dosage rate change of 2 mcg per min.

$$\frac{4\ \text{mcg/min}}{30\ \text{mL/h}} = \frac{2\ \text{mcg/min}}{x\ \text{mL/h}}$$

$$\frac{4x}{4} = \frac{60}{4}$$

$$x = \frac{60}{4}$$

$$x = 15\ \text{mL/h}$$

For each dosage change of 2 mcg per min, the incremental IV flow rate is 15 mL per hour. The titration table follows.

Titration Table	
Dosage Rate (mcg/min)	**IV Flow Rate (mL/h)**
4 mcg/min **(minimum)**	30 mL/h
6 mcg/min	45 mL/h
8 mcg/min	60 mL/h
10 mcg/min	75 mL/h
12 mcg/min **(maximum)**	90 mL/h

49. Step 1: Convert the weight from lb to kg
(2.2 lb = 1 kg).
127.2 lb ÷ 2.2 = 57.8 kg
Step 2: 10 mcg/kg × 57.8 kg = 578 mcg
Answer: 578 mcg

50. a. Select 500 000 units per mL. The medication is being administered IV, and will require further dilution before IV administration.
   b. 1 mL (once reconstituted, each mL will contain 500 000 units per mL).
   c.

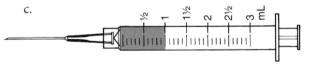

51. a. $20\ \text{mg} : 2\ \text{mL} = 5\ \text{mg} : x\ \text{mL}$

   or

$$\frac{5\ \text{mg}}{20\ \text{mg}} \times 2\ \text{mL} = x\ \text{mL}$$

$$x = 0.5\ \text{mL}$$

   Answer: 0.5 mL

   b.

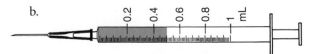

52. a. $75 \text{ mg} : 2 \text{ mL} = 32 \text{ mg} : x \text{ mL}$

or

$$\frac{32 \text{ mg}}{75 \text{ mg}} \times 2 \text{ mL} = x \text{ mL}$$

$$x = 0.85 = 0.9 \text{ mL}$$

Answer: 0.9 mL

b.

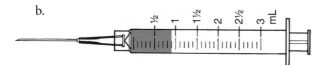

53. $150 \text{ mg} : 1 \text{ mL} = 900 \text{ mg} : x \text{ mL}$

or

$$\frac{900 \text{ mg}}{150 \text{ mg}} \times 1 \text{ mL} = x \text{ mL}$$

$$x = 6 \text{ mL}$$

Answer: 6 mL

54. a. The patient's routine bolus insulin at dinner is 6 units of rapid-acting insulin. BG is 13.1 mmol per litre, so 4 units will be added to the 6 units to make 10 units.

6 units + 4 units = 10 units of rapid-acting insulin

b. No extra units. BG is within target.

55. a. Morphine sulphate 4 mg SUBCUT q4h prn pain
b. Digoxin 0.375 mg PO daily

56. a. Since the child is 8 years old and has a respiratory tract infection, the nurse must choose the dosage category recommended for the 6-months to 12-year-old age group. Since dosages are indicated for children based on weight in kg, the child's weight must first be converted from lb to kg (55 lb ÷ 2.2 = 25 kg).
Recommended dosage: 7.5 mg/kg q12h.
7.5 mg × 25 kg = 187.5 mg q12h
Every 12 hours is 2 times per day; therefore, 187.5 mg × 2 = 375 mg/day
The recommended dosage for the child is 375 mg/day.

b. The recommended dosage for the child per dose is 375 mg ÷ 2 = 187.5 mg

c. $\dfrac{375 \text{ mg}}{125 \text{ mg}} \times 5 \text{ mL} = x \text{ mL} = 15 \text{ mL}$

d. No.

e. Call the prescriber and report that the dosage ordered is higher than the recommended dosage.

57. a. 187 ÷ 2.2 = 85 kg: 90 units × 85 kg = 7 650 units

b. $\dfrac{25\,000 \text{ units}}{5\,000 \text{ units}} \times 1 \text{ mL} = x \text{ mL} = 5 \text{ mL}$

c. 20 units × 85 kg × 1 h = 1 700 units/h

d. $\dfrac{1\,700 \text{ units}}{25\,000 \text{ units}} \times 500 \text{ mL} = x \text{ mL} = 34 \text{ mL/h}$

58. $\dfrac{x \text{ mL}}{1 \text{ h}} = \dfrac{750 \text{ mL}}{5 \text{ h}} = 150 \text{ mL/h}$

$$x \frac{\text{gtt}}{\text{min}} = \frac{150 \text{ mL}}{60 \text{ min}} \times 60 \text{ gtt/mL} = 150 \text{ gtt/min}$$

59. a. 0.1 unit/kg/h × 50 kg = 5 units/h

b. $\dfrac{5 \text{ units}}{50 \text{ units}} \times 250 \text{ mL} = 25 \text{ mL/h}$

60. a. The patient weighs 95 kg.
Therefore, 4 mL × 95 kg × 56 = 21 280 mL
b. 21 280 × 0.5 = 10 640 mL
c. 10 640 mL ÷ 8 h = 1 330 mL/h
d. 21 280 × 0.5 = 10 640 mL
e. 10 640 mL ÷ 16 h = 665 mL/h
f. 1 mL × 95 kg × 56 = 5 320 mL
g. 5 320 mL ÷ 24 h = 221.6 or 222 mL/h

Arabic Equivalents for Roman Numerals

Arabic Number	Roman Numeral	Arabic Number	Roman Numeral
$\frac{1}{2}$	ss or $\overline{ss}$	9	ix or $\overline{ix}$, IX
1	i or $\overline{i}$, I	10	x or $\overline{x}$, X
2	ii or $\overline{ii}$, II	15	xv or $\overline{xv}$, XV
3	iii or $\overline{iii}$, III	20	xx or $\overline{xx}$, XX
4	iv or $\overline{iv}$, IV	30	xxx or $\overline{xxx}$, XXX
5	v or $\overline{v}$, V	50	L(l)
6	vi or $\overline{vi}$, VI	100	C(c)
7	vii or $\overline{vii}$, VII	500	D(d)
8	viii or $\overline{viii}$, VIII	1 000	M(m)

Diabetes Management Record: Subcutaneous Insulin

HOSPITAL LOGO	**Diabetes Management Record** – Subcutaneous Insulin	FRONT SIDE
	Is patient on non-insulin anti-hyperglycemic agents? ☐ No ☐ Yes – *refer to MAR*	
	Is patient on corticosteroids? ☐ No ☐ Yes – *refer to MAR*	ADDRESSOGRAPH

Record 1

Date: / Time:	Pre-breakfast or Morning :	Additional Morning : :	Pre-lunch or Midday :	Additional Afternoon : :	Pre-supper or Early Evening :	Additional Evening : :	Bedtime or Late Evening :	Overnight : :
Blood Glucose Result:								
Basal Insulin:	units	units units	units	units units	units	units units	units	units units
Scheduled Bolus Insulin:	units	units units	units	units units	units	units units	units	units units
Correction Dose (*Same insulin as above*):	units	units units	units	units units	units	units units	units	units units
Pre-mixed Insulin:	units	units units	units	units units	units	units units	units	units units
Correction Dose:	units	units units	units	units units	units	units units	units	units units
RN / RPN *and* **Witness Initials:**								
Nutrition: (*greater or less than 50% of meal consumed, enteral feeds, TPN, NPO*)								

Hypoglycemic episodes: *time, BG value, treatment, response*   **Other events that may have impacted BG**

Record 2

Date: / Time:	Pre-breakfast or Morning :	Additional Morning : :	Pre-lunch or Midday :	Additional Afternoon : :	Pre-supper or Early Evening :	Additional Evening : :	Bedtime or Late Evening :	Overnight : :
Blood Glucose Result:								
Basal Insulin:	units	units units	units	units units	units	units units	units	units units
Scheduled Bolus Insulin:	units	units units	units	units units	units	units units	units	units units
Correction Dose (*Same insulin as above*):	units	units units	units	units units	units	units units	units	units units
Pre-mixed Insulin:	units	units units	units	units units	units	units units	units	units units
Correction Dose:	units	units units	units	units units	units	units units	units	units units
RN / RPN *and* **Witness Initials:**								
Nutrition: (*greater or less than 50% of meal consumed, enteral feeds, TPN, NPO*)								

Hypoglycemic episodes: *time, BG value, treatment, response*   **Other events that may have impacted BG**

Record 3

Date: / Time:	Pre-breakfast or Morning :	Additional Morning : :	Pre-lunch or Midday :	Additional Afternoon : :	Pre-supper or Early Evening :	Additional Evening : :	Bedtime or Late Evening :	Overnight : :
Blood Glucose Result:								
Basal Insulin:	units	units units	units	units units	units	units units	units	units units
Scheduled Bolus Insulin:	units	units units	units	units units	units	units units	units	units units
Correction Dose (*Same insulin as above*):	units	units units	units	units units	units	units units	units	units units
Pre-mixed Insulin:	units	units units	units	units units	units	units units	units	units units
Correction Dose:	units	units units	units	units units	units	units units	units	units units
RN / RPN *and* **Witness Initials:**								
Nutrition: (*greater or less than 50% of meal consumed, enteral feeds, TPN, NPO*)								

Hypoglycemic episodes: *time, BG value, treatment, response*   **Other events that may have impacted BG**

iSMP CANADA

Diabetes Management Record – Subcutaneous Insulin

HOW TO USE THIS FORM

1. Transcribe all intermittent subcutaneous insulin orders on the MAR. This form is **not** intended for intravenous insulin infusions or insulin pumps.
2. Indicate on top of the form if the patient is on oral non-insulin anti-hyperglycemic agents.
3. Indicate on top of the form if the patient is on corticosteroids.
4. Record the time of the blood glucose reading.
5. Record the name of the insulin given.
6. Record the number of units of insulin given in the appropriate box.
7. If patient requires correction dose insulin record the extra number of units given in the designated box.
8. The person who administered the dose should document their initials.
9. If your facility requires an independent double check the "witness" should document their initials beside that of the person who administered the insulin.
10. Indicate the nutritional status of the patient by indicating if greater or less than 50% of the meal has been consumed, if the patient is on parenteral or enteral feeds or if the patient is NPO.
11. If a patient experiences a hypoglycemic episode indicate the time it happened, the BG reading, the treatment that was given to correct it, the patient's response to the treatment and any other factors that may have contributed to the episode.
12. Document if any additional factors occurred to cause the BG to deviate from the normal range (e.g., starting corticosteroids).

INSULIN PRODUCTS

Brand (Generic) Name of Insulin	Onset	Peak (h)	Duration (h)
Bolus – Meal time and Correction* *Rapid Acting*			
Apidra (Glulisine)	10–15 min	1–1.5	3–5
Humalog (Lispro)	10–15 min	1–1.5	3–5
NovoRapid (Aspart)	10–15 min	1–1.5	3–5
Short Acting			
Humulin-R, Novolin ge Toronto (Regular)	30–60 min	2–3	6.5
Basal *Intermediate Acting*			
Humulin-N, Novolin ge NPH (NPH)	1–3 hours	5–8	Up to 18
Long Acting			
Lantus (Glargine)	1.5 hours	No peak	Up to 24
Levemir (Detemir)	1.5 hours	No peak	16–24
Pre-Mixed Insulin			
Humalog Mix25, Mix50 (Lispro/Lispro protamine)	10–15 min	1–8	Up to 18
NovoMix30 (Aspart/Aspart protamine)	10–15 min	1–8	Up to 18
Humulin 30/70, Novolin ge 30/70 (Regular, NPH)	30–60 min	2–8	Up to 18

Non-Insulin Anti-Hyperglycemic Agents

Acarbose (Glucobay)
Exenatide (Byetta)
Glicazide (Diamicron, Diamicron MR)
Glimepiride (Amaryl)
Glyburide (Diabeta)
Linagliptin (Trajenta)
Linagliptin + Metformin (Jentadueto)
Liraglutide (Victoza)
Metformin (Glucophage, Glumetza)
Metformin + Saxagliptin (Komboglyze)
Metformin + Sitagliptin (Janumet)
Nateglinide (Starlix)
Repaglinide (GlucoNorm)
Pioglitazone (Actos)
Rosiglitazone (Avandia)
Saxagliptin (Onglyza)
Sitagliptin (Januvia)

*Correction dosing – rapid or short acting insulin used to correct hyperglycemia.

© 2013 Institute for Safe Medication Practices Canada. Developed by ISMP Canada with Support from the Ontario Ministry of Health and Long-Term Care; http://www.ismp-canada.org/download/insulin/DiabetesManagementRecord_SubcutaneousInsulin.pdf. Reprinted with permission from ISMP Canada.

References

Accreditation Canada. (2013). *All Canadians have the right to safe, high-quality health services.* Retrieved from http://www.accreditation.ca/about-us

Accreditation Canada. Canadian Institute for Health Information., Canadian Patient Safety Institute., & Institute for Safe Medication Practices Canada. (2012). *Medication reconciliation in Canada: Raising the Bar – progress to date and the course ahead.* Ottawa, Canada: Author.

Brown, M., & Mulholland, J. (2008). *Drug calculations: Process and problems for clinical practice* (8th ed.). St. Louis, MO: Mosby.

Canada Health Infoway. (2010, July 13). *Health information technology: Innovation to improve health care quality, access and availability.* Retrieved from https://www.ic.gc.ca/eic/site/028.nsf/eng/00293.html

Canadian Diabetes Association Clinical Practice Guidelines Expert Committee. (2013). Canadian diabetes association 2013 clinical practice guidelines for the prevention and management of diabetes in Canada. *Canadian Journal of Diabetes, 37*(suppl 1), S1-S212.

Canadian Medication Incident Reporting and Prevention System. (2011). *What is CMIRPS?* Retrieved from http://www.cmirps-scdpim.ca/?p=14

Cancer Care Ontario. (2012). *Computerized Prescriber Order Entry (CPOE) for Systemic Treatment: Best Practice Guideline.* Toronto, Canada: Author.

Clayton, B. D., & Willihnganz, M. (2013). *Basic pharmacology for nurses* (16th ed.). St. Louis, MO: Mosby.

Cohen, M. R. (Ed.). (2010). *Medication errors* [Abridged ed.]. Washington, DC: American Pharmacists Association.

College of Nurses of Ontario. (2015). *Practice standard: Medication revised 2015.* Retrieved from http://www.cno.org/Global/docs/prac/41007_Medication.pdf

College of Registered Nurses of British Columbia. (2010). *Medication Administration: Principles.* Retrieved from https://www.crnbc.ca/Standards/PracticeStandards/Pages/medicationadmin.aspx

College of Registered Nurses of Nova Scotia. (2015). *Medication guidelines for registered nurses.* Retrieved from http://crnns.ca/wp-content/uploads/2015/05/Medication-Guidelines.pdf

Harkreader, H., & Hogan, M. A. (2007). *Fundamentals of nursing: Caring and clinical judgment* (3rd ed.). St. Louis, MO: Saunders.

Health Canada. (2015). *Drugs and health products: Health Canada's role in the in the management and prevention of harmful medication incidents.* Retrieved from http://www.hc-sc.gc.ca/dhp-mps/medeff/cmirps-scdpim-eng.php

Hockenberry, M. J., & Wilson, D. (2011). *Wong's nursing care of infants and children* (9th ed.). St. Louis, MO: Mosby.

Health Canada, & Institute for Safe Medication Practices Canada. (2015). *Document for industry: Draft good label and package practices guide.* Retrieved from <http://www.ismp-canada.org/download/LabellingPackaging/Draft-GoodLabelandPackagePracticesGuide-EN-2015-03.pdf>.

Houlden, R., Capes, S., Clement, M., & Miller, D. (2013). Canadian diabetes association 2013 clinical practice guidelines for the prevention and management of diabetes in Canada: In-hospital management of diabetes. *Canadian Journal of Diabetes 2013, 37*(suppl 1), S77-S81.

Institute for Medicine. (2006, July). Report brief: Preventing medication errors. *National academy of Sciences.* Retrieved from www.iom.edu/~/media/Files/Report%20Files/2006/Preventing-Medication-Errors-Quality-Chasm-Series/medicationerrorsnew.pdf

Institute for Safe Medication Practices. (2011a). *FDA and ISMP lists of look-alike drug names with recommended Tall Man letters.* Retrieved from https://www.ismp.org/tools/tallmanletters.pdf

Institute for Safe Medication Practices. (2011b). *ISMP Acute care guidelines for timely administration of scheduled medications.* Retrieved from http://www.ismp.org/tools/guidelines/acutecare/tasm.pdf

Institute for Safe Medication Practices. (2013, October). *As U-500 insulin safety concerns mount, it's time to rethink safe use of strength above U-100. Acute Care:* ISMP Medication Safety Alert. Retrieved from https://www.ismp.org/newsletters/acutecare/showarticle.aspx?id=62

Institute for Safe Medication Practices. (2015). *ISMP's list of confused drug names.* Retrieved from <http://www.ismp.org/tools/confuseddrugnames.pdf>.

Institute for Safe Medication Practices Canada (2000-2016). *Medication errors and risk management in hospitals.* Retrieved from https://www.ismp-canada.org/Riskmgm.htm

Institute for Safe Medication Practices Canada. (2003). Insulin errors. *ISMP Canada Safety Bulletin, 3*(4), 1-2.

Institute for Safe Medication Practices Canada. (2004, January). Infusion pump project: Survey results and time for action. *ISMP Canada Safety Bulletin 4*(1), 1-2.

Institute for Safe Medication Practices Canada. (2006a). *Do not use: Dangerous abbreviations, symbols and dose designations.* Retrieved from http://www.ismp-canada.org/download/ISMPC_List_of_Dangerous_Abbreviations.pdf

Institute for Safe Medication Practices Canada. (2006b). Eliminate use of dangerous abbreviations, symbols, and dose designations. *ISMP Canada Safety Bulletin, 6*(4), 1.

Institute for Safe Medication Practices Canada. (2010, November). Application of TALLman lettering for drugs used in oncology. *ISMP Canada Safety Bulletin, 10*(8), 1.

Institute for Safe Medication Practices Canada. (2010). Application of TALLman lettering for drugs used in oncology. *ISMP Canada Safety Bulletin, 10*(8), 1.

Institute for Safe Medication Practices Canada. (2012). *Knowledge translation of insulin use interventions/safeguards.* Toronto, Canada: Author.

Institute for Safe Medication Practices Canada. (2013a). *ISMP Canada guidelines for subcutaneous insulin order sets.* Retrieved from <http://www.ismp-canada.org/download/insulin/ISMP_Guidelines_SC_InsulinOrderSets.pdf>.

Institute of Safe Medication Practices Canada. (2013b). *Medication bar code system implementation planning: A resource guide.* Retrieved from http://www.ismp-canada.org/barcoding/

Institute for Safe Medication Practices Canada, & Healthcare Insurance Reciprocal of Canada. (2008, July 25). Enhancing safety with unfractionated heparin: A national and international area of focus. *ISMP Canada Safety Bulletin, 8*(5), 1-3.

Institute for Safe Medication Practices Canada, & Healthcare Insurance Reciprocal of Canada. (2012, March 6). Analysis of Harmful Medication Incidents Involving Psychotropic Medications. *ISMP Canada Safety Bulletin, 12*(2), 1-5.

Kee, J. L., & Marshall, S. M. (2013). *Clinical calculations: With applications to general and specialty areas* (7th ed.). St. Louis, MO: Saunders.

Kliegman, R. M., Stanton, B. F., St. Geme, J. W., & Schor, N.F. (2011). *Nelson textbook of pediatrics* (19th ed.). Philadelphia, PA: Saunders.

Lilley, L. L., Harrington, S., Snyder, J. S., & Swart, B. (2011). *Pharmacology for Canadian health care practice* (2nd ed.). Toronto, Canada: Elsevier.

MacKinnon, N. J., U, D., & Koczmara, C. (2008, September-October). Medication incidents involving heparin in Canada: "Flushing" out the problem. *Canadian Journal of Hospital Pharmacy 61*(5), 348-350.

Macklin, D., Chernecky, C., & Infortuna, H. (2011). *Math for clinical practice.* Maryland Heights, MO: Mosby Elsevier.

Meyers, R. S. (2009). Pediatric fluid and electrolyte therapy. *Journal of Pediatric Pharmacology and Therapeutics, 14*(4), 204-211.

Miller, D., Yu, C., Adams, L., Berard, L., Cheng, A. Y., Clarke C.,…Landry, E. (2014). *In-hospital management of diabetes: Clinical order sets. Blood glucose lowering working group, CPG dissemination & implementation Committee.* Retrieved from http://guidelines.diabetes.ca/CDACPG_resources/Summary_In-hospital_mgmt_of_diabetes_FINAL_July_8-2014.pdf

Mosby's drug consult 2007. (2007). St. Louis, MO: Mosby.

Mulholland, J. M. (2011). *The nurse, the math, the meds: Drug calculations using dimensional analysis* (2nd ed.). St. Louis, MO: Mosby.

National Council of State Boards of Nursing. (2015, Spring). Does the NCLEX use the metric or imperial system? *NCLEX Communiqué, 2.*

Ogden, S. G., & Fluharty, L. K. (2012). *Calculation of drug dosages* (9th ed.). St. Louis, MO: Mosby.

Ontario Ministry of Health and Long Term Care. (2000). *Mental health: Bill 68 (mental health legislative reform 2000.* Retrieved January 23, 2015 from http://www.health.gov.on.ca/en/public/publications/mental/treatment_order.aspx

Perry, A. G., Potter, P. A., & Elkin, M. K. (2012). *Nursing interventions and clinical skills* (5th ed.). St Louis, MO: Mosby.

Potter, P. A., Perry, A. G., Stockert, P., & Hall, A. (2011). *Basic nursing* (7th ed.). St. Louis, MO: Mosby.

Potter, P. A., Perry, A. G., Stockert, P., Hall, A. (2013). *Fundamentals of nursing* (8th ed.). St. Louis, MO: Mosby.

Sanofi Canada. (2015, June 1). *Toujeo: New basal insulin option for adults living with diabetes approved by Health Canada* [Press Release]. Retrieved from http://sanoficanada.mediaroom.com/

Skidmore-Roth, Linda. (2015). *Mosby's 2015 nursing drug reference.* St. Louis, MO: Mosby Elsevier.

Statistics Canada. (2014, September 26). Canada's population estimates: Age and sex 2014. *The Daily.* Retrieved from http://www.statcan.gc.ca/daily-quotidien/140926/dq140926b-eng.htm

The Joint Commission. (2016). *Speak up: Take medication safely.* Retrieved from http://www.jointcommission.org/topics/speak_up_preventing_medicine_errors.aspx

Williams, C. (2008). Fluid resuscitation in burn patients 1: Using formulas. *Nursing Times, 104*(14), 28-29.

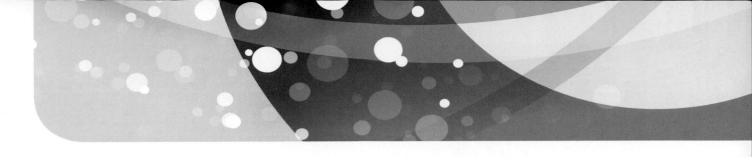

Drug Label Credits

We would like to thank the following copyright holders for providing us with their current drug label images. Please note that actual drug labels are subject to change at any time and any drug label image in this text is to be used only for the educational purpose of practicing dosage calculations. Readers are otherwise instructed to refer to the most recent product monograph.

AbbVie labels on pages 165, 169, 171, 182, 185, 319, 363, 364: Courtesy AbbVie Corporation.

Apotex labels on pages 164, 166, 168, 176, 184, 190, 194, 195. 196, 210, 213, 214, 215, 217, 220, 221, 227, 244, 245, 246, 253, 254, 256, 258, 259, 260, 272, 274, 275, 276, 280, 299, 305, 316, 323, 326, 328, 330, 331, 332, 333, 334, 335, 337, 338, 456, 683: Courtesy Apotex Inc.

GlaxoSmithKline labels on pages 319, 450, 682; current as of July 15, 2015: Courtesy GlaxoSmithKline Inc.

Hospira labels on pages 167, 180, 189, 230, 250, 251, 255, 273, 276, 365, 366, 367, 368, 370, 383, 385, 407, 422, 426, 453, 513, 514, 526, 666: Courtesy Hospira Healthcare Corporation.

Merck labels on pages 140, 165, 168, 174, 175, 191, 193, 215, 244, 258, 323: This drug label is reproduced with permission of Merck. All rights reserved.

Novo Nordisk labels on pages 216, 328, 370, 475, 477, 478, 479, 480, 496, 497, 500, 501, 502, 686, 687: Courtesy Novo Nordisk Canada Inc.

Omega labels on pages 80, 164, 170, 173, 180, 190, 225, 228, 230, 252, 274, 279, 361, 364, 369, 380, 381, 383, 385, 390, 392, 393, 394, 403, 406, 595, 635, 667: Courtesy Omega Laboratories Ltd.

Pfizer labels on pages 80, 164, 168, 169, 172, 179, 181, 191, 197, 215, 218, 222, 224, 227, 229, 231, 248, 249, 251, 256, 257, 279, 292, 303, 306, 324, 327, 329, 331, 334, 339, 340, 360, 365, 367, 384, 387, 393, 397, 399, 426, 429, 444, 459, 463, 543, 563, 565, 575, 576, 581, 602, 696: Courtesy Pfizer Inc.

Sandoz labels on pages 166, 171, 183, 186, 192, 194, 220, 224, 225, 248, 250, 255, 270, 307, 337, 360, 363, 366, 380, 386, 388, 389, 391, 395, 396, 401, 402, 404, 459, 574, 578, 627, 631, 632, 633, 671, 684, 690, 691, 692, 694, 695: © Sandoz Canada Inc. All rights reserved. For educational purposes only.

Sanofi labels on pages 140, 172, 193, 211, 214, 216, 257, 307, 334, 367, 400, 450, 477, 479, 563: Courtesy Sanofi Canada.

Taro label on page 300: Copyright Taro Pharmaceuticals Inc., All Rights Reserved.

Teva and Novopharm labels on pages 183, 193, 223, 249, 252, 301, 302, 304, 318, 325, 326, 350, 387, 392, 427, 443, 445, 447, 456, 462, 600, 603, 625, 635: The product labels and intellectual property of Teva Canada Limited are reproduced with the permission of Teva Canada Limited and used herein for educational purposes only.

Index

Page numbers followed by f, t, and b indicate figures, tables, and boxes, respectively.

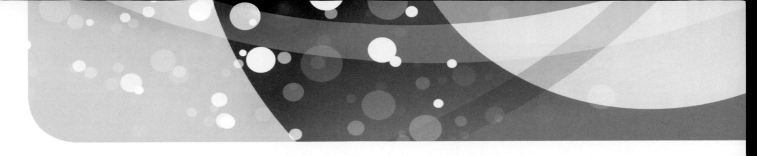

Drug Label Credits

We would like to thank the following copyright holders for providing us with their current drug label images. Please note that actual drug labels are subject to change at any time and any drug label image in this text is to be used only for the educational purpose of practicing dosage calculations. Readers are otherwise instructed to refer to the most recent product monograph.

AbbVie labels on pages 165, 169, 171, 182, 185, 319, 363, 364: Courtesy AbbVie Corporation.

Apotex labels on pages 164, 166, 168, 176, 184, 190, 194, 195. 196, 210, 213, 214, 215, 217, 220, 221, 227, 244, 245, 246, 253, 254, 256, 258, 259, 260, 272, 274, 275, 276, 280, 299, 305, 316, 323, 326, 328, 330, 331, 332, 333, 334, 335, 337, 338, 456, 683: Courtesy Apotex Inc.

GlaxoSmithKline labels on pages 319, 450, 682; current as of July 15, 2015: Courtesy GlaxoSmithKline Inc.

Hospira labels on pages 167, 180, 189, 230, 250, 251, 255, 273, 276, 365, 366, 367, 368, 370, 383, 385, 407, 422, 426, 453, 513, 514, 526, 666: Courtesy Hospira Healthcare Corporation.

Merck labels on pages 140, 165, 168, 174, 175, 191, 193, 215, 244, 258, 323: This drug label is reproduced with permission of Merck. All rights reserved.

Novo Nordisk labels on pages 216, 328, 370, 475, 477, 478, 479, 480, 496, 497, 500, 501, 502, 686, 687: Courtesy Novo Nordisk Canada Inc.

Omega labels on pages 80, 164, 170, 173, 180, 190, 225, 228, 230, 252, 274, 279, 361, 364, 369, 380, 381, 383, 385, 390, 392, 393, 394, 403, 406, 595, 635, 667: Courtesy Omega Laboratories Ltd.

Pfizer labels on pages 80, 164, 168, 169, 172, 179, 181, 191, 197, 215, 218, 222, 224, 227, 229, 231, 248, 249, 251, 256, 257, 279, 292, 303, 306, 324, 327, 329, 331, 334, 339, 340, 360, 365, 367, 384, 387, 393, 397, 399, 426, 429, 444, 459, 463, 543, 563, 565, 575, 576, 581, 602, 696: Courtesy Pfizer Inc.

Sandoz labels on pages 166, 171, 183, 186, 192, 194, 220, 224, 225, 248, 250, 255, 270, 307, 337, 360, 363, 366, 380, 386, 388, 389, 391, 395, 396, 401, 402, 404, 459, 574, 578, 627, 631, 632, 633, 671, 684, 690, 691, 692, 694, 695: © Sandoz Canada Inc. All rights reserved. For educational purposes only.

Sanofi labels on pages 140, 172, 193, 211, 214, 216, 257, 307, 334, 367, 400, 450, 477, 479, 563: Courtesy Sanofi Canada.

Taro label on page 300: Copyright Taro Pharmaceuticals Inc., All Rights Reserved.

Teva and Novopharm labels on pages 183, 193, 223, 249, 252, 301, 302, 304, 318, 325, 326, 350, 387, 392, 427, 443, 445, 447, 456, 462, 600, 603, 625, 635: The product labels and intellectual property of Teva Canada Limited are reproduced with the permission of Teva Canada Limited and used herein for educational purposes only.

Index

A

Abbreviations
  on medication labels, 174
  in medication orders, 137, 138b–139b
    commonly used, 138t
    "Do Not Use" list for, 139t
    for units of measurement, 138t
  in metric system, 72, 72b–73b
Activated partial thromboplastin time (APTT), 563
AcuDose Rx, 157
ad lib, in medication orders, 138t
ADCs (automated dispensing cabinets), 157, 158f
ADD-Vantage system, 517, 519f
Addition
  of decimals, 27–28, 27b
  of fractions, 11–12, 11b
Alerts, on medication labels, 171, 172f
am, in medication orders, 138t
Aminophylline, 667–668, 667f, 670
  dosage calculation for parenteral medications, 403f, 418f
  label of, 361, 361f
Amiodarone, label of, 366, 366f
amp, in medication orders, 138t
Ampules, 348–349, 349f
Ante meridian, 109
Antiarrhythmic, titrated medications and, 653
Apo-Procainamide, 667
Apothecary system, 77, 79b
  chapter review on, 81–83
    answers to, 84
  metric system vs., 70
  practice problems for, 80–81
    answers to, 83–84
APTT (activated partial thromboplastin time), 563
aq, in medication orders, 138t
Arabic equivalents for Roman numerals, 705
Atropine sulphate, dosage calculation according to syringe, 375–376, 375f
Automated dispensing cabinets (ADCs), 120, 157, 158f
AZT, 141

B

Bar code
  for medication delivery, 158–159, 159f
  for medication errors, 119
Bar-code symbols, on medication labels, 169
Barrel, of syringe, 351, 351f
Basal-bolus insulin therapy, 475–476, 487
Baxter Mini-Bag Plus, 517–518, 520f
Betamethasone, dosage calculation for parenteral medications, 403f, 417f
Bicillin, dosage calculation for parenteral medications, 387f, 412f
BID, in medication orders, 138t

Blood and blood products, IV administration of, 516, 516f
Body surface area (BSA), calculating pediatric dosage using, 604–606, 604b, 609–610, 610b
  formula for, 607–608
    from kilograms and centimetres, 607, 607b
    from pounds and inches, 608
    technological advances in, 608
  for IV therapy, 622
  points to remember, 609b, 612b
  practice problems for, 606–608, 610–612
    answers to, 639–644
  West nomogram chart for, 604–606, 605f, 606b
Body weight
  converting between units of, 107
  dosage calculation based on, 592–593, 592b, 604b
    for adults, 599–600, 599b, 599f
    converting grams to kilograms in, 592–593
    for dosages around the clock, 596–597
    key terms and concepts, 593–594
    practice problems for, 593–604
      answers to, 639–644
    for single dose medications, 594–596, 595f–596f
    for single-dose range medications, 596–599, 596f, 597b, 599b
Boiling point, 103
Bolus, IV, 550–551
Borrowing, subtracting fractions using, 13–14, 13b
Brand name
  on medication labels, 165, 165f, 166b
  on medication orders, 140–141, 140f
BSA. see Body surface area (BSA)
Buccal tablets, 290, 290f
  administration of, 129
Bumetanide, dosage calculation for parenteral medications, 402f, 417f
Burette, calibrated, 616, 617f
  calculating intravenous medications by, 619–622, 619b–620b
  with electronic controller or pump, 616–617, 621, 621b
Burn injury, fluid resuscitation after, 612–614, 612b
  calculation of, 613–614, 614b
  formula for, 613
  Parkland formula for, 612, 612b
  points to remember, 614b
  post-24-hour formula for, 612–613
  practice problems for, 615–616
    answers to, 639–644

C

c or C. see Cup
Calculation, dosage
  based on micrograms per kilogram per minute, 657–658

Calculation, dosage (Continued)
  critical care dosages per hour or per minute, 655–656, 656b
    dimensional analysis, 656
    ratio and proportion, 655–656
  dimensional analysis for, 266–269, 266b, 269b
    chapter review on, 272–281
      answers to, 283–285
    points to remember on, 269b
    practice problems on, 270–272
      answers to, 282
  formula method for, 237–262, 237b
    chapter review on, 243–260, 262b
      answers to, 262
    with different systems or units of measurement, 239b
    formula for, 237–238, 238b
    points to remember on, 241b
    practice problems on, 242–243
      answers to, 260–262
    steps for use of, 238–241, 238b–241b
  lower, in titration table, 661–663
  upper, in titration table, 661, 663
Calculation errors, 205
  dosage, 237b
Calibrated dropper
  for measuring liquid oral medications, 307, 307b, 308f
  for medication administration, 130–131, 131f
cap, in medication orders, 138t
Caplets, 288
Capsules
  administration of, 291
  calculating dosages of, 292–297
    chapter review on, 322–340
      answers to, 347
    different strengths in, 292
    with divided doses, 297
    maximum number in, 292–293
    number of capsules needed in, 296
    points to remember on, 292b–293b, 297b
    practice problems on, 298–306
      answers to, 341–346
    problem setup on, 293b–296b
  defined, 291
  gelatin, 291f
  sprinkle, 291
  timed-release, 291f
Carpuject, 350
Cartridges, 350, 350b, 351f
CBDA (computer-based drug administration), 159
cc. see Cubic centimetre (cc)
CD, in medication orders, 138t
Celsius, Fahrenheit and
  converting between, 103–105
    formulas for, 104–105, 104b–105b
  differentiating between, 103–104, 104f

Page numbers followed by f, t, and b indicate figures, tables, and boxes, respectively.

Notes

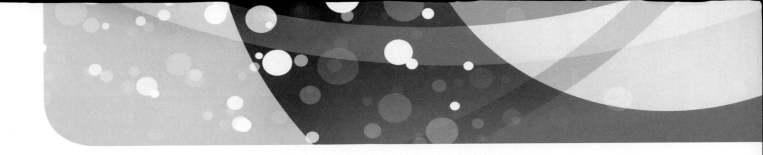

Notes

723

Notes